Handbook of Gerontology

Handbook of Gerontology

Editor: Oliver Fincher

AMERICAN
MEDICAL PUBLISHERS
www.americanmedicalpublishers.com

AMERICAN
MEDICAL PUBLISHERS
www.americanmedicalpublishers.com

Cataloging-in-Publication Data

Handbook of gerontology / edited by Oliver Fincher.
p. cm.
Includes bibliographical references and index.
ISBN 978-1-63927-008-8
1. Gerontology. 2. Geriatrics. 3. Older people--Diseases. 4. Older people--Health and hygiene.
5. Older people--Medical care. 6. Aging. I. Fincher, Oliver.
RC952 .H36 2022
618.97--dc23

American Medical Publishers,
41 Flatbush Avenue,
1st Floor, New York,
NY 11217, USA

ISBN 978-1-63927-008-8 (Hardback)

Contents

Preface

Gerontology is characterized as the scientific study of the phenomena of aging. The goal of gerontology is to trace the changes that take place in a cell, a tissue, an organ system, a group of organisms with the passage of time. Some of the common fields that fall under this domain are biogerontology, social gerontology, environmental gerontology, and jurisprudential gerontology. Gerontology utilizes the methodologies of many other scientific and medical disciplines and aims to learn about the aging process for the purpose of possibly minimizing the disabilities of old age. Geriatrics is a subset of gerontology that is concerned with the prevention and treatment of diseases in older people. This book provides comprehensive insights into the field of gerontology. It provides significant information of this discipline to help develop a good understanding of gerontology and related fields. Students and researchers actively engaged in this field will find this book full of crucial and unexplored concepts.

This book is a result of research of several months to collate the most relevant data in the field.

When I was approached with the idea of this book and the proposal to edit it, I was overwhelmed. It gave me an opportunity to reach out to all those who share a common interest with me in this field. I had 3 main parameters for editing this text:

1. Accuracy – The data and information provided in this book should be up-to-date and valuable to the readers.
2. Structure – The data must be presented in a structured format for easy understanding and better grasping of the readers.
3. Universal Approach – This book not only targets students but also experts and innovators in the field, thus my aim was to present topics which are of use to all.

Thus, it took me a couple of months to finish the editing of this book.

I would like to make a special mention of my publisher who considered me worthy of this opportunity and also supported me throughout the editing process. I would also like to thank the editing team at the back-end who extended their help whenever required.

Editor

1

Swimming as a Positive Moderator of Cognitive Aging

Amira Abou-Dest, Cédric T. Albinet, Geoffroy Boucard, and Michel Audiffren

UMR CNRS 7295, University of Poitiers, Sport Sciences Faculty, Bât. A5, 5 rue Théodore Lefebvre, 86000 Poitiers, France

Correspondence should be addressed to Cédric T. Albinet, cedric.albinet@univ-poitiers.fr

Academic Editor: Teresa Liu-Ambrose

This study examined whether regular swimming in older adults was related to better cognitive functioning and whether there were any global or selective positive effects of this physical activity (PA) on cognition. The cognitive performances of three groups of sixteen volunteer participants (young adults, sedentary older adults, and older adults who regularly practice swimming) were evaluated using a multitask approach. All participants performed a battery of ten tasks: two reaction time tasks assessing information processing speed and eight experimental tasks assessing three executive functions (EFs), (behavioral inhibition, working memory updating, and cognitive flexibility). The results showed that young adults performed significantly better than older adults on all examined cognitive functions. However, in older adults, regular swimming was related to better performance on the three EFs, but not on information processing speed. More precisely, five experimental tasks out of the eight tapping EFs were shown to be sensitive to positive effects from swimming practice. Finally, the demonstrated benefits of swimming on EFs were not necessarily linked to better cardiorespiratory fitness. The present findings illustrate the validity of using a multitask approach in examining the potential benefits of regular PA on cognitive aging.

1. Introduction

The growth of the proportion of the population aged 65 and older in the industrialized world, as well as in developing countries, has profound implications for public health and the economic costs of medical care. Cerebral and cognitive decline, as a function of aging, represents a predominant cause of autonomy loss in aging populations. According to the prefrontal-executive theory [1], executive functions (EFs) and their underpinning prefrontal and frontal brain structures are particularly sensitive to the effects of normal and pathological aging [2, 3]. Therefore, the preservation of these brain areas and their associated cognitive functions is of particular importance. Chronic physical activity (PA), aimed at improving cardiorespiratory health, has been proposed to be a good, practical, and powerful candidate to overcome cerebral and behavioral declines [4–6]. Accordingly, the principal aim of the present study was to examine the potential benefits of an understudied form of PA—regular swimming (one of the most popular and accessible forms of PA for older adults)—on EF performance in a population aged 65 to 80 years old.

Executive functions involve higher-order functions of control and coordination allowing behavioral adaptation to complex or novel situations for which automatisms or routines are inappropriate. As such, EFs refer to a set of cognitive processes involved in goal and strategy formulation, planning and monitoring, mental flexibility, and behavioral inhibition [7, 8]. This multicomponent or fractionated view implies that EFs may be composed of different executive processes that are at least partially independent, yet are sufficiently correlated to represent a unique construct. In this line, an authoritative model was developed by Miyake and colleagues [9], who proposed that EFs can be fractionated into at least three separable processes; cognitive flexibility (shifting between multiple tasks or mental sets), behavioral inhibition (suppression of dominant, automatic, or prepotent responses when necessary), and updating of working memory (substitution of old information by new more relevant information in working memory). This three-factor structure of EFs has been frequently postulated in the literature and replicated in older populations [2, 10, 11]. Although caution is still needed when choosing the tasks used to assess this construct, all three EFs have been quite constantly shown to be impaired in older people, even after having controlled for other confounders such as level of education and information processing speed [2].

In contrast to the prefrontal-executive theory, the processing speed theory [12] assumes that age-related cognitive declines are accounted for by generalized slowing of cognitive processing due to a diffuse or global deterioration of white matter integrity throughout the whole brain with aging. A meta-analysis by Colcombe and Kramer [13] showed that the effect size of the positive effects of chronic exercise is significantly smaller on information processing speed than on executive functions. It is then very interesting to compare the effects of aging and physical activity on these two functions in the same experiment.

In contrast to this negative view of cognitive aging, a new line of research has developed works that examine how keeping a physically active lifestyle can maintain or even improve cognition and brain functions. In recent years, using various methodologies, several studies have shown that older adults who maintain a physically active way of life by participating in regular PA or chronic exercise outperform their sedentary counterparts in cognitive performance, exhibit higher brain plasticity [14, 15] and are more efficiently protected against neurological diseases and dementia [16, 17]. Moreover, randomized controlled trials have demonstrated that short physical training programs (from 3 months to 1 year) improve cognitive performance, particularly EFs, in sedentary older adults with no pathology of the central nervous system [18–21] or dementia [22, 23]. Narrative and meta-analytic reviews tend to show that this positive effect may be particularly selective to attentional, controlled cognitive functions involving EFs (see [4, 13, 24]) and that the PA programs should involve a strong proportion of aerobic exercises (see [4, 13, 25]). Moderate-to-vigorous PA induces improvements in cardiorespiratory fitness (indexed by maximal oxygen uptake, VO_2max) and leads to a cascade of neurophysiological mechanisms such as the release of neurotrophic factors that facilitate neurogenesis and/or angiogenesis [19, 26–28], two mechanisms known to be associated with higher brain plasticity, which ultimately leads to improvements in cognitive performance. It is important to note that, on the one hand, the putative links between neurophysiological mechanisms and efficiency of cognitive processes are not yet fully understood and, on the other hand, the possible mechanisms explaining these links are most likely not exclusive. A number of reviews on this topic suggest a concomitant increase in cardiorespiratory fitness, brain plasticity, and cognitive performance, but inconsistent results have been reported concerning the last point. For instance, some authors have been unable to show cognitive improvements after an aerobic exercise program that was sufficient to increase VO_2max [29]. Others have shown that not all EFs are enhanced after a PA program and that the improvement in cognitive performance, when effective, was not related to the improvement in cardiorespiratory fitness [21, 25]. Finally, Liu-Ambrose et al. [30] recently reported the results of a randomized controlled study showing that a 12-month resistance training program (involving strength exercises twice a week) induced the same improvements in EF performance and functional plasticity as an aerobic program. These findings emphasize the need to further study the relationships between PA and cognitive performance in the aged population. In the present study, we were particularly interested in one understudied aerobic physical activity: swimming. To the best of our knowledge, only one study was designated to explicitly test the specific relationship between water aerobics and cognitive improvements in older adults [31]. In this study, Hawkins and collaborators examined the influence of a 10-week program of basic swimming skills on variations of two experimental tasks involving processing speed, attentional switching, and dual-task time-sharing. They found that subjects who trained in water aerobics showed significantly larger improvements on the executive control tasks than a nontrained control group. Interestingly, similar performance improvements were demonstrated for both groups in the nonexecutive tasks. Thus, it is important to verify whether this isolated finding can be generalized and to determine if swimming benefits are global or selective to some executive processes given the fractionated reality of EFs. To that end, we employed a clear theoretically driven framework to examine the potential mediator role of VO_2max in this relationship.

The objectives of the present study were twofold. First, we wanted to replicate our team's previous results on age-related declines in EF and processing speed performance [2] by comparing the performances of younger and older adults on various tasks that assess information processing speed and the three postulated EFs, inhibition, working memory updating, and shifting. Second, assuming these age-related cognitive declines, we wanted to determine the selectivity of the relationship between swimming and the three EFs and information processing speed, in our sample of older adults. An important feature of this experiment was to combine the use of two or three cognitive tasks that are well-known for tapping each of the cognitive functions of interest with a multivariate approach. This procedure was shown to accurately assess the construct of EF and to reveal age-related executive declines in a previous pool of participants [2]. Swimming was chosen for three main reasons. (1) It is an understudied aerobic activity in the field of cognitive aging, and it solicits all the muscle groups and increases cardiorespiratory fitness. (2) It is one of the most accessible and practiced PAs in the elderly and is rated as the second most popular PA in France for the age range 65 and older [32]. (3) It is less traumatic on joints than walking or jogging. Several reviews have described the beneficial effects of water-based exercise on physical fitness parameters, such as aerobic capacity and strength in the elderly [33–35]. The elderly take a particular interest in water activity because it reduces the fear of falling, limits tolerance for weight-bearing activities, and enhances adherence and participation [36].

2. Methods

2.1. Participants. Thirty-two older adults aged 65 to 80 years (16 sedentary people and 16 swimmers) and 16 younger adults (18–30 years), all of whom were free of neurological and cardiovascular disease, participated to this study. The older participants were recruited from senior community centers, civic groups, and aquatic centers through the use of flyers and newspapers. All the older participants were screened by their personal physicians who rated them as being in good health and signed a medical certificate indicating no contraindications for cardiorespiratory fitness testing. Younger participants were recruited from the University of Poitiers.

Inclusion criteria for older adults were as follows: (a) being aged between 65 and 80 years; (b) having adequate mental status as indicated by a score strictly greater than 25 on the Mini Mental State Examination (MMSE) [37]; (c) for the sedentary group, leading a sedentary lifestyle with no participation in any structured PA as assessed by a validated PA questionnaire, the Dijon Score of Physical Activity (DSPA) [38]; (d) for the active group, leading a physically active lifestyle as assessed first by a history of regularly swimming at least twice a week for at least two years but no other regular PA. Secondly, the DSPA was also administered for the active group to ensure a significant difference in the amount of physical activity between the two groups. Inclusion criteria for younger adults were being aged from 18 and 30 years. The exclusion criteria were the following: (a) using medication that could affect cardiovascular health or cognitive functions; (b) cardiorespiratory or neurological disease; (c) major surgery within one year prior to testing. All participants gave written informed consent and the study was approved by the local ethics committee. The demographic and physical characteristics of all participant groups are displayed in Table 1. The active older adults (swimmers) had been practicing swimming for two to 43 years (M = 2.56 years; SD = 0.79), two to five times a week. The mean session duration was between 45 and 100 minutes (M = 64.38 min; SD = 15.37).

2.2. Evaluation of Cardiorespiratory Fitness. For the older participants, VO_2max was estimated by the Rockport Fitness Walking test [39]. This submaximal field test has been shown to accurately estimate VO_2max in populations similar to the one in the present study [39, 40]. Participants were required to walk one mile (1609 m) as quickly as possible, and heart rate was continuously recorded by a Polar RS 800 beat-to-beat recorder (Polar Electro, Oy, Kempele, Finland). VO_2max was calculated using the equation developed by Kline and collaborators.

2.3. Evaluation of Information Processing Speed. Information processing speed was measured through two reaction time tasks: an auditory simple reaction time (SRT) task and a visual 2-Choice Reaction Time (CRT) task [2]. SRT and CRT were used as the main dependent variables and the error rate in the CRT task enabled checking for possible speed-accuracy tradeoffs.

2.4. Evaluation of Executive Functions. Each of the three EFs was assessed via 2 or 3 different experimental tasks. All tasks were the same as those used in a previous study from our laboratory that involved a different sample of younger and older adults [2]. We refer the reader to this paper for a full description of the procedure and tasks used.

2.4.1. Inhibition

The Stroop Task. In this computerized version of the Stroop task, the dependent variable was the difference in mean RTs (ms) between incongruent trials (e.g., the word RED written in blue) and neutral trials (e.g., XXXXX written in blue) for correct responses. The error rate in incongruent and neutral conditions was also controlled to check for any possible speed-accuracy tradeoffs.

The Stop-Signal Task. In this task, participants were required to respond as quickly as possible to a visual stimulus by pressing the corresponding key, unless an auditory tone rang out requiring to abort (or inhibit) the prepotent motor response. The dependent variable selected for the multivariate analyses of variance (MANOVAs) was the rate of successful inhibition calculated as the probability (P, between 0 and 1) of successful inhibition. The stop-signal reaction time (SSRT) has also been calculated according to Logan's race model [41]. This variable was not included in the MANOVAs for two reasons: (1) SSRT correlated moderately with SRT and CRT (r = .41 and .50, resp.), while $P(I)$ did not (see Table 2); (2) SSRT did not correlate with the interference score measured in the Stroop task and the adjacency score measured in the RNG task, two variables reflecting inhibition (r = .13 and r = −.06, resp.), while $P(I)$ correlated significantly with the adjacency score (see Table 2).

The Random Number Generation (RNG) Task. In this task, participants were required to generate and say aloud series of random numbers from one to nine at the rate of one digit per second. The dependent variable that reflected inhibition for this task was the Adjacency score (A in %), ranging from 0% (no neighboring pairs, i.e., good performance) to 100% (only neighboring pairs, i.e., poor performance). The RNG task necessitates inhibiting counting in ascendant or descendant series, and the Adjacency score measures the tendency of the participants to count by one.

2.4.2. Updating

The Verbal Running Span Task. In this computerized task, participants were required to recall serially the last four letters of a list of six, eight, ten, or twelve consonants that were presented visually. The dependent variable was the number of letters correctly recalled in the right order (max. = 48).

The spatial Running Span Task. Like for the previous task, in this computerized task, participants were required to recall serially the last four spatial locations of a dot in a 4 × 4

Table 1: Characteristics of the three groups of participants.

Characteristics	Young adults	Active older adults	Sedentary older adults	Young versus older adults	Active versus Sedentary
n	16	16	16	$P = 1$	$P = 1$
Gender M/F	9/7	9/7	9/7	$P = 1$	$P = 1$
Age (years)	23.56 (2.56)	69.13 (3.88)	69.25 (3.25)	$P < .05$	$P = .92$
MMSE (max = 30)	29.31 (0.01)	28.75 (0.93)	28.69 (1.08)	$P = .06$	$P = .86$
Education (years)	16.09 (1.25)	13.75 (3.11)	13.56 (1.93)	$P < .05$	$P = .84$
DPAS (max = 30)	—	24.25 (1.48)	15.17 (4.37)	—	$P < .05$
VO_2max (mL/min/kg)	—	29.35 (5.13)	25.27 (4.94)	—	$P < .05$

Note. M: Male, F: Female, MMSE: Mini Mental State Examination, DPAS: Dijon Physical Activity Score.

matrix. The dependent variable was the number of dots correctly recalled in the right order (max. = 48).

2.4.3. Shifting

The Dimension-Switching Task. In this computerized task, participants watched on the computer screen the French words for LEFT or RIGHT enclosed in a left or right arrow, and displayed above or below the center of the white screen. Depending on instructions, they were required to respond to the word or to the direction of the arrow by pressing the correct corresponding key. The dependent variable selected for this task was the global switch cost for correct responses, calculated as the difference in RT (ms) between trials from the simple blocks and task-repeat trials from the mixed blocks. The error rate in simple and mixed blocks of trials was calculated to check for any possible speed-accuracy tradeoffs. The local switch cost was also calculated but was not included for further analyses because it did not correlate with the number of perseverative errors in the Wisconsin Card Sorting Task ($r = .18$) while the global switch cost did ($r = .32$, see Table 2).

Stimulus-Response Compatibility Switching Task. In this computerized task, participants watched an arrow pointing left or right, surrounded by a frame on the computer screen. Depending on the color of the frame, participants were to press the response key located either on the side pointed by the arrow (green or blue frame), or on the opposite side (red or orange frame). The dependent measure for this task was the local switch cost for correct responses, calculated as the difference in RT (ms) between task-repeat trials and task-switch trials during the mixed blocks. The error rate for repetition and alternation trials was also computed to check for any possible speed-accuracy tradeoffs. The global switch cost has not been computed in this task because the number of trials in the simple blocks was too small; the simple blocks have only been used to familiarize participants to the rules of mapping between stimuli and responses.

The Wisconsin Card Sorting Test (WCST). In this computerized version of the WCST, participants were required to sort a set of cards according to three different rules that changed periodically. The dependent variable that reflected shifting for this task was the number of perseverative errors.

For the processing speed construct and for each EF component, a standardized Cronbach alpha was computed to assess how well the selected tasks measured a latent construct. Alphas for each postulated cognitive function were low to good (standardized Cronbach alphas were .77, .60, .78, and .59 for Information processing speed, Inhibition, Updating, and Shifting, resp.). Table 2 presents the results of the bivariate correlations between all cognitive tasks within the whole sample.

2.5. Procedure. After careful screening for inclusion and exclusion criteria, older participants were first evaluated for cardiorespiratory fitness on one day. Second, each participant was tested individually in a quiet experimental room in two sessions on different days separated by a minimum of two days and a maximum of seven days. Each session lasted approximately 1.5–2 hours. The two sessions were counterbalanced across participants and, within each session, all tasks were counterbalanced across participants. Participants were given short breaks between each experimental task.

2.6. Statistical Analyses. The data on cognitive performance were analyzed in three ways. First, a series of one-way multivariate planned analyses of covariance (MANCOVAs) was conducted on each set of dependent variables reflecting a specific cognitive function (speed of information processing, behavioral inhibition, updating of working memory, and shifting), contrasting young adults and seniors with level of education (number of years) as a covariate. This first series of planned MANCOVAs was conducted in order to test the effect of age on each cognitive function. The level of education was entered as a covariate because younger adults showed a higher level of education than older adults (see Table 1). When the effect of age on a cognitive function was significant, we conducted a series of planned analyses of covariance (ANCOVAs) on each cognitive function task, contrasting young adults and seniors with level of education as a covariate. Second, a series of one-way multivariate planned analyses of variance (MANOVAs) was conducted on the same sets of dependent variables only in older adults, contrasting regular swimmers and sedentary people. This second series of planned MANOVAs was conducted in order

TABLE 2: Matrix of correlations between the indices of cognitive performance, one index per cognitive task, for the whole sample.

Dependent variable/Task	1	2	3	4	5	6	7	8	9	10
(1) Auditory SRT	1.00									
(2) Visual CRT	**.63***	1.00								
(3) *P*(*I*)	−.05	−.02	1.00							
(4) Interference cost	.42*	.43*	**.18**	1.00						
(5) Adjacency score	.16	.34*	**.31***	**.51***	1.00					
(6) NO correct letters	−.18	−.29*	.10	−.26	−.56*	1.00				
(7) NO correct locations	−.30*	−.69*	−.03	−.51*	−.63*	**.64***	1.00			
(8) NO perseverative errors	.23	.30*	.04	.40*	.58*	−.52*	−.55*	1.00		
(9) Global switching cost	.08	.54*	−.03	.20	.49*	−.51*	−.69*	**.32***	1.00	
(10) Local switching cost	.25	.46*	.01	.20	.46*	−.40*	−.44*	**.22**	**.42***	1.00

Note. SRT: Simple reaction time, CRT: Choice reaction time, *P*(*I*): Rate of successful inhibitions, *: $P < .05$, bold : Correlations within the same cognitive function.

to test the effect of physical activity level on each cognitive function. When the result of the MANOVA was significant, we performed a series of planned analyses of variance (ANOVAs) on each of the individual tasks composing cognitive function. Finally, for the older adult sample, simple regression analyses were performed between VO_2max and EF scores when there was a significant correlation between these variables. The level of significance was set at $P < .05$ and Cohen's d was reported for pairwise comparisons as a measure of effect size. As proposed by Cohen [42], a "small" effect is when $d = 0.2$, a "medium" effect when $d = 0.5$, and a "large" effect when $d = 0.8$. For the MANOVAs and MANCOVAs, partial eta squared (Partial η^2) was also reported as a measure of the percentage (when multiplied by 100) of variance explained by the treatment factors.

3. Results

3.1. Group Differences in Demographics and Global Cognition. As seen in Table 1, young adults attended more years of education than older participants ($F(1, 46) = 12.97$; $P < 0.05$). In addition, as expected, older active participants were more physically active than their sedentary counterparts as revealed by a higher score on the DPAS ($F(1, 30) = 60.75$; $P < 0.05$), and a higher level of VO_2max ($F(1, 29) = 5.13$; $P < 0.05$), but the two groups did not differ in MMSE scores.

3.2. Effects of Chronological Age on Cognitive Functions. Results of the statistical analyses and behavioral performance as a function of age group for each cognitive function and each cognitive task are detailed in Table 3. As seen, there was a significant effect of age on each cognitive function, even after having controlled for the level of education. Subsequent ANCOVAs on each individual dependent measure revealed that the age-related effect was significant for each experimental task (see Table 3) except for three: the stop-signal task, the letter running-span, and the WCST, for which there was no significant difference between younger and older adults after having controlled for education level.

The effect of age was also examined on error rate for all the tasks that included choice reaction time measurements. A first ANOVA was conducted on error rate in the CRT task with age as between-subjects factor. There was no significant effect of age ($F(1, 45) = 0.22$; $P > .63$); error rate = 2.81% and 2.44% for younger and older adults, respectively. A second ANOVA with age as between-subjects factor and type of trials (neutral versus incongruent) as within-subjects factor was then conducted on error rate in the Stroop task. The interaction between age and type of trials was close to significance ($F(1, 45) = 3.40$; $P > .07$), the simple effect of age was not significant ($F(1, 45) = 0.98$; $P > .32$) while the simple effect of type of trials reached significance ($F(1, 45) = 12.10$; $P < .002$). Participants made significantly more errors in the incongruent condition (2.43%) than in the neutral condition (0.35%). A third ANOVA with age as between-subjects factor and type of block of trials (simple versus mixed) as within-subjects factor was conducted on error rate in the dimension-switching task. The interaction between age and type of block of trials was close to significance ($F(1, 45) = 3.60$; $P > .06$), as well as the simple effect of age ($F(1, 45) = 3.18$; $P > .08$), but the effect of type of block of trials reached significance ($F(1, 45) = 26.25$; $P < .0001$). Participants made significantly more errors in the mixed block of trials (5.07%) than in the simple block of trials (1.61%). A fourth and last ANOVA with age as between-subjects factor and type of trials (alternation versus repetition) as within-subjects factor was conducted on error rate in the mixed blocks of trials of the stimulus-response compatibility switching task. The interaction between age and type of transition did not reach significance ($F(1, 45) = 1.89$; $P > .17$), but the simple effects of age and type of transition did ($F(1, 45) = 6.07$; $P < .02$ and $F(1, 45) = 37.10$; $P < .0001$, resp.). All participants made more errors when they had to alternate (9.27%) rather than when they had to repeat the stimulus-response mapping (3.33%) and older adults (7.63%) made more errors than younger adults (3.63%). These results on error rate and those concerning RTs (see Table 3) showed that there was no speed-accuracy tradeoffs for the effect of age on cognitive functions assessed through RT tasks.

3.3. Effects of Swimming Practice on Cognitive Functions Performance in Older Adults. The results of the statistical

Table 3: Results of the MANCOVAs, ANCOVAs, and effect-sizes contrasting young and older participants on cognitive performance, with level of education as covariate, and mean behavioral performance for each age group (SD).

Cognitive functions	Cognitive tasks	Dependent variables	MANCOVA F	ddl	Wilk's λ	Partial η^2	ANCOVA F(1,44)	Cohen's d	Young adults M (SD)	Older adults M (SD)
Speed of information processing	**Auditory simple reaction time task**	**Reaction time (ms)**	**47.98** ($P < .0001$)	**2, 43**	**.31**	**.69**	**23.06** ($P < .0001$)	**1.51**	**194 (26)**	**257 (52)**
	Visual choice reaction time task	**Reaction time (ms)**					**94.89** ($P < .0001$)	**3.34**	**335 (28)**	**475 (53)**
Behavioral inhibition	Stop-signal task	Rate of successful inhibition	**4.29** ($P < .001$)	**3, 42**	**.77**	**.23**	1.13 ($P = .29$)	0.16	0.41 (0.15)	0.44 (0.21)
	Stroop task	**Interference cost (ms)**					**12.46** ($P < .001$)	**1.10**	**189 (63)**	**291 (115)**
	RNG task	**Adjacency score**					**5.96** ($P < .02$)	**0.93**	**33.50 (7.04)**	**42.27 (11.29)**
Updating of working memory	Letter running-span task	NO correct responses	**19.77** ($P < .0001$)	**2, 43**	**.52**	**.48**	2.69 ($P = .11$)	0.80	39.19 (4.62)	34.28 (7.35)
	Spatial running-span task	**NO correct responses**					**36.81** ($P < .0001$)	**2.23**	**41.25 (4.84)**	**23.31 (10.30)**
Shifting	Wisconsin card sorting test	NO perseverative errors	**8.37** ($P < .0002$)	**3, 42**	**.63**	**.37**	3.69 ($P = .06$)	0.79	8.50 (2.68)	12.81 (7.22)
	Dimension switching task	**Global switch cost (ms)**					**15.65** ($P < .0003$)	**1.74**	**192 (154)**	**606 (299)**
	Stimulus-Response switching task	**Local switch cost (ms)**					**9.86** ($P < .0031$)	**1.09**	**71 (57)**	**184 (135)**

Note. RNG: Random Number Generation, in bold: Significant effect.

analyses and behavioral performance as a function of level of activity for each cognitive function and each experimental task are detailed in Table 4. The MANOVAs revealed a significant effect of swimming activity on each of the three EF components but no significant effect on information processing speed. Subsequent ANOVAs on each task tapping EFs showed that older participants who swim regularly performed significantly better in five out of eight tests. More precisely, swimmers outperformed sedentary participants on the two tasks tapping Updating, on two of three tasks tapping Shifting, and on the RNG task tapping Inhibition. When it was significant, the effect size of swimming was large (mean Cohen's $d = 1.05$).

The effect of swimming was examined on error rate for all the tasks that included choice reaction time measurements. A first ANOVA was conducted on error rate in the CRT task with PA level as between-subjects factor. There was a significant effect of PA level on error rate ($F(1, 45) = 8.24$; $P < .007$); sedentary older adults made more errors in the CRT task (3.75%) than older swimmers (1.13%). A second ANOVA with PA level as between-subjects factor and type of trials (neutral versus incongruent) as within-subjects factor was conducted on error rate in the Stroop task. There was a significant interaction between these two factors ($F(1, 45) = 8.07$; $P < .007$). A post hoc test showed that sedentary older adults made more errors in the incongruent condition than in the neutral condition (3.39% versus 0%, respectively; $P < .02$) while older adults who practiced swimming did not (1.24% versus 0.26% resp.; $P > .45$). A third ANOVA with PA level as between-subjects factor and type of block of trials (simple versus mixed) as within-subjects factor was conducted on error rate in the dimension-switching task. The interaction between PA level and the type of block of trials was significant ($F(1, 45) = 10.81$; $P = .002$). A post hoc test showed that older swimmers made more errors in the mixed than in the simple block of trials (8.68% versus 1.61%; $P < .0002$) while sedentary older adults did not (3.26% versus 1.67%; $P > .34$). The examination of RT and error data in the dimension-switching task suggests that the two groups of older adults did not use the same strategy in the more difficult condition: swimmers preferred to emphasize speed whereas sedentary people preferred to emphasize accuracy. A fourth and last ANOVA with PA level as between-subjects factor and type of trials (alternation versus repetition) as within-subjects factor was conducted on error rate in the mixed blocks of trials of the stimulus-response compatibility switching task. The interaction between PA level and type of transition did not reach significance ($F(1, 45) = 0.61$; $P > .43$), but the simple effects of PA level and type of transition did ($F(1, 45) = 12.43$; $P < .001$ and $F(1, 45) = 33.25$; $P < .0001$, resp.). Older adults made more errors when they had to alternate (11.07%) rather than when they had to repeat the stimulus-response mapping (4.19%) and, overall, older swimmers (10.94%) made more errors than sedentary older adults (4.33%). One more time, swimmers preferred to emphasize speed while sedentary participants preferred to emphasize accuracy in the more difficult condition.

3.4. Relationship between Cardiorespiratory Fitness and Executive Function. To examine the relationships between cardiorespiratory fitness and EF performance in older adults, we performed a series of bivariate correlations (Spearman coefficients of correlation) between each cognitive task performance and VO_2max level. The performance of only two tasks significantly correlated with VO_2max level: the updating of verbal information ($r = .56$; $P < .05$) and the global switch cost ($r = .46$; $P < .05$). Figure 1 depicts the scatter plots of executive performance on these tasks with VO_2max level with their respective coefficients of determination (R^2).

4. Discussion

As has been extensively documented, age-related cerebral and cognitive declines are not uniform but quite differentiated (see [43, 44] for reviews). Similarly, most of the recent literature on aging, fitness, and cognition has shown that chronic exercise would result in selective improvements in executive functions rather than general benefits [13, 20, 21]. However, contemporary theoretical models of executive functions posit that the construct of EF is not uniform but encompasses fractionated executive subprocesses [2, 8, 9]. It is then important to examine whether chronic exercise benefits are homogeneous or selective to some particular executive subprocesses. Using this established theoretical and methodological framework, the aim of this study was to examine differences in cognitive performance as a function of chronological age and long-term regular practice of swimming by measuring younger and older adults' information processing speed and performance on three well-known EFs, inhibition, updating, and shifting. Globally, the results revealed a clear pattern of age-related decline in all cognitive functions. On the other hand, older adults who practice regular swimming were shown to have a positive relation with improved performance on five of eight experimental tasks and all EF components. VO_2max level was only positively related to executive performance for two tasks. These results provide a clear argument for the use of a multitask approach when studying the effects of chronic exercise on cognitive functions.

Before examining the effects of aging and swimming practice on cognitive performance, it is important to discuss the multitask approach used in this study. Because it is impossible to find a "pure" task to assess an isolated cognitive function, particularly an EF, multiple measures were used to rule out "task impurity" (see [2, 7–9]). As such, we wanted to assess the EF construct at the level of a general or latent variable, which reflects the postulated cognitive function more strongly than each individual experimental task alone. However, as revealed by the standardized Cronbach alphas and the matrix of correlations displayed in Table 2, it appears that the construct validity of our three EFs was quite low. Indeed, the correlations between tasks supposed to reflect a particular EF component were often low or even nonsignificant and sometimes smaller than the correlations between two tasks thought to assess different EF components. Such

TABLE 4: Results of the MANOVAs, ANOVAs, and effect-sizes contrasting active and sedentary older participants on cognitive performance and mean behavioral performance for each age group (SD).

Cognitive function	Cognitive task	Dependent variable	MANOVA F	ddl	Wilk's λ	Partial η^2	ANOVA F(1,45)	Cohen's d	Sedentary older adults M (SD)	Active older adults M (SD)
Speed of information processing	Auditory simple reaction time task	Reaction time (ms)	0.43 ($P = .73$)	2, 44	.98	.02	—	—	252 (40)	262 (64)
	Visual choice reaction time task	Reaction time (ms)					—	—	468 (49)	482 (57)
Behavioral inhibition	Stop-signal task	Rate of successful inhibition	**2.79 (P= .05)**	**3, 43**	**.84**	**.16**	0.00 ($P = .96$)	0.02	0.44 (0.23)	0.44 (0.20)
	Stroop task	Interference cost (ms)					0.10 ($P = .76$)	0.10	297 (132)	285 (99)
	RNG task	**Adjacency score**					**7.04 ($P < .011$)**	**0.85**	**46.72 (11.09)**	**37.82 (9.91)**
Updating of working memory	**Letter running-span task**	**NO correct responses**	**9.61 ($P < .0004$)**	2, 44	.70	.30	**19.50 ($P < .0001$)**	**1.45**	**29.94 (6.08)**	**38.63 (5.88)**
	Spatial running-span task	**NO correct responses**					**7.04 ($P < .013$)**	**0.80**	**19.44 (8.39)**	**27.19 (10.80)**
Shifting	**Wisconsin card sorting test**	**NO perseverative errors**	**10.24 ($P < .0001$)**	3, 43	.58	.42	**21.70 ($P < .0001$)**	**1.41**	**17.00 (8.05)**	**8.63 (2.36)**
	Dimension switching task	Global switch cost (ms)					2.65 ($P = .11$)	0.68	704 (267)	508 (306)
	Stimulus-Response switching task	**Local switch cost (ms)**					**6.24 ($P < .017$)**	**0.76**	**232 (129)**	**135 (126)**

Note. RNG: Random Number Generation, in Bold: Significant effect.

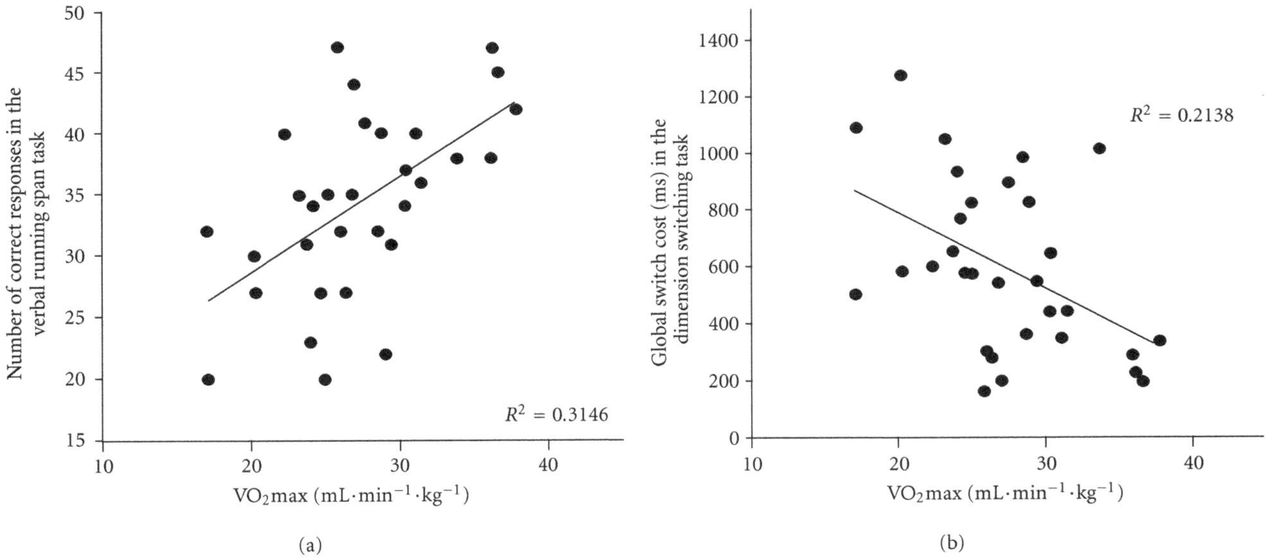

Figure 1: Scatter plots relating VO_2max level and updating performance of verbal information (a) and global switch cost (b) in the older participants.

results have already been reported by previous studies from our own team [2] and others [11, 45] and raise a question of the low specificity of the tasks used to assess EFs, which will be discussed in the limitations section.

Consistent with a large body of research on cognitive and cerebral aging, we found that chronological age has a detrimental effect on information processing speed and on the three evaluated EFs. The age-related decline in the RT tasks is in agreement with numerous studies on the effect of aging on processing speed [2, 12]. The performance deficits observed in our older adults in the three EF domains also agree with the literature examining this question with a similar approach [2, 10, 11]. Our results also suggest that the deleterious effects of aging are more pronounced for processing speed (69% of the explained variance, see partial η^2 in Table 3) than for updating (48% of the explained variance), shifting (37% of the explained variance), and inhibition (23% of the explained variance). However, it is important to note that taking into account the educational level (as measured by the number of years of academic education) decreased the age-related effects on all the cognitive tasks and even eliminated the effects of chronological age on the letter running-span task and the WCST. This finding strengthens the importance of taking into account education as an important moderator of cognitive aging which can be interpreted in the more general context of cognitive reserve [46, 47]. As we will discuss below, it may be that PA (in the present study, swimming) could also be viewed as a proxy of cognitive reserve beyond educational level.

In the older population, the differences in cognitive performance between swimmers and sedentary people were not homogeneous across all the studied cognitive processes. First, there was no significant difference between active and sedentary participants in the measures of information processing speed, as assessed by the SRT and the CRT tasks (see Table 4). This result contrasts with some previous results [48, 49] but agrees with others [20, 21, 24], particularly with those of Hawkins and coworkers [31] in the same context of swimming practice. These contradicting findings may be due to specific differences between particular PAs practiced by different samples of participants. The impact on processing speed may be different between racket sports or hand-ball, such as in Spirduso's study [49], and swimming such as in our study. Another, more likely possibility is linked to the assertion that chronic exercise exerts selective effects on cognitive processes involving executive control and not on less-controlled processes, such as the stimulus-driven information processing involved in basic reaction time tasks (see [13, 20, 24]). Our results favor this second possibility and strengthen this selective benefit of PA on EF processes.

Second, our results indicate prima facie that the impact of swimming practice was quite homogeneous across all three EF components, assuming that our groups only differed at the level of swimming practice. All three MANOVAs contrasting the performance between older swimmers and sedentary participants were significant for these cognitive functions. However, the percentage of variance explained by swimming practice was more important for Shifting (42%) than for Updating (30%) and Inhibition (16%), as revealed by partial eta squared (see partial η^2 in Table 4). Our results of a strong relationship between swimming practice and Shifting confirm the previous conclusions of Hawkins et al. [31] on the positive effect of water aerobics on attentional flexibility. However, as pointed out in the Results section, the examination of speed and accuracy measures in the two switching tasks underscores that the two groups of participants may not have used the same strategies to perform these tasks. The swimmers made more errors and emphasized speed to the detriment of accuracy. Consequently, the speed-accuracy tradeoffs observed in the two switching tasks weaken the strength of the positive relationship between swimming practice and Shifting.

Moreover, five out of eight tasks were strongly sensitive to differences between swimmers and sedentary participants, but the performance of two tasks out of three (Stroop task and signal-stop task) assessing inhibition and one task out of three (dimension-switching task) assessing shifting did not significantly differ between regular swimmers and sedentary participants. As previously stated, we think that this result underscores the importance of using a multitask approach when studying the effects of chronic exercise on cognitive functions and may help to resolve some discrepant results in this domain. For example, the absence of significant effect of exercise training reported by other researchers on some cognitive tasks [21, 29, 50] may not reflect an absence of real effects but instead a lack of sensitivity of the experimental tasks. For instance, our results conflict with those reported by Smiley-Oyen et al. [21], because they found an effect of aerobic exercise on the Stroop task and no effect on the WCST. Several reasons can be hypothesized to explain the discrepancies, such as differences in study design, experimental tasks, modes of response, and selected dependent measures, but it is always difficult to definitively conclude which is the correct explanation. One of the strengths of the present study is to combine the use of several different experimental tasks to examine the influence of PA within the same sample not only at the level of individual tasks but also at the more general level of the explored cognitive functions. This procedure allowed us to show that regular swimming was clearly related to better executive performance on the three examined EFs, despite the absence of significant effect on three of the eight tasks. This may indicate that some tasks could be more sensitive to the effects of PA than other tasks. Additional work should verify the consistency of our results, as our findings are far from conclusive. A recent study from our group [51] used different measures of PA and explored the same executive functions with different tasks or variations of the same tasks as used in the present study and showed that PA exerted a selective effect on inhibition but not on updating or shifting and only for the oldest adults of the sample (71 years and older). These different results highlight the lability of the effects of exercise on cognitive performance according to tasks and characteristics of the participants. Clearly, more work is needed to draw a definitive conclusion on the selectivity of the effects of chronic exercise effects on EFs.

The role of cardiorespiratory fitness in the relationship between PA and cognitive performance in older adults remains under debate (see [4, 21, 25]). Accordingly, we were interested in examining the relationships between VO_2max level and cognitive performance. As shown in Figure 1, only performance on the verbal running span task and the dimension-switching task was significantly correlated with VO_2max level. Of particular interest, one must remember that there was no significant effect of PA on the global switch cost of the dimension-switching task ($P = .11$, see Table 4). Thus, there is only one task (the verbal running span task) showing PA-related benefits that could be mediated by cardiorespiratory fitness level and one task (the dimension-switching task) showing no relationship with swimming practice but a significant relationship with VO_2max level. These results underscore the differences between a behavioral measure assessed through questionnaires (PA) and an estimated physiological measure assessed through field test (VO_2max), and their different influences on different cognitive functions [21, 25, 51]. Distinguishing between PA and cardiorespiratory fitness, which were weakly related ($r = .35$; $P = .054$) in the present study, seems of particular importance because they may exert their influence on cognitive functioning by different mechanisms. A challenge for future studies will be to understand and characterize the mechanisms underlying these selective effects. One may hypothesize that PA could be viewed qualitatively as a proxy of cognitive reserve, as defined by Stern and collaborators [46, 47], allowing physically active older adults to make flexible and efficient use of available brain reserve and to demonstrate better cognitive performance. In other respects, better cardiorespiratory fitness could induce anatomical and neurophysiological changes in the brain [6, 14, 26–28] that could reflect and enhance brain reserve [46, 47].

There are potential limitations in the present study that should be addressed. First, the low specificity of the tasks used to assess the construct of EF in this study limits the generalizability of our conclusions and strengthens the importance of looking for and using well-designed tasks to reflect the postulated cognitive functions. Second, our cross-sectional design precludes inferences about causality in the relationship between chronic engagement in swimming and executive performance. Well-designed randomized-controlled trials are now needed, using the same multitask approach, before a definitive conclusion can be made. Third, the level of education of the participants has been taken into account as a covariate in the statistical analyses of the present study. However, other important moderators of aging related to lifestyle, such as income, socioeconomic status, food habits, previous careers, and lifelong leisure activities, have not been measured in our experiment. These different variables can explain part of the variance in cognitive aging and may lead to an overestimation of the relationship between present level of physical activity and cognitive performance in cross-sectional designs, as could have been the case in the present study.

To summarize the principal findings, this study demonstrated the validity of using a multitask approach in examining the potential benefits of regular swimming on the aging of cognitive function. Such a theoretical and methodological approach allowed us to show that chronic swimming practice is related to better executive functions in older adults and that these benefits are seen on the three EFs studied but that some tasks are less sensitive to detecting these benefits. Finally, the demonstrated benefits of PA were not necessarily linked to better cardiorespiratory fitness, showing the potential relative independence of these behavioral or physiological moderators on executive performance.

Acknowledgment

This work was supported by grants from Regional Council of Poitou-Charentes, University of Poitiers (France) and University of Tishreen (Syria). The authors greatly thank Professor Cedric A. Bouquet for his help on designing some of the experimental tasks and Professor Phillip D. Tomporowski for his valuables comments on an earlier version of this paper.

References

[1] R. L. West, "An application of prefrontal cortex function theory to cognitive aging," *Psychological Bulletin*, vol. 120, no. 2, pp. 272–292, 1996.

[2] C. T. Albinet, G. Boucard, C. A. Bouquet, and M. Audiffren, "Processing speed and executive functions in cognitive aging: how to disentangle their mutual relationship?" *Brain and Cognition*, vol. 79, no. 1, pp. 1–11, 2012.

[3] L. H. Phillips and J. D. Henry, "Adult aging and executive functioning," in *Executive Functions and the Frontal Lobes: A Lifespan Perspective*, V. Anderson, R. Jacobs, and P. J. Anderson, Eds., pp. 57–79, Taylor & Francis, New York, NY, USA, 2008.

[4] M. Audiffren, N. André, and C. T. Albinet, "Effects of chronic exercise on cognitive functions in older adults: assessment and prospects," *Revue de Neuropsychologie*, vol. 3, no. 4, pp. 207–225, 2011.

[5] C. H. Hillman, K. I. Erickson, and A. F. Kramer, "Be smart, exercise your heart: exercise effects on brain and cognition," *Nature Reviews Neuroscience*, vol. 9, no. 1, pp. 58–65, 2008.

[6] A. F. Kramer and K. I. Erickson, "Capitalizing on cortical plasticity: influence of physical activity on cognition and brain function," *Trends in Cognitive Sciences*, vol. 11, no. 8, pp. 342–348, 2007.

[7] V. Anderson, R. Jacobs, and P. J. Anderson, Eds., *Executive Functions and the Frontal Lobes: A Lifespan Perspective*, Taylor & Francis, New York, NY, USA, 2008.

[8] M. B. Jurado and M. Rosselli, "The elusive nature of executive functions: a review of our current understanding," *Neuropsychology Review*, vol. 17, no. 3, pp. 213–233, 2007.

[9] A. Miyake, N. P. Friedman, M. J. Emerson, A. H. Witzki, A. Howerter, and T. D. Wager, "The unity and diversity of executive functions and their contributions to complex "frontal lobe" tasks: A latent variable analysis," *Cognitive Psychology*, vol. 41, no. 1, pp. 49–100, 2000.

[10] J. E. Fisk and C. A. Sharp, "Age-related impairment in executive functioning: updating, inhibition, shifting, and access," *Journal of Clinical and Experimental Neuropsychology*, vol. 26, no. 7, pp. 874–890, 2004.

[11] L. Vaughan and K. Giovanello, "Executive function in daily life: age-related influences of executive processes on instrumental activities of daily living," *Psychology and Aging*, vol. 25, no. 2, pp. 343–355, 2010.

[12] T. A. Salthouse, "The processing-speed theory of adult age differences in cognition," *Psychological Review*, vol. 103, no. 3, pp. 403–428, 1996.

[13] S. Colcombe and A. F. Kramer, "Fitness effects on the cognitive function of older adults: a meta-analytic study," *Psychological Science*, vol. 14, no. 2, pp. 125–130, 2003.

[14] S. J. Colcombe, K. I. Erickson, N. Raz et al., "Aerobic fitness reduces brain tissue loss in aging humans," *Journals of Gerontology A*, vol. 58, no. 2, pp. 176–180, 2003.

[15] C. Voelcker-Rehage, B. Godde, and U. M. Staudinger, "Physical and motor fitness are both related to cognition in old age," *European Journal of Neuroscience*, vol. 31, no. 1, pp. 167–176, 2010.

[16] L. Fratiglioni, S. Paillard-Borg, and B. Winblad, "An active and socially integrated lifestyle in late life might protect against dementia," *Lancet Neurology*, vol. 3, no. 6, pp. 343–353, 2004.

[17] E. B. Larson, L. Wang, J. D. Bowen et al., "Exercise is associated with reduced risk for incident dementia among persons 65 years of age and older," *Annals of Internal Medicine*, vol. 144, no. 2, pp. 73–81, 2006.

[18] C. T. Albinet, G. Boucard, C. A. Bouquet, and M. Audiffren, "Increased heart rate variability and executive performance after aerobic training in the elderly," *European Journal of Applied Physiology*, vol. 109, no. 4, pp. 617–624, 2010.

[19] S. J. Colcombe, A. F. Kramer, K. I. Erickson et al., "Cardiovascular fitness, cortical plasticity, and aging," *Proceedings of the National Academy of Sciences of the United States of America*, vol. 101, no. 9, pp. 3316–3321, 2004.

[20] A. F. Kramer, S. Hahn, N. J. Cohen et al., "Ageing, fitness and neurocognitive function," *Nature*, vol. 400, no. 6743, pp. 418–419, 1999.

[21] A. L. Smiley-Oyen, K. A. Lowry, S. J. Francois, M. L. Kohut, and P. Ekkekakis, "Exercise, fitness, and neurocognitive function in older adults: the "selective improvement" and "cardiovascular fitness" hypotheses," *Annals of Behavioral Medicine*, vol. 36, no. 3, pp. 280–291, 2008.

[22] G. Kemoun, M. Thibaud, N. Roumagne et al., "Effects of a physical training programme on cognitive function and walking efficiency in elderly persons with dementia," *Dementia and Geriatric Cognitive Disorders*, vol. 29, no. 2, pp. 109–114, 2010.

[23] N. T. Lautenschlager, K. L. Cox, L. Flicker et al., "Effect of physical activity on cognitive function in older adults at risk for Alzheimer disease: a randomized trial," *Journal of the American Medical Association*, vol. 300, no. 9, pp. 1027–1037, 2008.

[24] C. D. Hall, A. L. Smith, and S. W. Keele, "The impact of aerobic activity on cognitive function in older adults: a new synthesis based on the concept of executive control," *European Journal of Cognitive Psychology*, vol. 13, no. 1-2, pp. 279–300, 2001.

[25] J. L. Etnier, P. M. Nowell, D. M. Landers, and B. A. Sibley, "A meta-regression to examine the relationship between aerobic fitness and cognitive performance," *Brain Research Reviews*, vol. 52, no. 1, pp. 119–130, 2006.

[26] S. J. Colcombe, K. I. Erickson, P. E. Scalf et al., "Aerobic exercise training increases brain volume in aging humans," *Journals of Gerontology A*, vol. 61, no. 11, pp. 1166–1170, 2006.

[27] A. D. Brown, C. A. McMorris, R. S. Longman et al., "Effects of cardiorespiratory fitness and cerebral blood flow on cognitive outcomes in older women," *Neurobiology of Aging*, vol. 31, no. 12, pp. 2047–2057, 2010.

[28] A. C. Pereira, D. E. Huddleston, A. M. Brickman et al., "An in vivo correlate of exercise-induced neurogenesis in the adult dentate gyrus," *Proceedings of the National Academy of Sciences of the United States of America*, vol. 104, no. 13, pp. 5638–5643, 2007.

[29] D. J. Madden, J. A. Blumenthal, P. A. Allen, and C. F. Emery, "Improving aerobic capacity in healthy older adults does not necessarily lead to improved cognitive performance," *Psychology and Aging*, vol. 4, no. 3, pp. 307–320, 1989.

[30] T. Liu-Ambrose, L. S. Nagamatsu, P. Graf, B. L. Beattie, M. C. Ashe, and T. C. Handy, "Resistance training and executive

functions: a 12-month randomized controlled trial," *Archives of Internal Medicine*, vol. 170, no. 2, pp. 170–178, 2010.

[31] H. L. Hawkins, A. F. Kramer, and D. Capaldi, "Aging, exercise, and attention," *Psychology and aging*, vol. 7, no. 4, pp. 643–653, 1992.

[32] L. Muller, *Participation culturelle et sportive: Tableaux issus de l'enquête PCV de mai 2003*, Ministère de la Jeunesse, des Sports et de la Vie Associative, Paris, 2005.

[33] Y. Katsura, T. Yoshikawa, S. Y. Ueda et al., "Effects of aquatic exercise training using water-resistance equipment in elderly," *European Journal of Applied Physiology*, vol. 108, no. 5, pp. 957–964, 2010.

[34] J. E. Taunton, E. C. Rhodes, L. A. Wolski et al., "Effect of land-based and water-based fitness programs on the cardiovascular fitness, strength and flexibility of women aged 65–75 years," *Gerontology*, vol. 42, no. 4, pp. 204–210, 1996.

[35] M. Bergamin, S. Zanuso, B. A. Alvar, A. Ermolao, and M. Zaccaria, "Is water-based exercise training sufficient to improve physical fitness in the elderly," *European Review of Aging and Physical Activity*, vol. 9, no. 2, pp. 129–141, 2012.

[36] K. Hauer, N. Specht, M. Schuler, P. Bärtsch, and P. Oster, "Intensive physical training in geriatric patients after severe falls and hip surgery," *Age and Ageing*, vol. 31, no. 1, pp. 49–57, 2002.

[37] M. F. Folstein, S. E. Folstein, and P. R. McHugh, "'Mini mental state': a practical method for grading the cognitive state of patients for the clinician," *Journal of Psychiatric Research*, vol. 12, no. 3, pp. 189–198, 1975.

[38] H. Robert, J. M. Casillas, M. Iskandar et al., "Le Score d'activité physique de Dijon: reproductibilité et corrélations avec l'aptitude physique de sujets sains âgés," *Annales de Réadaptation et de Médecine Physique*, vol. 47, no. 8, pp. 546–554, 2004.

[39] G. M. Kline, J. P. Porcari, and R. Hintermeister, "Estimation of VO2max from a one-mile track walk, gender, age, and body weight," *Medicine and Science in Sports and Exercise*, vol. 19, no. 3, pp. 253–259, 1987.

[40] E. McAuley, A. N. Szabo, E. L. Mailey et al., "Non-exercise estimated cardiorespiratory fitness: associations with brain structure, cognition, and memory complaints in older adults," *Mental Health and Physical Activity*, vol. 4, no. 1, pp. 5–11, 2011.

[41] G. D. Logan, W. B. Cowan, and K. A. Davis, "On the ability to inhibit simple and choice reaction time responses: a model and a method," *Journal of Experimental Psychology*, vol. 10, no. 2, pp. 276–291, 1984.

[42] J. Cohen, *Statistical Power Analysis for the Behavioral Sciences*, Lawrence Erlbaum Associates, Hillsdale, NJ, USA, 2nd edition, 1988.

[43] T. A. Salthouse, *Theoretical Perspectives on Cognitive Aging*, Lawrence Erlbaum Associates, Hillsdale, NJ, USA, 1991.

[44] K. W. Schaie and S. L. Willis, *Handbook of the Psychology of Aging*, vol. 7, Elsevier, Amsterdam, The Netherlands, 2011.

[45] T. A. Salthouse, T. M. Atkinson, and D. E. Berish, "Executive functioning as a potential mediator of age-related cognitive decline in normal adults," *Journal of Experimental Psychology*, vol. 132, no. 4, pp. 566–594, 2003.

[46] J. Steffener and Y. Stern, "Exploring the neural basis of cognitive reserve in aging," *Biochimica & Biophysica Acta*, vol. 1822, no. 3, pp. 467–473, 2012.

[47] Y. Stern, "Cognitive reserve," *Neuropsychologia*, vol. 47, no. 10, pp. 2015–2028, 2009.

[48] M. Renaud, L. Bherer, and F. Maquestiaux, "A high level of physical fitness is associated with more efficient response preparation in older adults," *Journals of Gerontology B*, vol. 65, no. 3, pp. 317–322, 2010.

[49] W. W. Spirduso, "Reaction and movement time as a function of age and physical activity level," *Journals of Gerontology*, vol. 30, no. 4, pp. 435–440, 1975.

[50] J. A. Blumenthal, C. F. Emery, D. J. Madden et al., "Long-term effects of exercise on psychological functioning in older men and women," *Journals of Gerontology*, vol. 46, no. 6, pp. P352–P361, 1991.

[51] G. K. Boucard, C. T. Albinet, A. Bugaiska, C. Bouquet, D. Clarys, and M. Audiffren, "Impact of physical activity on executive functions in aging: a selective effect on inhibition among old adults," *Journal of Sport and Exercise Psychology*, vol. 34, pp. 808–827, 2012.

2

Effects of Multicomponent Exercise on Functional and Cognitive Parameters of Hypertensive Patients

Hélio José Coelho Junior,[1] Bruno Rodrigues,[1] Daniele Jardim Feriani,[1] Ivan de Oliveira Gonçalves,[2] Ricardo Yukio Asano,[3] Samuel da Silva Aguiar,[4] and Marco Carlos Uchida[1]

[1]*School of Physical Education, University of Campinas, Campinas, SP, Brazil*
[2]*Center of Health Sciences, University of Mogi das Cruzes, Mogi das Cruzes, SP, Brazil*
[3]*School of Arts, Sciences and Humanities, University of São Paulo, São Paulo, SP, Brazil*
[4]*Brazil School of Physical Education, Catholic University of Brasília, Brasília, DF, Brazil*

Correspondence should be addressed to Hélio José Coelho Junior; coelhojunior@hotmail.com.br

Academic Editor: F. R. Ferraro

Purpose. The present study aimed to investigate the impact of a 6-month multicomponent exercise program (MCEP) on physical function and cognitive parameters of normotensive (NTS) and hypertensive (HTS) older patients and verify if age can influence the adaptations in response to the exercise. *Methods.* A total of 218 subjects, 101 NTS and 117 HTS, were recruited and underwent functional and cognitive evaluations before and after six months of a MCEP. The program of exercise was performed twice a week, for 26 weeks. The physical exercises were thought to mimic the activities of daily living and, therefore, aggregated functional and walking exercises. Exercise sessions were performed at moderate intensity. *Results.* Data indicated that HTS and NST patients showed a similar increase in the performance of walking speed test and one-leg stand test after the MCEP. Regarding age, results did not show differences in the magnitude of adaptations between old and young HTS and NTS patients. *Conclusions.* Data of the present study indicated that a 6-month MCEP was able to increase equally balance and mobility in NTS and HTS patients. Moreover, data demonstrated that aging did not seem to impair the capacity to adapt in response to exercise in both groups.

1. Introduction

The aging process is a continuous phenomenon accompanied by alterations in some physiological systems, collaborating with the development of geriatric syndromes and chronical diseases, such as hypertension (HTN) [1–3]. In fact, HTN has higher prevalence in older people (~70%), which leads to a poor prognosis in this population because patients with high blood pressure show increased risk for stroke and myocardial infarction [4, 5].

However, several evidences have been indicating that HTN not only is strongly associated with cardiovascular risk factors, but also can lead to physical and cognitive impairments in older adults in a time-dependent fashion [6–8]. In turn, aging process per se is already accompanied by marked decrease on physical functioning and on cognitive capacities [9]. Thus, aggregate HTN and aging can potentialize physical and cognitive decline. This phenomenon is a public health problem, once physical functioning and cognitive capacities compose two largest domains: independence and autonomy, respectively, which are analogous to the concept of health in older population [9].

Multicomponent exercise programs (MCEP) emerge as a possible type of physical exercise able to prevent the deleterious effects of aging on the organic system, improving physical functioning, and cognitive capacities [10, 11]. This occurs, since a mix of different exercise regimes are offered in the same exercise routine, thereby not requiring sessions of physical exercise with long duration while developing several physical capacities and skills [11], which can collaborate with exercise adherence in the hypertensive population [12].

Nevertheless, just one study, which was performed with a low-sample size, recorded the effects of a MCEP on functional parameters of hypertensive patients [13]. Moreover, cognitive capacities have not been studied in this context.

Therefore, the present study aimed to investigate the impact of a 6-month MCEP on physical function and cognitive parameters of normotensive (NTS) and hypertensive (HTS) older patients and verify if age can influence the adaptations in response to the exercise.

Based on aforementioned data, the alternative hypothesis *(H1)* of the present study is that MCEP is capable of inducing significant improvements in functional and cognitive parameters of NTS and HTS older adults, regardless of age.

2. Materials and Methods

The present study has a quasi-experimental design, which aimed to investigate the effects of a 6-month multicomponent exercise program (MCEP) in the functional and cognitive parameters of normotensive (NTS) and hypertensive (HTS) older patients. Therefore, patients were undergoing functional and cognitive evaluations before and after 6 months of MCEP. All volunteers signed the informed consent form and completed all measurements. This study was approved by the Research Ethics Committee of the University of Campinas (UNICAMP). This study was developed in accordance with the Declaration of Helsinki and according to Resolution 196/96 of the National Health Council.

2.1. Subjects. A total of 101 NTS and 117 HTS untrained patients were recruited from two specialized healthcare centers for older adults in a town located in the metropolitan area of São Paulo, Brazil. Volunteers were recruited by convenience and asked verbally by the medical team and researchers about their participation in the study. All subjects provided informed consent before enrolment.

The exclusion criteria were use of hormone replacement and/or psychotropic drugs, cerebrovascular disease (e.g., stroke), pulmonary disease, neurological or psychiatric disease (e.g., Parkinson's or Alzheimer's disease), musculoskeletal disorders, comorbidities associated with greater risk of falls and any kind of dizziness, and blurred vision or lightheadedness when rising or remaining standing for long, which could indicate orthostatic hypertension and/or labyrinthitis. The inclusion criterion was age ≥60 years. Patients of both genders were accepted in the present study. After the application of the exclusion and inclusion criteria, 218 older women were included in the analyses.

The volunteers were subdivided into NTS and HTS groups according to previous clinical diagnosis of HTN. Since both healthcare centers serve a large number of patients and the medical team (i.e., nurse, physician, and physical educator) is of limited size, the pathological conditions were simply recorded by the head physician and head nurse of each center. A specialist (i.e., cardiologist) who was not affiliated to and was outside the center then made the diagnosis of HTN, according to the guidelines [14].

In summary, before the participants began the activities in the centers where they were recruited, a medical consultation was conducted and an extensive list of medical exams was required (e.g., fasting blood glucose, fasting blood insulin). If the patient showed any signal of HTN, such as high blood pressure levels during the first visits in the centers, he/she was invited to measure blood pressure levels, at least, three times, during different periods of the day at home. If her/his blood pressure evaluations remained elevated, he/she was referred to a cardiologist. After they underwent specific medical consultation (i.e., cardiologist) and perform all specific exams (i.e., 24-hour ambulatory blood pressure monitoring [ABPM], home blood pressure) [14], patients should return to the centers with a letter signed by the specialist confirming or not the diagnosis of HTN. It is important to mention that the criteria adopted in HTN diagnosis (i.e., stage 1) proposed by the Brazilian Society of Cardiology (BSC) was based on systolic blood pressure (SBP) values among 140–159 mmHg and/or diastolic blood pressure (DBP) values among 90-90 mmHg [14]. Moreover, repeated measurements in different places were proposed by the cardiologist to confirm the clinical diagnosis of HTN. Final diagnosis was signed by the head physician of the center and a nurse updated the medical records each 6 month. Patients of the present study were recruited one week after the update of the medical records.

All volunteers were instructed to refrain from physical exercise for the 96 hours, as well as drinking coffee, alcoholic, and energy drinks during the 24 hours before all evaluations. Although alimentary ingestion was not controlled, subjects were instructed to maintain the habitual food intake throughout the period of the protocol. All volunteers ensure that these parameters were not altered during the protocol. Evaluations (pre and post) were performed 120 hours before and after the beginning and the end of the physical exercise program, respectively.

2.2. Functional Evaluations. Before the performance of the tests, an experienced researcher detailed the procedures of each test. The volunteers performed all tests twice and the higher value recorded in each test was used in the analysis. During all tests, verbal encouragement was provided to ensure that volunteers reached the best performance possible. The present protocol was used by our group elsewhere [42].

2.2.1. Sit-to-Stand Test. Volunteers were requested to rise from a chair five times as fast as possible with their arms crossed in front of the body. The stopwatch was activated when the volunteer raised their buttocks off the chair and was stopped when the volunteer seated back.

2.2.2. One-Leg Stand Test. The one-leg stand test was performed with the volunteers standing in a unipodal stance with the dominant lower limb, the contralateral knee remaining flexed at 90°, the arms remaining crossed in front of the chest, and the head being straight. A stopwatch (Moure Jar®, China) was activated when the volunteer raised their contralateral foot off the floor and was stopped when the contralateral foot touched the floor again.

2.2.3. Usual and Maximal Walking Speed Test. To measure walking speed, a three-meter walking speed test was performed. Volunteers were required to walk a distance of five meters at their usual and fastest possible cadences (without running). Before the evaluation, both feet of each volunteer were to remain on the starting line. Measurement was initiated when a foot reached the one-meter line and was stopped when a foot reached the four-meter line. The one-meter intervals at the beginning and end were used to avoid early acceleration and/or deceleration.

2.2.4. Time Up and Go (TUG) Test. The Time Up and Go (TUG) test involved getting up from a chair without the help of the arms, walking a distance of three meters around a marker placed on the floor, coming back to the same position, and sitting back on the chair. The test began when a researcher shouted a "go!" command. The stopwatch was activated when the volunteers got up from the chair and was stopped when they were seated again.

2.3. Cognitive Evaluation-Executive Function (EF)

2.3.1. TUG Cognitive Test. TUG cognitive test was accomplished to evaluate EF. This test is performed equally to the conventional TUG; however, a cognitive task (verbal fluency, animal category) must be accomplished during the motor task. Therefore, after the signal of the evaluator, the volunteer performed the route—stand up from the chair, walk three meters, turn around, walk three meters back, and sit down again—naming as many animals as he/she could remember. This task was performed out loud, allowing the evaluators to confirm if the volunteers were, in fact, accomplishing the task. The time spent to perform the task was recorded for evaluation [15].

2.4. Multicomponent Exercise Program (MCEP). The MCEP was performed twice a week, on nonconsecutive days, during 26 weeks at the fitness center of an institutional center for elderly care and living (Centro de Convivência do Idoso [CCI]), Poá, Brazil. The program was designed to offer exercises that would mimic activities of daily live (ADL) gestures, thereby inducing neuromuscular adaptations to maintain the subjects able to perform the ADL. Each exercise session was composed of twelve different exercises stations. The structure of each exercise session was defined by the sequence of one functional exercise followed, immediately, by a brief walk. Therefore, exercise session was composed of approximately 12 minutes of functional exercises, 24 minutes of walk, and 12 minutes of rest. Approximately each session of exercise was composed of 50 patients. A physical trainer professional with larger expertise on exercise training to older people supervised all sessions (OI). Volunteers were instructed to avoid the Valsalva maneuver during the performance of exercises.

The functional exercises were changed during the whole program. However, they always represented ADL with a large necessity of the activity of the lower limbs, as, for example, standing and sitting on the chair, picking up a weight off the floor and putting it on top of a structure, and transferring a weight from one place to another. Balance and proprioception exercises were also composed of functional exercises, as one-leg stand. At most three balance and/or proprioception exercises were used in each session. To complete the list of physical exercises, upper limbs resistance exercises were added.

All functional exercises were performed for one minute. The brief walk was performed for two minutes. Thus, after the end of each functional exercise, volunteers must walk from one point to another (30 m), around a cone, come back to the initial line (30 m), and start the path again until completing the two minutes. A rest interval of 60 seconds was adopted between the stations.

2.5. Exercise Intensity Control. The control of exercise intensity was accomplished by the rating of perceived exertion (RPE) method using the adapted Borg scale (2001) (i.e., CR-10) [16], which was used to ensure that volunteers performed the exercises in the aimed intensity. This scale is composed by eleven numbers (i.e., 0, 1, 2, 3, 4, and so on) and eight descriptors (i.e., rest; very, very easy; easy; moderate; somewhat hard; hard; very hard; and maximal), which represents the perception of effort of the subject in front of an exercise load. The higher the reported number, the greater the sensation of effort [16]. During the performance of functional—except for balance exercises—and resistance exercises, volunteers were instructed to maintain the physical activity intensity in 3–5—which represents moderate (i.e., 3), somewhat hard (i.e., 4), and hard (i.e., 5) descriptors. To that, a large picture of RPE scale (i.e., 4 meters high and 1.30 meters wide) was positioned on the wall in the gym's room. The increase in the exercise intensity was based on alterations in the cadence of the performance (i.e., faster), for functional exercises and walk. Moreover, for resistance exercises, volunteers could use elastic bands (EXTEX Sports, São Paulo, Brazil) and dumbbells to reach the intensity prescribed.

Determination of the Prevalence of Pathologies and Use of Medications. The prevalence of pathologies and consumption of medications was determined by reviewing the medical records of each subject. As aforementioned, the head physician and the head nurse of the medical centers recorded the pathological conditions, and a specialist not affiliated with the centers made the pathologic diagnoses. Records were reviewed by two researchers (HJCJ and SSA), and data were compared.

2.6. Statistical Analyses. Normality of data was tested using the *Kolmogorov-Smirnov* test. Since data did not demonstrate normal distribution, nonparametric statistics were performed. Baseline comparisons between the groups for age and morphological (i.e., body mass, height, and body mass index [BMI]) and hemodynamic (i.e., systolic blood pressure [SBP], diastolic blood pressure [DBP], and mean

TABLE 1: Comparison between the groups regarding the morphological and hemodynamic parameters.

Variables	NTS (n = 101)	HTS (n = 117)
Subjects characteristics		
Age (years)	64.1 ± 6.8	66.3 ± 6.9*
Body mass (kg)	65.0 ± 12.1	71.5 ± 13.3*
Height (cm)	156.3 ± 0.1	158.4 ± 0.6
Body mass index (kg/m^2)	26.1 ± 5.0	28.5 ± 4.8*
Hemodynamic parameters		
SBP (mmHg)	124.9 ± 16.2	135.2 ± 18.1*
DBP (mmHg)	72.9 ± 11.1	79.2 ± 10.4*
MAP (mmHg)	89.8 ± 17.0	96.2 ± 17.0*

Data are presented as mean ± SD. NTS = normotensive group; HTS = hypertensive group; SBP = systolic blood pressure; DBP = diastolic blood pressure; MAP = mean arterial pressure.
*$P < 0.05$ versus NTS.

arterial pressure [MAP]) parameters were performed using two-sided Mann–Whitney test for unpaired samples. Intragroup comparisons in the different periods *(pre, post)* were performed using Wilcoxon matched-pairs. Kruskal-Wallis test was performed to compare the differences of intergroup (mean and delta [% Δ]). Cohen's effect size (ES) d was calculated to assess the magnitude of the results. Cohen's effect size d was calculated to assess the magnitude of the results. The effect size was classified according to Rhea, 2004 [17] for untrained volunteers [17]. The level of significance was 5% ($P < 0.05$) and all procedures were performed using the GraphPad Prism 6.0. (San Diego, California, USA).

3. Results

Subjects did not show adverse events during exercise sessions and evaluations, and they were not absent for more than three exercise sessions. There were no dropouts during the study, so that the adherence to the physical exercise program was 100%. Volunteers did not report any changes in food intake and in the number or class of medications use during the whole course of the present study.

Table 1 shows the comparison between the groups regarding morphological and hemodynamic parameters. Data demonstrated that HTS patients were older and heavier and had higher BMI, SBP, DBP, and MAP than NTS patients.

Table 2 shows the effects of multicomponent physical exercise on functional and cognitive parameters, as well as the ES, in NTS and HTS patients. One-leg stand and usual and maximal walking speed tests showed significant increase after exercise (pre-post) in both groups. ES classification was *small* for one-leg stand test and *trivial* for usual and maximal walking speed tests in NTS. Similarly, alterations on one-leg stand and usual walking speed tests were classified as *trivial*, whereas maximal walking speed test received *small* classification in HTS. Therefore, ES results indicate that improvements in functional parameters were similar in NTS and HTS.

On the other hand, sit-to-stand, TUG, and TUG with a cognitive task did not show significant alterations. Qualitative analyses are in concordance with the hypothesis test, once the ES for sit-to-stand, TUG, and TUG with a cognitive task were near zero in NTS and HTS patients.

Table 3 shows the comparison between the magnitudes of alterations (% Δ) on functional and cognitive tests after multicomponent physical exercise in NTS and HTS patients. The results are congruent with the ES shown in Table 1, since there were no significant differences among the groups in relation to the magnitude of alterations after the MCEP.

The effects of multicomponent physical exercise on functional and cognitive parameters of NTS and HTS patients adjusted by age (<75 and ≥75) are shown in Table 4. All groups, except NTS ≥75, showed significant increase in the performance of one-leg stand and on maximal walking speed tests. In relation to one-leg stand, ES classification was *small* for all groups that showed a significant increase after MCEP (i.e., NTS < 75, HTS < 75, and HTS ≥ 75), whereas the alterations shown in NTS ≥75 were just classified as *trivial*, confirming the results observed in the hypothesis test. Interestingly, ES classification of maximal walking speed test was not in concordance with the hypothesis test. In fact, alterations after MCEP on NTS <75 were classified as *moderate*. On the other hand, alterations on HTS <75 and HTS ≥75—which demonstrated significant increase in one-leg stand performance—and on NTS ≥75—which did not demonstrate significant alterations—were classified as *trivial*.

In turn, time to perform usual walking speed test was decreased in the youngest groups (i.e., NTS < 75 and HTS < 75), but not in the oldest groups (i.e., NTS ≥ 75 and HTS ≥ 75). Similar with the results from the maximal walking speed test, ES classification was not congruent with the hypothesis test, and ES classification was *small* for HTS <75 and *trivial* for NTS < 75, NTS ≥ 75, and HTS ≥ 75. Taken together, ES classifications in the usual and maximal walking speed tests could indicate that young groups showed a larger magnitude of alterations after the MCEP in comparison with the oldest groups.

The comparison between the magnitudes of alterations (% Δ) after multicomponent physical exercise in NTS and HTS patients adjusted by age is shown in the Table 5. Data refuted the hypothesis created by ES classification and did not indicate significant differences between the groups.

4. Discussion

The present study aimed to investigate and compare the effects of 6 months of a MCEP on the functional and cognitive parameters of NTS and HTS patients. Furthermore, we wished to verify if age was a confounding factor in this phenomenon, affecting the capacity of HTS patients to adapt to physical stimulus.

We hypothesized that the MCEP would be able to improve functional and cognitive parameters of NTS and HTS patients, regardless of age. Nevertheless, data of the present study partially refuted our *H1*, since improved functional capacity was observed (i.e., balance and mobility) in both, NTS and HTS patients, after the MCEP. However, cognitive capacities were not altered in any of the groups. In addition, when a new set of analyses were performed with

TABLE 2: Effect size and its classification of behavior of functional parameters after the experimental session.

Variable		NTS	HTS
	Pre	10.8 ± 2.8	10.4 ± 2.1
Sit-to-stand (repetitions)	Post	10.6 ± 2.7	10.2 ± 2.8
	ES	0.07 (trivial)	0.08 (trivial)
	Pre	17.6 ± 13.2	14.9 ± 12.3
One-leg stand (s)	Post	25.6 ± 7.5*	22.5 ± 9.1*
	ES	−0.74 (small)	0.15 (trivial)
	Pre	0.88 ± 0.62	0.83 ± 0.24
Usual walking speed (m/s)	Post	0.70 ± 0.11*	0.73 ± 0.19*
	ES	0.40 (trivial)	0.46 (trivial)
	Pre	1.06 ± 1.26	0.94 ± 0.55
Maximal walking speed (m/s)	Post	0.55 ± 0.8*	0.56 ± 0.12*
	ES	0.48 (trivial)	0.95 (small)
	Pre	6.5 ± 1.3	6.9 ± 1.1
TUG (s)	Post	6.6 ± 1.2	6.8 ± 1.6
	ES	−0.07 (trivial)	0.07 (trivial)
	Pre	7.5 ± 2.1	7.8 ± 1.8
TUG with a cognitive task (s)	Post	7.6 ± 1.8	8.1 ± 2.2
	ES	−0.05 (trivial)	−0.14 (trivial)

*$P < 0.05$ versus pre; NTS = normotensive; HTS = hypertensive; TUG = Time Up and Go; ES = effect size.

TABLE 3: Magnitude (% Δ) of effect in both groups.

Variable		NTS	HTS
One-leg stand (s)	% Δ	45.4	51.0
Usual walking speed (m/s)	% Δ	−20.4	−12.0
Maximal walking speed (m/s)	% Δ	−48.1	−40.4
Sit-to-stand (repetitions)	% Δ	−1.5	−1.9
TUG (s)	% Δ	1.5	−1.4
TUG with a cognitive task (s)	% Δ	1.3	3.8

NTS = normotensive; HTS = hypertensive; TUG = Time Up and Go.

the subgroups of the NTS and HTS, <75 and ≥75, results did not demonstrate decreased functional adaptations on HTS ≥75 subgroup. However, significant results observed in NTS groups (Table 2) were reversed in NTS ≥75.

Regarding functional capacities (Tables 2 and 3), NTS and HTS patients increased similarly the time in the balance test (i.e., one-leg stand), 73% and 88%, concomitantly with decreased time spent to perform usual walking speed, −9.8% and −7.8%, and maximal walking speed tests, −32.4% and −36.5%, respectively, after 6 months of MCEP. Several evidences in the literature have confirmed our data, demonstrating improvements in balance and mobility in NTS patients after MCEP, even after short-term exercise programs (e.g., 4 weeks) and in frailty older adults [18–20].

However, despite these beneficial results of MCEP in NTS patients, just one study [13] investigated the effects of MCEP on a sample composed exclusively by hypertensive patients. In this experiment, de Moraes et al. [13] made 32 HTS patients undergo 60 minutes of MCEP, two days per week, for 3 months. Similar to the present study, the sessions of exercise were composed by walk and resistance exercises, at moderate to vigorous intensity. However, authors added dance exercises. Results demonstrated that MCEP was able to elicit significant improvement in lower-*limb muscle strength*, balance, and mobility [13].

Even if the present study also observed improvements in balance and mobility after MCEP, indicated by one-leg stand and walking speed, respectively, increase in lower-limb muscle strength was not shown by NTS and HTS patients. Interestingly, the time of intervention in the experiment performed by de Moraes et al. [13] was shorter than in the present study (3 months versus 6 months). An interference of pathological condition (i.e., hypertension) is unlikely, since results were not observed in NTS patients. An initial hypothesis to explain different outcomes among the studies could be differences on baseline physical levels between the samples. However, scores on sit-to-stand test—performed in both groups for lower-limb muscle strength evaluation—were similar in both studies, even after division of the groups by age.

In turn, the dissimilarities among the protocols of MCEP can be indicated as a possible factor responsible for different results observed in the comparison. In fact, muscle strength is composed basically of a morphological (i.e., muscle mass) and a neural component (i.e., muscle recruitment) [21, 22]. During aging, several mechanisms (e.g., hormonal, neural, and immunological) lead to marked decrease in muscle mass, muscle atrophy, and muscle strength—dynapenia—collaborating to development of sarcopenic phenotype, which is closely associated with poor prognosis (e.g., increase in sedentary behavior, low functionality, risk of falls, and diseases prevalence) [1, 23]. Maintenance or improvement of muscle strength during aging in response

TABLE 4: Effect size and its classification of behavior of functional parameters after the experimental session adjusted by age.

Variable		NTS < 75 (n = 96)	NTS ≥ 75 (n = 5)	HTS < 75 (n = 102)	HTS ≥ 75 (n = 15)
Sit-to-stand (repetitions)	Pre	10.7 ± 2.8	10.8 ± 1.0	10.2 ± 2.0	11.7 ± 2.5
	Post	10.5 ± 2.7	12.8 ± 1.5	9.9 ± 2.0	12.1 ± 2.7
	ES	0.07 (trivial)	−1.56 (moderate)	0.14 (trivial)	−0.15 (trivial)
One-leg stand (s)	Pre	17.5 ± 13.3	18.5 ± 10.3	15.8 ± 2.5	7.5 ± 6.0
	Post	26.2 ± 7.0*	15.7 ± 2.6	22.8 ± 9.2*	18.3 ± 9.6*
	ES	−0.81 (small)	0.37 (trivial)	−1.03 (small)	−1.34 (small)
Usual walking speed (m/s)	Pre	0.88 ± 0.64	0.80 ± 0.18	0.83 ± 0.24	0.89 ± 0.30
	Post	0.69 ± 0.11*	0.77 ± 0.18	0.71 ± 0.18*	0.85 ± 0.19
	ES	0.41 (trivial)	0.16 (trivial)	0.56 (small)	0.15 (trivial)
Maximal walking speed (m/s)	Pre	0.89 ± 0.36	0.92 ± 0.38	1.06 ± 1.24	0.93 ± 0.39
	Post	0.54 ± 0.08*	0.57 ± 0.11	0.54 ± 0.11*	0.62 ± 0.11*
	ES	1.34 (moderate)	1.25 (small)	0.59 (small)	1.08 (small)
TUG (s)	Pre	6.5 ± 1.3	6.6 ± 1.0	6.7 ± 1.0	8.0 ± 1.4
	Post	6.6 ± 1.3	6.8 ± 0.8	6.6 ± 1.4	7.6 ± 1.9
	ES	−0.07 (trivial)	−0.22 (trivial)	0.08 (trivial)	1.19 (moderate)
TUG with a cognitive task (s)	Pre	7.5 ± 2.1	7.9 ± 1.0	7.6 ± 1.7	9.2 ± 1.8
	Post	7.5 ± 1.8	9.2 ± 1.6	7.9 ± 2.1	9.5 ± 2.2
	ES	0 (trivial)	−0.97 (small)	−0.15 (trivial)	−0.14 (trivial)

*$P < 0.05$ versus pre; NTS = normotensive; HTS = hypertensive; TUG = Time Up and Go; ES = effect size.

TABLE 5: Magnitude (% Δ) of effect in both groups adjusted by age.

Variable		NTS < 75	NTS ≥ 75	HTS < 75	HTS ≥ 75
One-leg stand (s)	% Δ	80.7	29.3	182.9	179.9
Usual walking speed (m/s)	% Δ	−9.9	−3.6	−9.0	−5.1
Maximal walking speed (m/s)	% Δ	−32.16	−32.9	−35.2	−30.4
Sit-to-stand (repetitions)	% Δ	3.7	19.3	2.6	7.7
TUG (s)	% Δ	−3.4	−3.3	−1.3	2.5
TUG with a cognitive task (s)	% Δ	6.3	17.3	7.2	8.4

NTS = normotensive; HTS = hypertensive; TUG = Time Up and Go.

to physical exercise is generally associated with increase in muscle mass [24–26], but not exclusively, once evidences demonstrate increase in muscle strength even in the absence of apparent muscular hypertrophy [27, 28], which occur predominately in response to neuromuscular adaptations [25–28]. Yet, both factors can occur in response to physical exercise and collaborate to increase in muscle strength [25, 26]. Moreover, some authors suggest that the increase in muscle strength after programs of physical exercise is dependent on muscular tension generated during muscular contractions, which is associated with external load (e.g., intensity, during muscle contraction) [24].

In the present study, each session of MCEP (~48 minutes) was composed predominantly by an aerobic component, due the time of walk performed between functional exercises (~ 24 minutes [50%]) and the time of walk performed inside the functional exercises, since some exercises required that the volunteer translocase from one location to another for one minute. This characteristic is a possible explanation for the lack of changes in muscle strength in the present study, since aerobic stimulus requires the predominant action of slow-twitch muscle fibers (type I), which have a high capacity to keep muscle working for a long time, avoiding muscular fatigue, considering that the resistance imposed to skeletal muscle contraction occurs in a low and/or low to moderate levels. However, these fibers have low capacity to generate tension, which impairs their capacity to cause large improvement in muscle strength and muscle mass. Indeed, evidences indicate that older adults who engaged for a long time in physical exercise programs with high aerobic component show muscle strength and muscle mass values similar to sedentary matched-controls [29].

Furthermore, both studies, the present study and the study of de Moraes et al. [13], showed different relative time of functional exercises on MCEP, 25% and 33.3%, respectively. Yet, the present protocol of MCEP was composed of just a single set of each functional exercise, which was characterized predominantly by resistance exercises (66,6%) and also by balance and proprioceptive exercises (33,3%). Regarding resistance exercises, which is more associated with muscle mass and muscle strength development than balance and proprioceptive exercises, several evidences from original studies, corroborated by meta-analytic regressions, have been indicating that programs composed of single sets, even at high intensity, are limited to elicit improvement in muscle mass and strength, including in older adults [30–32].

Therefore, taken together, these data indicate that, due to the prevalence of aerobic components in the exercise session, added to an inappropriate resistance component, the protocol of MCEP used in the present study was not a profitable stimulus to elicit morphological changes in muscular architecture, as well as being able to reach a threshold necessary to cause adaptations of the neuromuscular components associated with improvement in muscle strength. However, interestingly, the lack of changes in muscle strength did not impair the improvements in the performance of usual and maximal walking speed, as well as on balance test, observed in both groups after MCEP.

In this sense, it is known that muscle power, compared with muscle strength, seems to decrease early and in a larger magnitude during aging [33, 34] and it seems to be the main functional limitation predictor in older adults [35]. Several evidences have been demonstrating that muscle power can be more associated with functional and physical capacities in older adults, including walking speed and balance, than muscle strength [33, 36]. Moreover, increase in muscle power has been observed after programs of exercise with different intensities (e.g., low, moderate, and high), since this kind of adaptation is closely associated with the velocity of muscle contraction, and muscle tension is not a determinant factor to induce its alterations [37–39]. Thus, it is possible to infer that patients of the present study could show increase in muscle power, even without changes in muscle strength, after 6 months of MCEP. However, more studies assessing this capacity are necessary to confirm our hypothesis.

Besides the functional tests, the present study also investigated the effects of MCEP on EF in NTS and HTS patients, through dual task (TUG associated with a cognitive task). EF is a cognitive capacity composed of other cognitive domains (e.g., shifting, working memory, and inhibition), which allow the subject to create, develop, and perform a strategy to perform an aim, evaluate the outcomes, and, if necessary, change the strategy during or at the end of the task, creating new strategies for the future [40]. Therefore, EF is an essential cognitive domain for maintenance of autonomy and independence during aging, and its impairment is observed in intermediate conditions (e.g., mild cognitive impairment), as well as during several psychopathological conditions, including Alzheimer's disease [15].

Just few evidences evaluated the effect of MCEP on cognitive domains in older adults [20, 41]. However, protocols investigated different samples (i.e., frailty) and in the study developed by Tarazona-Santabalbina et al. [20], volunteers also underwent nutritional supplementation, which can impair comparisons and inferences. Different from the present study, Eggenberger et al. [41] observed significant increase in EF after 6 months of MCEP. The cognitive regulatory mechanisms behind the modulation of physical exercise variables are still unclear and limit our inferences. However, different volumes of MCEP (48 minutes versus 60 minutes) and exercise resistance component are plausible explanations. Yet, different evaluation tools can help to explain dissimilarities, since EF in the aforementioned study was evaluated by a questionnaire test (i.e., Trail Making Test, Part B), while the present study added a verbal fluency test to a motor test. Therefore, more studies are still necessary.

This study was also developed to verify if age plus pathological condition (i.e., hypertension) could be a confounding factor in the magnitude of adaptations after MCEP. Our data accepted null hypothesis and show that age did not seem to alter the response of HTS patients after MCEP. Cross-sectional studies have been discussing the possibility that HTS patients present impairment on physical function [7, 8, 42]. However, results have been shown to be controversial.

Plausibility besides its theory is based on the continuous vascular damage in the arteries responsible for the transport of blood to the brain areas accountable for mobility (e.g., motor cortex), which could impair muscle movement throughout time and, consequently, muscle adaptations in response to physical exercise [7]. Moreover, evidences suggest that hypertensive patients could present a higher prevalence and magnitude of progression of white matter hyperintensities (WMHs) in comparison with normotensive patients [6, 43]. Yet, this phenomenon seems to be associated with decline in physical functioning [6]. Therefore, data of the present study (Tables 4 and 5) added evidences to cross-sectional studies and, for the first time, demonstrated that aged HTS patients did not present impairment in the capacity of adaptation in response to physical stimulus.

However, it is important to mention that a Mann–Whitney test was performed between HTS < 75 and HTS > 75 groups to evaluate differences between functional and cognitive tests. Again, data did not demonstrate significant differences between the magnitudes of alterations. Nonetheless, the P value for balance test was equal to 0.05. Interestingly, in the seminal study from Hausdorff et al. [8], the authors observed lower performance in the balance test in hypertensive patients being ~75 years old. Moreover, an association among high blood pressure values and poor balance performance was recorded [8]. Rosano et al. [6] showed an age-dependent association between WMHs, well-functioning hypertensive patients, and physical declining [6]. Therefore, it is possible that the results of the present study are not observed in patients with secondary morbidities (e.g., stroke) and older patients and in response to other kinds of physical exercise. Future studies should explore these factors.

On the other hand, NTS ≥ 75 patients did not present significant improvement in performance after MCEP. These data are complicated to be discussed, since scientific literature pointed out the possibility that HTS patients show impairment in adaptations, but not NTS. In our view, the sample size ($n = 5$) of the present study is a limitation factor and probably responsible for this absence of alterations. Thus, we encourage future studies with larger samples of NTS ≥ 75.

Other potential limitations of our study should be mentioned. The present study has a quasi-experimental design. Therefore, inherent characteristics of this kind of approach, as the lack of randomization and the absence of a control group (sedentary NTS and HTS), must be assumed. Moreover, future studies that aim to use MCEP should increase the number of sets of resistance training in the protocol, since this approach can collaborate to increase in the magnitude of alterations after MCEP, mainly in muscle strength. Due to all the aforementioned data, which highlight the importance of muscle power in the context of aging and functional capacity, the measurement of dynamic muscle power should be added in the methodology. However, the present study indicates that this model of MCEP should be studied in better design models of scientific studies (i.e., clinical randomized trial). Lastly, more information about the cognitive status and level of education of the volunteers of the present study was not collected. These data are important and could collaborate to a better explanation about the results shown in the present study.

Therefore, the present study indicates that a 6-month MCEP is able to increase equally balance (i.e., one-leg stand test) and mobility (i.e., usual and maximal walking speed test) in NTS and HTN adults. Therefore, aging did not seem to be a confounding factor, impairing the capacity of older HTS patients to adapt to physical stimulus. Thus, the current data indicate that this MCEP can be used to improve muscle functionality of several hypertensive patients, independently of age. This seems to be a good option to public health programs that have the necessity to offer short-time services to several patients in the same time.

Conflicts of Interest

The authors report no conflicts of interest.

Authors' Contributions

All authors participated in the development of the research project, analysis and interpretation of the data, and preparation of the manuscript.

Acknowledgments

The authors are grateful to the Conselho Nacional de Desenvolvimento Científico e Tecnológico (CNPq) for funding this research via scholarships to Hélio José Coelho Junior and Ricardo Yukio Asano. Bruno Rodrigues had financial support from the Fundação de Amparo à Pesquisa do Estado de São Paulo (FAPESP) and CNPq (BPQ). The authors are also grateful to Daisy dos Reis and Flávio Romano of the facility for older adults and all researchers of the Research Group on Chronic-Degenerative Diseases of Mogi das Cruzes University (Grupo de Pesquisa em Doenças Crônico-Degenerativas da Universidade de Mogi das Cruzes (GEDCD/UMC)) for their support.

References

[1] H. J. Coelho Júnior, S. D. S. Aguiar, I. D. O. Gonçalves et al., "Sarcopenia is associated with high pulse pressure in older women," *Journal of Aging Research*, vol. 2015, Article ID 109824, 6 pages, 2015.

[2] R. A. C. Sampaio, P. Y. Sewo Sampaio, M. Yamada et al., "Arterial stiffness is associated with low skeletal muscle mass in Japanese community-dwelling older adults," *Geriatrics and Gerontology International*, vol. 14, no. 1, pp. 109–114, 2014.

[3] P. Y. Sewo Sampaio, R. A. C. Sampaio, H. J. Coelho Júnior et al., "Differences in lifestyle, physical performance and quality of life between frail and robust Brazilian community-dwelling elderly women," *Geriatrics and Gerontology International*, vol. 16, no. 7, pp. 829–835, 2016.

[4] A. S. Go, D. Mozaffarian, V. L. Roger et al., "Heart disease and stroke statistics-2014 update," *Circulation*, vol. 128, no. 3, 2014.

[5] World Health Organization, *Global Health Risks: Mortality and Burden of Disease Attributable to Selected Major Risks*, World Health Organization, 2009.

[6] C. Rosano, W. T. Longstreth Jr., R. Boudreau et al., "High blood pressure accelerates gait slowing in well-functioning older adults over 18-years of follow-up," *Journal of the American Geriatrics Society*, vol. 59, no. 3, pp. 390–397, 2011.

[7] S. Acar, İ. Demirbüken, C. Algun, M. Malkoç, and N. Tekın, "Is hypertension a risk factor for poor balance control in elderly adults?" *Journal of Physical Therapy Science*, vol. 27, no. 3, pp. 901–904, 2015.

[8] J. M. Hausdorff, T. Herman, R. Baltadjieva, T. Gurevich, and N. Giladi, "Balance and gait in older adults with systemic hypertension," *American Journal of Cardiology*, vol. 91, no. 5, pp. 643–645, 2003.

[9] E. N. Moraes, *Atenção à Saúde do Idoso: Aspectos Conceituais*, Organização Pan-Americana da Saúde, Brasília, Brazil, 2012.

[10] C. E. Garber, B. Blissmer, M. R. Deschenes et al., "American College of Sports Medicine position stand. Quantity and quality of exercise for developing and maintaining cardiorespiratory, musculoskeletal, and neuromotor fitness in apparently healthy adults: guidance for prescribing exercise," *Medicine and Science in Sports and Exercise*, vol. 43, no. 7, pp. 1334–1359, 2011.

[11] E. L. Cadore, L. Rodríguez-Mañas, A. Sinclair, and M. Izquierdo, "Effects of different exercise interventions on risk of falls, gait ability, and balance in physically frail older adults: A systematic review," *Rejuvenation Research*, vol. 16, no. 2, pp. 105–114, 2013.

[12] R. Y. Asano, N. F. Moraes, V. P. Oliveira et al., "Fatores que afetam o perfil sedentário em pacientes com hipertensão arterial sistêmica," *Revista Brasileira de Ciência e Movimento*, vol. 24, no. 1, pp. 5–15, 2015.

[13] W. M. de Moraes, P. R. M. Souza, M. H. N. P. Pinheiro, M. C. Irigoyen, A. Medeiros, and M. K. Koike, "Exercise training program based on minimum weekly frequencies: effects on blood pressure and physical fitness in elderly hypertensive patients," *Brazilian Journal of Physical Therapy*, vol. 16, no. 2, pp. 114–121, 2012.

[14] Sociedade, Brasileira de Hipertensão, Sociedade Brasileira de Cardiologia, and Sociedade Brasileira de Nefrologia, "VI Brazilian guidelines on hypertension," *Arquivos Brasileiros de Cardiologia*, vol. 95, no. 1, 2010.

[15] S. M. Borges, M. Radanovic, and O. V. Forlenza, "Functional mobility in a divided attention task in older adults with cognitive impairment," *Journal of Motor Behavior*, vol. 47, no. 5, pp. 378–385, 2015.

[16] C. Foster, J. A. Florhaug, J. Franklin et al., "A new approach to monitoring exercise training," *Journal of Strength and Conditioning Research*, vol. 15, no. 1, pp. 109–115, 2001.

[17] M. R. Rhea, "Determining the magnitude of treatment effects in strength training research through the use of the effect size," *Journal of Strength and Conditioning Research*, vol. 18, no. 4, pp. 918–920, 2004.

[18] S. Karinkanta, A. Heinonen, H. Sievänen et al., "A multi-component exercise regimen to prevent functional decline and bone fragility in home-dwelling elderly women: randomized, controlled trial," *Osteoporosis International*, vol. 18, no. 4, pp. 453–462, 2007.

[19] S. Kang, S. Hwang, A. B. Klein, and S. H. Kim, "Multicomponent exercise for physical fitness of community-dwelling elderly women," *Journal of Physical Therapy Science*, vol. 27, no. 3, pp. 911–915, 2015.

[20] F. J. Tarazona-Santabalbina, M. C. Gómez-Cabrera, P. Pérez-Ros et al., "A multicomponent exercise intervention that reverses frailty and improves cognition, emotion, and social networking in the community-dwelling frail elderly: a randomized clinical trial," *Journal of the American Medical Directors Association*, vol. 17, no. 5, pp. 426–433, 2016.

[21] T. M. Manini and B. C. Clark, "Dynapenia and aging: an update," *Journals of Gerontology—Series A Biological Sciences and Medical Sciences*, vol. 67, no. 1, pp. 28–40, 2012.

[22] S. B. Ballak, H. Degens, A. de Haan, and R. T. Jaspers, "Aging related changes in determinants of muscle force generating capacity: a comparison of muscle aging in men and male rodents," *Ageing Research Reviews*, vol. 14, no. 1, pp. 43–55, 2014.

[23] A. J. Cruz-Jentoft, J. P. Baeyens, J. M. Bauer et al., "Sarcopenia: European consensus on definition and diagnosis: Report of the European Working Group on Sarcopenia in Older People," *Age and Ageing*, vol. 39, no. 4, pp. 412–423, 2010.

[24] V. I. Kalapotharakos, M. Michalopoulou, G. Godolias, S. P. Tokmakidis, P. V. Malliou, and V. Gourgoulis, "The effects of high- and moderate-resistance training on muscle function in the elderly," *Journal of Aging and Physical Activity*, vol. 12, no. 2, pp. 131–143, 2004.

[25] K. Häkkinen, M. Kallinen, M. Izquierdo et al., "Changes in agonist-antagonist EMG, muscle CSA, and force during strength training in middle-aged and older people," *Journal of Applied Physiology*, vol. 84, no. 4, pp. 1341–1349, 1998.

[26] K. A. Häkkinen, A. Pakarinen, W. J. Kraemer, A. Häkkinen, H. Valkeinen, and M. Alen, "Selective muscle hypertrophy, changes in EMG and force, and serum hormones during strength training in older women," *Journal of Applied Physiology*, vol. 91, no. 2, pp. 569–580, 2001.

[27] T. Moritani and H. A. DeVries, "Potential for gross muscle hypertrophy in older men," *Journals of Gerontology*, vol. 35, no. 5, pp. 672–682, 1980.

[28] K. R. Vincent, R. W. Braith, R. A. Feldman et al., "Resistance exercise and physical performance in adults aged 60 to 83," *Journal of the American Geriatrics Society*, vol. 50, no. 6, pp. 1100–1107, 2002.

[29] H. Klitgaard, M. Mantoni, S. Schiaffino et al., "Function, morphology and protein expression of ageing skeletal muscle: a cross-sectional study of elderly men with different training backgrounds," *Acta Physiologica Scandinavica*, vol. 140, no. 1, pp. 41–54, 1990.

[30] D. A. Galvão and D. R. Taaffe, "Resistance exercise dosage in older adults: Single-versus multiset effects on physical performance and body composition," *Journal of the American Geriatrics Society*, vol. 53, no. 12, pp. 2090–2097, 2005.

[31] J. W. Krieger, "Single vs. multiple sets of resistance exercise for muscle hypertrophy: a meta-analysis," *Journal of Strength and Conditioning Research*, vol. 24, no. 4, pp. 1150–1159, 2010.

[32] W. K. Kemmler, D. Lauber, K. Engelke, and J. Weineck, "Effects of single-vs. multiple-set resistance training on maximum strength and body composition in trained postmenopausal women," *Journal of Strength and Conditioning Research*, vol. 18, no. 4, pp. 689–694, 2004.

[33] M. Izquierdo, X. Aguado, R. Gonzalez, J. L. López, and K. Häkkinen, "Maximal and explosive force production capacity and balance performance in men of different ages," *European Journal of Applied Physiology and Occupational Physiology*, vol. 79, no. 3, pp. 260–267, 1999.

[34] F. Lauretani, C. R. Russo, S. Bandinelli et al., "Age-associated changes in skeletal muscles and their effect on mobility: an operational diagnosis of sarcopenia," *Journal of Applied Physiology*, vol. 95, no. 5, pp. 1851–1860, 2003.

[35] K. F. Reid and R. A. Fielding, "Skeletal muscle power: a critical determinant of physical functioning in older adults," *Exercise and Sport Sciences Reviews*, vol. 40, no. 1, pp. 4–12, 2012.

[36] J. F. Bean, S. G. Leveille, D. K. Kiely, S. Bandinelli, J. M. Guralnik, and L. Ferrucci, "A comparison of leg power and leg strength within the inCHIANTI study: which influences mobility more?" *Journals of Gerontology. Series A Biological Sciences and Medical Sciences*, vol. 58, no. 8, pp. 728–733, 2003.

[37] T. R. Henwood, S. Riek, and D. R. Taaffe, "Strength versus muscle power-specific resistance training in community-dwelling older adults," *Journals of Gerontology, Series A: Biological Sciences and Medical Sciences*, vol. 63, no. 1, pp. 83–91, 2008.

[38] R. A. Fielding, N. K. LeBrasseur, A. Cuoco, J. Bean, K. Mizer, and M. A. Fiatarone Singh, "High-velocity resistance training increases skeletal muscle peak power in older women," *Journal of the American Geriatrics Society*, vol. 50, no. 4, pp. 655–662, 2002.

[39] S. P. Sayers, K. Gibson, and C. R. Cook, "Effect of high-speed power training on muscle performance, function, and pain in older adults with knee osteoarthritis: a pilot investigation," *Arthritis Care and Research*, vol. 64, no. 1, pp. 46–53, 2012.

[40] H. R. Snyder, A. Miyake, and B. L. Hankin, "Advancing understanding of executive function impairments and psychopathology: bridging the gap between clinical and cognitive approaches," *Frontiers in Psychology*, vol. 6, article 328, 2015.

[41] P. Eggenberger, N. Theill, S. Holenstein, V. Schumacher, and E. D. de Bruin, "Multicomponent physical exercise with simultaneous cognitive training to enhance dual-task walking of older adults: a secondary analysis of a 6-month randomized controlled trial with I-year follow-up," *Clinical Interventions in Aging*, vol. 10, pp. 1711–1732, 2015.

[42] H. J. Coelho-Junior, B. Rodrigues, S. S. A. Aguiar, I. O. Gonçalvez, F. O. Pires, and R. Y. Asano, "Hyperntesion and functional capatities in community-dwelling older women: a croos-sectional study," *Blood Press*, vol. 26, no. 3, pp. 156–165, 2017.

[43] C. Dufouil, A. De Kersaint-Gilly, V. Besançon et al., "Longitudinal study of blood pressure and white matter hyperintensities: The EVA MRI cohort," *Neurology*, vol. 56, no. 7, pp. 921–926, 2001.

3

Physical Inactivity and Related Barriers: A Study in a Community Dwelling of Older Brazilians

Sebastião Gobbi,[1] Emerson Sebastião,[2] Camila Bosquiero Papini,[1] Priscila Missaki Nakamura,[1] Américo Valdanha Netto,[1] Lilian Teresa Bucken Gobbi,[1] and Eduardo Kokubun[1]

[1] *Department of Physical Education, Universidade Estadual Paulista (UNESP), Avenida 24-A, 1515 Bela Vista, 13506-900 Rio Claro, SP, Brazil*
[2] *Department of Kinesiology and Community Health, University of Illinois at Urbana-Champaign, 906 South Goodwin Avenue, Urbana, IL 61801, USA*

Correspondence should be addressed to Emerson Sebastião, decounesp@yahoo.com.br

Academic Editor: Wojtek Chodzko-Zajko

This study sought to investigate the prevalence of physical inactivity and related barriers in older Brazilian adults. A cross-sectional, population-based study was conducted, and a stratified random sampling procedure was used. A total of 359 older adults were interviewed. The long version of the International Physical Activity Questionnaire (IPAQ) and the Questionnaire of Barriers to Physical Activity Practice were used to assess physical activity level and barriers, respectively. No statistically significant difference was observed on the prevalence of physical inactivity in either gender or age groups. Regarding barriers, the proportion of 9 out of 22 barriers was statistically significant between men and women. Self-reported physical inactivity/activity in older Brazilian adults continues to be a concern. Uncommonly, older males reported a higher prevalence of physical inactivity compared to their counterparts. Additionally, physical inactivity prevalence continued to increase with the aging process. Yet, personal barriers such as lack of time and poor health were strongly associated with physical inactivity. The results of this study may help health professionals and public policy makers to better address the issues related to a healthy lifestyle among older adults and promote physical activity among Brazilian older adults and in other countries with similar characteristics.

1. Introduction

The benefits of physical activity have been widely published in the literature. The many advantages of physical activity include promoting health and well-being, delaying or preventing the onset of chronic disease and disability, and reducing mortality [1, 2]. Despite the well-known benefits of physical activity and the public health efforts to promote physical activity, physical inactivity remains a concern throughout the world [3, 4]. Compared to younger age groups, older adults present the highest prevalence of physical inactivity [5, 6]. For instance, Florindo and colleagues [6], examining the physical inactivity epidemiology in a Brazilian capital, observed that older adults present the highest prevalence of insufficient physical activity compared to their younger counterparts [6]. Similar findings can be observed in several other studies [5, 7–9].

Several factors have been associated with decreased physical activity levels during the lifespan. Chronic diseases and other conditions frequently related to the aging process and poor health have been commonly reported as barriers to physical activity. For instance, Dawson and colleagues [10, 11] observed that around 53% of the individuals in their sample reported at least one barrier to engaging in walking, with poor health being the most cited. Similar findings were observed by Rasinaho and colleagues [12].

Physical activity and barriers to participation are strongly influenced by socioeconomic, demographic, environmental factors and exercise mode. Therefore, it is important to understand such behavior in different settings and contexts.

For instance, Benedetti and colleagues [13] investigated physical activity and health conditions in a sample of 1,062 older adults living in Florianopolis, Brazil, either engaged or not engaged in social welfare groups. The authors observed no difference in the prevalence of physical inactivity (nearly 40%) for both groups. In addition, 74% of the participants reported illness; however the presence of illness was not associated with physical activity level (active and insufficient active). Siqueira and colleagues [14] explored physical activity level in over 4,000 older adults living in areas attended by primary healthcare units in the south and northeast of Brazil. The authors observed that 58% of their sample was considered physically inactive according to international recommendations (<150 minutes/week). Although using a large sample size and the same instrument and procedures to assess physical activity (IPAQ) the previous mentioned studies did not seek to include an instrument aiming to explore in depth possible barriers to physical activity. Reichert and colleagues [15] investigated barriers regarding adults in general (>18 years old); however the authors investigated only barriers related to leisure-time physical activity. Regarding older adults, it is known that all physical activity domains are important in order to achieve the current recommendation of 150 minutes/week [16]. In addition, most studies tend to collapse older individuals into only one category (e.g., 70 years and over or 65 years and over), which limits the findings about possible age differences. The purpose of this study was to examine the prevalence of physical inactivity and perceived barriers to physical activity in a community dwelling of older adults living in Brazil. Additionally, this study focused on different age groups and on gender in an attempt to determine whether or not age and gender modulate these variables. Physical activity behavior is a dynamic process influenced by many factors; therefore, the present study will be grounded in the social ecological theory of health behavior [17]. This theory suggests that individual behavior occurs in the interaction between the individuals and the environment and community in which they live [18].

Studies trying to identify factors associated with physical inactivity in different settings are important in order to address the wide array of differences between countries, environment, and individuals and for the development of strategies and interventions tailored specifically for each population. It is particularly important regarding the older adult population, which presents the highest prevalence of physical inactivity. Factors associated with physical activity barriers have received large attention from investigators in developed countries; however, Brazil is an emerging nation, where large transformations in the economy and health field have been seen in the last few years. The main perceived barriers for physical activity remain unclear in a developing country such as Brazil, especially regarding older adults. Studies, to date, that addressed this issued have used small samples, which limit the generalization of the findings. Therefore, the present study adds knowledge to current literature by investigating physical activity as a whole (occupation, transportation, housework, and leisure time) and related barriers in a representative sample of Brazilian older adults—using a broad instrument with 22 barrier-options and by attempting to analyze the participants in different older age groups.

2. Methods

A cross-sectional, population-based study was conducted in Rio Claro, São Paulo, Brazil, a midsized city (190,000 inhabitants) in central-southern Brazil. The physical activity level of the participants was measured using the long version of the International Physical Activity Questionnaire (IPAQ) [19], which is also validated for Brazilian older adults [20], and barriers to the practice of physical activity were assessed by means of a specially designed questionnaire [21]. Studies in the literature have recommended the use of accelerometers when measuring physical activity level, once it is a more direct measure, and can provide more reliable information. However, the use of accelerometers may not be afforded in all studies especially large-scale studies. Therefore, in order to accomplish our aim we conducted our investigation using the well-known IPAQ questionnaire, although aware of its limitations. The São Paulo State University Ethical Committee approved the research protocol, and informed consent was obtained from each subject before data collection.

3. Participants

A stratified random sampling procedure was used to select a representative sample of adults living in Rio Claro. From a total number of geographic census tracts ($n = 200$), half were randomly selected for inclusion in the study, and eight households within each tract were randomly chosen to be interviewed. This yielded a total of 800 households. All residents over 20 years of age in each home in the selected tracts, and who were able to walk independently, were eligible for inclusion in the study. This procedure resulted in a sample of 1,572 individuals who were interviewed. However, for the purposes of the present study, only the data related to older adults 60 years and over ($n = 359$) were analyzed.

4. Measures

Physical activity level was assessed using the IPAQ long form, version 8. The IPAQ questionnaire estimates physical activity levels in four domains (occupation, transportation, housework, and leisure time). A total physical activity score was calculated following procedures reported by Hallal and colleagues [22] and used in several other different studies [6, 15, 22]. The score was calculated using the sum of the number of minutes of total moderate activity (including walking), plus two times the number of minutes of vigorous activity. The IPAQ defines moderate activity as an activity, performed for at least 10 minutes, that produces an increase in respiration and heart rate and causes sweating. Vigorous activities are defined as those activities that, performed for at least 10 minutes, produce even greater increases in breathing, heart rate, and sweating. For the purpose of this study, we defined insufficient physical activity in accordance with the

Department of Health and Human Services of the United States Guidelines [16]. Individuals who reported less than 150 minutes per week of combined moderate and vigorous physical activity were considered to be insufficiently active. Similarly, people who reported at least 150 minutes per week of combined moderate and vigorous physical activity were considered to be active.

Barriers to physical activity engagement were assessed using the Questionnaire of Barriers to Physical Activity Practice (QBPAP) [21], which was developed based on barriers reported in scientific literature [23, 24]. This questionnaire was developed by Hirayama [21] to attend the purpose of his thesis. The first version of the QBPAP questionnaire was developed using the Likert scale and it was composed of 22 factors/barriers. According to the author, the Likert scale, was very difficult to understand by older adults, especially by clinical patients. To attend the purpose of the present study (epidemiologic approach) the QBPAP was modified in a list of 22 dichotomous (yes/no) factors and was previously tested in a pilot study. The pilot study consisted in the application of the QBPAP questionnaire in a sample of older adults living in a census tract sector not selected to be included in the study. After the pilot study, a few questions (barriers) were readjusted in order to provide better clarification. Following data collection, the internal consistency of the QBPAP questionnaire was tested by means of Cronbach's Alpha Coefficient, which returns 0.61 of standardized values, which means that the questionnaire met the conditions to be used for the proposed objective.

5. Data Collection

Questionnaires were administered face to face by trained interviewers who had at least a high school education. The interviewers received 40 hours of training to correctly administer and code the questionnaires and were not aware of the aims of the study. The training sections were led by the investigators and used a manual developed specifically for this purpose, which included interview techniques with dramatizations about how to appropriately administer the questionnaire. The interviewers also were instructed with regard to terminology and how to interpret terms such as moderate and vigorous physical activity and were shown examples of common activities. Following the training procedures, a total of 17 interviewers were selected for data collection.

Fieldwork supervisors (research staff) were responsible for checking the questionnaires completed by the interviewers. Fieldwork supervisors checked 40% of the questionnaires that each interviewer completed in order to ensure the reliability and validity of the data. They checked 30% by telephone and the remaining 10% by returning to the participant's home less than a week after the initial interview. The supervisors checked the questionnaires using a miniquestionnaire that was specifically developed for this purpose with key questions that were compared to the original questionnaires. When inconsistencies occurred, the interview was repeated by a different interviewer. This process identified inconsistencies in about 3% of the interviews, which were replicated.

After data collection the physical activity data was controlled for possible outliers. Such control was done by means of total day time (24 hours). According to the physical activity data provided, individuals that did not present at least 8 hours of sleep were excluded from the analysis with the assumption that they may overestimate their physical activity level. This procedure resulted in zero subjects excluded from the sample.

Table 1: Number of individuals, mean age, and standard deviation of older men and women, in different age groups, Rio Claro, São Paulo, Brazil.

Age groups (years)	Men		Women	
	N	Mean ± SD (years)	N	Mean ± SD (years)
60–69	69	64 ± 3.07	108	64 ± 2.64
70–79	53	74 ± 2.81	85	74 ± 2.97
≥80	12	83 ± 3.29	32	84 ± 4.51

6. Statistical Analysis

Statistical descriptive analyses (mean, standard deviation, and percentage) were performed. Differences between groups in the categorical variables were calculated using the chi-square for testing differences in proportions, *u* Mann Whitney, and Kruskal Wallis tests, at $P < 0.05$. Logistic regression was performed to observe a possible existence of association between physical inactivity and reported barriers adopting a 95% confidence interval.

7. Results

The final sample was comprised of 359 individuals, aged 60 years and over (females: $n = 225$, 62.7%; males: $n = 134$), with women constituting the majority even when the participants were distributed in age groups (Table 1). For the entire group of participants, the average body mass index was 26.2 kg/m^2, which resulted in a classification as overweight. Around 65% reported good health; 58% were married, and 71% had completed high school.

In general 50.7% of the older adults interviewed did not meet the physical activity guidelines of 150 minutes per week of moderate physical activity and were considered insufficiently active. Examined by gender, men reported higher levels of physical inactivity (60.74%) compared to women (45.53%); however, such differences were not statistically significant ($\chi^2 = 1.867$; df $= 1$; $P = 0.17$). Physical activity data were also compared between age groups. The oldest group (80 years and over) reported the highest prevalence of physical inactivity (61.36%) compared to their younger counterparts; however, the prevalence observed in the oldest age group was not statistically significant compared to others

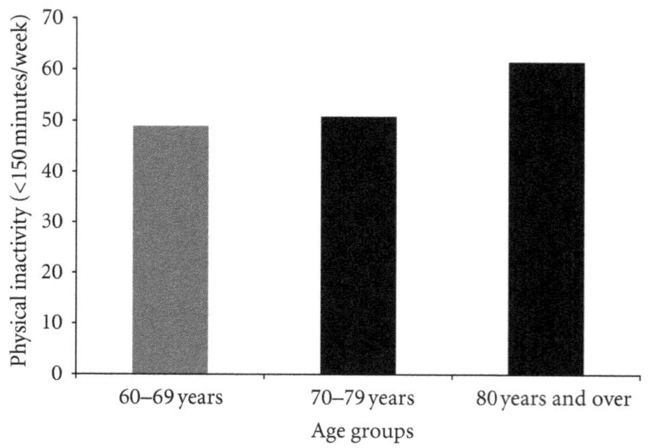

Figure 1: Prevalence of physical inactivity in Brazilian older adults according to age group.

($\chi^2 = 1.540$; df = 2; $P = 0.46$). Details are presented in Figure 1.

Regarding barriers to physical activity, 100% of the participants, regardless of age group and gender, reported at least one barrier. The most frequently reported barriers for men were "Feel already active enough" and "need to relax during free time." For women, "fear of falling and being hurt" and also "need to relax during free time" were among the most reported. The proportion of perception of barriers was significantly different ($P < 0.05$) between the men and women for nine out of 22 barriers (Table 2).

The mean number of barriers reported was significantly ($P < 0.05$) higher for women compared to men in the 60–69 year age groups and marginally significant in the 70–79 and 80 years and over groups ($P = 0.08$). Detailed information regarding the mean number of barriers is depicted in Table 3.

The perceptions of barriers were quite similar among older males regardless of age group. Notably, 91% of the oldest women group reported barriers associated with a lack of environmental safety.

Although 22 barriers were investigated in the present sample, only poor health and fear of injury were positively associated with physical inactivity, whilst being active enough was negatively associated with the outcome. The associations remain after adequate adjustments. Table 4 displays the associations observed.

8. Discussion

This study sought to investigate physical inactivity rates and related barriers in older adults living in the city of Rio Claro, São Paulo, Brazil. To our knowledge the study is the first in Brazil using a representative sample of older adults addressing barriers and physical activity. Previous investigations in Brazil using a representative sample of older adults did not include an instrument to assess barriers in depth [13, 14], and studies using adults in general include older adults just as a subset in their analysis [15].

The present findings revealed that older adults living in Rio Claro, Brazil, reported high levels of physical inactivity (50.7%). Additionally, increased physical inactivity levels tended to increase through age groups (please report to Figure 1). Regarding gender, men in our study reported higher levels of physical inactivity compared to their counterparts; however differences were not statistically significant. These findings are in line with the literature [3, 22, 25, 26]. For example, Knuth and colleagues [25] investigated changes in physical activity over a five-year period in adults using the short version of the IPAQ questionnaire. In general, the authors observed an increase in physical inactivity among the participants (41 to 52%). Regarding older adults, Knuth and colleagues [25] observed higher prevalence of physical inactivity compared to our study. Despite differences in prevalence, both studies observed that physical inactivity increases as a function of the aging process. Regarding gender differences in physical activity level, Hallal and colleagues [22] verified that women in their study presented lower levels of physical inactivity compared to men. Similar findings were also observed in our study. According to Hallal and colleagues [22] household-related physical activity is an important part of the total amount of physical activity for women. In the present study only 18% of the women reported zero minutes per week in household-related physical activity compared to 42% of men. Such common patterns in Latin America regarding household tasks appear to play an important role in the total physical activity for women.

Regarding physical activity barriers, 100% of the assessed sample reported at least one barrier to engaging in physical activity. This finding differs somewhat from those reported by Reichert and colleagues [15] and Dawson and colleagues [10, 11]. Of the mentioned studies, 85% and 53% of the samples, respectively, reported at least one barrier. Possibly, methodological differences in both studies could explain, at least in part, the different findings. Reichert and colleagues [15], for example, assessed individuals 20 years of age and older; therefore, the younger population might be counted to reduce the prevalence of barriers observed. Younger populations appear to have different perceptions of health compared to older adults [27] and generally have wider social networks as well. The current social emphasis on the physical esthetic helps motivate young people to be engaged in physical activities. A lower prevalence of barriers in the Dawson et al. study [10, 11] may be explained by the fact that the authors focus only on barriers related to walking. However, the present study assessed barriers that could be related to any kind of physical activity.

Differently, Stathi and colleagues [28] performing a mixed method to assess physical activity and barriers in older adults (70 years and over) observed functional limitations, lack of intrinsic motivation, and not having an activity companion as the highest impact on barriers in their study. Albeit intrinsic motivation was not included in our questionnaire, our sample revealed high prevalence in the barriers "need to relax," "too lazy," and "lack of energy." These barriers are strongly related to lack of motivation [29, 30]. In addition, the barrier need to relax during the free time, reveals that older Brazilian adults may think physical activity in some sort of "old fashion" types of exercises when

TABLE 2: Barriers to being engaged in physical activity as reported by older Brazilians, according to gender, Rio Claro, São Paulo, Brazil.

Barriers	Men ($n = 134$) n (%)	Women ($n = 225$) n (%)	χ^2	P
Lack of time	37 (27.8)	81 (36.2)	2.624	0.10
Feel active enough	80 (59.7)	107 (48.2)	4.434	0.03
Lack of company	38 (28.4)	92 (40.9)	5.709	0.02
Lack of money	53 (39.6)	93 (41.7)	0.160	0.68
Too old	30 (22.4)	59 (26.2)	0.662	0.41
Have a disease	30 (22.6)	86 (38.2)	9.366	0.02
Poor health	21 (15.7)	52 (23.1)	2.869	0.09
Too shy	26 (19.4)	76 (33.9)	8.683	0.03
Bad experience	11 (8.2)	26 (11.6)	1.045	0.30
Lack of nearby facilities	56 (41.8)	91 (41.0)	1.139	0.56
Need to relax	75 (56.4)	129 (58.1)	0.100	0.75
Lazy	56 (41.8)	99 (44.0)	0.167	0.68
Fear of injury	34 (25.6)	124 (55.1)	29.598	0.01
Dislike exercise	43 (32.1)	69 (30.9)	0.051	0.82
Lack of appropriate clothes	27 (20.6)	36 (16.1)	1.126	0.30
Give up soon	37 (28.0)	72 (32.1)	1.298	0.52
Feel too fat/thin	21 (15.7)	52 (23.3)	3.009	0.01
Lack of energy	34 (25.6)	94 (41.8)	9.566	0.02
Do not believe in physical activity	1 (0.7)	6 (2.7)	1.646	0.20
Lack of security	33 (24.6)	79 (35.3)	4.416	0.04
Bad weather	42 (32.1)	99 (44.8)	5.556	0.02
Urinary incontinence	6 (4.5)	21 (9.5)	2.936	0.08

TABLE 3: Number of barriers (means) reported by older adults, by gender, and by age groups, Rio Claro, São Paulo, Brazil.

Age group (years)	Men	Women	P UMW
60–69	5.3[a]	6.5[d]	0.01
70–79	6.8[b]	7.8[e]	0.08
80-and-over	6.8[c]	9.3[f]	0.05

UMW: U Mann-Whitney test. Kruskal Wallis test: (a) significantly different from (b) ($P < 0.02$); (d) significantly different from (f) ($P < 0.01$) and (e) ($P < 0.04$); (e) significantly different from (f) ($P < 0.015$).

severe intensity would be required. Nowadays, exercise may also be performed as a way of relaxation. It could be the cause of lack of health literacy or even the fact that as older adults they have done a lot of physical activity throughout their lives and they believe no more is needed, as most of them reported to be already physically active enough. Regarding functional limitation, it was included in our study as "disease or disability," which was reported by 50% of men and 69% of women in the oldest age group. Interestingly, not having an activity companion, described in our study as "lack of company," appears as an important barrier to the youngest old group (60–69 years old). The prevalence of the barrier, "fear of injury," seems noteworthy. Despite the strong association observed in the present study, 91% of the women in the 80-year-old group reported it as a barrier. Such prevalence suggests either a self-perception of frailty or a reduced self-efficacy in this age group. The barrier "active enough" appears to affect approximately 53% of men and women (60 to 79 years old), however, not the oldest group. In fact, this barrier revealed to be negatively associated with physical inactivity. It may suggest a false positive perception of being active for health benefits. According to Costello and colleagues [31], people who are physically inactive perceived themselves to be physically active, mostly due to their perception of physical activity being grounded in a social context, which may not represent a real physical activity behavior that benefits health. That is a concern, because compelling evidence demonstrated that health benefits from physical activity are achieved if the individual performs at least 150 minutes per week of moderate physical activity [32]. If physically inactive persons' perception of physical activity is grounded in social context, public health makers should attempt for this aspect to develop public policies, strategies, and interventions, and health professionals need to be aware of the role that social context background has in older adults in order to recommend physical activity.

In general, there are many similarities in the barriers, both for men and women, regardless of age groups. Barriers like "need to relax" and "lack of energy," which are strongly related to lack of motivation, were common in our sample. Additionally, these barriers are comparable to barriers related to health status, such as "poor health" and "have a disease or disability." These findings suggest that public health strategies and interventions should address programs to improve self-efficacy and programs to empower older adults to self-manage their disease and disabilities, which can highly contribute to frailty. These findings also can support health

TABLE 4: Multiple logistic regression. Barriers to physical activity and insufficient physical activity.

Barriers	Crude analysis OR (IC 95%)	P	Adjusted analysis* OR (IC 95%)	P
Lack of time	0.78 (0.637–0.966)	0.022	0.81 (0.649–1.012)	0.063
Feel enough active**	0.74 (0.604–0.910)	0.004	0.75 (0.601–0.944)	0.014
Poor health	1.98 (1.351–2.909)	0.001	1.69 (1.067–2.702)	0.026
Fear of injury	1.49 (1.154–1.936)	0.002	1.37 (1.020–1.852)	0.037

*Adjusted for socioeconomic variables and all other barriers.
**Protection factor for physical inactivity.

professional's use of physical activity as part of the treatment plan.

The high prevalence of physical inactivity observed in the present study is a public health concern due to the well-known negative effects of physical inactivity. Despite the negative effects on physical and mental health, and consecutively quality of life, physical inactivity is an economic burden to the government [33, 34]. For countries in which health services are supported by the government, for example, Brazil, Canada, and France, it is extremely important. Billions of dollars can be saved per year if the population increased their level of physical activity. Moreover, compelling evidence in the literature clearly states the benefits of physical activity for older adults [1].

To our knowledge, the present study is the first population-based investigation of older adults, and therefore, producing more robust evidence regarding physical activity and barriers of this population in Brazil. These findings have enabled us to develop a better insight of older adult's physical inactivity and a better understanding of the obstacles that prevent older adults from engaging in physical activity on a regular basis in an emerging country. The incidence of diseases in older adults can be worsened by physical inactivity, and overall health may be improved by regular participation in physical activity. Taken together, the findings of the present and similar studies can be a support for the development of public health policies and strategies, specifically tailored for older adults. In addition, these findings can support health professionals, such as physicians, if physical activity is addressed during medical consultation.

Rio Claro presents, relatively, one of the largest older adult populations in Brazil, being 13.5% aged 60 years and over [35]. The findings of the study, combined with the population characteristics, provide an opportunity for public health interventions in Rio Claro. The generalization of these findings may be questionable, because Rio Claro presents some characteristics that most other Brazilian cities do not have (e.g., inner midsized city 112 miles from the capital São Paulo; one campus of a top Brazilian University; Rio Claro was the first city to elaborate a specific elderly county law, etc.). Another important aspect of the present findings, in terms of public health, lies in the lack of national data on this topic. Brazil has one national survey dedicated to monitoring health behaviors (physical activity, alcohol consumption, food intake, prevalence of obesity, type 2 diabetes, etc.), named "Vigilância de Fatores de Risco e Proteção para Doenças Crônicas por Inquérito Telefônico." The first publication of the survey occurred in 2002 and has been published every two years since then. Although important, the survey does not provide any information about possible barriers that could play a role in physical inactivity. Additionally, the survey takes place only in the capitals, which presents an entirely different dynamic compared to inner cities, especially regarding behaviors.

Albeit important, our findings should be interpreted with caution due to study limitations. First, we use a cross-sectional design, and it does not provide information on causal effect. Additionally, we divided our sample by age group, and the oldest-old group (80 years and over), especially for men, yielded only 12 individuals, which could bias the results. In addition, we assessed physical activity level using a self-reported physical activity questionnaire. Although the IPAQ questionnaire is a valid instrument and used worldwide, some studies have reported concerns about its accuracy in estimating physical activity level [36, 37], due to problems related to overestimation of the results. Therefore, although the prevalence of physical inactivity observed in our study is in consonance with the literature, it is important to highlight that our sample was found to be quite active (generally nearly 50% was considered active for health benefits; physical activity ≥ 150 minutes/week), which probably reflects the difficulties associated with the use of IPAQ questionnaire to accurately assess physical activity levels. Thus, such information supports the idea that although the IPAQ is validated for different countries, some sort of cultural validation is still needed to improve the sensibility of such an instrument to measure physical activity among populations. Furthermore, although we controlled the IPAQ data for outliers using a daytime cut-off, as aforementioned, we did not verify our data based on more accurate statistical procedures (Skews and kurtosis), so possible outliers could exist in our sample. Future studies should attempt, whenever possible, for the use of more direct measures, such as accelerometry. Despite the criticism related to the use of the IPAQ questionnaire, useful information can be drawn from the data provided. It is important to mention that this study is part of a larger one that was conducted in the city of Rio Claro, São Paulo, Brazil, where we aim to investigate the prevalence of physical inactivity and associated factors in adults over the age of 18 years. Therefore, as the first large study that took place in the city, this data represents the first "snapshot" of the physical inactivity prevalence of the adult population. In such case the use of self-reported questionnaire is understandable, as in the cases of monitoring, such as in national surveillances. However, when using self-reported information related to physical activity, by means of IPAQ, or other ones, it should be advised to include other studies results and also with different health information before proceeding with interventions and strategies to promote tailored physical activity. Second, although we used a large barrier questionnaire, it certainly does not cover all possible barriers that may exist, especially regarding environmental barriers. The present study included only three possibilities. It is possible that participants have other barriers that were not addressed. Thereby, studies using a mixed method design (qualitative and quantitative), in different settings, are important throughout in order to monitor both physical activity level and perceived barriers to physical activity for older adults in order to provide strategies and interventions if needed.

In short, a high prevalence of physical inactivity was observed in older Brazilian adults living in a midsized city. It was observed that men reported higher levels of physical inactivity compared to women. Additionally, physical inactivity keeps increasing as adults age after 60. Consistent with these findings, high prevalence of barriers was reported by the participants, with those participants 80 years and over reporting significantly greater numbers of barriers than younger age groups. Despite the lower physical inactivity level compared to men, women reported significantly higher numbers of barriers compared to their counterparts. This suggests that, although perceiving greater number of barriers compared to men, women are more likely to overcome these barriers and be active, or the barriers reported by women in the present study are more temporal. Regarding physical activity barriers, "poor health," "have a disease and disability," low self-efficacy, diagnosed by "fear of injury" and barriers related to lack of motivation were mostly reported. Yet, despite the large number of barriers addressed, only poor health and fear of injury were positively associated with physical inactivity.

These findings should be a concern to the government and public health policy makers, due to the negative effects of physical inactivity in physical and mental health and economic costs. Several studies have demonstrated a strong association between physical inactivity and chronic diseases, such as type two diabetes, hypertension, and cognitive decline. Therefore, the results of this study may help public policy makers to better address the issues of active lifestyle among the older population and promote physical activity.

Acknowledgments

This paper was supported by Brazilian Funding Agencies CNPq, FAPESP (2007/02229-4), and FUNDUNESP; Rio Claro Health Foundation; CREF-4-SP.

References

[1] W. J. Chodzko-Zajko, D. N. Proctor, M. A. Fiatarone Singh et al., "Exercise and physical activity for older adults," *Medicine and Science in Sports and Exercise*, vol. 41, no. 7, pp. 1510–1530, 2009.

[2] H. B. Hubert, D. A. Bloch, J. W. Oehlert, and J. F. Fries, "Lifestyle habits and compression of morbidity," *Journals of Gerontology A*, vol. 57, no. 6, pp. M347–M351, 2002.

[3] S. C. Dumith, P. C. Hallal, R. S. Reis, and H. W. Kohl, "Worldwide prevalence of physical inactivity and its association with human development index in 76 countries," *Preventive Medicine*, vol. 53, no. 1-2, pp. 24–28, 2011.

[4] R. Guthold, T. Ono, K. L. Strong, S. Chatterji, and A. Morabia, "Worldwide variability in physical inactivity. A 51-country survey," *American Journal of Preventive Medicine*, vol. 34, no. 6, pp. 486–494, 2008.

[5] G. Zhao, E. S. Ford, C. Li, and L. S. Balluz, "Physical activity in U.S. Older adults with diabetes mellitus: prevalence and correlates of meeting physical activity recommendations," *Journal of the American Geriatrics Society*, vol. 59, no. 1, pp. 132–137, 2011.

[6] A. A. Florindo, V. V. Guimarães, C. L. G. Cesar, M. B. De Azevedo Barros, M. C. G. P. Alves, and M. Goldbaum, "Epidemiology of leisure, transportation, occupational, and household physical activity: prevalence and associated factors," *Journal of Physical Activity and Health*, vol. 6, no. 5, pp. 625–632, 2009.

[7] A. Shibata, K. Oka, K. Harada, Y. Nakamura, and I. Muraoka, "Psychological, social, and environmental factors to meeting physical activity recommendations among Japanese adults," *International Journal of Behavioral Nutrition and Physical Activity*, vol. 6, article 1479, p. 60, 2009.

[8] S. J. Marshall, D. A. Jones, B. E. Ainsworth, J. P. Reis, S. S. Levy, and C. A. Macera, "Race/ethnicity, social class, and leisure-time physical inactivity," *Medicine and Science in Sports and Exercise*, vol. 39, no. 1, pp. 44–51, 2007.

[9] J. Sims, K. Hill, S. Davidson, J. Gunn, and N. Huang, "A snapshot of the prevalence of physical activity amongst older, community dwelling people in Victoria, Australia: patterns across the "young-old" and 'fold-old'," *BMC Geriatrics*, vol. 7, article 4, 2007.

[10] J. Dawson, M. Hillsdon, I. Boller, and C. Foster, "Perceived barriers to walking in the neighbourhood environment and change in physical activity levels over 12 months," *British Journal of Sports Medicine*, vol. 41, no. 9, pp. 562–568, 2007.

[11] J. Dawson, M. Hillsdon, I. Boller, and C. Foster, "Perceived barriers to walking in the neighborhood environment: a survey of middle-aged and older adults," *Journal of Aging and Physical Activity*, vol. 15, no. 3, pp. 318–335, 2007.

[12] M. Rasinaho, M. Hirvensalo, R. Leinonen, T. Lintunen, and T. Rantanen, "Motives for and barriers to physical activity among older adults with mobility limitations," *Journal of Aging and Physical Activity*, vol. 15, no. 1, pp. 90–102, 2007.

[13] T. R. B. Benedetti, E. d'Orsi, A. Schwingel, and W. J. Chodzko-Zajko, "Convivência groups: building active and healthy communities of older adults in Brazil," *Journal of Aging Research*, vol. 2012, 7 pages, 2012.

[14] F. V. Siqueira, L. A. Facchini, R. X. Piccini et al., "Physical activity in young adults and the elderly in areas covered by primary health care units in municipalities in the South and Northeast of Brazil," *Cadernos de Saude Publica*, vol. 24, no. 1, pp. 39–54, 2008.

[15] F. F. Reichert, A. J. D. Barros, M. R. Domingues, and P. C. Hallal, "The role of perceived personal barriers to engagement in leisure-time physical activity," *American Journal of Public Health*, vol. 97, no. 3, pp. 515–519, 2007.

[16] DHHS. Physical Activity Guidelines Advisory Committee Report, 2008.

[17] D. Stokols, J. Allen, and R. L. Bellingham, "The social ecology of health promotion: implications for research and practice," *American Journal of Health Promotion*, vol. 10, no. 4, pp. 247–251, 1996.

[18] J. F. Sallis, R. B. Cervero, W. Ascher, K. A. Henderson, M. K. Kraft, and J. Kerr, "An ecological approach to creating active living communities," *Annual Review of Public Health*, vol. 27, pp. 297–322, 2006.

[19] C. L. Craig, A. L. Marshall, M. Sjöström et al., "International physical activity questionnaire: 12-Country reliability and validity," *Medicine and Science in Sports and Exercise*, vol. 35, no. 8, pp. 1381–1395, 2003.

[20] T. R. B. Benedetti, P. D. C. Antunes, C. R. Rodriguez-Añez, G. Z. Mazo, and E. L. Petroski, "Reproducibility and validity of the International Physical Activity Questionnaire (IPAQ) in elderly men," *Revista Brasileira de Medicina do Esporte*, vol. 13, no. 1, 2007.

[21] M. S. Hirayama, "Physical Activity and Parkinson disease: behavior change, self-efficacy and perceived barriers," Rio Claro, Brazil, Institute of Bioscience—Department of Physical Education, Sao Paulo State University, 2006.

[22] P. C. Hallal, C. G. Victora, J. C. K. Wells, and R. C. Lima, "Physical inactivity: prevalence and associated variables in Brazilian adults," *Medicine and Science in Sports and Exercise*, vol. 35, no. 11, pp. 1894–1900, 2003.

[23] M. L. Booth, A. Bauman, N. Owen, and C. J. Gore, "Physical activity preferences, preferred sources of assistance, and perceived barriers to increased activity among physically inactive Australians," *Preventive Medicine*, vol. 26, no. 1, pp. 131–137, 1997.

[24] W. J. Brown and Y. D. Miller, "Too wet to exercise? Leaking urine as a barrier to physical activity in women," *Journal of Science and Medicine in Sport*, vol. 4, no. 4, pp. 373–378, 2001.

[25] A. G. Knuth, G. Bacchieri, C. G. Victora, and P. C. Hallal, "Changes in physical activity among Brazilian adults over a 5-year period," *Journal of Epidemiology and Community Health*, vol. 64, no. 7, pp. 591–595, 2010.

[26] A. Shibata, K. Oka, Y. Nakamura, and I. Muraoka, "Prevalence and demographic correlates of meeting the physical activity recommendation among Japanese adults," *Journal of Physical Activity and Health*, vol. 6, no. 1, pp. 24–32, 2009.

[27] E. L. Idler and Y. Benyamini, "Self-rated health and mortality: a review of twenty-seven community studies," *Journal of Health and Social Behavior*, vol. 38, no. 1, pp. 21–37, 1997.

[28] A. Stathi, H. Gilbert, K. R. Fox, J. Coulson, M. Davis, and J. L. Thompson, "Determinants of neighborhood activity of adults aged 70 and over: a mixed methods study," *Journal of Aging and Physical Activity*, vol. 20, no. 2, pp. 148–170, 2012.

[29] H. R. Bowles, J. R. Morrow, B. L. Leonard, M. Hawkins, and P. M. Couzelis, "The association between physical activity behavior and commonly reported barriers in a worksite population," *Research Quarterly for Exercise and Sport*, vol. 73, no. 4, pp. 464–470, 2002.

[30] S. G. Trost, N. Owen, A. E. Bauman, J. F. Sallis, and W. Brown, "Correlates of adults' participation in physical activity: review and update," *Medicine and Science in Sports and Exercise*, vol. 34, no. 12, pp. 1996–2001, 2002.

[31] E. Costello, M. Kafchinski, J. Vrazel, and P. Sullivan, "Motivators, barriers, and beliefs regarding physical activity in an older adult population," *Journal of Geriatrics and Physical Therapy*, vol. 34, no. 3, pp. 138–147, 2011.

[32] P. C. Hallal, S. M. Matsudo, V. K. Matsudo, T. L. Araújo, D. R. Andrade, and A. D. Bertoldi, "Physical activity in adults from two Brazilian areas: similarities and differences," *Cadernos de Saude Publica*, vol. 21, no. 2, pp. 573–580, 2005.

[33] L. H. Anderson, B. C. Martinson, A. L. Crain et al., "Health care charges associated with physical inactivity, overweight, and obesity," *Preventing Chronic Disease*, vol. 2, no. 4, p. A09, 2005.

[34] R. R. Pate, M. Pratt, S. N. Blair et al., "Physical activity and public health: a recommendation from the Centers for Disease Control and Prevention and the American College of Sports Medicine," *Journal of the American Medical Association*, vol. 273, no. 5, pp. 402–407, 1995.

[35] IBGE—Brazilian Institute of Geography and Statistics, Demographic Census 2010, http://www.ibge.gov.br/cidadesat/topwindow.htm.

[36] P. C. Hallal, L. F. Gomez, D. C. Parra et al., "Lessons learned after 10 years of IPAQ use in Brazil and Colombia," *Journal of Physical Activity & Health*, vol. 7, supplement 2, pp. S259–264, 2010.

[37] R. Rzewnicki, Y. Vanden Auweele, and I. De Bourdeaudhuij, "Addressing overreporting on the International Physical Activity Questionnaire (IPAQ) telephone survey with a population sample," *Public Health Nutrition*, vol. 6, no. 3, pp. 299–305, 2003.

4

Sources of Life Strengths Appraisal Scale: A Multidimensional Approach to Assessing Older Adults' Perceived Sources of Life Strengths

Prem S. Fry[1] and Dominique L. Debats[2]

[1] *Graduate Psychology Program, Trinity Western University, 7600 Glover Road, Langley, BC, Canada V2Y 1Y1*
[2] *Private Practice, 9711 RS 2E4 Groningen, The Netherlands*

Correspondence should be addressed to Prem S. Fry; fry@twu.ca

Academic Editor: Kee Lee Chou

Both cognitive and psychosocial theories of adult development stress the fundamental role of older adults' appraisals of the diverse sources of cognitive and social-emotional strengths. This study reports the development of a new self-appraisal measure that incorporates key theoretical dimensions of internal and external sources of life strengths, as identified in the gerontological literature. Using a pilot study sample and three other independent samples to examine older adults' appraisals of their sources of life strengths which helped them in their daily functioning and to combat life challenges, adversity, and losses, a psychometric instrument having appropriate reliability and validity properties was developed. A 24-month followup of a randomly selected sample confirmed that the nine-scale appraisal measure (SLSAS) is a promising instrument for appraising older adults' sources of life strengths in dealing with stresses of daily life's functioning and also a robust measure for predicting outcomes of resilience, autonomy, and well-being for this age group. A unique strength of the appraisal instrument is its critically relevant features of brevity, simplicity of language, and ease of administration to frail older adults.

1. Introduction

Given the resurgence of interest in the field of positive psychology [1], both gerontologists (e.g., [2, 3]) and social psychologists (e.g., [4]) concur that older adults' appraisals of their life strengths are at the very basis of older adults' identity development and contribute significantly to their perceptions of empowerment.

In recent years, an approach known as the "life strengths perspective" has emerged both in the theoretical literature (e.g., [5]) and in the practice literature as extended to the treatment and clinical approach to older adults ([6, 7]). The life strengths perspective recognizes that, even in the most difficult circumstances, there is reciprocity between older adults' personally constructed views of reality and their social environment (see [8, 9]). Another conceptual framework that is related to the life strengths perspective, in collaboration with the resilience theory perspective, is Maslow's self-actualization perspective [10]. It is reasoned that internal and external sources of life strengths that older adults identify within themselves reinforce personal identity and actualization, factors which are the cornerstone of resilience in older adults (see [5, 7]). The life strengths perspective represents a paradigm shift in clinical practice wherein practitioners focus on assessing and magnifying the worth, dignity, and uniqueness of older adults by helping them identify strengths and resources that facilitate and promote the actualization and achievement of client goals and plans for success [11] in contrast to highlighting disabilities.

Accordingly, what is urgently needed by professionals and by older adults themselves is a *self-report assessment scale* that enables older clients to identify, appraise, and take stock of various aspects of the sources of social, emotional, and cognitive strengths that may assist them in facing both problems of daily life functioning and also life's challenges, crises, and struggles (see [11–14]). In the present research we describe various stages in the development of a psychometrically valid instrument targeted to assess older adults' appraisals of important dimensions of internal and external sources of strengths and capabilities. We subsequently demonstrate through a 24-month followup of a selected group of study participants, how individuals' self-assessments of their various sources of life strengths are a robust measure for predicting outcomes of resilience as defined previously by authors of earlier standardized scales of well-being in terms of constructs such as perceived challenge, control, and engagement [15] and in terms of perseverance, equanimity, meaningfulness, self-reliance, and existential aloneness [16].

2. Conceptual Framework for the Study of Life Strengths

Our assumptions and hypotheses concerning older adults' appraisals of the sources of life strengths are embedded within three distinct conceptual frameworks which we sum up as follows.

(1) *The existential theory framework* which argues that the search for new and emerging sources of life strengths is continual throughout life but greatly accelerated in late life as individuals move toward seeking and defining their meaning for life and achieving some measure of self-transcendence over the stress and pain of physical and emotional losses [17–20]. Hoffman [21] suggests that "the attainment of meaning is one of the most central aspects of human existence and necessary to address in existential therapy" (p. 49). From the perspective of existential theorists, individuals' appraisals of the sources of life strengths will vary in terms of the personal maturity and depth of meaning they perceive themselves to have achieved. These are assumed to enhance both physical and psychological well-being and to predict resilience and autonomy in overcoming adversity (see [17, 22, 23]).

(2) *The social-cognitive framework* originally proposed by Bandura [4] stresses the primacy of the human agency and the acquisition of empowerment through self-efficacy beliefs and beliefs about control. This perspective embraces a broad ecological view of human growth which argues that individuals' strength and persistence in the face of challenges and adversity come from their self-efficacy beliefs and positive perceptions of their own knowledge, competence, and expertise to resolve problems and dilemmas. A number of empirical studies in the aging literature (e.g., [24–26]) show how self-efficacy beliefs provide the foundations for higher levels of life satisfaction and self-esteem (see [27]) and are sound predictors of older adults' psychological resilience.

(3) *The psychosocial framework* posits that thematic strengths in old age functioning are directly linked to unique socioeconomic challenges that older adults encounter, which are embedded in the changing social, economic, and political structures of Western society [28]. This framework is closely tied in with the psychological framework of successful aging (e.g., [29, 30]) to include older adults' personal needs to achieve maximum optimization and resilience in late-life functioning within the social, economic, and political structures of society [31], and to pursue goals in late life that allow for autonomy and continuity of personal commitments and aspirations that were developed in earlier life stages [32].

Throughout the literature (starting with Maslow [10] and continuing into the current literature detailed in Ungar [9] and Vaillant [14], there is agreement that the search for various sources of life strengths is embedded in multidimensional contexts and contributes significantly to individuals' appraisals of their self-worth and sense of well-being. However, it is recognized that individuals might differ in the extent to which they appraise internal sources of strengths, as distinguished from external sources of strength, more positively or vice versa in facing life stressors (see [13]).

2.1. Sources and Determinants of Life Strengths and Their Relationship to Constructs of Vulnerability and Resilience. Based on theoretical dimensions of sources of life strengths we reviewed in the existential, social-cognitive, and psychosocial frameworks, it is reasonable to define the global construct of life strengths as a constellation of inner resources including skills, habits, beliefs, values, goals, behaviors, commitments, and expert knowledge, as well as the ability and resourcefulness to draw on resources in the external environment (e.g., social support and monetary gains) in order to adapt to changing circumstances. These agentic factors are a powerful source of personal strength and protective power and contribute to resilience which is conceptualized in terms of protective factors within the individual. Resilience defined as a "defense mechanism which enables people to thrive in the face of adversity" [33] is instrumental in both the individual's recovery and flourishing after the recovery [34]. However, resilience is not necessarily innate to the individual, but is largely contingent on the individual having sufficient inner and external resources that capacitate the person to endure, bounce back, and grow in the midst of adversities and existential anxieties [34, 35]. The underlying research and science-based assumption is that the adaptive processes underlying resilience development are intrinsically embedded in the vast expanse of life strengths that individuals have in their repertoire of learning and development. The greater the number of sources of life strengths, the greater the number of protective factors within the individual leading to higher levels of resilience and related positive health outcomes in the face of significant challenge, adversity, and stressful circumstances [36, 37]. Recently, Ungar and his associates [38, 39] have broadened resilience to include ecological and cultural factors. They define resilience as the development and application of science-based knowledge pertaining to positive development, positive adjustment, and thriving across the life-span. Thus, the construct of sources of life strengths is intrinsically linked to the concept of resilience in that they are acknowledged to be both intrapersonal and process-oriented and have a reciprocal relationship. Briefly stated, the "sources of life strengths" construct is a multidimensional and multifaceted dynamic construct assumed to have a reciprocal relationship with a number of other primary constructs, such as resilience and persistence, and other internal sources of self-regulatory controls such as self-efficacy, maturity, and sense of control, and external sources (such as social support and socioeconomic resources) that may impact positively or negatively on social, emotional, and intellectual well-being [40–42].

There is agreement that, while each framework we have considered in our review of the gerontological literature emphasizes a different set of independent structures and pathways for the emergence of life strengths, we postulate that collectively they all contribute to the maintenance and enhancement of resilience. Thus, our major assumption for the instrument development was the potential for plasticity in older adults. In developing our instrument on older adults' perceived sources of life strengths we worked from the basic assumption that older adults' appraisals of their internal strengths are protective mechanisms that are robust predictors of dispositional resilience in late life functioning [43].

A search of the literature revealed that, although there is a range of existing screening instruments that assess individuals' perceptions of their life strengths, each measure focuses narrowly on one single dimension only, for example, purpose for life (e.g., [22]), global self-efficacy beliefs (e.g., [44]), sense of control measure (e.g., [45]), and social support (e.g., [46]). Although these measures are widely accepted as screening instruments, their usefulness with respect to assessing older adults' sources of strengths is limited for a number of reasons. First, the measures, as noted, are not validated exclusively on samples of older adults. Second, their usefulness as a general measure of sources of life strengths of older adults is limited in that the focus is on one single (unitary) dimension, structure, or source of life strengths. Third, many items of the self-report measures are not easily understood by older adults themselves, and frequently must be interpreted to them by professionals. Accordingly, there is a strongly felt need for the development and validation of one easily comprehensible and reliable self-report instrument that takes into account multidimensional and multifaceted internal and external sources of life strengths of older adults.

3. Overall Objectives of the Study

Specific aims of the current study were fourfold: (1) to design an instrument "*sources of life strengths appraisal scale (SLSAS)*" specifically aimed at identifying a number of relevant cognitive and social-emotional dimensions of life strengths critical to late-life functioning; (2) to establish evidence of its factorial validity; (3) to assess the reliability of this instrument; and (4) to present evidence of the concurrent and predictive validity of the SLSAS measure with respect to ascertaining resilience potential of the study participants.

4. Method

4.1. Sample Pool for Study. The sample pool for this study was comprised of a total of 540 older adults, including a sample of 110 randomly selected volunteers for the pilot phase of the study, and another 430 older adults who were subsequently recruited as three independent samples (sample 1, $n = 120$; sample 2, $n = 120$; sample 3, $n = 190$) as used in the study. All participants in the pilot sample and three study samples were between the ages of 65 to 89 years residing in three large cities and semirural communities in Southern Alberta and British Columbia. Participants were recruited from a variety of civic, social, recreational, and semi-institutional settings and consisted of an almost equal number of females (51.3%) and males (48.7%). The mean age was 72.6 years, with all years between 65 and 89 represented. Participants were predominantly Caucasian/White (78.7%). Level of education ranged between a minimum of a junior high school certificate (17%) to a university degree (21%). A majority of the adults (42%) had a high school level education. At the time of recruitment of participants, 36% reported that they were in "excellent" health, 40% in "fair to good" health, and 24% in "poor" health. Participants were from all walks of life, ranging from being "unskilled" to "blue collar" workers, to "white collar professionals", and "competent executives".

Our systematic plan was to examine the concurrent validity of the SLSAS measure by comparing various SLSAS factor scores with other existing measures of mental health, depression, or other forms of vulnerability. In accordance with this plan, we administered a number of other test measures against which we could assess the concurrent validity of the SLSAS measure.

4.2. Measures. All study samples were administered the following measures that are well-reputed standardized measures developed by earlier researchers. They were included in a counterbalanced order in the questionnaire booklet. Participants were given the choice to complete the measures at their own pace, at their permanent home, or in their place of temporary residence (such as assisted living quarters or group homes). Participants arranged to return the materials at their earliest convenience to a designated research assistant. Participants who did not return the response materials within the first two weeks were recontacted by the research assistant who offered to give any additional help, if needed, for pickup of the materials, or for any difficulty in responding to the research questionnaires.

(1) Sources of Life Strengths Measure (SLSAS). (For a description of this measure and its development, see details in Section 4.)

(2) Sense of Control [45]. In this standardized measure, the sense of control is operationalized with two dimensions: personal mastery and personal constraints. Following Lachman and Weaver [45], we selected two items measuring Personal mastery: "I can do just about anything I really set my mind to" and "When I really want to do something, I usually find a way to succeed at it." "Perceived constraints" were measured using four items (e.g., "Other people determine most of what I can do to change many of the important things in my life," "I often feel helpless in dealing with problems in my life"). A 4-point rating scale (ranging from 1 = a lot to 4 = not at all) was used for both dimensions. Using this scale, we derived a global score of internal control. Cronbach's alphas for respondents in the three samples of the present study ranged from .73 to .76 and from 70 to .73 for men and women, respectively. With respect to this measure of control, our hypothesis was that the SLSAS measures would correlate positively with high internal control.

(3) Measure of Self-Esteem (SEI: [47]). This inventory was used to measure self-esteem as a global and stable disposition. The inventory has 10 items, 5 positively keyed and 5 negatively keyed. Each item is rated on a 4-point Likert type scale. Cronbach's alphas for respondents in the three samples of the present study ranged from .83 to .85 and from .79 to .82 for men and women, respectively. With respect to the measure of self-esteem, our hypothesis was that the SLSAS measure would correlate positively with high self-esteem on the SEI.

(4) Life Satisfaction Was Assessed by Means of the Five-Item Satisfaction with Life Scale (SLS: [48]). Each item is rated on a 5-point Likert type scale, yielding a score range of 5 to 25. The measure assumes that participants compare their current circumstances against subjective standards to arrive at a global appraisal of life satisfaction (e.g., "In most ways my life is close to ideal"). Cronbach's alphas for respondents in the three samples of the present study ranged from .81 to .86 and from 79 to .82 for men and women, respectively. With respect to the measure of life satisfaction (SLS), our hypothesis was that the SLSAS measure would correlate positively with high self-esteem on the SLS.

(5) Measure of Vulnerability [49]. This is a 12-item screening test to measure older adults' state of vulnerability in terms of anxiety, dependence, helplessness, and rejection. In the present study, each item was scored on a 4-point Likert type scale with scores ranging between 12 and 48. Responses were summed to give a total vulnerability score. In the context of this scale, vulnerability is conceptualized as being the opposite of resilience. Vulnerable individuals are characterized as being low in resilience and reserve capacity. Psychological vulnerability from the perspective of this scale is viewed as morbidity, depression, and psychological distress. Cronbach's alphas for respondents in the three samples of the present study ranged from .80 to .86 and from .79 to .83 for men and women, respectively. Our hypothesis with respect to this measure of vulnerability was that the SLSAS measure would correlate negatively with vulnerability dimensions of stress, anxiety, and depression.

(6) Depression. Depression was measured by the Zung self-rating depression scale (SDS: [50]) covering depressive symptoms relating to somatic, psychological, psychomotor, and mood areas. A total depression score was calculated for each respondent by summing scores in the four domains. Cronbach's alphas for respondents in the three samples of the present study ranged from .80 to .84 and from .78 to .81 for men and women, respectively. With respect to the measure of depression (SDS), our hypothesis was that the SLSAS measure would correlate negatively with the depression measure on the SDS.

4.3. Two Outcome Measures Administered at 24-Month Longitudinal Followup of Respondents Procedures Related to Predictive and Concurrent Validity of SLSAS. Additionally, we also planned on conducting a 24-month (two years) followup of respondents from the time of baseline assessments to obtain evidence of the predictive validity of the SLSAS with respect to ascertaining resilience potential of the study participants.

Thus, following baseline assessment of the SLSAS, a group of 150 respondents were randomly selected from the overall sample of 540 older adults for a 24-month followup. The purpose of the followup was to assess the predictive validity of the SLSAS with respect to outcome measures of resilience. The randomly selected sample of 150, who at the time of baseline agreed to a 24-month followup, was administered with the following two additional measures of resilience.

(1) Dispositional Resilience Scale (DRS: [15]). This measure is composed of 45 items with 15 items each assessing *commitment to living* (e.g.,most days life is interesting and exciting for me), *control* and *focused engagement* (e.g.,planning ahead can help me avoid most future problems), and *challenge* (e.g., changes in routine are interesting to me). The DRS was originally developed as a measure of hardiness. In the context of this scale, resilience in later adulthood is a form of hardiness or mindset that facilitates recovery from risk and adversity (see [35, 43]). Those who typify psychological hardiness espouse a commitment to living; they enjoy challenge and believe that change rather than stability is normal. Also they manifest a pervasive belief that they can and will respond effectively under stress [51]. Internal consistency of responses as measured by Cronbach's alpha was .82 and .83 for men and women, respectively, in our sample.

Our hypothesis was that the greater the number of internal and external sources of life strengths that are identified by the SLSAS scale, the stronger the association with the three domains of resilience in the DRS, at the time of the 24-month followup. Internal consistency of responses as measured by

Cronbach's alpha for the DRS *Scale* was .79 and .82 for men and women, respectively.

(2) *The Resilience Scale* [16]. We used the 50-item version of the resilience scale as originally constructed [16] to measure the potential for resilience. The construct of resilience is defined in terms of five characteristics: *perseverance* (act of persistence despite adversity or discouragement), *equanimity* (balanced perspective of life and experiences that moderate the extreme responses to adversity), *meaningfulness* (the realization that life has a purpose and recognition that there is always something for which to live), *self-reliance* (the ability to believe in one's self and to rely on one's personal strengths and capabilities in the face of adverse circumstances to guide one's actions), and *existential aloneness* (the realization that each person is unique and that, while some experiences can be shared, others must be faced alone). These five characteristics form the conceptual foundation for the *resilience scale* (TRS) [16]. Internal consistency of responses as measured by Cronbach's alpha for the *resilience scale* was .82 and .83 for men and women, respectively.

Our hypothesis was that the greater the number of internal and external sources of life strengths that are identified by the SLSAS scale, the stronger the association with the five components of resilience as detailed in the *resilience scale* (TRS) [16] at the time of the 24-month followup.

5. Construction of the Preliminary SLSAS

5.1. Use of Focus Groups for Generating Items and Item Selection. We resorted to focus group methodology that other recent researchers have found particularly useful for the purpose of generating items for preliminary scale development and for ensuring that a diversity of theoretical constructs and dimensions are considered in the scale development (see [52]). There were 48 focus group members assigned in equal numbers to four subgroups of 12 individuals (6 men and 6 women). Each subgroup included both lay persons and professionals. Assisted by two graduate student researchers who searched the psychology literature, each focus group participated in four discussion sessions of approximately 1- to 1.25-hour duration. They brain-stormed and explored the core focus and key concepts of internal and external sources of life strengths as identified in the literature, and delineated several constructs relevant to the major themes. Collectively, the focus group teams drew attention to the major theoretical constructs that might serve as the bases for generating items for the current scale development. Key dimensions that were suggested and discussed for item generation included the following areas of focus:

(1) factors conducive to coping with normative losses in old age (see [31]),

(2) factors conducive to personal resilience (i.e., factors conducive to recovery from risk and adversity and factors conducive to the maintenance of developmental capacities in the face of cumulating threat and challenge);

(3) factors conducive to development of social identity and social well-being (i.e., factors conducive to the attainment of stability and structure in one's social life) (see [14]); factors conducive to the expansion of the self and/or self-knowledge (i.e., perception of continuity in one's life, provision of meaning in life, perceptions of positive self-regard, a sense that life is purposeful, a sense of continuing growth, and a general sense of life satisfaction) [30, 53]; and actualization of self and life goals [10];

(4) factors conducive to a sense of altruism and morality (i.e., factors conducive to the ability to follow inner convictions and to live life in the context of giving, sharing, and receiving) [54];

(5) factors conducive to a sense of affiliation and belongingness (i.e., factors conducive to perceptions of having good quality relationships with family and others) [10, 12];

(6) factors conducive to a sense of stimulation, challenge, and excitement/enjoyment (i.e., factors conducive to the provision of novelty and exciting and meaningful experiences);

(7) factors conducive to a sense of accomplishment and competence (i.e., having perceptions of goals in life);

(8) factors conducive to a sense of social superiority by comparison and competition with others (i.e., reflection of one's achievement over others and a sense of victory) (see [26]);

(9) factors conducive to a sense of power, influence, and control (i.e., the provision of opportunity to exert effect on others' lives) [4] (see also discussion by [5, 12]).

Each of the focus group sessions lasted on average for 1 to 1.25 hours and the sessions collectively generated an initial multiple item pool of 85 items that tapped individuals' perceptions of sources of life strengths that are valued most in different situations of stress, challenge, adversity, success, victory, and flourishing. Five to 7 items operationalizing each of the selected key theoretically relevant dimensions were generated by members of the focus group, based on their understanding of key themes drawn from the literature on developmental aging that were suggested to them by the graduate research assistants. The 85 items were submitted to three contents experts (a recently retired university professor, one experienced social worker, and one geriatric practitioner) for judging the importance of each item (YES-NO) with respect to its relevance to an identifiable key construct or a key dimension of strengths identified in the literature. All 85 items were judged to be of importance. A satisfactory level of interrater agreement was obtained if two of the three raters agreed on the classification of the item to a construct domain that had been identified during item generation.

All components judged by focus group experts as being important and relevant to the "sources of internal strengths" construct were picked out and expanded into complete sentences that allowed respondent(s) to rate the extent to which they believe the item component "*as being a source of strength for me during times of difficulty, or generally contributing to my overall sense of psychological well-being*" was "very important" = 5 to "not important" = 1.

Based on interrater agreement ratings, 60 items out of the original 85 items were judged to be "important" and were retained. The remaining 25 items were discarded. Based on the preceding item selection procedures, the preliminary SLSAS was defined as a 60-item instrument and subsequently administered to one pilot group of 110 members and subsequently to three sample groups (sample 1, n = 120; sample 2, n = 120; sample 3, n = 190) for further reliability.

6. Results

6.1. Instrument Evaluation on a Pilot Group. The condition of the data matrix was evaluated, first, by testing the adequacy of the sample correlation matrix on a pilot group of 110 persons for the 60 items of our scale by using the Kaiser-Meyer Olin (KMO) measure for sampling adequacy [55]. This was calculated to be .90, attesting that the sample size was large enough to evaluate the factor structure [55]. Second, we tested the factorability of the data set using Bartlett's test of sphericity, χ^2 (528/3 = 3711.72) that was significant at the .0001 level indicating further that the data matrix approximates an identity matrix and that the factor model was appropriate for a principal components analysis [56].

6.2. Factorial Validity. To empirically test the validity of the SLSAS items that were developed, two separate factor analyses were conducted (see Table 1).

6.2.1. Primary Analysis: Exploratory Factor Analysis (EFA) (See EFA, Table 1). A preliminary (exploratory) factor analysis using the method of factorial components with Varimax rotation was performed to determine the factor structure of the preliminary SLSAS items. Data used in the exploratory factor analysis were obtained from the administration of the preliminary SLSAS items to 240 respondents (samples 1 and 2 combined) from the total sample (see Table 1). Factors that yielded an eigenvalue greater than one were deemed to merit further consideration. Because we desired a relatively brief instrument, we used the loading criteria suggested by Stevens [57]. Accordingly, we decided that there must be a minimum of five items, with factor loadings of .40 or higher within a factor, for the factor to be considered for interpretation. Furthermore, it was decided that, if an item loaded on more than one factor, then the factor with the highest loadings would be selected.

Thirteen component factors with eigenvalues greater than one emerged from the preliminary factor analysis (EFA) (see Table 1). We agreed that, in addition to the "eigenvalue-one" criteria, we consider two other criteria to decide how many component factors to retain. First, we examined the scree plot [58] and observed the break between components with large eigenvalues and those with small eigenvalues (but not less than one). In our data, we observed a major and notable break which occurred at 10 components that accounted for a cumulative percentage of 70% of the explained variance that is deemed appropriate for initial scale development (see [57, 59]). This 10-factor solution, which could be considered as a relatively conservative representation of the data, was rotated to a Varimax criterion for further interpretation. The first component had an explained variance of 38% followed by five more accounting for a cumulative variance of 20% and the last four providing a cumulative variance of 12% (see footnote in Table 1). Based on the relative strengths of factors as determined by the percentage of the explained variance, the definition and labeling of the first six factors was as follows: (1) personal commitment; (2) self-efficacy beliefs; (3) personal maturity; (4) attitudes toward life; (5) continuity in mid-life roles; (6) personal achievements. These six factors accounted for 54% of the total cumulative variance, with the remaining variance of 16% accounted for by the four factors that we labeled and defined as follows: (7) informal social support; (8) monetary status; (9) personal traits; and (10) self-care routines.

6.2.2. Second Analysis: Principal Components Factor Analysis (PCA) (See PCA, Table 1). A second principal component factor analysis with Varimax rotation was performed on the data derived from the administration of the preliminary SLSAS to 190 new respondents. It is important to note that these 190 individuals were new respondents who had not participated in any of the earlier stages of item generation, nor had been involved in any reliability assessment of the SLSAM research. Therefore, they had no familiarity with the SLSAM items or subscales that had been generated to this point. The purpose of the second factor analysis was to replicate the factor structure identified in the primary (exploratory) factor analysis (EFA) and to estimate the relative independence of the established factors in the context of a new independent study sample. Thus, the second principal component analysis was intended to serve a confirmatory function (PCA). In this analysis, the first component had an explained variance of 32% followed by five more accounting for a cumulative variance of 23% and the last three providing a cumulative variance of 15% (total explained variance = 70%) (see footnote in Table 1). Results of the PCA showed nine factors with factor loadings of .40 or higher (see Table 1: PCA).

With the exception of the personal achievement factor, the factor structures that emerged in the PCA strongly confirmed the strength of the original factor structures reported in the exploratory factor analysis (EFA). The total amount of variance explained by the six most salient factors in the PCA was 52%, compared with 54% in the EFA. In both factor analyses, the communalities ranged from .77 to .25 and from .74 to .22, respectively, indicating that items shared a reasonable amount of variance with all other items (see [60]). The finding of an overall close correspondence between the factors identified in the two sets of factorial analysis provides robust evidence that the factor structure within the SLSAS items is relatively stable across samples.

Table 1: Factor structure of the SLSAS for exploratory factorial analysis (EFA) with samples one and two ($N = 240$) combined and principal component analysis (PCA) with sample three ($N = 190$).

SLSAS scale items[a]	I		II		III		IV		V		VI (Factor loadings[b])		VII		VIII		IX		X		Factor VIII Factor IX
	EFA	PCA	EFA	PCA	EFA	PCA	EFA	PCA	EFA	PCA	EFA	PCA	EFA	PCA	EFA	PCA	EFA	PCA	EFA	PFA	
Personal self-efficacy beliefs																					
Ability to overcome problems	.85	.79																			
Ability to succeed	.76	.74																			
High motivation to excel	.72	.77																			
Excellent knowledge	.77	.82																			
Ability to obtain information	.69	.67																			
Personal maturity																					
Strong meaning for life			.78	.82																	
Awareness of limitations			.82	.79																	
Well-defined goals	.47		.61	.51																	
Desire for spirituality			.70	.73																	
Accepting of negative consequences			.79	.75																	
Personal traits																					
Courageous					.46	.50															
Truthfulness and honesty					.75	.75															
Autonomous and self-reliant					.81	.81															
Responsible					.59	.56															
Faithful and loyal					.79	.77															
Self-care routines																					
Diligent							.81	.76													
Follow sound diet regimen							.69	.69													
Persistent in task completion							.79	.75													
Exercise regularly							.69	.77													
Devotional prayer regularly							.70	.76													
Personal commitments																					
Desire to make a positive social impact									.77	.75											
Committed to personal mission									.70	.72											
Committed to leaving legacy									.70	.70											
Committed to life of service									.79	.77											
Committed to imparting education to the young									.69	.63											
Personal achievements																					
Achieved important career/life goals											.61	.48									
Achieved social success											.49										
Achieved family respect											.60	.54									
Achieved financial success											.49										

Table 1: Continued.

SLSAS scale items[a]	I		II		III		IV		V		VI		VII		VIII		IX		X		Factor VIII Factor IX
	Factor loadings[b]																				
	EFA	PCA	EFA	PCA	EFA	PCA	EFA	PCA	EFA	PCA	EFA	PCA	EFA	PCA	EFA	PCA	EFA	PCA	EFA	PFA	
Achieved outside (external) recognition											.47	.42									
Attitudes toward Life																					
Optimistic and hopeful for future													.72	.78							
Life is a challenge	.46												.69	.72							
Life is an adventure													.73	.74							
Believe there is solution to all problems													.81	.74							
Believe human nature is good													.88	.80							
Social support: informal sources																					
Intimate relationships															.88	.83					
Friends and associates															.75	.72					
Formal social service agency															.69	.66					
Seniors' associations and clubs															.70	.69					
Religious institutions															.72	.71					
Monetary status																					
Having sound investments																	.81	.87			
Having stable credit rating																	.69	.71			
Having good prospects for inheritance																	.72	.69			
Having steady income from pension																	.71	.75			
Having means for more earnings																	.69	.62			
Continuity in mid-life roles																					
Opportunity to continue in mid-life careers and positions																			.74	.72	
Continuing opportunity for achieving recognition and awards for past achievements																			.90	.87	
Continuing opportunity to be involved in parenting function																			.79	.79	
Continuing opportunity to pursue mid-life hobbies/interest.																			.73	.77	
Continuing opportunity to pursue mid-life friendships																			.81	.87	

[a]SLSAS items are identified by key words in item. [b]All loadings > 0.40 are shown.

EFA was conducted on 60 items: ten items were subsequently dropped because of unacceptably high item-total correlations above 0.80. The first component had an explained variance of 38% followed by five more components accounting for a cumulative variance of 20% and the last four providing a cumulative variance of 12% (total percent of explained variance is 70).

PCA was conducted on 50 items: the first component had an explained variance of 32% followed by five more accounting for a cumulative variance of 23% and the last four providing a cumulative variance of 15% (total percent of explained variance = 70).

Note: Table 1 shows factor loadings for only those 50 items that were used in both the EFA and PCA.

Table 2: Intercorrelations between subscale factors of the SLSAS ($N = 430$).

Subscales	(1)	(2)	(3)	(4)	(5)	(6)	(7)	(8)	(9)	(10)
(1) Personal efficacy	—	$.24^{**}$	$.20^{**}$	$.25^{**}$	$.21^{**}$	$.18^{*}$	$.27^{**}$	$-.12^{*}$	$-.24^{**}$	$.25^{**}$
(2) Personal maturity		—	$.22^{**}$	$.34^{**}$	.16	.18	$.21^{**}$	$.21^{*}$	−.16	$-.19^{*}$
(3) Personal traits			—	$.25^{**}$	.17	$.21^{*}$	$.26^{**}$	−.15	$-.21^{*}$	.14
(4) Self-care routines				—	$.23^{**}$	$.24^{**}$	.13	$.19^{*}$	$.24^{**}$	$-.20^{*}$
(5) Personal commitments					—	−.12	.17	$.27^{**}$	−.12	$.26^{**}$
(6) Personal achievements						—	$.27^{**}$	.14	$.22^{*}$	$.27^{**}$
(7) Attitudes toward life							—	.17	.16	.13
(8) Social support: informal								—	.15	.17
(9) Monetary status									—	$.28^{**}$
(10) Continuity in mid-life roles										—

$^{*}P < 0.05$; $^{**}P < 0.001$.

6.3. Composite Description of the SLSAS. Based on the findings of the two independent factor analyses, the structures of the SLSAS were described as follows.

Internal sources of life strength were (1) *personal self-efficacy* (five items) which includes beliefs of one's competence to handle life's situations and motivation to overcome problems; (2) *personal maturity* (five items) which includes such components as meaning for life, purposes and goals for living, a sense of spirituality, acceptance of one's limitations and acceptance of negative consequences; (3) *personal traits* (five items) which includes dispositional characteristics such as courage, self-confidence, sense of personal responsibility, and accountability; (4) *self-care routines* (five items) such as habits of diligence, persistence and determination in task performance, sound dietary habits, and other habits such as physical exercise, devotional prayer, and relaxation; (5) *personal commitments* (five items) which include the individual's commitments to make a positive impact on others, or to support and advocate causes in the public interest; (6) *attitudes toward life* (five items) which include elements such as the individual's positive outlook on life, viewing life to be a challenge and adventure, and believing in the goodness of human nature.

External sources of life strengths were (7) *social support: informal sources* (five items) representing support coming from intimate relationships, friends, and associates; (8) *monetary status* (five items) which includes monetary advantage such as a steady income in terms of retirement and old age security benefits, financial investments, and inherited assets; (9) *continuity in mid-life roles* (five items) which refers to opportunities available to continue in employment after retirement age, opportunities to preserve and sustain long-term relationships from the mid-life years, and opportunities to gain recognition for new and past activity and functions.

It should be noted that the factor of "personal achievement" ratified in the first EFA did not get commensurate factor loadings in the second confirmatory PCA, and accordingly it was dropped from further consideration in the instrument development (specimen items from each structure that were retained in the final version of the 45-item SLSAS are included in the Appendix).

6.4. Reliability Assessments of the SLSAS Measure. In order to investigate the psychometric quality of the SLSAS scales that were created to correspond with factors identified in the preliminary factor analyses and cross-validated with another confirmatory factor analysis, we pursued a number of other preliminary but vitally important steps. *First,* following Nunnally [61], we set a predetermined standard for internal reliability (Cronbach's α) at .70. Cronbach's alphas were calculated and these ranged from .71 to .81 for ten scales that were derived from the EFA analysis. Cronbach's alphas ranging from .82 to .89 were observed for nine scales derived from the PCA, indicating moderate to very good internal reliability appropriate for a relatively brief screening instrument [62].

Second, we examined the correlations among the SLSAS subscales themselves (Table 2).

Findings showed that they were moderately correlated, with correlations ranging from .12 to .28. The mean intercorrelation was .21. This suggests that these scales, despite the potential for some overlap, are tapping relatively independent appraisal dimensions.

Third, we conducted an inspection of item-total correlations of all the items, factor matrix, and communalities. Out of the original 60 items, only 45 items showing interitem correlations ranging from .15 to .20, and subscale correlations ranging from .18 to .22, were retained as being acceptable [63]. As a final step, the reliability of the final SLSAS was assessed using internal consistency estimates (Cronbach's alpha) for the separate samples. With a few exceptions, alphas for six of the "*internal sources of strength*" scales and three of the "*external sources of strength*" scales were good, ranging from .73 to .94. Cronbach's alphas for three scales were lower than our predetermined criterion of .70, and therefore these scales (personal achievement, social support from formal sources, and monetary stability) were dropped from further analysis.

Test-retest reliability over a 6-month interval was fully acceptable with test-retest reliability coefficients ranging from .79 to .82 for the nine subscales. Internal consistency of responses ranged from $\alpha = .79$ to $\alpha = .85$ (*further raw data details about item-total correlations, factor matrix, communalities, and retest reliability data are available from the authors*).

TABLE 3: Correlations of SLSAS scales with measures of internal control, self-esteem, life satisfaction, vulnerability, and depression.

	Internal control	Self-esteem	Life satisfaction	Vulnerability	Depression
SLSAS Scales					
Personal self-efficacy beliefs	.65***	.69***	.48***	−.48***	−.50***
Personal maturity	.41***	.26**	.38***	−.49***	−.33**
Personal traits	.33**	.35**	.29**	−.22*	−.21*
Self-care routines	.21*	.24**	.22*	.14	−.29**
Personal commitments	.59***	.57***	.52***	−.36**	−.49***
Attitudes toward life	.46**	.54***	.37**	−.45***	−.31**
Personal achievements	.37**	.36**	.31**	−.42**	−.1.4
Social supports: informal sources	−.21*	−.34**	.12	−.08	−.18
Monetary status	.12	.20*	.48***	−.27*	−.24*
Continuity in mid-life roles	.28**	.58***	.48***	−.32**	−.26*

High scores indicate high levels of personal control, self-esteem, life satisfaction, vulnerability, and depression.
$^{*}P < 0.05$; $^{**}P < 0.01$; $^{***}P < 0.001$.

Examination of the mean scores showed that, in most of the scales, the mean scores were approximately in the middle range, with reasonably high mean appraisal scores assigned to personal commitments, personal self-efficacy beliefs, personal maturity, personal traits, self-care routines, life attitudes, social support (informal), monetary status, and continuity in mid-life roles.

Based on the results of the preceding reliability procedures and the results of two factor analyses (EFA and PCA), more specific definitions were arrived at for the nine scales of the final 45-item version of the SLSAS. The Principal components factor analysis of the SLSAS reported that the factors also belong to a latent construct of the overall sources of life strengths and this score can be achieved by a summation of the nine subscale scores. Cronbach's alpha for the summed scale is .81, now being a summated rating scale employing a 5-point response format (ranging from *Not At All Important* to *Very Important*). In its final form, the SLSAS is scored by summing the responses to all 45 items, with subscale scores obtained by summing the responses to five items within each subscale (i.e., structure).

6.5. Further Evidence of Concurrent Validity of SLSAS. Further evidence of concurrent validity for the SLSAS was obtained by examining the correlations between the SLSAS scales and other related psychological variables, notably variables of internal control, self-esteem, life satisfaction, vulnerability, and depression. Examination of the correlations of the SLSAS factor structures with various measures (see Table 3) shows that almost all of the correlations are at a significant level (ranging from .21 to .69).

Consistent with our hypothesis, we observed a positive correlation between the subscale scores on the SLSAS and variables of internal control, self-esteem, and life-satisfaction. Conversely, consistent with our hypotheses, we observed a negative association between most of the subscale scores on the SLSAS and variables of vulnerability and depression. These findings provide further evidence of the concurrent validity of the SLSAS life strength structures corresponding with key theoretical dimensions of mental health fitness (e.g., internal control, self-esteem, and life satisfaction) as underscored in the recent gerontological literature. Also, the negative association of the SLSAS subscales and the measures of vulnerability and depression is consistent with the trends reported in the gerontological literature.

6.6. SLSAS as a Predictor of Outcomes Measures of Dispositional Resilience (Control, Challenge, and Commitment) and Resilience Characteristics (Perseverance, Equanimity, Meaningfulness, Self-Reliance, and Existential Aloneness) at the 24-Month Followup. The predictive validity of the SLSAS measure was further established by conducting a 24-month follow-up study of 150 randomly selected respondents, commencing from the time of baseline administration of the final SLSAS measure and two measures of resilience: (1) Bartone et al.'s measure of dispositional resilience (DRS) and (2) the resilience scale ([16] further modified in 2009), These instruments were readministered at the time of the 24-month followup. Correlation coefficients of the SLSAS subscales with three subscales of dispositional resilience (DRS) (i.e., perceived challenge, control processing, and commitment to Living) were examined (Table 4). Similarly, correlation coefficients of the SLSAS nine subscales with five subscales of the Wagnild and Young [16] resilience scale (further modified in 2009) (i.e., perseverance; equanimity; meaningfulness; self-reliance; existential aloneness) were examined (Table 5).

The results clearly demonstrate that there were robust correlations (all in the hypothesized direction) between the nine SLSAS subscales and the three subscales and the total of the dispositional resilience scale (with correlations ranging between .21 and .69) (see Table 4). Similarly, there are robust correlations (all in the hypothesized direction) between the five dimensions of the Wagnild and Young [16] resilience scale and nine SLSAS subscales (i.e., correlations ranging from .41 to .69).

Subsequent multiple regression analyses conducted for predictors of resilience showed that, after controlling for demographic variables, subscales of personal self-efficacy, personal commitments, attitudes toward life, and continuity in-mid-life roles in the SLSAS were the most significant

TABLE 4: Correlation coefficients of SLSAM scales with outcome measures of global resilience and its four subscales of perceived challenge, controlled processing, commitment to living (DRS: dispositional resilience scale, Bartone et al., 1989 [15]) administered at 24-month followup from date of baseline assessments of the SLSAS measure (sample = 150).

	Global	Perceived challenge	Controlled processing	Commitment to living
SLSAS Scale				
Personal self-efficacy beliefs	.51***	.56***	.53***	.67***
Personal maturity	.31**	.29**	.26**	.31**
Personal traits	.39***	.43***	.29*	.27**
Self-care routines	.21*	.21*	.15	.29**
Personal commitments	.49***	.47***	.46***	.51***
Attitudes toward life	.46**	.54***	.45***	.31**
Personal achievements	.17	.16	.21*	.16
Social supports: informal sources	.21*	.23*	.22*	.25*
Monetary status	.22*	.26*	.22*	.20*
Continuity in mid-life roles	.28*	.46***	.38***	.40***

High scores indicate high global resilience, high level of perceived challenge, high level of controlled processing, and high level of commitment to living.
$^{*}P < 0.05$; $^{**}P < 0.01$; $^{***}P < 0.001$.

TABLE 5: Correlation coefficients of SLSAS scales with outcome measures of total resilience, perseverance, equanimity, meaningfulness, self-reliance, and existential aloneness administered at 24-month followup from date of baseline assessment (sample = 150).

	Total resilience	Perseverance	Equanimity	Meaningfulness	Self-reliance	Existential aloneness
SLSAS Scale						
Personal self-efficacy beliefs	.55***	.69***	.52***	.51***	.34***	.43***
Personal maturity	.41***	.29**	.38***	.46***	.43**	.36**
Personal traits	.38***	.41***	.29**	.23*	.21*	.41***
Self-care routines	.21*	.24*	.22*	.14	.39**	.21*
Personal commitments	.59***	.57***	.52***	.36***	.59***	.32**
Attitudes toward life	.46**	.54***	.37***	.45***	.31**	.28*
Personal achievements	.31**	.16	.31**	.22*	.34**	.37**
Social supports: informal sources	.21*	.24*	.12	.08	.18	.21*
Monetary status	.32**	.20*	.22*	.27*	.44***	.48***
Continuity in mid-life roles	.48***	.56***	.46***	.22*	.46***	.32**

High scores indicate high levels of total resilience; perseverance; personal equanimity; meaningfulness; self-reliance; existential aloneness.
$P < 0.05$;$^{**}P < 0.01$; $^{***}P < 0.001$.

predictors of resilience (as defined in the two resilience scales that were administered in the 24-month followup), accounting for a significant proportion of the variance (76% and 79%, resp.). These data attest further to the fact that the SLSAS has the potential to predict outcomes of challenge, control, and commitment as defined in the *dispositional resilience scale*. Similarly, the SLSAS has the potential to predict outcomes of perseverance, equanimity, self-reliance meaningfulness and existential aloneness as defined in *the resilience scale* [16].

7. Discussion

7.1. Strengths of the SLSAS Measure. In terms of unique strengths, the SLSAS is among the first of validated measures to provide support for the notion that what keeps a majority of older individuals strong in the face of both daily life stresses and obstacles and adversity is a balance of perceived life strength resources, both internal and external. The major strengths of the instrument can be observed in terms of the multidimensional internal and external resources it taps, and its capability to integrate, as parsimoniously as possible, several useful constructs that have hitherto been embedded in a multiplicity of single construct assessment scales and measures. While the present study is cross-sectional and causal directionality, therefore, cannot be imputed, our results from the SLSAS measure show, at the least, a significant relationship between various dimensions of the "life strengths" construct, such as personal self-efficacy beliefs, personal maturity, personal traits, self-care routines, personal commitment, personal achievements, positive attitudes toward life, social support, monetary status, and continuity in mid-life roles, and older adults' subsequent self-appraisals of resilience/hardiness, internal control, self-esteem, and life satisfaction when encountering situations of stern challenges, threat and uncertainty.

The final version of the 45-item SLSAS is derived from two rounds of exploratory factor analysis and principal factor analysis centered on nine appraisal dimensions (structures) comprised of 5 items per structure. It should be noted that the SLSAS measure was validated on four samples of older adults (one nonrandom pilot sample and three randomly selected samples) ranging in age from 65 to 87 years. Within the predetermined scope of the present study, we were able to establish the concurrent validity by assessing the association of the structures of the SLSAS with other related measures of self-esteem, life satisfaction, vulnerability, and depression. Additionally, it should be noted that concurrent validity of the instrument was based on a postbaseline followup of 25% of individuals drawn randomly from the original Pilot sample and samples 1, 2, and 3. Another unique feature of the SLSAS is that we were able to establish the predictive validity of the SLSAS measure over a 24-month followup, specifically with respect to predicting older adults' resilience as measured by other well-reputed standardized scales of resilience. It is important to note that the sample of 540 older participants, involved in various phases of the validity and reliability procedures, is representative of individuals who reported a range of health statuses, a range of educational levels, and a range of occupational backgrounds and financial status. The SLSAM was thus validated on a sample of older adults appropriately representative of individuals from various walks of life.

Another significant feature of the instrument is that it is brief, requiring, on average, about 10 to 12 min. response time as opposed to a multiplicity of single dimension measures which are commonly used to assess the same nine factors, and which are reported to be extremely time-consuming for the average older adult. Thus, it has ease of administration to frail older adults who have trouble responding to lengthy questionnaires frequently precipitating fatigue and unreliability in response ratings (see [64]).

To conclude, the SLSAS instrument meets stringent criteria of reliability, construct, and predictive validity essential to the development of new screening instruments (see [62] for discussion of practical and theoretical considerations in developing brief screening instruments). The SLSAS is a valid omnibus measure of older adults' life strengths described variously as a constellation of beliefs about the self, one's values and commitments, one's perceptions of competence, abilities and controls, and one's perspective of social domains outside the self.

7.2. Implications and Applications of the SLSAS for Counseling Practice with Older Adults. As a relatively brief assessment instrument, the SLSAS maybe useful to geriatric professionals and health professionals who wish to obtain a multidimensional picture or profile of their elderly clients' highly valued sources of strengths with the aim of predicting their future psychological well-being and resilience capacity. In short, the SLSAS instrument offers counseling psychologists and other geriatric service providers a reliable and valid, but also sensitive, approach to assessing older adults' self-appraisals of a diversity of internal and external sources of life strengths. This is important client information for counseling psychologists to consider. Mounting evidence points to the importance of older adults' perceived personal strengths as a valid indicator of their overall resilience with respect to psychological health and well-being [9, 65]. Also there is increasing evidence suggesting that older adults' self-perceptions and self-appraisals of their life strengths and sources of strength have an important influence on their objective health and well-being, with poor appraisals and negative perceptions of internal strengths leading to greater helplessness and loss of control, and positive appraisals and positive perceptions of internal strengths leading to higher motivation to preserve and maintain resilience in late life [66]. By using the SLSAS measure with older clients, counseling psychologists may be able to assist clients to develop a realistic self profile of their sources of life strengths in relation to self-growth and control over every day life situation. Conversely, counseling psychologists' own understanding of their older clients' perceived sources of strengths may serve as a basis for encouraging clients to develop new areas of strength and, where relevant, to draw on internal sources of strengths such as reflecting on meaning and purpose for life, maintaining social ties, and finding satisfaction through continuing pursuit of earlier life goals and plans [32]. Counselors may be able to help clients develop existing sources of life strengths by reflecting on prior experience of having overcome negative conditions, and thereby seeking to harness the positive potentials (see [67]). The SLSAS also has considerable potential for predicting psychological resilience if used with middle-aged individuals who are concerned about the prospects for successful aging in their later years.

7.3. Limitations of the Present Research. The sample in the current study was predominantly Caucasian and this factor may limit the generalizability of the findings. As is the case with most contemporary scientific approaches, the theoretical and measurement models we employed in the development of the SLSAS measure are, by and large, embedded within a Western culture that places an emphasis on individualistic and personal values such as personal achievement, self-efficacy, and self-directed competence (see [68]). It is reasonable to assume that in a non-Western collectivistic sample, a sense of community relatedness and personal meaning and belongingness may figure more predominantly than appears to be the case in our present Caucasian sample. Earlier research in a number of other contexts (see [67]) has indicated that people in strong collectivistic cultures may be more concerned about securing a better life for their family than for themselves. Also their life satisfactions may come more from interpersonal harmonious relationships, group morale, and collaborative success as contrasted with a predominance of intrapersonal factors such as factors of self-reliance, financial independence and self-care activities which were important to the Caucasian samples we used in the present study. It now remains for future cross-cultural researchers to compare the SLSAS factorial structures with those derived from the responses of older adults from non-Caucasian backgrounds in order to establish further the universality of the "sources of life strengths" construct(s). Suffice it to say that the SLSAS has the potential to stimulate further research along a number of other cross-cultural dimensions.

Another issue that needs to be addressed in future studies of the SLSAS has to do with the potential of the SLSAS to predict resilience when conceptualized within a process-oriented framework, as distinguished from an intrapersonal framework. In our present delineation and definition of "life strengths" and "resilience," our conceptualization of both of these constructs was that they involve a combination of intrapersonal and interpersonal processes. However, both scales of resilience [15, 16] that we used against which to establish the concurrent validity of the SLSAS viewed resilience to be a stable dispositional intrapersonal trait and not an ongoing process. Unfortunately, within the time constraints of our study and the predetermined scope of our research (where the primary goal was to construct a scale for appraising sources of life strengths with the potential to predict resilience) we were obliged, at the time of the 24-month followup, to use the best available standardized scales of resilience. Future research using the SLSAS should consider its potential to predict resilience as being more process-oriented rather than a dispositional intrapersonal trait.

Appendix

Specimen items for nine structures of the SLSAS measure, each structure carrying five items,

I believe my strength to overcome problems and to sustain my present sense of well-being comes from (each rated *very important = 5—not at all important = 1*):

structure one items:

(i) from my beliefs and self-confidence that I can continue to succeed in the future,

(ii) from my very good understanding of the people around me;

structure two items:

(i) from my strong sense of meaning and purpose for my life,

(ii) from my having well-defined goals and plans for living;

structure three items:

(i) from my desire to be independent and self-reliant under most circumstances,

(ii) from my desire to be faithful and honest in most of my life's functions and roles;

structure four items:

(i) from my habit of engaging in regular devotional prayer and worship,

(ii) from my strong desire to be regular and persevering in most tasks assigned to me;

structure five items:

(i) from my desire to make a positive social impact on people around me,

(ii) from my commitment to lead a life of service to others;

structure six items:

(i) from my optimistic and cheerful attitude to life,

(ii) from the fact that I see life as being a pleasurable adventure;

structure seven items:

(i) from the knowledge that I have a circle of intimate friends and relationships,

(ii) from my association with social net works who have high moral and religious principles;

structure eight items:

(i) from the knowledge that I have a solid income source,

(ii) from the knowledge that I am not, nor need to be, financially dependent on anyone else;

structure nine items:

(i) from the opportunities I have to continue with my life goals, roles, and activities from my earlier years of life,

(ii) from continuing opportunities to gain and receive respect and acknowledgment from others for contributions I made during my earlier years of life.

Conflict of Interests

The authors declared no conflict of interests.

Acknowledgments

The research was supported, in part, by a Population Aging Research Grant (P. S. Fry, File no. 492-93-0006) awarded to the first author by the Social Sciences and Humanities Research Council of Canada (SSHRC) while she was on Faculty at the University of Calgary, Calgary, Alberta. The research was further implemented and conducted with funds from Strategic Research Grant Award (P. S. Fry, File no. 816-97-009). Completion of the study was facilitated, in part, by a Standard Senior Scholars' Research Grant (P. S. Fry, File no. 410-2004-0152) awarded to the first author by the SSHRC. The authors greatly appreciate the assistance of Shaun Fry and Dr. Mark Kolodziej in data tabulation.

References

[1] M. E. Seligman and M. Csikszentmihalyi, "Positive psychology. An introduction," *The American Psychologist*, vol. 55, no. 1, pp. 5–14, 2000.

[2] L. G. Aspinwall and U. M. Staudinger, Eds., *A Psychology of Strengths: Fundamental Questions and Future Directions for a Positive Psychology*, American Psychological Association, Washington, DC, USA, 2003.

[3] J. Brandtstädter, D. Wentura, and K. Rothermund, "Intentional self-development through adulthood and later life: tenacious pursuit and flexible adjustment of goals," in *Action and Self-Development: Theory and Research Through the Life-Span*, J. Brandtstädter and R. M. Lerner, Eds., pp. 373–400, Sage, Thousand Oaks, Calif, USA, 1999.

[4] A. Bandura, *Self-Efficacy: The Exercise of Control*, W.H. Freeman, New York, NY, USA, 1997.

[5] P. S. Fry and D. L. Debats, "Sources of human life-strengths, resilience, and health," in *New Frontiers in Resilient Aging: Life Strengths and Well-Being in Late Life*, P. S. Fry and C. L. M. Keyes, Eds., pp. 15–59, Cambridge University Press, Cambridge, UK, 2010.

[6] R. Chapin, "Social policy development: the strength perspective," *Social Work*, vol. 40, pp. 506–514, 1995.

[7] R. Chapin, H. Nelson-Becker, and K. MacMillion, "Strength-based and solution-focused approaches to practice," in *Handbook of Social Work in Health and Aging*, B. Berkman, Ed., pp. 789–796, Oxford University Press, New York, NY, USA, 2006.

[8] R. J. Schlegel and J. A. Hicks, "The true self and psychological health: emerging evidence and future directions," *Social and Personality Psychology Compass*, vol. 5, no. 12, pp. 989–1003, 2011.

[9] M. Ungar, Ed., *The Social Ecology of Resilience*, Springer, New York, NY, USA, 2012.

[10] A. H. Maslow, *Toward a Psychology of Being*, Van Nostrand, Princeton, NJ, USA, 1968.

[11] D. Saleeby, *The Strength Perspective in Social Work Practice*, Longman, New York, NY, USA, 2nd edition, 1997.

[12] H. Q. Kivnick, "Through the life cycle: psychological thoughts on old age," in *The Course of Life*, G. H. Pollock and S. J. Greenspan, Eds., vol. 7, International Universities Press, Madison, Wis, USA, 1998.

[13] S. E. Hobfoll, "Social and psychological resources and adaptation," *Review of General Psychology*, vol. 6, no. 4, pp. 307–324, 2002.

[14] G. Vaillant, *Aging Well*, Little, Brown and Co, Boston, Mass, USA, 2002.

[15] P. T. Bartone, R. J. Ursano, K. M. Wright, and L. H. Ingraham, "The impact of a military air disaster on the health of assistance workers: a prospective study," *Journal of Nervous and Mental Disease*, vol. 177, no. 6, pp. 317–328, 1989.

[16] G. M. Wagnild and H. M. Young, "Development and psychometric evaluation of the Resilience Scale," *Journal of Nursing Measurement*, vol. 1, no. 2, pp. 165–178, 1993.

[17] R. F. Baumeister, *Meanings of Life*, Guilford Press, New York, NY, USA, 1991.

[18] P. S. Fry, "The unique contribution of key existential factors to the prediction of psychological well-being of older adults following spousal loss," *Gerontologist*, vol. 41, no. 1, pp. 69–81, 2001.

[19] P. S. Fry, "Religious involvement, spirituality and personal meaning for life: existential predictors of psychological wellbeing in community-residing and institutional care elders," *Aging and Mental Health*, vol. 4, no. 4, pp. 375–387, 2000.

[20] M. A. Steger, S. Oishi, and T. B. Kashdan, "Meaning in life across the life span: levels and correlates of meaning in life from emerging adulthood to older adulthood," *Journal of Positive Psychology*, vol. 4, no. 1, pp. 43–52, 2009.

[21] L. Hoffman, "Introduction to existential psychology in a cross-cultural context: an east-west dialogue," in *Existential Psychology East-West*, L. Hoffman, M. Yang, F. J. Kaklauskas, and A. Chan, Eds., pp. 1–67, University of the Rockies Press, Colorado Springs, Colo, USA, 2009.

[22] D. L. Debats, "Measurement of personal meaning: the psychometric properties of the life regard index," in *The Human Quest for Meaning: A Handbook of Psychological Research and Clinical Applications*, P. T. P. Wong and P. S. Fry, Eds., pp. 237–261, Lawrence Erlbaum, Mahwah, NJ, USA, 1998.

[23] G. T. Reker and L. C. Woo, "Personal meaning orientations and psychosocial adaptation in older adults," *SAGE Open*, pp. 1–10, 2011.

[24] P. S. Fry, "Predictors of health-related quality of life perspectives, self-esteem, and life satisfactions of older adults following spousal loss: an 18-month follow-up study of widows and widowers," *Gerontologist*, vol. 41, no. 6, pp. 787–798, 2001.

[25] P. S. Fry, "Perceived self-efficacy domains as predictors of fear of the unknown and fear of dying among older adults," *Psychology and Aging*, vol. 18, no. 3, pp. 474–486, 2003.

[26] P. S. Fry and D. L. Debats, "Domain-specific social comparison orientations as predictors of health-related quality of life, life satisfaction, and general optimism in late life functioning," *Journal of Mental Health and Aging*, vol. 9, no. 4, pp. 243–268, 2003.

[27] G. J. McAvay, T. E. Seeman, and J. Rodin, "A longitudinal study of change in domain-specific self-efficacy among older adults," *Journals of Gerontology B*, vol. 51, no. 5, pp. P243–P253, 1996.

[28] D. L. Featherman, J. Smith, and J. G. Peterson, "Successful aging in a post-retired society," in *Successful Aging: Perspectives from the Behavioral Sciences*, P. B. Baltes and M. M. Baltes, Eds., pp. 50–93, Cambridge University Press, New York, NY, USA, 1990.

[29] J. W. Rowe and R. L. Kahn, "Human aging: usual and successful," *Science*, vol. 237, no. 4811, pp. 143–149, 1987.

[30] C. D. Ryff and B. Singer, "Understanding healthy aging: key components and their integration," in *Handbook of Theories of Aging*, V. L. Bengston, D. Gans, N. M. Pulney, and M. Silverstein, Eds., pp. 117–144, Springer, New York, NY, USA, 2nd edition, 2009.

[31] P. B. Baltes and M. M. Baltes, "Psychological perspectives on successful aging: the model of selective optimization with compensation," in *Successful Aging: Perspectives from the Behavioral Sciences*, P. B. Baltes and M. M. Baltes, Eds., pp. 1–34, Cambridge University Press, New York, NY, USA, 1990.

[32] R. C. Atchley, *Continuity and Adaptation in Aging*, Johns Hopkins University Press, Baltimore, Md, USA, 1999.

[33] D. M. Davydov, R. Stewart, K. Ritchie, and I. Chaudieu, "Resilience and mental health," *Clinical Psychology Review*, vol. 30, no. 5, pp. 479–495, 2010.

[34] C. L. Keyes and S. J. Lopez, "Toward a science of mental health: positive directions in diagnosis and interventions," in *Handbook of Positive Psychology*, C. R. Snyder and S. J. Lopez, Eds., pp. 45–62, Oxford University Press, New York, NY, USA, 2002.

[35] U. M. Staudinger, M. Marsiske, and P. B. Baltes, "Resilience and reserve capacity in later adulthood: potentials and limits of development across the life span," in *Developmental Psychopathology: Vol. 2, Risk, Disorder, and Adaptation*, D. Cicchetti and D. J. Cohen, Eds., pp. 801–847, Wiley, New York, NY, USA, 1995.

[36] R. J. Davidson, D. C. Jackson, and N. H. Kalin, "Emotion, plasticity, context, and regulation: perspectives from affective neuroscience," *Psychological Bulletin*, vol. 126, no. 6, pp. 890–909, 2000.

[37] A. S. Waterman, "On the importance of distinguishing hedonia and eudaimonia when contemplating the hedonic treadmill," *American Psychologist*, vol. 62, no. 6, pp. 612–613, 2007.

[38] M. Ungar and R. M. Lemer, "Introduction to a special issue of research on human development: resilience and positive development across the life span: a view of the issues," *Research in Human Development*, vol. 5, pp. 135–138, 2008.

[39] M. Ungar and L. Liebenberg, "Cross-cultural consultation leading to the development of a valid measure of youth resilience: the international resilience project," *Studia Psychologica*, vol. 51, no. 2-3, pp. 259–268, 2009.

[40] Canadian Index of Well-being, "Measuring what matters," 2009.

[41] V. Huta and R. M. Ryan, "Pursuing pleasure or virtue: the differential and overlapping well-being benefits of hedonic and eudaimonic motives," *Journal of Happiness Studies*, vol. 11, no. 6, pp. 735–762, 2010.

[42] P. Martin, "Individual and social resources predicting well-being and functioning in later years: conceptual models, research, and practice," *Ageing International*, vol. 27, no. 2, pp. 3–29, 2002.

[43] A. D. Ong and C. S. Bergeman, "Resilience and adaptation to stress in later life: empirical perspectives and conceptual implications," *Ageing International*, vol. 29, pp. 219–246, 2004.

[44] M. Sherer, R. W. Maddux, B. Mercandante, S. Prentice-Duce, B. Jacobs, and R. W. Rogers, "The self-efficacy scale: construction and validation," *Psychological Reports*, vol. 51, pp. 5–14, 1982.

[45] M. E. Lachman and S. L. Weaver, "The sense of control as a moderator of social class differences in health and well-being," *Journal of Personality and Social Psychology*, vol. 74, no. 3, pp. 763–773, 1997.

[46] T. C. Antonucci, "Social relations: an examination of social networks, social support and sense of control," in *Handbook of the Psychology of Aging*, J. E. Birren and K. W. Schaie, Eds., pp. 427–453, Academic Press, San Diego, Calif, USA, 5th edition, 2001.

[47] M. Rosenberg, C. Schooler, C. Schoenbach, and F. Rosenberg, "Global self-esteem and specific self-esteem: different concepts, different outcomes," *American Sociological Review*, vol. 60, pp. 141–156, 1995.

[48] E. Diener, R. A. Emmons, R. J. Larsen, and S. Griffin, "The satisfaction with life scale," *Journal of Personality Assessment*, vol. 49, no. 1, pp. 71–75, 1985.

[49] M. J. Schofield, R. Reynolds, G. D. Mishra, J. R. Powers, and A. J. Dobson, "Screening for vulnerability to abuse among older women: women's Health Australia Study," *Journal of Applied Gerontology*, vol. 21, no. 1, pp. 24–39, 2002.

[50] W. W. Zung, "A self-rating depression scale," *Archives of General Psychiatry*, vol. 12, pp. 63–70, 1965.

[51] S. R. Maddi and S. C. Kobasa, *The Hardy Executive: Health Under Stress*, Dow Jones, Irwin, Homewood, Ill, USA, 1984.

[52] S. S. Travis, M. A. Bernard, W. J. McAuley, M. Thornton, and T. Kole, "Development of the family caregiver medication administration hassles scale," *Gerontologist*, vol. 43, no. 3, pp. 360–368, 2003.

[53] C. L. M. Keyes, D. Shmotkin, and C. D. Ryff, "Optimizing well-being: the empirical encounter of two traditions," *Journal of Personality and Social Psychology*, vol. 82, no. 6, pp. 1007–1022, 2002.

[54] R. F. Baumeister and M. R. Leary, "The need to belong: desire for interpersonal attachments as a fundamental human motivation," *Psychological Bulletin*, vol. 117, no. 3, pp. 497–529, 1995.

[55] H. F. Kaiser, "A second generation little jiffy," *Psychometrika*, vol. 35, no. 4, pp. 401–415, 1970.

[56] H. F. Kaiser, "An index of factorial simplicity," *Psychometrika*, vol. 39, no. 1, pp. 31–36, 1974.

[57] J. Stevens, *Applied Multivariate Statistics for the Social Sciences*, Erlbaum, Hillsdale, NJ, USA, 1996.

[58] R. B. Cattell, "The scree test for the number of factors," *Multivariate Behavioral Research*, vol. 1, pp. 245–276, 1966.

[59] L. A. Clark and D. Watson, "Constructing validity: basic issues in objective scale development," *Psychological Assessment*, vol. 7, no. 3, pp. 309–319, 1995.

[60] S. E. Pollock and M. E. Duffy, "The health-related hardiness scale: development and psychometric analysis," *Nursing Research*, vol. 39, no. 4, pp. 218–222, 1990.

[61] J. C. Nunnally, *Psychometric Theory*, McGraw-Hill, New York, NY, USA, 2nd edition, 1978.

[62] D. L. Streiner and G. R. Norman, *Health Management Scales: A Practical Guide to their Development and Use*, Oxford University Press, Oxford, UK, 1995.

[63] D. C. Miller, *Handbook of Research Design and Social Measurement*, Sage, Newbury Park, Calif, USA, 5th edition, 1991.

[64] M. P. Lawton, M. Moss, C. Hoffman, R. Grant, T. T. Have, and M. H. Kleban, "Health, valuation of life, and the wish to live," *Gerontologist*, vol. 39, no. 4, pp. 406–416, 1999.

[65] D. L. McGee, Y. Liao, G. Cao, and R. S. Cooper, "Self-reported health status and mortality in a multiethnic cohort," *American Journal of Epidemiology*, vol. 149, no. 1, pp. 41–46, 1999.

[66] R. J. Schlegel, J. A. Hicks, L. A. King, and J. Arndt, "Feeling like you know who you are: perceived true self-knowledge and meaning in life," *Personality and Social Psychology Bulletin*, vol. 37, no. 6, pp. 745–756, 2011.

[67] P. T. P. Wong, "Positive psychology 2.0: towards a balanced interactive model of the good life," *Canadian Psychology*, vol. 52, no. 2, pp. 69–81, 2011.

[68] S. H. Schwartz and W. Bilsky, "Toward a theory of the universal content and structure of values: extensions and cross-cultural replications," *Journal of Personality and Social Psychology*, vol. 58, no. 5, pp. 878–891, 1990.

5

Caudate Nucleus Volume Mediates the Link between Cardiorespiratory Fitness and Cognitive Flexibility in Older Adults

Timothy D. Verstynen,[1,2] Brighid Lynch,[3] Destiny L. Miller,[3] Michelle W. Voss,[4] Ruchika Shaurya Prakash,[5] Laura Chaddock,[6,7] Chandramallika Basak,[8] Amanda Szabo,[9] Erin A. Olson,[9] Thomas R. Wojcicki,[9] Jason Fanning,[9] Neha P. Gothe,[9] Edward McAuley,[7,9] Arthur F. Kramer,[6,7] and Kirk I. Erickson[2,3]

[1] *Department of Psychology, Carnegie Mellon University, Pittsburgh, PA 15213, USA*
[2] *Center for the Neural Basis of Cognition, Carnegie Mellon University, Pittsburgh, PA 15213, USA*
[3] *Department of Psychology, University of Pittsburgh, 3107 Sennott Square, 210 South Bouquet Street, Pittsburgh, PA 15260, USA*
[4] *Department of Psychology, University of Iowa, Iowa city, IA 52242, USA*
[5] *Department of Psychology, The Ohio State University City, Columbus, OH 43210, USA*
[6] *Department of Psychology, University of Illinois, Champaign-Urbana at Champaign, IL 61820, USA*
[7] *Beckman Institute for Advanced Science and Technology, University of Illinois at Champaign-Urbana, Champaign, IL, USA*
[8] *Department of Psychology, The University of Texas at Dallas, Dallas, TX 75080, USA*
[9] *Department of Kinesiology and Community Health, University of Illinois, Champaign-Urbana at Champaign, IL 61820, USA*

Correspondence should be addressed to Kirk I. Erickson, kiericks@pitt.edu

Academic Editor: Denis Gerstorf

The basal ganglia play a central role in regulating the response selection abilities that are critical for mental flexibility. In neocortical areas, higher cardiorespiratory fitness levels are associated with increased gray matter volume, and these volumetric differences mediate enhanced cognitive performance in a variety of tasks. Here we examine whether cardiorespiratory fitness correlates with the volume of the subcortical nuclei that make up the basal ganglia and whether this relationship predicts cognitive flexibility in older adults. Structural MRI was used to determine the volume of the basal ganglia nuclei in a group of older, neurologically healthy individuals (mean age 66 years, $N = 179$). Measures of cardiorespiratory fitness (VO_{2max}), cognitive flexibility (task switching), and attentional control (flanker task) were also collected. Higher fitness levels were correlated with higher accuracy rates in the Task Switching paradigm. In addition, the volume of the caudate nucleus, putamen, and globus pallidus positively correlated with Task Switching accuracy. Nested regression modeling revealed that caudate nucleus volume was a significant mediator of the relationship between cardiorespiratory fitness, and task switching performance. These findings indicate that higher cardiorespiratory fitness predicts better cognitive flexibility in older adults through greater grey matter volume in the dorsal striatum.

1. Introduction

Age-related cognitive decline is an unfortunate, but nearly ubiquitous, characteristic of late life that is preceded by atrophy of several brain regions including the prefrontal cortex, medial temporal lobe, and basal ganglia [1, 2]. Because of the expected increase in the proportion of adults over the age of 65 in the next forty years, it has become a major public health initiative to identify methods to prevent or reverse regional brain atrophy with the hope that this might concurrently improve cognitive performance [3]. Randomized trials of aerobic exercise have proven promising from this regard, with participation in exercise programs leading to greater prefrontal [4] and hippocampal volumes [5]. Nonrandomized longitudinal studies of physical activity [6, 7] and cross-sectional studies of cardiorespiratory fitness [8–10] have shown similar results, with more physical activity and higher fitness levels associated with greater volumes.

Unfortunately, few studies have examined whether cardiorespiratory fitness levels in older adult humans are associated with brain areas other than the prefrontal cortex and hippocampus [4–6, 8–10]. The striatum is of particular interest because it shows relatively early and rapid age-related atrophy, [2, 11] is a critical node in motor circuitry, supports task coordination and attentional control processes, and disruption of its dopamine circuits is linked to common age-related disorders such as Parkinson's disease [12, 13]. Yet, there is emerging evidence that exercise directly influences dopamine circuitry, angiogenesis, and cell signaling cascades in the striatum. For example, rodent research has found that voluntary wheel running increases the production of dopamine and brain-derived neurotrophic factor in the dorsal striatum [14–16]. Exercise is also considered to be one of the more promising treatments for attenuating dopamine deficiency in 6-hydroxydopamine models of Parkinson's disease [17, 18]. In concert with this, exercise ameliorates motor and cognitive deficits in adults with Parkinson's disease [19, 20]. Finally, higher cardiorespiratory fitness levels are associated with larger caudate nucleus and putamen volumes in children and these volume differences were in turn associated with better performance on a measure of attentional control [21]. Yet, the possible link between fitness levels and basal ganglia structure in older adults has not been investigated despite the accumulation of research suggesting an association.

In this study, we examined the association between the volume of basal ganglia and cardiorespiratory fitness levels in older adults. Given the extant rodent literature and one study in humans [21], we predicted that the size of the dorsal striatum, including the caudate nucleus and putamen, and the size of the ventral striatum (i.e., nucleus accumbens) would be positively associated with cardiorespiratory fitness compared to the output nucleus of this system, the globus pallidum, which has been less frequently associated with exercise. Furthermore, we predicted that any association between fitness and dorsal striatum volume would have implications on cognitive tasks that are supported by these structures. Specifically, cognitive flexibility and attentional control paradigms have been closely linked to the function of the dorsal striatum [21–23]. Therefore, using mediation modeling, we predicted that the volume of the dorsal striatum, but not the ventral striatum, would mediate the association between higher cardiorespiratory fitness levels and elevated performance on attentional control and task switching paradigms.

2. Methods

2.1. Participants. One hundred and seventy-nine older adults (109 females; 56 males) between 59 and 81 yrs of age (mean age = 66.6 years; standard deviation = 5.6 years) participated in this study. Participants were recruited for a 1-year randomized controlled trial examining the effect of aerobic training on brain and cognition. We report here results from the initial baseline MR session. Subjects were recruited through community advertisements and physician referrals and were screened for dementia by the revised and modified Mini-Mental Status Examination [24]. Participants were excluded from participation if they did not reach the required cutoff of 51 (high score of 57).

Additional inclusion criteria have been described elsewhere [5, 9, 25–27]. In brief, participants were required to be 60+ years of age during the trial, capable of performing physical exercise, successfully complete a graded exercise test, have normal or corrected-to-normal vision, absence of clinical depression (as measured by the Geriatric Depression Scale [28]), and a low-active lifestyle at time of baseline assessment. All participants have received a physician's clearance to engage in a maximal graded exercise test and signed an informed consent approved by the University of Illinois.

In addition to these criteria, all participants met or surpassed criteria for participating in a magnetic resonance imaging (MRI) study including no previous head trauma, no previous head or neck surgery, no diagnosis of diabetes, no neuropsychiatric or neurological condition including brain tumors, and no metallic implants that could interfere with or cause injury due to the magnetic field.

The current study focused on participants that had both high-resolution MRI data and completed the cognitive assessments described below. All analyses were performed in a pairwise manner with the subjects who had relevant data points. The specific degrees of freedom are reported for each test.

2.2. Cardiorespiratory Assessment. Aerobic fitness (VO_{2max}) was assessed by graded maximal exercise testing on a motor-driven treadmill. The participant walked at a speed slightly faster than their normal walking pace (approximately 30–100 m/min) with increasing grade increments of 2% every 2 min. A cardiologist and nurse continuously monitored measurements of oxygen uptake, heart rate and blood pressure. Oxygen uptake was measured from expired air samples taken at 30 s intervals until a maximal VO_2 was attained or to the point of test termination due to symptom limitation and/or volitional exhaustion. VO_{2max} was defined as the highest recorded VO_2 value when two of three criteria were satisfied: (1) a plateau in VO_2 peak between two or more workloads; (2) a respiratory exchange ratio >1.00; (3) a heart rate equivalent to their age predicted maximum (i.e., 220-age).

2.3. Body Mass Index (BMI). Height and weight were measured using a Seca electronic scale and stadiometer (model 763 1321139). Participants were measured while wearing light clothing and without shoes. BMI was calculated using the standard formula of weight (kg)/[height (m)]^2.

2.4. MRI Acquisition and Volumetric Analysis. High-resolution T1-weighted brain images were acquired within two weeks of the cardiorespiratory fitness tests using a 3D Magnetization Prepared Rapid Gradient Echo Imaging (MPRAGE) protocol with 144 contiguous axial slices, collected in ascending fashion parallel to the anterior and posterior

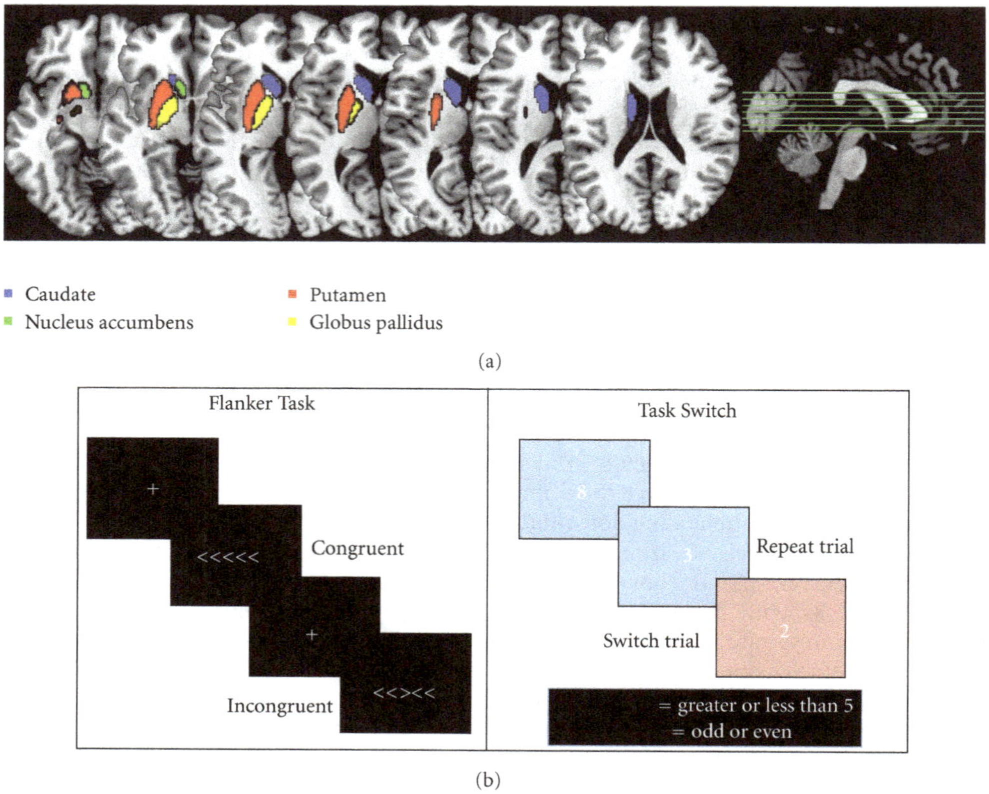

Figure 1: (a) Template maps for the four regions of interest used in this study. While only left hemisphere regions are shown here, data from both hemispheres was collapsed together in the final analyses. (b) Illustration of the two behavioral paradigms tested.

commissures, echo time (TE) = 3.87 ms, repetition time (TR) = 1800 ms, field of view (FOV) = 256 mm, acquisition matrix 192 mm × 192 mm, slice thickness = 1.3 mm, and flip angle = 8. All images were collected on a 3T head-only Siemens Allegra MRI scanner.

For segmentation and volumetric analysis of the basal ganglia we employed FMRIB's Integrated Registration and Segmentation Tool (FIRST) in FMRIB's Software Library (FSL) version 4.1. FIRST is a semiautomated model-based subcortical segmentation tool utilizing a Bayesian framework from shape and appearance models obtained from manually segmented images from the Center for Morphometric Analysis, Massachusetts General Hospital, Boston, MA, USA. Structural and landmark information was obtained from 317 manually segmented and labeled T1 weighted images of the brain from normal children, adults, and pathological populations (including schizophrenia and Alzheimer's disease) and were modeled as a point distribution model in which the geometry and variation of the shape of the structure are submitted as priors. Volumetric labels are parameterized by a 3D deformation of a surface model based on multivariate Gaussian assumptions. FIRST then searches through linear combinations of shape modes of variation for the most probable shape given the intensity distribution in the T1-weighted image (see Patenaude et al. [29], for further description of this method).

This method first runs a two-stage affine registration to a standard space template (MNI space) with 1 mm resolution using 12 degrees of freedom and a subcortical mask to exclude voxels outside the subcortical regions. Second, the left and right basal ganglia including the caudate nucleus, putamen, pallidum, and nucleus accumbens are segmented with 30, 40, 40, and 50 modes of variation, respectively. The modes of variation are optimized based on leave-one-out cross-validation on the training set and increase the robustness and reliability of the results [29]. Finally, boundary correction takes place for each structure that classifies the boundary voxels as belonging to the structure or not based on a statistical probability (z-score > 3.00; $P < 0.001$). Figure 1(a) shows the template masks for these nucleus volumes in the left hemisphere. Although volumes were estimated separately for the left and right hemispheres the volumetric estimates were highly correlated between the hemispheres for the nucleus accumbens ($r(139) = 0.552$, $P < 0.001$), caudate nucleus ($r(151) = 0.638$, $P < 0.001$), putamen ($r(151) = 0.542$, $P < 0.001$), and globus pallidus ($r(151) = 0.806$, $P < 0.001$). Therefore, a total volume estimate was generated for each nucleus by summing the values for the two hemispheres together.

Intracranial volume (ICV) is frequently used to adjust the regional volumes for sex and height (e.g., [1]). Here, we calculated ICV as the sum of gray, white, and cerebrospinal fluid using FMRIB's automated segmentation tool in FSL version 4.1 [30, 31]. In accordance with other volumetric studies, ICV was used as a covariate in all analyses reported below [5, 9, 32].

2.5. Behavioral Tasks. Figure 1(b) shows the time line of each trial for the two behavioral paradigms utilized in this study. Results from the full battery of cognitive tasks have been reported in previous studies [5, 9, 25–27]. Given the *a priori* interest in the basal ganglia, we analyzed the flanker and task switching batteries because they both have been associated with basal ganglia function in animal and human studies. Cognitive tasks for which we did not predict *a priori* to be associated with the basal ganglia were not analyzed in this study.

2.5.1. Task Switching. This task provided a measure of executive function by testing participants' abilities to flexibly switch their focus of attention between multiple task sets. In this task participants had to switch between judging whether a number (1, 2, 3, 4, 6, 7, 8, or 9) was odd or even and judging whether it was low or high (i.e., smaller or larger than 5). Numbers were presented individually for 1500 ms against a pink or blue background at the center of the screen, with the constraint that the same number did not appear twice in succession (see Figure 1(b)).

If the background was blue, participants used one hand to report as quickly as possible whether the letter was high ("*X*" key) or low ("*Z*" key). If the background was pink, participants used their other hand to report as quickly as possible whether the number was odd ("*N*" key) or even ("*M*" key). Participants completed four single task blocks (2 blocks of odd/even and 2 blocks of high/low) of 24 trials each. Due to the difficulty of this task, participants were provided with a practice block in which they switched from one task to the other for 120 trials. This practice block allowed participants to become acquainted with the switching block and ensured compliance with task instructions. Finally, they completed a switching block of 120 trials during which the task for each trial was chosen randomly.

For the current study, we examined local switch cost, which refers to the difference in performance for trials when the preceding trial involved the same task (nonswitch trial) and those when the preceding trial was of the other task (switch trial), and represents a measure of attentional set reconfiguration and inhibition, two subcomponents of executive function [33]. Reaction time measures (based on mean reaction time) were used for computing local switch cost. Consistent with prior studies using this paradigm [27], we used accuracy rates (percent correct) as an outcome measure and also calculated an accuracy cost score that reflects the difference in accuracy rates between switch and repeat conditions within the switching block.

2.5.2. Flanker Task. A modified flanker paradigm required participants to identify the orientation of a central arrow cue that was flanked by arrows that were in either a congruent (e.g., >>>>>) or incongruent (e.g., >><>>) orientation. We used reaction times for both conditions in addition to proportional cost. Cost was calculated by subtracting the reaction times of congruent trials from those of incongruent trials and dividing by the reaction time of congruent trials. Such an approach accounts for individual differences in perceptual speed (see Figure 1(b)).

2.6. Data Analysis

2.6.1. Partial Correlations. Initial analyses examined the distribution of the variables for skew using Q-Q plots. All variables were confirmed to be normally distributed by both visual inspection of the Q-Q plots and a resulting r-squared value to the simulated distribution of >0.95. Any missing values were eliminated from calculations. This resulted in degrees of freedom ranging from 139 to 178 in this sample, depending on the variables used in each analytical comparison. Bivariate analyses examined the correlation between VO_{2max} and age, sex, education, ICV, and BMI using Pearson's correlation coefficients. These variables were then used as covariates in all subsequent analyses looking at VO_{2max}, task and brain volume relationships.

Once the covariate relationships were determined, partial correlations were then used to test the relationship between VO_{2max} and pallidum, putamen, nucleus accumbens, and caudate nucleus volumes. Next, the direct effect of VO_{2max} on the cognitive tasks described above was estimated. Partial correlations were then conducted to assess the association between basal ganglia volumes and cognitive tasks.

2.6.2. Mediation Analysis. To determine indirect pathways, we conducted a bootstrapped mediation analysis. The main requirement for mediation is that the *indirect effect* of the independent variable (VO_{2max}) through the mediator (e.g., caudate nucleus volume) on the dependent variable (e.g., task switch % accuracy) be significant.

Mediation analyses were conducted using the *indirect macro* designed for SPSS [34]. This macro uses bootstrapped sampling to estimate the indirect mediation effect of volume on the relationship between VO_{2max} and Flanker Task or task switching performance. In this analysis, 5,000 bootstrapped samples were drawn with replacement from the dataset to estimate a sampling distribution for the indirect mediation pathway. Indirect effects and 95% confidence intervals are reported. Mediation indirect effects can be interpreted as the strength of the relationship between the independent variable (VO_{2max}) and dependent variable (e.g., Task Switching performance) when accounting for the mediating pathway [35]. We report adjusted R^2 values for an estimate of the effect size. Each outcome measure was used as a dependent variable in separate analyses. All models controlled for the variance from age, education, BMI, ICV, and sex.

3. Results

3.1. Covariate Effects. We first examined the association between cardiorespiratory fitness and other factors that may act as sources of noise in the analyses. These relationships are illustrated in Figure 2 (Covariates section). As expected, there were significant negative correlations between VO_{2max} and BMI ($r(178) = -0.242$, $P = 0.001$), sex (logistic beta = -1.034, $r(178) = -0.480$, $P < 0.001$), and age ($r(178) = -0.391$, $P < 0.001$). Thus, cardiorespiratory fitness levels were lower in overweight and obese subjects, lower in women than men, and lower in older aged participants. We also found positive correlations between VO_{2max} and years of

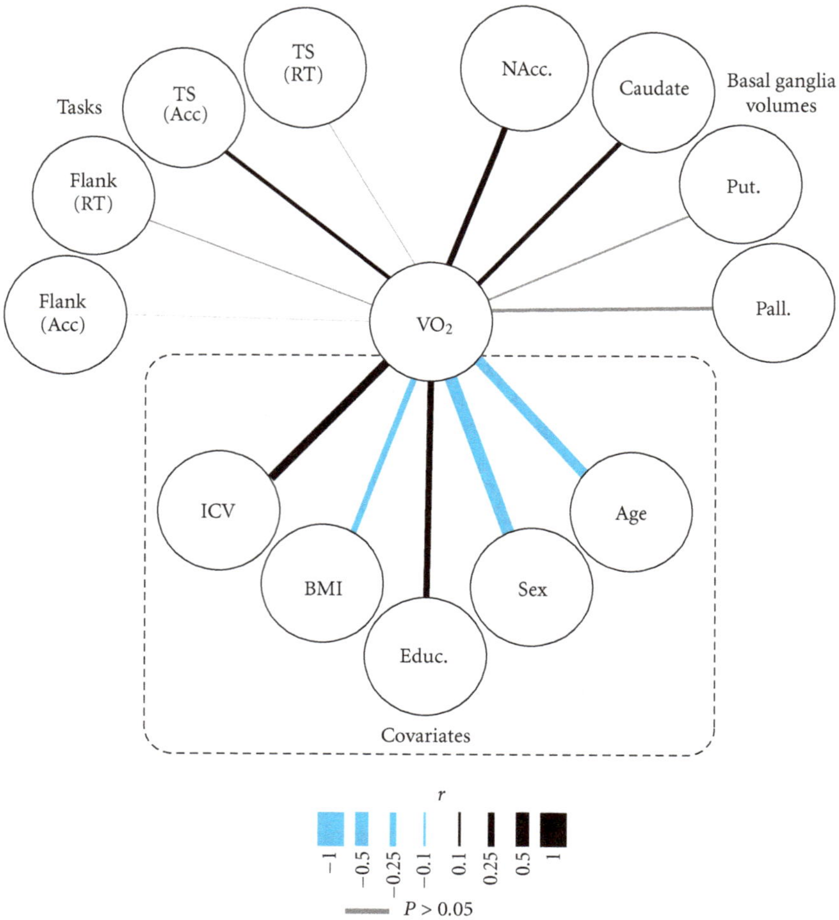

FIGURE 2: Correlation paths relating directly to measures of cardiorespiratory integrity (VO_{2max}). Colored lines show significant correlations and the width of the line reflects the strength of the relationship. All correlation values are reported in the text. Variables highlighted in the "Covariates" section were used as control factors in the partial correlation analyses for the other pathways. Behavioral results reflect between condition changes in performance (i.e., costs). VO_{2max}: VO_2, Task Switching: TS, Flanker Task: Flank, accuracy: Acc, reaction time: RT, nucleus accumbens: NAcc., putamen: Put. globus pallidus: Pall. education: Educ., body mass index: BMI, intracranial volume: ICV.

education ($r(178) = 0.234$, $P = 0.002$) as well as intracranial volume ($r(178) = 0.322$, $P < 0.001$). Thus, cardiorespiratory fitness increased with educational attainment and overall body size. This latter association is presumably driven by the sex effects since men had significantly larger intracranial volumes than women ($t(156) = 7.86$, $P < 0.001$). These five factors were included in all subsequent analyses as covariates.

3.2. Associations between Cardiorespiratory Fitness and Task Performance. Next, we examined relationships between cardiorespiratory fitness and performance in the two behavioral tasks. These relationships are illustrated in Figure 2 (Tasks region). To get a full appreciation of relationships to the behavioral tasks, Table 1 shows the simple bivariate correlations between all demographic variables, cardiorespiratory fitness, and behavioral task performance. However, our core analysis centers on relationships specific to cardiorespiratory fitness, therefore we used a partial correlation analysis to control for noncardiorespiratory effects (see Section 2).

Unlike the results from previous studies [15, 21, 36, 37], we did not see an association between cardiorespiratory fitness and performance in the Flanker Task. After adjusting for covariate effects, there was no significant correlation between VO_{2max} scores and percent interference for reaction times in the Flanker Task ($r(149) = 0.049$, $P = 0.546$). We also failed to detect a significant association between VO_{2max} and response times on either the congruent ($r(149) = 0.035$, $P = 0.669$) or incongruent ($r(149) = 0.001$, $P = 0.994$) conditions. This effect does not appear to be due to a lack of sensitivity in the overall behavioral responses, as there was a significant group-level increase in response times to incongruent trials, compared to congruent trials (mean percent interference = 14.9%, std = 10.4, $t(166) = 18.55$, $P < 0.001$).

We also failed to detect a significant association between fitness levels and accuracy rates in the Flanker Task. After controlling for covariate effects, there was no significant correlation between VO_{2max} scores and differences in accuracy between the incongruent and congruent conditions

Table 1: Simple bivariate Pearson correlations between demographic variables, cardiorespiratory fitness, and behavioral data. *Significant at $P < .05$; **significant at $P < .01$.

	VO_2	Age	Sex	Education	BMI
Flanker					
Con RT	−.178*	.283**	.207**	.009	−.036
Inc RT	−.144	.162*	.211**	.042	−.056
Cost (RT)	.020	−.179*	.064	.023	−.034
Con Acc	.199**	−.277**	−.133	.092	.060
Inc Acc	.112	−.168*	−.022	.052	.009
Cost (Acc)	−.055	.099	.084	−.015	−.060
Task-switch					
Repeat RT	−.021	.006	.135	−.034	.005
Switch RT	−.082	−.011	.173*	−.105	.020
Cost (RT)	−.071	−.004	.151	−.088	.025
Repeat Acc	.174*	−.224**	.001	.040	.135
Switch Acc	.231**	−.270**	−.032	.061	.130
Cost (Acc)	.190*	−.281**	−.027	.022	.154

($r(149) = 0.008$, $P = 0.925$). As with response times, there was no significant association between VO_{2max} scores and response accuracy during either the congruent ($r(149) = 0.053$, $P = 0.521$) or incongruent conditions ($r(149) = 0.041$, $P = 0.648$). However, these null effects may be driven by a ceiling effect in accuracy rates in this sample (congruent: mean = 95.89%, std = 9.40%; incongruent: mean = 93.43%, 13.00%).

We also failed to detect significant associations between cardiorespiratory fitness and local switch costs in the Task Switching experiment. That is, after adjusting for covariate effects, VO_{2max} was not significantly correlated with the delayed reaction times that result from switching between trial types ($r(150) = 0.025$, $P = 0.398$). Although, there was a significant positive correlation between VO_{2max} and response times for the repeat condition such that individuals with higher VO_{2max} had slightly slower response times ($r(150) = 0.312$, $P < 0.001$). This correlation was not seen with response times during switch trials ($r(150) = 0.019$, $P = 0.815$). The lack of a correlation between fitness and switch costs does not appear to be due to a floor effect in the switching costs because across all subjects the average response times were significantly slower after a switch relative to a repeat condition (mean difference = 530.5, std = 225.94, $t(162) = 29.976$, $P < 0.001$).

In contrast to response times, we did observe a small, but significant, association between cardiorespiratory fitness and accuracy in the Task Switching experiment. After adjusting for covariate effects, VO_{2max} scores were positively correlated with task-switch accuracy for switch trials after subtracting the accuracy rates from repeat trials ($r(150) = 0.160$, $P = 0.048$). In general, switching accuracies were negative (mean $= -0.167$, std $= 0.228$, $t(165) = -9.42, P < 0.001$) meaning that more errors occurred on switch trials compared to repeat trials. Within each condition used to calculate the accuracy cost, we also found a positive correlation between VO_{2max} scores and accuracy rates for repeat trials ($r(150) = 0.176$, $P = 0.030$) and switch trials ($r(150) = 0.177$, $P = 0.029$). Thus, individuals with higher VO_{2max} scores were both more accurate in general and were better able to maintain accurate responses immediately following a change in task goals.

3.2.1. Associations between Cardiorespiratory Fitness and Basal Ganglia Volumes. We next set out to identify relationships between cardiorespiratory fitness and volumetric measures of the subcortical nuclei that compose the basal ganglia system. These relationships are illustrated in the "Basal Ganglia Volumes" region of Figure 2.

Our first analysis focused on the nuclei that compose the major input of the basal ganglia system, the striatal nuclei. Partial correlations, after adjusting for covariate effects, revealed significant associations between cardiorespiratory fitness and the volume of nuclei that compose the caudal sections of the striatum. Specifically, VO_{2max} scores positively correlated with the volume of the nucleus accumbens ($r(138) = 0.232$, $P = 0.006$) and caudate nucleus ($r(151) = 0.186$, $P = 0.022$). In both cases, individuals with higher cardiorespiratory fitness also had larger volumes of these striatal nuclei. In contrast, we did not observe this same correlation with the volume of the putamen ($r(151) = 0.085$, $P = 0.296$).

We next looked at the principal output nucleus of the basal ganglia, the globus pallidus. Although we found a trend for a positive association between VO_{2max} scores and pallidal volume, this relationship did not reach statistical significance ($r(151) = 0.139$, $P = 0.086$). Thus, although VO_{2max} had significant associations with sections of the input to the basal ganglia, the relationship between cardiorespiratory fitness and the globus pallidus remains uncertain.

3.2.2. Associations between Basal Ganglia Volumes and Task Performance. According to current methods of mediation analysis, detecting direct pathway effects (i.e., VO_{2max} to task performance) is not a necessary condition for indirect pathway effects (i.e., VO_{2max} to brain volume to task performance) [34]. However, in order to identify possible indirect mediating pathways between cardiorespiratory fitness and task performance through basal ganglia volumes, the direct pathways between brain volumes and behavior must also be established. These pathways are illustrated in Figure 3.

For performance in the Flanker Task, we failed to observe any significant associations between basal ganglia volume and task performance. Specifically, the partial correlation analysis failed to detect a significant relationship between response interference in the Flanker Task and the volume of either the nucleus accumbens ($r(138) = 0.031$, $P = 0.721$), caudate nucleus ($r(150) = 0.062$, $P = 0.446$), putamen ($r(150) = 0.131$, $P = 0.106$), or globus pallidus ($r(150) = 0.087$, $P = 0.284$). There was also a lack of significant relationships between accuracy in the Flanker Task and the volume of either the nucleus accumbens ($r(138) = 0.078$, $P = 0.361$), caudate nucleus ($r(149) = -0.074$, $P = 0.368$), putamen ($r(149) = 0.028$, $P = 0.732$), or globus pallidus ($r(149) = 0.054$, $P = 0.511$). This same pattern was also present when the partial correlations were run against

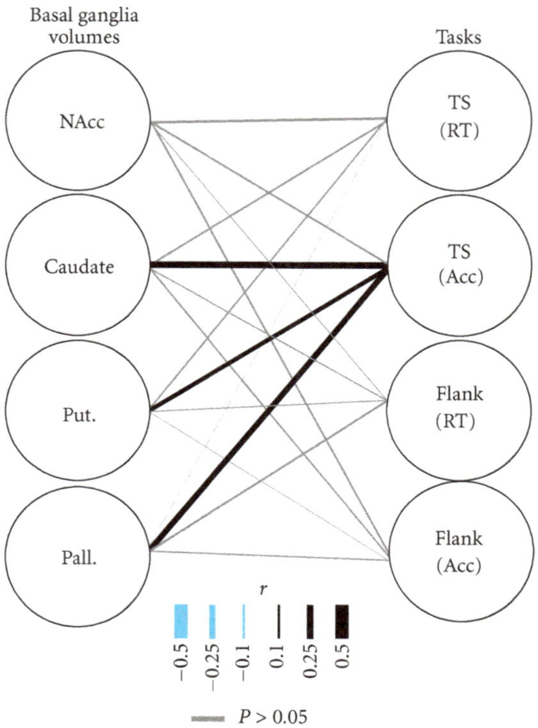

FIGURE 3: Correlation paths between basal ganglia regions of interest volume and behavioral costs for both tasks. Same plotting convention as Figure 2.

TABLE 2: Partial correlations between nuclear volumes and components of the behavioral scores.

	Nucleus accumbens	Caudate nucleus	Putamen	Pallidum
Flanker				
Con RT	−.114	−.015	−.054	.013
Inc RT	−.096	−.037	−.127	−.035
Cost (RT)	.031	.062	.131	.087
Con Acc	.132	.122	.045	−.034
Inc Acc	.176	.013	.069	−.012
Cost (Acc)	.078	−.074	.028	.054
Task-switch				
Repeat RT	.010	−.238**	−.018	.089
Switch RT	.079	−.103	.081	.016
Cost (RT)	.107	−.069	.058	−.003
Repeat Acc	.120	.286**	.115	.176*
Switch Acc	.133	.274**	.153	.217**
Cost (Acc)	.089	.247**	.164*	.218**

the congruent and incongruent scores in the Flanker Task separately (Table 2). Therefore, we can rule out any possible indirect pathway effects in the Flanker Task in our sample.

Similarly, we failed to detect any significant associations between Task Switching costs in response times and basal ganglia volumes. The partial correlation analysis failed to detect a significant correlation between switching and the volume of the nucleus accumbens ($r(138) = 0.102$, $P = 0.209$), caudate nucleus ($r(148) = -0.069$, $P = 0.398$), the putamen ($r(148) = 0.059$, $P = 0.477$), or the globus pallidus ($r(148) = -0.003$, $P = 0.973$). We did detect a negative correlation between caudate volume and reaction times in the repeat trial condition (see Table 2), suggesting that greater caudate nucleus volume predicted overall faster reaction times in the simpler condition. However, the speed cost of changing between conditions was not predicted by caudate volume. Therefore, similar to performance in the Flanker Task, we can rule out the possibility of indirect mediating pathways between cardiorespiratory fitness and response times in the Task Switching experiment in our sample.

We did, however, observe significant associations between the volume of basal ganglia nuclei and accuracy in the Task Switching experiment. While the volume of the nucleus accumbens failed to have a significant partial correlation ($r(138) = 0.089$, $P = 0.293$), we observed significant positive correlations between the volumes of the caudate nucleus ($r(150) = 0.247$, $P = 0.002$), the putamen ($r(150) = 0.164$, $P = 0.044$) and the globus pallidus ($r(150) = 0.218$, $P = 0.007$) with accuracy rates in the switch condition. When we look at the components of the accuracy cost score, we see that both repeat and switching trials were negatively correlated with the volume of the caudate nucleus and the globus pallidus, but not the putamen (see Table 2). Thus, these two nuclei had predictive value for both overall accuracy rates

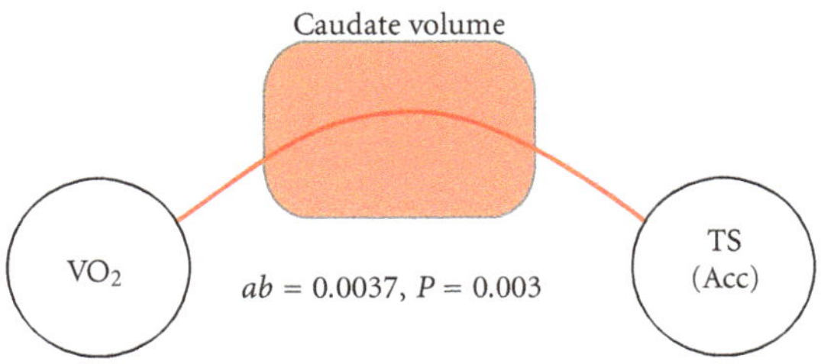

FIGURE 4: Indirect mediating pathway between cardiorespiratory fitness and Task Switching performance via the volume of the caudate nucleus.

and accuracy costs in switching between conditions. Taken together, these results suggest that, in our sample, the size of the two largest striatal nuclei and the output nucleus of the basal ganglia were predictive of better accuracy during Task Switching conditions. This leaves open the possibility of indirect mediating pathways of the basal ganglia in the relationship between cardiorespiratory fitness and accuracy in the Task Switching experiment.

3.2.3. Mediating Pathways. The presence of significant relationships between (a) VO_{2max} and caudate nucleus volume and (b) caudate nucleus volume and accuracy in the Task Switching experiment, suggests that the caudate nucleus may be a candidate mediator for the relationship between cardiorespiratory fitness and task switch performance. We set out to determine the degree to which the caudate nucleus volume mediated the relationship between VO_{2max} and task performance. We tested this using a bootstrapped mediation analysis approach [34] and included all the covariate terms in the regression model. This analysis revealed a significant indirect mediation pathway between VO_{2max} and accuracy through caudate nucleus volume (Figure 4; *ab* coefficient = 0.0037, $P = 0.003$, 95%CI = 0.0009–0.0085, df = 150). The effect size of this mediation effect was small ($R^2 = 0.1661$), however including the caudate volume in the calculation of the direct pathway from VO_{2max} to Task Switching accuracy accounted for approximately 33% of the total effect (*c* coefficient = 0.0106, *c′* coefficient = 0.0070). Thus, caudate nucleus volume was a significant, partial mediator of the relationship between cardiorespiratory fitness and task performance.

4. Discussion

Our results show that similar to our previous findings in cortical regions [5, 9], increased cardiorespiratory fitness, that is, higher VO_{2max}, in older adults is associated with larger volumes of several core basal ganglia nuclei, specifically the caudate nucleus and nucleus accumbens. The putamen and globus pallidus were not significantly associated with VO_{2max}. Cardiorespiratory fitness levels were also positively associated with accuracy rates in a Task Switching paradigm that assesses cognitive flexibility. While several basal ganglia nuclei were positively associated with Task Switching accuracy, only the caudate nucleus met the assumptions necessary to perform subsequent mediation analyses. This subsequent analysis found that the caudate nucleus volume was a partial mediator of the relationship between fitness and Task Switching accuracy. These results highlight a key candidate pathway by which differences in cardiorespiratory fitness may regulate cognitive flexibility in older adults.

Our results are consistent with previous studies demonstrating that dopamine receptor pathways in the nucleus accumbens and mesolimbic circuitry mediate the rewarding aspects of exercise in rodents [38–40]. In addition, rodents that are provided access to running wheels show attenuated effects of methamphetamine and cocaine in the nucleus accumbens [41–43] and increased gene expression in both the dorsal and ventral striatum for D1 and D2 receptors and associated G-proteins [40]. Exercise attenuates the neurotoxic effects of 6-hydroxydopamine on dopaminergic circuitry in the dorsal striatum [16, 44], possibly through BDNF pathways [44]. Hence, results from rodent studies of exercise are in line with our finding that cardiorespiratory fitness levels in humans are positively associated with the size of basal ganglia. The results from rodent models also provide potential molecular mechanisms by which fitness is associated with greater volume of the basal ganglia. Although the cellular and molecular correlates of MRI-based volumetric estimates remain unknown, our finding of larger volumes as a function of cardiorespiratory fitness is interesting in the light of this previous literature in rodents.

To the extent that cardiorespiratory fitness is modifiable by participation in regular aerobic exercise [5], our results suggest that age-related loss in volume of the caudate nucleus and nucleus accumbens may be remediable by exercise. In relation to this, however, a recent study by our group [5] reported that a randomized 1-year aerobic exercise intervention failed to significantly increase caudate nucleus volume, despite a significant increase in the size of the hippocampus. Hence, the results from the cross-sectional analysis reported here are not in line with the results from the randomized exercise intervention. There are several potential explanations for this apparent discrepancy. First, the sample size in the current study ($N = 179$) was larger than the results from the Erickson et al. [5] study ($N = 60$ per group) suggesting that the intervention might have been underpowered to detect exercise-induced changes in volume of the caudate nucleus. Such a conclusion is strengthened by a closer examination of the Erickson et al. [5] intervention results that showed a trend for the volume of the caudate nucleus to be different between the exercise and stretching groups at post-assessment, but the difference did not reach significance. Longer randomized trials with larger sample sizes are needed to confirm whether an exercise intervention is capable of increasing the size of the caudate nucleus and nucleus accumbens.

A second explanation for the apparent discrepancy between our results and those of Erickson et al. [5] is the inherent limitation in all cross-sectional study designs. Specifically, it is possible that an uncontrolled third variable, correlated with both cardiorespiratory fitness and caudate nucleus volume, but not with exercise participation *per se*, explains the discrepancy between our results and those of Erickson et al. [5]. In fact, there is a genetic component to VO_{2max} [45] that might explain both the link to the volume of the basal ganglia and cognitive flexibility. Again, these results suggest that randomized trials with larger sample sizes and longer periods of an exercise treatment are necessary to disentangle the possible explanations for the discrepancy between the cross-sectional results reported here and the intervention results reported in Erickson et al. [5]. In fact, a larger scale intervention study could attempt to replicate the cross-sectional results that we describe here in addition to testing whether an exercise regimen could alter the size of the basal ganglia. Another method of testing these hypotheses would be to recruit individuals with dysfunction or deficits of the basal ganglia into an exercise intervention to examine whether volume could be altered in these at-risk or impaired populations.

To our knowledge, there is only one other cross-sectional neuroimaging study examining the volume of the basal ganglia in relation to cardiorespiratory fitness levels [21]. In that study of 55 preadolescent children (9-10 years old) higher fitness levels were associated with greater volume of the caudate nucleus, putamen, and globus pallidus, but not the nucleus accumbens. Interestingly, the volume of the putamen and globus pallidus was also correlated with performance on a Flanker Task. The results we report here are clearly only partially consistent with the results from Chaddock et al. [21]. First, we failed to find any associations with Flanker Task performance and the size of the basal ganglia, and second, we only find associations with fitness for the caudate nucleus and nucleus accumbens, not the putamen or pallidum. One possible explanation for the inconsistency between our study and that of Chaddock et al. [21] is that there are maturational differences in the growth and later atrophy of the basal ganglia [46] such that fitness effects emerge on different brain structures at different time points throughout the lifespan. In fact, such an explanation is likely given developmental trajectories of brain growth, pruning, and myelination [47] earlier in development in contrast to atrophy and volumetric loss late in life [2]. Of course another possible explanation for these between-study differences could simply result from the inter-subject variability inherent in all cross-sectional experimental designs.

Here we were able to demonstrate that greater volume of the caudate nucleus is a significant indirect pathway between cardiorespiratory fitness and cognitive flexibility as assessed by a Task Switching paradigm. Switching abilities and reversal learning are supported by the basal ganglia, medial frontal cortex, and dorsolateral prefrontal cortex in both rodents and humans [48, 49]. Our results, therefore, are consistent with this literature and suggest that variation in cardiorespiratory fitness levels might explain significant individual variability in correlations between volume and task-switch performance. Interestingly, we failed to find associations with performance on the Flanker Task, despite previous studies showing links with attentional control and function of the basal ganglia circuits [21, 50]. This dissociation between the task-switch and flanker paradigms suggests some specificity of the function of the basal ganglia circuits in late adulthood. One explanation might be that tasks involving attentional control and response conflict, like the flanker paradigm, might be more dependent on prefrontal structures than basal ganglia in late life. This hypothesis is supported by a recent study demonstrating that older adults had less activity in the dorsal striatum during performance of a Stroop task compared to a younger group [50]. Given the presence of cortico-striatum loops, it is likely that a distributed circuit of frontal, parietal, and striatum is involved in mediating both attentional and switching behaviors, but that the relative importance of these structures changes with age.

In addition, we failed to find significant associations between Flanker Task performance and fitness levels despite numerous other studies finding significant associations throughout the lifespan [15, 21, 36, 37, 51–53]. It is likely that our limited range of cardiorespiratory fitness levels precluded our ability to detect significant associations and that the correlations with Task Switching performance are more robustly associated with fitness levels. In any case, it will be important for future studies with a wider range of fitness levels to examine the links between Flanker performance and caudate nucleus volume.

Finally, as alluded to earlier, there are several limitations to the current study that warrant further exploration in future work. First, our study was cross-sectional in nature so causal conclusions about how increased cardiorespiratory fitness might influence the size of the basal ganglia are inherently limited. It will be critical for randomized exercise interventions conducted with a large well-characterized cohort to determine whether it is possible to alter the size of these structures. Second, we did not have any tasks (i.e., reward-based) that might be considered to be dependent on the nucleus accumbens, so we were unable to examine the behavioral importance of greater nucleus accumbens volume with higher fitness levels. However, despite these limitations we were able to detect associations using a relatively large and homogeneous sample of older adults and cognitive tasks that have been previously linked to the function of the dorsal striatum. In sum, we find that cardiorespiratory fitness levels are positively associated with volume of the caudate nucleus and nucleus accumbens in late adulthood and that the size of the caudate nucleus is a significant mediator between fitness and performance in the Task Switch paradigm.

Authors' Contribution

T. D. Verstynen, B. Lynch, and K. I. Erickson equally contributed to this work.

Acknowledgments

This work was supported by National Institutes of Aging, National Institutes of Health Grants RO1 AG25667 and RO1 AG25032. K. I. Erickson was supported by a Junior Scholar Award (P30 AG024827) from the Pittsburgh Claude D. Pepper Older Americans Independence Center.

References

[1] N. Raz, U. Lindenberger, K. M. Rodrigue et al., "Regional brain changes in aging healthy adults: general trends, individual differences and modifiers," *Cerebral Cortex*, vol. 15, no. 11, pp. 1676–1689, 2005.

[2] K. B. Walhovd, A. M. Fjell, A. M. Dale et al., "Multi-modal imaging predicts memory performance in normal aging and cognitive decline," *Neurobiology of Aging*, vol. 31, no. 7, pp. 1107–1121, 2010.

[3] S. C. Cramer, M. Sur, B. H. Dobkin et al., "Harnessing neuroplasticity for clinical applications," *Brain*, vol. 134, no. 6, pp. 1591–1609, 2011.

[4] S. J. Colcombe, K. I. Erickson, P. E. Scalf et al., "Aerobic exercise training increases brain volume in aging humans," *Journals of Gerontology A*, vol. 61, no. 11, pp. 1166–1170, 2006.

[5] K. I. Erickson, M. W. Voss, R. S. Prakash et al., "Exercise training increases size of hippocampus and improves memory," *Proceedings of the National Academy of Sciences of the United States of America*, vol. 108, no. 7, pp. 3017–3022, 2011.

[6] K. I. Erickson, C. A. Raji, O. L. Lopez et al., "Physical activity predicts gray matter volume in late adulthood: the Cardiovascular Health Study," *Neurology*, vol. 75, no. 16, pp. 1415–1422, 2010.

[7] S. Rovio, G. Spulber, L. J. Nieminen et al., "The effect of midlife physical activity on structural brain changes in the elderly," *Neurobiology of Aging*, vol. 31, no. 11, pp. 1927–1936, 2010.

[8] S. J. Colcombe, K. I. Erickson, N. Raz et al., "Aerobic fitness reduces brain tissue loss in aging humans," *Journals of Gerontology A*, vol. 58, no. 2, pp. 176–180, 2003.

[9] K. I. Erickson, R. S. Prakash, M. W. Voss et al., "Aerobic fitness is associated with hippocampal volume in elderly humans," *Hippocampus*, vol. 19, no. 10, pp. 1030–1039, 2009.

[10] A. M. Weinstein, M. W. Voss, R. S. Prakash et al., "The association between aerobic fitness and executive function is mediated by prefrontal cortex volume," *Brain, Behavior, and Immunity*, vol. 2, no. 1, pp. 32–41, 2012.

[11] A. M. Fjell and K. B. Walhovd, "Structural brain changes in aging: courses, causes and cognitive consequences," *Reviews in the Neurosciences*, vol. 21, no. 3, pp. 187–221, 2010.

[12] E. Aarts, M. Van Holstein, and R. Cools, "Striatal dopamine and the interface between motivation and cognition," *Frontiers in Psychology*, vol. 2, p. 163, 2011.

[13] R. Cools, L. Clark, and T. W. Robbins, "Differential responses in human striatum and prefrontal cortex to changes in object and rule relevance," *Journal of Neuroscience*, vol. 24, no. 5, pp. 1129–1135, 2004.

[14] L. Marais, D. J. Stein, and W. M. U. Daniels, "Exercise increases BDNF levels in the striatum and decreases depressive-like behavior in chronically stressed rats," *Metabolic Brain Disease*, vol. 24, no. 4, pp. 587–597, 2009.

[15] C. T. Wu, M. B. Pontifex, L. B. Raine et al., "Aerobic fitness and response variability in preadolescent children performing a cognitive control task," *Neuropsychology*, vol. 25, no. 3, pp. 333–341, 2011.

[16] M. J. Zigmond, J. L. Cameron, R. K. Leak et al., "Triggering endogenous neuroprotective processes through exercise in models of dopamine deficiency," *Parkinsonism and Related Disorders*, vol. 15, no. 3, pp. S42–S45, 2009.

[17] J. Y. F. Lau, D. Goldman, B. Buzas et al., "BDNF gene polymorphism (Val66Met) predicts amygdala and anterior hippocampus responses to emotional faces in anxious and depressed adolescents," *NeuroImage*, vol. 53, no. 3, pp. 952–961, 2010.

[18] N. Tajiri, T. Yasuhara, T. Shingo et al., "Exercise exerts neuroprotective effects on Parkinson's disease model of rats," *Brain Research*, vol. 1310, pp. 200–207, 2010.

[19] J. E. Ahlskog, "Does vigorous exercise have a neuroprotective effect in Parkinson disease?" *Neurology*, vol. 77, no. 3, pp. 288–294, 2011.

[20] A. D. Speelman, M. van Nimwegen, G. F. Borm, B. R. Bloem, and M. Munneke, "Monitoring of walking in Parkinson's disease: validation of an ambulatory activity monitor," *Parkinsonism and Related Disorders*, vol. 17, no. 5, pp. 402–404, 2011.

[21] L. Chaddock, K. I. Erickson, R. S. Prakash et al., "Basal ganglia volume is associated with aerobic fitness in preadolescent children," *Developmental Neuroscience*, vol. 32, no. 3, pp. 249–256, 2010.

[22] A. A. Kehagia, R. A. Barker, and T. W. Robbins, "Neuropsychological and clinical heterogeneity of cognitive impairment and dementia in patients with Parkinson's disease," *The Lancet Neurology*, vol. 9, no. 12, pp. 1200–1213, 2010.

[23] C. Stelzel, U. Basten, C. Montag, M. Reuter, and C. J. Fiebach, "Frontostriatal involvement in task switching depends on genetic differences in D2 receptor density," *Journal of Neuroscience*, vol. 30, no. 42, pp. 14205–14212, 2010.

[24] Y. Stern, M. Sano, J. Paulsen, and R. Mayeux, "Modified mini-mental state examination: validity and reliability," *Neurology*, vol. 37, p. 179, 1987.

[25] E. McAuley, A. N. Szabo, E. L. Mailey et al., "Non-exercise estimated cardiorespiratory fitness: associations with brain structure, cognition, and memory complaints in older adults," *Mental Health and Physical Activity*, vol. 4, no. 1, pp. 5–11, 2011.

[26] R. S. Prakash, M. W. Voss, K. I. Erickson et al., "Cardiorespiratory fitness and attentional control in the aging brain," *Frontiers in Human Neuroscience*, vol. 4, article 229, 2010.

[27] M. W. Voss, K. I. Erickson, R. S. Prakash et al., "Functional connectivity: a source of variance in the association between cardiorespiratory fitness and cognition?" *Neuropsychologia*, vol. 48, no. 5, pp. 1394–1406, 2010.

[28] J. I. Sheikh and J. A. Yesavage, "Geriatric Depression Scale (GDS): recent evidence and development of a shorter version," *Clinical Gerontologist*, vol. 5, no. 1-2, pp. 165–173, 1986.

[29] B. Patenaude, S. M. Smith, D. N. Kennedy, and M. Jenkinson, "A Bayesian model of shape and appearance for subcortical brain segmentation," *NeuroImage*, vol. 56, no. 3, pp. 907–922, 2011.

[30] Y. Zhang, M. Brady, and S. Smith, "Segmentation of brain MR images through a hidden Markov random field model and the expectation-maximization algorithm," *IEEE Transactions on Medical Imaging*, vol. 20, no. 1, pp. 45–57, 2001.

[31] S. M. Smith, M. Jenkinson, M. W. Woolrich et al., "Advances in functional and structural MR image analysis and implementation as FSL," *NeuroImage*, vol. 23, supplement 1, pp. S208–S219, 2004.

[32] K. M. Kennedy, K. I. Erickson, K. M. Rodrigue et al., "Age-related differences in regional brain volumes: a comparison of optimized voxel-based morphometry to manual volumetry," *Neurobiology of Aging*, vol. 30, no. 10, pp. 1657–1676, 2009.

[33] A. Miyake, N. P. Friedman, M. J. Emerson, A. H. Witzki, A. Howerter, and T. D. Wager, "The unity and diversity of executive functions and their contributions to complex "frontal lobe" tasks: a latent variable analysis," *Cognitive Psychology*, vol. 41, no. 1, pp. 49–100, 2000.

[34] K. J. Preacher and A. F. Hayes, "Asymptotic and resampling strategies for assessing and comparing indirect effects in multiple mediator models," *Behavior Research Methods*, vol. 40, no. 3, pp. 879–891, 2008.

[35] A. F. Hayes, "Beyond Baron and Kenny: statistical mediation analysis in the new millennium," *Communication Monographs*, vol. 76, no. 4, pp. 408–420, 2009.

[36] S. J. Colcombe, A. F. Kramer, K. I. Erickson et al., "Cardiovascular fitness, cortical plasticity, and aging," *Proceedings of the National Academy of Sciences of the United States of America*, vol. 101, no. 9, pp. 3316–3321, 2004.

[37] A. F. Kramer, S. Hahn, N. J. Cohen et al., "Ageing, fitness and neurocognitive function," *Nature*, vol. 400, no. 6743, pp. 418–419, 1999.

[38] B. N. Greenwood, T. E. Foley, T. V. Le et al., "Long-term voluntary wheel running is rewarding and produces plasticity in the mesolimbic reward pathway," *Behavioural Brain Research*, vol. 217, no. 2, pp. 354–362, 2011.

[39] M. D. Roberts, L. Gilpin, K. E. Parker, T. E. Childs, M. J. Will, and F. W. Booth, "Dopamine D1 receptor modulation in nucleus accumbens lowers voluntary wheel running in rats bred to run high distances," *Physiology & Behavior*, vol. 105, no. 3, pp. 661–668, 2012.

[40] W. F. Mathes, D. L. Nehrenberg, R. Gordon, K. Hua, T. Garland Jr., and D. Pomp, "Dopaminergic dysregulation in mice selectively bred for excessive exercise or obesity," *Behavioural Brain Research*, vol. 210, no. 2, pp. 155–163, 2010.

[41] C. A. Fontes-Ribeiro, E. Marques, F. C. Pereira, A. P. Silva, and T. R. A. Macedo, "May exercise prevent addiction?" *Current Neuropharmacology*, vol. 9, no. 1, pp. 45–48, 2011.

[42] S. J. O'Dell, B. A. Galvez, A. J. Ball, and J. F. Marshall, "Running wheel exercise ameliorates methamphetamine-induced damage to dopamine and serotonin terminals," *Synapse*, vol. 66, pp. 71–80, 2012.

[43] M. L. Mustroph, D. J. Stobaugh, D. S. Miller, E. K. DeYoung, and J. S. Rhodes, "Wheel running can accelerate or delay extinction of conditioned place preference for cocaine in male C57BL/6J mice, depending on timing of wheel access," *European Journal of Neuroscience*, vol. 34, pp. 1161–1169, 2011.

[44] N. Tajiri, T. Yasuhara, T. Shingo et al., "Exercise exerts neuroprotective effects on Parkinson's disease model of rats," *Brain Research*, vol. 1310, pp. 200–207, 2010.

[45] J. Rico-Sanz, T. Rankinen, T. Rice et al., "Quantitative trait loci for maximal exercise capacity phenotypes and their responses to training in the HERITAGE Family Study," *Physiological Genomics*, vol. 16, pp. 256–260, 2004.

[46] D. P. Casey, B. D. Madery, T. B. Curry, J. H. Eisenach, B. W. Wilkins, and M. J. Joyner, "Nitric oxide contributes to the augmented vasodilatation during hypoxic exercise," *Journal of Physiology*, vol. 588, no. 2, pp. 373–385, 2010.

[47] E. S. Anderson, "Morphology of early developing oligodendrocytes in the ventrolateral spinal cord of the chicken," *Journal of Neurocytology*, vol. 32, no. 9, pp. 1045–1053, 2003.

[48] E. Dahlin, A. S. Neely, A. Larsson, L. Bäckman, and L. Nyberg, "Transfer of learning after updating training mediated by the striatum," *Science*, vol. 320, no. 5882, pp. 1510–1512, 2008.

[49] L. Chaddock, K. I. Erickson, R. S. Prskash et al., "A functional MRI investigation of the association between childhood aerobic fitness and neurocognitive control," " *Biological Psychology*, vol. 89, no. 1, pp. 260–268, 2012.

[50] C. H. Hillman, S. M. Buck, J. R. Themanson, M. B. Pontifex and D. M. Castelli, "Aerobic fitness and cognitive development: event-related brain potential and task performance indices of executive control in preadolescent children," *Developmental Psychology*, vol. 45, no. 1, pp. 114–129, 2009.

[51] M. B. Pontifex, M. R. Scudder, M. L. Brown et al., "On the number of trials necessary for stabilization of error-related brain activity across the life span," *Psychophysiology*, vol. 47, no. 4, pp. 767–773, 2010.

[52] J. R. Themanson, C. H. Hillman, E. McAuley et al., "Self-efficacy effects on neuroelectric and behavioral indices of action monitoring in older adults," *Neurobiology of Aging*, vol. 29, no. 7, pp. 1111–1122, 2008.

[53] S. Stroth, S. Kubesch, K. Dieterle, M. Ruchsow, R. Heim, and M. Kiefer, "Physical fitness, but not acute exercise modulates event-related potential indices for executive control in healthy adolescents," *Brain Research*, vol. 1269, pp. 114–124, 2009.

6

Older Adults Making End of Life Decisions: An Application of Roy's Adaptation Model

Weihua Zhang

Nell Hodgson Woodruff School of Nursing Emory University, 1520 Clifton Road, Atlanta, GA 30322-4207, USA

Correspondence should be addressed to Weihua Zhang; wzhang3@emory.edu

Academic Editor: Barbara Shukitt-Hale

Purpose. The purpose of this study was to identify variables that influenced completion of advanced directives in the context of adaptation from national data in older adults. Knowledge gained from this study would help us identify factors that might influence end of life discussions and shed light on strategies on effective communication on advance care planning. *Design and Method.* A model-testing design and path analysis were used to examine secondary data from 938 participants. Items were extracted from the data set to correspond to variables for this study. Scales were constructed and reliabilities were tested. *Results.* The final path model showed that physical impairment, self-rated health, continuing to work, and family structure had direct and indirect effects on completion of advanced directives. Five percent of the variance was accounted for by the path analysis. *Conclusion.* The variance accounted for by the model was small. This could have been due to the use of secondary data and limitations imposed for measurement. However, health care providers and families should explore patient's perception of self-health as well as their family and work situation in order to strategize a motivational discussion on advance directive or end of life care planning.

1. Introduction

Those aged 65 and older represented 35.9 million or 12.3% of the US population in 2003, and this number will reach 19% by the year 2030 [1]. The great majority of deaths (80–85%) occur in this population, and most die from chronic conditions such as heart failure, cancer, obstructive pulmonary disease, diabetes, Alzheimer's disease, and renal failure [2]. The Institute of Medicine (IOM) noted that while technology continues to increase life expectancy, the quality of life of dying patients has not kept the same pace [3]. Studies indicate that patients' families are still dissatisfied with end of life care [4–7]. Advance directives (ADs) were seen as a way for individuals to decide on and communicate their end of life care wishes to those who care for them to ensure, more in a legal term, that individuals' wishes for end of life care are followed. ADs include durable power of attorney and a living will. However, more than 2 decades after passage of the 1991 Patient Self-Determination Act (PSDA) requiring AD discussion on admission to health care institutions, the rate of completion of ADs remains at approximately 29% of the population [8]. Advance care planning is starting to replace the term "advance directives" to make its slow transitioning from a legal model to a tool to enhance communication [8]. However, factors learned from those who have completed the advance directives could help us identify factors that might influence end of life discussions [9–12] and shed lights on strategies on effective communication on advance care planning. The intent of this study was to identify and analyze factors influencing AD completion in an older population.

2. Literature Review

The literature on outcomes of end of life communication is focused on AD completion for this study. Those studies explore the influence of demographic factors such as age, gender, family relationships, and health issues on the completion of ADs.

Studies indicate that older white women with more education who perceive themselves to be in poor health are more likely to have signed an AD [13–16]. Douglas and Brown [17] also reported that women were more likely than men to have completed ADs. However, Cooper and colleagues [18] found that gender was not related to AD completion.

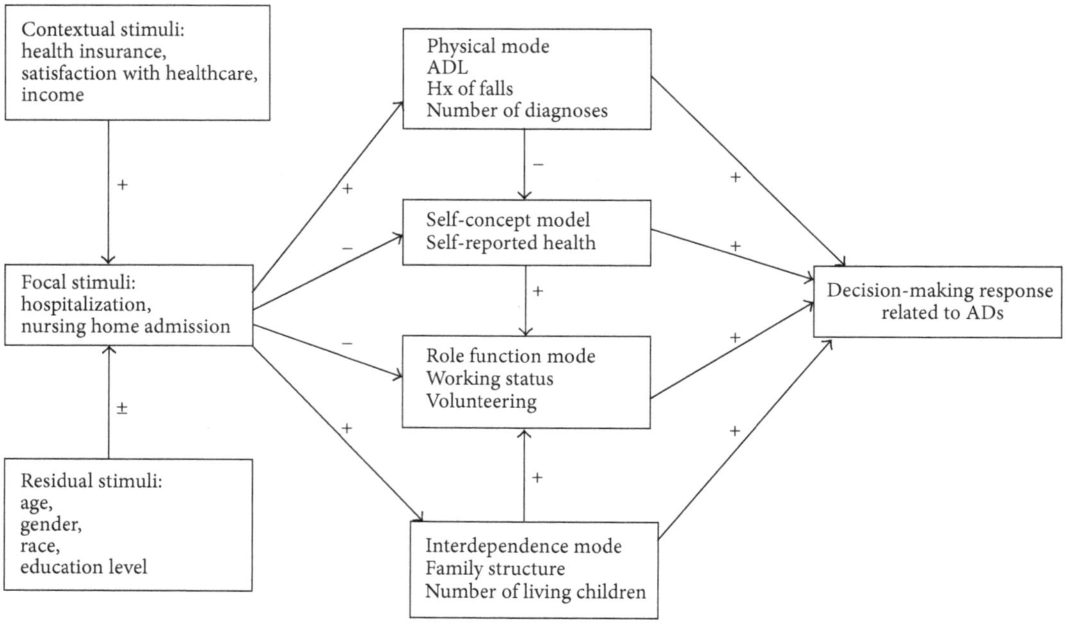

FIGURE 1: Application of the RAM to AD Completion.

Race may also be related to AD completion. Study reported that African-Americans were significantly more likely to choose aggressive life-saving interventions and less likely than Caucasians and Asians to complete ADs [19, 20]. Eleazer and associates also noted that Hispanics were more likely to refuse to complete any form of ADs [19]. In support of Eleazer et al.'s finding, Degenholtz et al. [21] also found that African-Americans and Hispanics were less likely than Caucasians to have living wills. However, Morrison and associates [22] reported that race was not significantly related to the signing of a durable power of attorney. Nolan et al. reported that gender, race, and health status are not significantly related to AD completion [23].

Investigators in two studies found that those with higher incomes, health insurance, and more trust in the medical system were more likely to complete ADs [24, 25]. Findings from other studies note that those with less education were significantly less likely to sign ADs and more likely to desire life-sustaining treatment [26, 27]. It is evident that studies examining demographic variables have diverse findings. Overall, age, income, health insurance, and more trust in medical system are positively related to AD completion. However, age-related variables, such as poor health and more physical impairment, could complicate the relationship between age and AD completion.

In Gerald's [14] study, neither diagnosis nor marital status was significantly related to AD completion. However, more widows or widowers had signed an AD than those who were married, single, or divorced. Colenda et al. [28] reported that those who lived close to their children and those who with large social networks had lower AD completion rates. Studies indicated that those had close relationships with their families [29] or have family members living nearby [30] tended to desire less aggressive life-saving interventions than those who did not have close relationships.

Although the completion rate for ADs is about 15% to 25% in adults [10], hospitalization or perception of poor self-health may precipitate completion of ADs. Studies indicate that those who had a recent hospitalization completed ADs more than those who had not been hospitalized [25, 31]. McAuley and associates reported that after a 12-month nursing home admission, AD completion rates increased by 18% from the baseline [32]. Morrison et al. [22] and Salmond and David [10] found that poorer self-reported health status was significantly related to AD completion. Hospital admission, suffering an illness, and decline of health status could prompt more AD completion. Being informed about ADS at admission during a health care crisis could also contribute to more completion upon hospitalization.

The relationships among age, gender, race, education level, family structure, and health factors to AD completion have been studied separately. Variables that influence decision making on AD completion can be analyzed in a contextual model. How those external and internal factors (stimuli), modes of adaption, and decision-making factors working together to influence AD completion has yet to be examined. The purpose of this study is to apply Roy's Adaptation Model to analyze the influence of demographic, family structure, and health status variables on AD completion.

Roy's Adaptation Model (RAM) [33] provides a framework for identifying variables that influence individuals' responses to stressful situations (Figure 1).

According to Roy, individuals mobilize all possible ways to adapt to a stressful situation. An individual's ability to adapt to situations varies depending on the nature of the stimuli confronting the person. Stimuli are focal, contextual, or residual. Focal stimuli are influenced by contextual and residual stimuli. Contextual stimuli are internal or external factors that influence how the individual reacts to the focal stimuli but do not require direct and immediate attention or energy. Residual stimuli are factors affecting the person with an uncertain effect.

Focal stimuli exert a direct and immediate effect on the individual and become the focus of attention for the person. The person mobilizes control processes which consist of regulator and cognator processes [34]. Neural, chemical, and endocrine coping processes (physiological) are termed regulator processes, while cognator processes result from cognitive-emotive channels. The person spends energy to mobilize four adaptive modes: physical, self-concept, role-function, and interdependence mode in dealing with the focal stimuli in order to maintain or restore adaptation through stressful event [33]. The assumption of using this theory is that each individual under any stressful situation would attempt to balance the interrelationship of physical, self-concept, role function, and interdependence mode in order to maintain or restore adaptation.

As shown in Figure 1, incorporating variables identified by the literature and placing them in the RAM provided the framework for this study. The focal stimulus was the number of hospitalization and nursing home admissions. Contextual stimuli for this study were health insurance, household income, and satisfaction with health care because those variables have shown relevance to AD completion. The residual stimuli were age, gender, race, and education level because those variables' relationships to the AD completion are not consistent. The contextual and residual stimuli were expected to have direct effects on focal stimuli (having a stressful event with AD completion status inquiry prompted by each hospitalization is operationalized as number of hospital and nursing home admissions) and indirect effects on the adaptive modes (physical, self-concept, role function, and interdependence mode) and, finally, on the decision-making responses (having signed ADs or not). Adaptive modes were expected to have direct or indirect effects on signing ADs. The regulator and cognator control processes were not measured in this study.

3. Design and Methods

A model-testing design based on the RAM and path analysis was selected for this study. This allowed examination of the predictive effects from one concept to the next one as identified in Figure 1. Secondary data containing information on AD completion were used for the study.

3.1. Sample. Noninstitutionalized US citizens aged 55 or older participated in the 1984 Longitudinal Study of Aging (LSOA) which included the 1984 National Health Interview Survey, the 1984 Health Insurance Supplement, and the 1984 baseline Supplement on Aging (SOA). The LSOA was followed by three follow-up interviews. The first follow-up interview was the 1994 Second Supplement on Aging (SOA II), which included those who had participated in the National Health Interview Survey and added a new cohort of those over the age of 70. The second follow-up interview (1997-1998) included data on those who had died since 1994. Information on those who had died (the decedent interview file) was collected from family members of the deceased. Data from the 1994 SOA II and the 1998 decedent file were extracted and merged for this study since these data are termed relevant to AD completion and also contain baseline information on demographics, physical function, working status, and family relationships. The sample consisted of the 938 participants in the merged dataset.

3.2. Instruments. Instruments were constructed from items identified as appropriate to the concepts of interest. The reliability of each constructed instrument with more than one item was then tested [35]. Instruments with less than a Cronbach's alpha of 0.70 were revised.

Focal, Contextual, and Residual Stimuli. The number of admissions to the hospital and the number of nursing home admissions were originally designed to measure the focal stimulus. These were selected as the focal stimuli because they would reflect the number of times persons were asked about AD completion status. The low Cronbach's alpha for these two items (0.31) and the fact that 732 participants had missing data on the number of nursing home admissions led to the decision that only the number of hospital admissions would be used to measure the focal stimulus.

The contextual stimuli were defined as health insurance status, household income, and satisfaction with health care. Health insurance and income were selected because they are closely related and affect both the quality and extent of health care delivery. Satisfaction with health care was chosen as an indicator of trust in the correctness of the healthcare provider's decisions and advice, and higher scores meant greater satisfaction. Age, gender, race, and education were considered as residual stimuli.

The Adaptive Modes. The physical mode was measured by summing up the activities of daily living (ADLs), the number of falls, and the total number of diseases. Higher scores indicated more physical impairment. Reliability for the constructed physical mode scale was 0.72. The self-concept mode was operationalized as self-rated health status. Working status and/or doing volunteer work were measuring role function. Working or engaging in volunteer activities was assumed to provide more opportunities for social engagement. Living arrangement and size of the family were chosen to measure the interdependence mode. The higher the score, the more emotional support provided to the participants. This constructed scale had a Cronbach's alpha of 0.75.

Adaptive Response. Having a completed AD indicates either having had an end of life discussion with family or a health provider or having given at least some thoughts to end of life care planning. The adaptive response for this study was having signed or not signed either a living will, a durable power of attorney, or both.

4. Results

4.1. Sample Characteristics. As shown in Table 1, the mean age of the 938 participants was 80 years old. Of the 938

TABLE 1: Demographic characteristics (N = 938).

Characteristic	N	(Percent)
Age (range = 70–99, M = 80, SD = 6.84)	938	
Gender		
Male	460	(49.0)
Female	478	(51.0)
Race		
White	828	(88.3)
Black	93	(9.9)
Others	17	(1.8)
Education level		
Less than 12 years	413	(44)
12 or more years	497	(53)
Unknown	28	(3)
Marital status and living arrangement		
Married, living with spouse	481	(51.3)
Widowed	357	(38.0)
Living alone	295	(31.4)
Household income		
Less than 20,000	396	(58.1)
More than 20,000	286	(41.9)
Health insurance		
No insurance	4	(0.4)
Medicaid only	3	(0.3)
Medicare only	722	(76.9)
Private insurance or more than one	209	(22.2)

participants, about half were women and most were Caucasian. More than half had at least a high school education. About half were married and lived with their spouses, and about a third lived alone. Roughly half had household incomes below $20,000 in 1994, and 256 participants did not report income. Virtually all had Medicare, and about a fourth had some other type of health insurance in addition to Medicare.

4.2. Descriptive Statistics for Variables in the Model. All variables except race and gender were continuous and normally distributed. Table 2 shows the mean, standard deviation, possible range, and obtained range for each variable or constructed scale. A total of 5% had never been hospitalized and 37% had been hospitalized once, with the remainder being two or more times hospitalized from 1994 to 1997. Only 22% of the sample responded to the item on number of nursing home admissions. Of these, 80% had one nursing home admission, and 16% had more than one nursing home admission. Most (93%) ranked satisfaction with their health care provider as good or excellent. A total of 78% had a high school education or less. The majority (60%) scored 6 or less on activities of daily living 6 months prior to death, and 53% reported no falls for the four-year period. About 65% reported having been diagnosed with three or more diseases. More than half (54%) considered themselves in good or excellent health. Only 4.5% were working, and 8% were doing some volunteer work. About half (51%) lived with their spouses. A living will had been completed by 52% of the participants.

4.3. Path Analyses

Procedures. The assumptions of normal distribution, homoscedasticity, and linear relationships were met for analyses using multiple regressions. Six endogenous variables (the focal stimulus; the physical, self-concept, rolefunction, and interdependence modes; and AD completion) along with seven exogenous variables (insurance, household income, satisfaction with healthcare, age, gender, race, and education level) were included in the initial model. First, bivariate correlations were examined to give a sense of which variables might be important. Next, preliminary multiple regressions analyses were done with each of the dependent endogenous variables in turn as predicted by the theoretical model. Using results from the preliminary multiple regressions, spurious relationships were identified and eliminated. Another set of multiple regression analyses were performed with only the significant independent variables as identified in the preliminary regression analyses entered. The results from that set of analyses provided the path coefficients for the final model.

Path Analysis Results. From the left of the theoretical framework to the right (Figure 2), Pearson's correlation coefficients were calculated to assess bivariate relationships between the independent variables (contextual and residual stimuli) and the dependent variable (focal stimulus). Only age ($r = -0.09$, $P = .01$) was statistically significantly related to the focal stimulus. Munro [36] stated that r-values less than 0.49 were low and an r-value less than 0.25 indicates that little if any correlation exists.

Bivariate relationships between the focal stimulus and the four adaptive modes were examined next. These showed that the focal stimulus was significantly related to the physical mode ($r = 0.29$, $P = 0.00$) and the self-concept mode ($r = -0.10$, $P = 0.01$). The physical mode was also significantly related to the self-concept mode ($r = -0.24$, $P = 0.00$) and the rolefunction mode ($r = -0.16$, $P = 0.00$). The self-concept mode was significantly related to both the role function mode ($r = 0.16$, $P = 0.00$) and the interdependence mode ($r = -0.14$, $P = 0.00$).

The bivariate relationships of the four adaptive modes to AD completion indicated that only the physical mode ($r = 0.17$, $P = 0.00$) and the interdependence mode ($r = -0.15$, $P = 0.00$) were significantly related to AD completion.

The preliminary multiple regression analysis, with number of hospitalizations (the focal stimulus) as the dependent variable, showed that only age was a significant predictor ($\beta = -0.10$, $P = 0.01$).

The next set of multiple regressions assessed the predictive (independent) effect of the focal stimulus on each of the four adaptive modes and then the paths from one mode to the next mode. These results showed that the focal stimulus significantly predicted only the physical mode ($\beta = 0.29$, $P = 0.00$). The physical mode had a predictive inverse relationship with the self-concept mode ($\beta = -0.24$, $P = 0.00$). The role

TABLE 2: Descriptive statistics for variables in the model.

Variable	M	(SD)	Possible range	Obtained range
Focal stimulus				
Number of hospitalizations	2.30	(2.00)	NA	0–24
Contextual stimuli				
Health insurance	2.34	(0.80)	0–8	0–6
Household income	5.22	(2.15)	1–9	1–9
Satisfaction with HC	3.45	(0.64)	1–4	1–4
Residual stimuli				
Education	3.60	(1.40)	1–7	1–7
Physical mode				
ADL score	6.07	(3.48)	3–15	3–15
Fall score	1.78	(0.89)	1–3	1–3
No. of diseases	3.19	(1.53)	0–10	0–8
Total	**10.89**	**(4.42)**	**4–28**	**4–25**
Self-concept mode	2.62	(1.17)	1–5	1–5
Role function mode	1.12	(0.32)	1-2	1-2
Interdependence mode				
Family structure	6.92	(3.62)	NA	2–7
AD completion	1.57	(0.49)	1-2	1-2

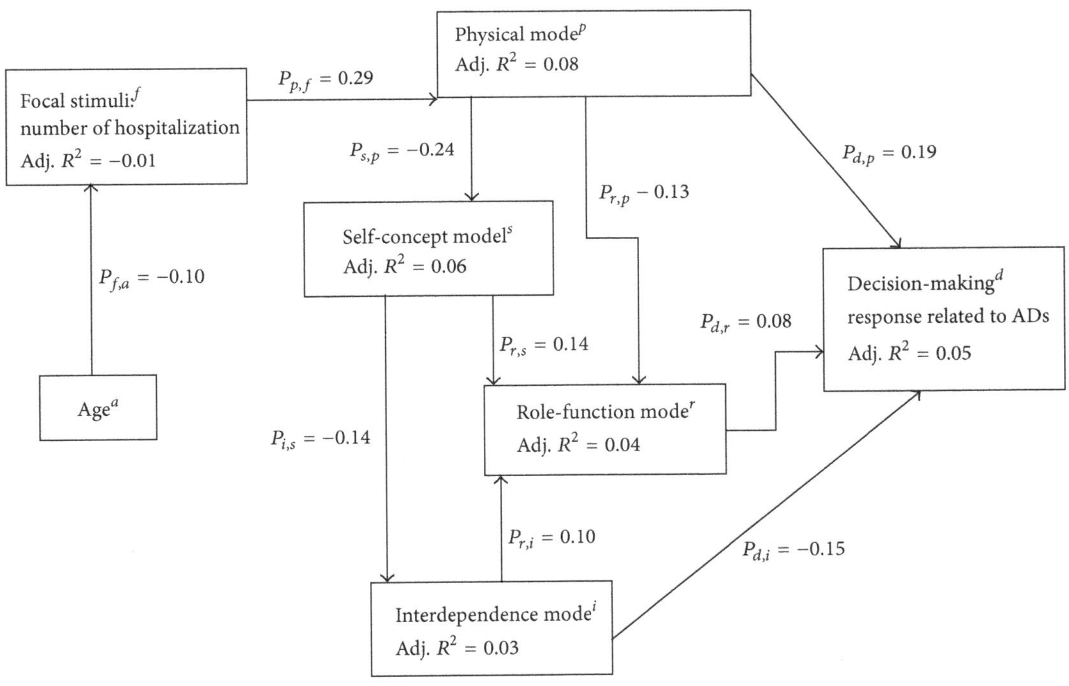

FIGURE 2: Final path model for AD Completion.

function mode was significantly predicted by the physical (β = −0.13, P = 0.00), self-concept (β = 0.14, P = 0.00), and interdependence modes (β = 0.10, P = 0.00). The results suggested a potentially significant path between the self-concept and interdependence modes, thus an additional multiple regression was done. Self-concept was identified as a significant predictor to the interdependence mode (β = −0.14, P = 0.00).

The last set of multiple regressions assessed the predictive effects of the four modes on the decision-making response. Three of the four modes were significant: they are the physical mode (β = 0.19, P = 0.00), role function mode (β = 0.08, P = 0.02), and the interdependence mode (β = −0.15, P = 0.00).

The final path model is presented in Figure 2. The physical, role, and interdependence modes jointly explained 5% of the variance in AD completion (adjusted R^2 = 0.05).

The physical mode explained 6% of the variance in the self-concept mode. The physical and self-concept modes together explained 4% of the variance in the rolefunction mode. The self-concept and rolefunction modes explained 3% of the variance in the interdependence mode. The focal stimulus explained 7% of the variance in the physical mode, and age explained 1% of the variance in the focal stimulus. These findings indicate that the variance explained by application of the RAM to the study variables was not very strong. However, the soundness of the final path model was confirmed by decomposition of the bivariate correlations [37].

5. Discussion and Conclusion

The RAM helped to put the concepts of the interest of this study into perspective and guided the analysis of how each variable influenced other variables. However, physical impairment, remaining working, and family structure explained only a small percent of the variance in decision making on AD completion. It might be that the constructed instruments did not completely operationalize the concepts which is a disadvantage to using secondary data sets [38]. Or it can also suggest the complexity of the AD completion process. Conducting a study with instruments to fully operationalize the concepts would be helpful or an AD completion process could be a decision-making process beyond reasonable decision making.

There was no significant path from contextual stimuli and residual stimuli to the focal stimuli except for age, and age had a very small path coefficient. Contrary to the RAM, this suggests a direct path between the contextual and residual stimuli to the adaptive response. This also suggests that a possible theoretical framework modification for future research is needed. This same proposition was pointed out by a study done by Robinson [39] where a direct path from the contextual stimuli to the adaptive response was proposed.

This study supports other reports where hospitalization precipitates AD completion but only where there are decrements in physical function as well. The greater the physical impairment, the more the were completed. Participants in this study were relatively older and noninstitutionalized, so the AD completion rate of more than 50% suggests that ADs are more acceptable to this population. It is also logical to deduce that hospitalization reflects more physical impairment, and more physical impairment should make individuals more aware of the issues related to end of life care and more receptive to AD information. The path model showed that the physical mode had the greatest positive influence on decision making on ADs. This is supported by the literature [40, 41]. The paths also indicated that those who stayed connected with society were more likely to have AD completed. It is possible that those who were connected with society through work had opportunities to discuss a variety of health concerns with others, including end of life care. It may also be attributed to those who were still working or doing volunteer work wanted to maintain their independence through making their own end of life decisions. Those living in close proximity to their family were less likely to complete an AD. Such individuals may expect family members to decide on end of life care under the assumption that family members know what they would want rather than complete a legal document.

It is also worth noting that those who had discussion on ADs with their family and healthcare providers did not necessarily complete ADs. Decision making on AD completion is an ensemble of processes and cannot be predicted by a single variable or a single process. Recent literature has focused on effectiveness of discussion on end of life care planning [8]. This study provided some variables (such as physical impairment, self-rated health status, family closeness, and social involvement) that could help to design a motivational interview model for advance care planning discussion [42]. Healthcare workers should provide information in a sensitive way, without causing undue stress. Advance care planning discussions in settings other than hospitals might be more natural and less stressful. Recent study also supports this model of care and stated that early discussion should emphasize managing symptoms, strengthening coping, and cultivating illness understanding [43]. Education programs should encourage patients and families to actively participate in this discussion as early as possible. Those who received health care provider's personal request on initiating advance care planning have high completion rates on advance directives [44]. Health care workers in any health care setting should assess each individual's physical function, personal perception of the illness, family, and social factors and determine the right approach to promote adaptation. Further studies are needed to develop reliable instruments to study variables that promote adaptation and improve quality of life at the end of life by introducing a motivational discussion actively participated by patients and family.

Acknowledgments

The author acknowledge the mentoring from Dr. Carolyn Kee, Professor at Georgia State University, and Bidu Viswanathan, Statistician at Emory University.

References

[1] U.S. National Library of Medicine, NIoH, "Aging Population Issues," U.S. National Library of Medicine, National Institutes of Health, 2013, http://www.nlm.nih.gov/hsrinfo/aging_population_issues.html.

[2] National Vital Statistics Reports, "Deaths: Preliminary Data for 2011," 2011, http://www.cdc.gov/nchs/data/nvsr/nvsr61/nvsr61_06.pdf.

[3] M. J. Field and C. K. Cassel, *Approaching Death: Improving Care at the End of Life*, National Academy Press, Washington, DC, USA, 1997.

[4] N. A. Desbiens, N. Mueller-Rizner, A. F. Connors Jr., N. S. Wenger, and J. Lynn, "The symptom burden of seriously ill hospitalized patients," *Journal of Pain & Symptom Management*, vol. 17, no. 4, pp. 248–255, 1999.

[5] W. K. H. Fakhoury, M. McCarthy, and J. Addington-Hall, "The effects of the clinical characteristics of dying cancer patients on informal caregivers' satisfaction with palliative care," *Palliative Medicine*, vol. 11, no. 2, pp. 107–115, 1997.

[6] L. C. Hanson, M. Danis, and J. Garrett, "What is wrong with end-of-life care? Opinions of bereaved family members," *Journal of the American Geriatrics Society*, vol. 45, no. 11, pp. 1339–1344, 1997.

[7] G. N. Thompson, S. E. McClement, V. H. Menec, and H. M. Chochinov, "Understanding bereaved family members' dissatisfaction with end-of-life care in nursing homes," *Journal of Gerontological Nursing*, vol. 38, no. 10, pp. 49–60, 2012.

[8] C. P. Sabatino, "The evolution of health care advance planning law and policy," *Milbank Quarterly*, vol. 88, no. 2, pp. 211–239, 2010.

[9] S. Hazelett, K. R. Baughman, B. R. Palmisano, M. Sanders, and R. E. Ludwick, "Factors associated with advance care planning discussions by area agency on aging care managers," *American Journal of Hospice and Palliative Medicine*, vol. 30, no. 8, pp. 759–763, 2013.

[10] S. W. Salmond and E. David, "Attitudes toward advance directives and advance directive completion rates," *Orthopaedic Nursing*, vol. 24, no. 2, pp. 117–129, 2005.

[11] C. White, "An exploration of decision-making factors regarding advance directives in a long-term care facility," *Journal of the American Academy of Nurse Practitioners*, vol. 17, no. 1, pp. 14–20, 2005.

[12] G. S. Winzelberg, L. C. Hanson, and J. A. Tulsky, "Beyond autonomy: diversifying end-of-life decision-making approaches to serve patients and families," *Journal of the American Geriatrics Society*, vol. 53, no. 6, pp. 1046–1050, 2005.

[13] E. H. Elpern, S. B. Yellen, and L. A. Burton, "A preliminary investigation of opinions and behaviors regarding advance directives for medical care," *American Journal of Critical Care*, vol. 2, no. 2, pp. 161–167, 1993.

[14] L. B. Gerald, B. Sanderson, L. Fish et al., "Advance directives in cardiac and pulmonary rehabilitation patients," *Journal of Cardiopulmonary Rehabilitation*, vol. 20, no. 6, pp. 340–345, 2000.

[15] J. R. Levin, N. S. Wenger, J. G. Ouslander et al., "Life-sustaining treatment decisions for nursing home residents: who discusses, who decides and what is decided?" *Journal of the American Geriatrics Society*, vol. 47, no. 1, pp. 82–87, 1999.

[16] K. R. Waite, A. D. Federman, D. M. McCarthy et al., "Literacy and race as risk factors for low rates of advance directives in older adults," *Journal of American Geriatric Society*, vol. 61, no. 3, pp. 403–406, 2013.

[17] R. Douglas and H. N. Brown, "Patients' attitudes toward advance directives," *Journal of Nursing Scholarship*, vol. 34, no. 1, pp. 61–65, 2002.

[18] J. K. Cooper, J. A. Weber, P. Evans, and K. Juozapavicius, "End-of-life decisions: physicians as advocates for advance directives," *Journal of the American Osteopathic Association*, vol. 101, no. 10, pp. 571–575, 2001.

[19] G. P. Eleazer, C. A. Hornung, C. B. Egbert et al., "The relationship between ethnicity and advance directives in a frail older population," *Journal of the American Geriatrics Society*, vol. 44, no. 8, pp. 938–943, 1996.

[20] G. B. Zaide, R. Pekmezaris, C. N. Nouryan et al., "Ethnicity, race, and advance directives in an inpatient palliative care consultation service," *Palliat Support Care*, vol. 11, no. 1, pp. 5–11, 2013.

[21] H. B. Degenholtz, R. A. Arnold, A. Meisel, and J. R. Lave, "Persistence of racial disparities in advance care plan documents among nursing home residents," *Journal of the American Geriatrics Society*, vol. 50, no. 2, pp. 378–381, 2002.

[22] R. S. Morrison, L. H. Zayas, M. Mulvihill, S. A. Baskin, and D. E. Meier, "Barriers to completion of health care proxies: an examination of ethnic differences," *Archives of Internal Medicine*, vol. 158, no. 22, pp. 2493–2497, 1998.

[23] M. T. Nolan, M. Hughes, D. P. Narendra et al., "When patients lack capacity: the roles that patients with terminal diagnoses would choose for their physicians and loved ones in making medical decisions," *Journal of Pain & Symptom Management*, vol. 30, no. 4, pp. 342–353, 2005.

[24] E. H. Bradley, L. C. Walker, T. T. Wetle, and S. M. Horwitz, "Advance directives and the role of health beliefs," *Journal of Mental Health and Aging*, vol. 4, no. 3, pp. 379–392, 1998.

[25] J. E. Heffner and C. Barbieri, "End-of-life care preferences of patients enrolled in cardiovascular rehabilitation programs," *Chest*, vol. 117, no. 5, pp. 1474–1481, 2000.

[26] P. H. Ditto, W. D. Smucker, J. H. Danks et al., "Stability of older adults' preferences for life-sustaining medical treatment," *Health Psychology*, vol. 22, no. 6, pp. 605–615, 2003.

[27] M. D. Mezey, R. Leitman, E. L. Mitty, M. M. Bottrell, and G. C. Ramsey, "Why hospital patients do and do not execute an advance directive," *Nursing Outlook*, vol. 48, no. 4, pp. 165–171, 2000.

[28] C. Colenda, M. Jensen, J. Foster, B. Kendrick, K. Mewhinney, and C. Messick, "Variables predicting the completion of an advance directive by older adults," *Annals of Long-Term Care*, vol. 6, no. 3, 1998.

[29] M. L. Rurup, B. D. Onwuteaka-Philipsen, A. Van Der Heide, G. Van Der Wal, and D. J. H. Deeg, "Frequency and determinants of advance directives concerning end-of-life care in The Netherlands," *Social Science and Medicine*, vol. 62, no. 6, pp. 1552–1563, 2006.

[30] K. Bullock, "Promoting advance directives among African Americans: a faith-based model," *Journal of Palliative Medicine*, vol. 9, no. 1, pp. 183–195, 2006.

[31] E. B. Lamont and M. Siegler, "Paradoxes in cancer patients' advance care planning," *Journal of Palliative Medicine*, vol. 3, no. 1, pp. 27–34, 2000.

[32] W. J. McAuley, R. J. Buchanan, S. S. Travis, S. Wang, and M. Kim, "Recent trends in advance directives at nursing home admission and one year after admission," *Gerontologist*, vol. 46, no. 3, pp. 377–381, 2006.

[33] H. A. Andrews and C. Roy, *Essentials of the Roy Adaptation Model*, Appleton-Century-Crofts, Norwalk, Conn, USA, 1986.

[34] C. Roy and H. A. Andrews, *Overview of the Adaptive Modes. The Roy Adaptation Model*, Appleton & Lange, Stamford, Conn, USA, 1999.

[35] UCLA Academic Technology Services, "What does Cronbach's alpha mean?" 2004, http://www.ats.ucla.edu/stat/spss/faq/alpha.html.

[36] B. H. Munro, "Path analysis," in *Statistical Methods for Health Care Research*, B. H. Munro, Ed., Lippincott, Philadelphia, PA, USA, 2000.

[37] S. Wright, "The method of path coefficients," *Annals of Mathematical Statistics*, vol. 5, pp. 161–215, 1934.

[38] H. J. Moriarty, J. A. Deatrick, M. M. Mahon et al., "Issues to consider when choosing and using large national databases for research of families," *Western Journal of Nursing Research*, vol. 21, no. 2, pp. 143–153, 1999.

[39] J. H. Robinson, "Grief responses, coping processes, and social support of widows: research with Roy's model," *Nursing Science Quarterly*, vol. 8, no. 4, pp. 158–164, 1995.

[40] R. S. Phillips, N. S. Wenger, J. Teno et al., "Choices of seriously ill patients about cardiopulmonary resuscitation: correlates and outcomes. SUPPORT Investigators. Study to Understand Prognoses and Preferences for Outcomes and Risks of Treatments," *American Journal of Medicine*, vol. 100, no. 2, pp. 128–137, 1996.

[41] M. B. Scott, "Exploration of factors that impact mode of death in the hemodialysis patient," *ANNA Journal*, vol. 26, no. 6, pp. 577–585, 1999.

[42] R. A. Pearlman, H. Starks, K. C. Cain, and W. G. Cole, "Improvements in advance care planning in the Veterans Affairs System: results of a multifaceted intervention," *Archives of Internal Medicine*, vol. 165, no. 6, pp. 667–674, 2005.

[43] J. Yoong, E. R. Park, J. A. Greer et al., "Early palliative care in advanced lung cancer: a qualitative study," *JAMA Internal Medicine*, vol. 173, no. 4, pp. 283–290, 2013.

[44] G. J. Alano, R. Pekmezaris, J. Y. Tai et al., "Factors influencing older adults to complete advance directives," *Palliative and Supportive Care*, vol. 8, no. 3, pp. 267–275, 2010.

7

Positive Mental Attitude Associated with Lower 35-Year Mortality: The Leisure World Cohort Study

Annlia Paganini-Hill,[1] **Claudia H. Kawas**,[1,2,3] **and María M. Corrada**[1,3,4]

[1]*Department of Neurology, School of Medicine, University of California, Irvine, California, USA*
[2]*Department of Neurobiology & Behavior, School of Biological Sciences, University of California, Irvine, California, USA*
[3]*Institute for Memory Impairments and Neurological Disorders, University of California, Irvine, California, USA*
[4]*Department of Epidemiology, School of Medicine, University of California, Irvine, California, USA*

Correspondence should be addressed to Annlia Paganini-Hill; annliahi@usc.edu

Academic Editor: Carmela R. Balistreri

Background. Although emerging research has suggested that "positive psychological well-being" is associated with better health outcomes, studies of long-term health and mortality in the elderly are limited. This study assessed the relationship of mental attitude and mortality in older adults followed up for 35 years. *Methods.* In the 1980s, the Leisure World Cohort Study recruited residents of a California retirement community to a prospective cohort study of health promotion and disease prevention. Participants completed a postal survey including seven positively worded items from the Zung self-rating depression scale. Age-adjusted and multivariable-adjusted (for lifestyle behaviors and disease conditions) hazard ratios (HRs) for death were calculated using Cox regression for 8682 women and 4992 men (median age at entry, 74 years). During follow-up (1981–2016), 13,405 participants died (median age at death, 88 years). *Results.* In both women and men, HRs for death were significantly related to mental attitude with increasing risk with decreasing positive responses for total attitude and the seven individual items. The multivariable-adjusted HR (95% CI) for death for individuals in the lowest vs. highest quarter of total attitude was 1.24 (1.16, 1.32) for women and 1.30 (1.19, 1.41) for men. Some attenuation in the observed associations occurred after adjustment for potential confounders and after elimination of the first five years of follow-up. *Conclusions.* Our study suggests that persons with negative attitude have an increased risk of death even after many years of follow-up. Research into strategies to improve mental outlook may help improve the quantity as well as the quality of life.

1. Introduction

The number of elderly adults continues to increase as does the need for them to lead lives in good mental and physical condition. Although "positive mental attitude," "psychological well-being," "life satisfaction," and "happiness" are vague concepts, emerging research suggests that they are associated with better health outcomes [1–5] while their opposites "negative mental attitude," "life dissatisfaction," "pessimism," and "depression and depressive symptoms" are associated with poorer outcomes [6–9].

Studies of mental attitude and long-term health (including mortality) in the elderly are limited by sample size and length of follow-up. Four prospective cohort studies of all-cause mortality in the elderly have included more than 10,000 participants [10–13], and only one of these included both sexes [10]. Follow-up has been greater than 10 years in only three studies [10, 14, 15]. Thus, little is known about whether positive mental attitude has any predictive value in old age over a long-time span.

In 1981, we undertook a prospective cohort study of nearly 14,000 elderly women and men in a California retirement community with the aim of studying factors associated with longevity and successful aging. We report here the results of positive mental attitude (seven items from the Zung self-rating depression scale [16]) on all-cause mortality with 35 years of follow-up. To determine whether mental attitude is associated with mortality independently of known predictors of mortality, we adjusted for medical history (hypertension, angina, heart attack, stroke, cancer, diabetes, and arthritis), body mass index, and lifestyle practices (smoking, alcohol consumption, caffeine intake, and exercise). In addition, the large size of our cohort allowed us to analyze the two sexes separately. As those with health problems may have a poorer mental attitude in the time immediately preceding death, the elimination of early deaths permitted us to determine the long-term effect of mental attitude. Thus, our study adds to the existing knowledge on well-being and mortality in the aged.

2. Methods

2.1. Participants and Vital Status. The Leisure World Cohort Study was established in the early 1980s when 13,978 residents (8,877 women and 5,101 men) of a California retirement community (Leisure World Laguna Hills) completed a postal health survey. Recruitment procedures have been previously described [17, 18]. Briefly, residents were recruited in 4 waves: those who owned homes in Leisure World on June 1, 1981, and new residents who had moved into the community and were living there on June 1, 1982, June 1, 1983, and October 1, 1985. Recruitment included mailing the survey with simultaneous advertisements describing the study in the local community newspaper, second and third mailings to nonrespondents, and then telephoning nonrespondents (if a local phone number was listed). The baseline survey asked for information on demographic characteristics (sex, marital status, height, and weight), basic medical history (high blood pressure, heart attack, angina, stroke, diabetes, rheumatoid arthritis, glaucoma, fractures, and cancer), and several personal habits (smoking, alcohol consumption, caffeine intake, vitamin supplement use, and physical activity). The Leisure World population and the cohort are predominantly Caucasian, well-educated, and upper-middle class. Vital status of cohort members was determined by periodic resurvey, annual mailings, search of death indexes, and ascertainment of death certificates. Participants were followed to death or December, 31, 2016, whichever came first. To date, 25 cohort members have been lost to follow-up, including 5 who moved out of the country.

This study was approved by the Institutional Review Boards of the University of Southern California and the University of California, Irvine.

2.2. Mental Attitude Variables. The survey included only the seven positively worded items from the 20-item Zung self-rating depression scale [16]; the other 13 items were not asked. Participants were asked to read the seven items (Table 1) and to indicate "how much of the time the statement describes how you have been feeling during the past week." Possible responses were "none or a little of the time, some of the time, a good part of the time, most or all of the time" and were scored 1 through 4, respectively. A total attitude score (7–28) was calculated by summing the seven responses. A score of 7 indicates that the subject selected "none or a little of the time" as a response to all items and represents the poorest possible mental outlook. A score of 28 indicates that all responses were "most or all of the time" and represents the most positive mental outlook. To account for items with missing responses, we calculated the total attitude score in three ways: (1) calculating the total score only for participants without missing responses, (2) assigning a nonresponse item the lowest score of 1 and including it in the total attitude score, and (3) assigning a nonresponse item the highest score of 4 and including it in the total attitude score. For analyses of individual items, those with missing responses were excluded from the analyses.

2.3. Potential Confounding Variables. Several factors asked on the same survey with the mental attitude variables were previously found to be related to mortality in this cohort. We included these in analyses as potential confounders. *Medical history* was elicited in response to a question "Has a doctor ever told you that you have any of these conditions?" *Smoking* refers to cigarette use [19]. We estimated *daily caffeine intake* by summing the frequency of consumption of each beverage and chocolate multiplied by its average caffeine content (milligrams/standard unit) as 115, 3, 50, 50, and 6 for regular coffee, decaffeinated coffee, tea, cola soft drinks, and chocolate, respectively [20]. Consumption of *alcoholic beverages* was asked separately for wine, beer, and hard liquor and combined into number of alcoholic drinks per day [21]. *Body mass index* (BMI) (weight (kilograms)/height^2 (meters)) was calculated based on self-reported height and weight at baseline and categorized according to federal guidelines: underweight (<18.5), normal weight (18.5–24.9), overweight (25–29.9), and obese (30+) [22]. *Exercise* included active outdoor activities (e.g., swimming, biking, jogging, tennis, and vigorous walking) and active indoor activities (e.g., exercising and dancing). The time spent per day in active activities was calculated by summing the reported times spent in active outdoor and active indoor activities [23]. Previous reports present details of data collection [17–24].

2.4. Statistical Analysis. Differences between women and men were tested using *t*-tests for continuous variables and chi-squared tests for categorical variables. Hazard ratios (HRs) for the association between mental attitude and mortality were calculated separately for women and men using Cox regression analysis [25] with age as the time scale. Participants contributed person-years from age at baseline survey (delayed entry) to age at death or December 31, 2016, whichever occurred first. Total attitude (continuous and quartile categories) as well as the seven individual items were analyzed as independent variables. The reference category for the HRs was "good mental attitude," i.e., response of "most or all of the time" for the seven individual items and

TABLE 1: Attitude questions from the Zung self-rated depression scale in the Leisure World Cohort Study, 1980s, $N = 13,674$.

Attitude statement	No response *N* (%)	None or a little of the time (1) *N* (%)	Some of the time (2) *N* (%)	A good part of the time (3) *N* (%)	Most or all of the time (4) *N* (%)
My mind is as clear as it used to be	104 (0.8%)	233 (1.7%)	823 (6.0%)	3139 (23%)	9375 (69%)
I find it easy to do the things I used to do	156 (1.1%)	969 (7.1%)	3080 (23%)	5214 (38%)	4255 (31%)
I feel hopeful about the future	263 (1.9%)	530 (3.9%)	1438 (11%)	3170 (23%)	8273 (61%)
I find it easy to make decisions	124 (0.9%)	444 (3.2%)	1596 (12%)	4198 (31%)	7312 (53%)
I feel that I am useful and needed	178 (1.3%)	594 (4.3%)	1573 (12%)	2895 (21%)	8434 (62%)
My life is pretty full	157 (1.1%)	540 (3.9%)	1321 (9.7%)	3286 (24%)	8370 (61%)
I still enjoy the things I used to	120 (0.9%)	514 (3.8%)	1662 (12%)	3374 (25%)	8004 (59%)
Quarters of total attitude (sum of scores for the above seven items)		Q1 7–20	Q2 21–24	Q3 25–26	Q4 27–28
All persons: those with no response on any of the seven items included in no response category	657 (4.8%)	2646 (19%)	3421 (25%)	2757 (20%)	4193 (31%)
All persons: if no response on any item that response recoded as 1 = "none or a little of the time"		3057 (22%)	3633 (27%)	2791 (20%)	4193 (31%)
All persons: if no response on any item that response recoded as 4 = "most or all of the time"		2789 (20%)	3617 (26%)	2917 (21%)	4357 (32%)

a total attitude score of 27-28. To control for potential confounders, we performed analysis adjusting for factors previously found to be related to mortality in this cohort: smoking (never, past, and current), alcohol intake (0, ≤1, 2-3, and 4+ drinks/day), caffeine (<50, 50–99, 100–199, 200–399, and 400+ mg/day), exercise (0, ¼, ½, ¾-1¾, and 2+ hour/day), BMI (underweight, normal, overweight, and obese), and histories (yes/no) of hypertension, angina, heart attack, stroke, diabetes, rheumatoid arthritis, and cancer [19–23]. To account for the possibility that recent disease development may have altered attitude as well as be related to mortality, we repeated the analyses after excluding the first five years of follow-up. We performed sensitivity analyses to explore how results would change if the total attitude score on the Zung scale was computed with missing items assigned to either the lowest value (1 = none or little of the time) or alternatively to the highest value (4 = all or most of the time). Statistical analyses were performed using SAS® version 9.4 (SAS Institute Inc., Cary, NC). All tests were two-sided, and no adjustment in the *p*-values was made for multiple comparisons.

3. Results

After excluding 89 subjects with missing information on all seven attitude items and an additional 215 with missing information on potential confounding variables, data on 8682 women and 4992 men were analyzed. At study entry, the participants ranged in age from 44 to 101 years (median, 74 years). By December 31, 2016, 13,405 (98%) had died at ages 59 to 110 years (median, 88 years).

Table 1 presents the responses to the seven individual attitude questions. While 13,017 (95%) participants answered all seven questions, 443 did not answer one, 123 two, 28 three, 20 four, 9 five, and 34 six. The distributions of responses differed among the seven statements. The statement "I find it easy to do the things I used to do" had the least number of "most or all of the time" responses (31%) and far fewer than the other statements (53–69%).

Table 2 gives selected characteristics of the participants by sex. Men were on average older than women at study entry (74 vs. 73 years), and a smaller proportion were alive at the end of follow-up (0.9% vs. 2.7%). Men also had on average a greater BMI, exercised more, and consumed more alcohol and caffeine than women, but a smaller proportion never smoked. More men had a history of angina, heart attack, stroke, and diabetes, while more women had high blood pressure, cancer, and rheumatoid arthritis. Women were more likely to have a higher attitude score than men (score ≥25: 52% vs. 50%). All differences were statistically significant ($p < 0.02$).

HRs of mortality for the seven individual attitude items and for the total attitude score are shown in Table 3 for women and in Table 4 for men. Analysis of total attitude score by quartiles showed higher mortality with lower scores (more negative attitude) in both women and men (Figure 1). In the model fully adjusted for age and potential confounders, women with scores of <21 had 24% greater risk of death and men had a 30% greater risk of death compared with persons with scores of 27-28; these risks were 22% and 24% after exclusion of the first five years of follow-up including 854 deaths in women and 1102 deaths in men. As a continuous variable, risk of death significantly increased 2% (women) and 4% (men) for each unit decrease in the total attitude score. In sensitivity analyses that calculated the total score by assigning either the lowest value (1 = none or little of the time) or the highest value (4 = all or most of the time) to the missing items, the results were very similar to those where individuals with missing items were excluded when computing the total score (Tables 3 and 4).

The seven attitude items similarly showed a higher risk of death with increasing level of negative attitude. Adjustment for potential confounders resulted in modest attenuation of risks (less than 20%), and the HRs for poor mental attitude (responses of "none or little of the time" and "some of the time") remained statistically significant for all items except "I find it easy to make decisions" in

TABLE 2: Baseline characteristics in the Leisure World Cohort Study, 1980s.

Characteristic	Total (N = 13,674)	Men (N = 4992)	Women (N = 8682)
		Mean ± SD	
Age at baseline, years	73.6 ± 7.3	74.3 ± 7.2	73.2 ± 7.4
Age at last follow-up, years	87.6 ± 7.4	86.1 ± 7.1	88.5 ± 7.4
Follow-up years	14.0 ± 8.3	11.7 ± 7.7	15.3 ± 8.3
Body mass index, kg/m^2	23.5 ± 3.3	24.2 ± 2.9	23.1 ± 3.4
Exercise, hours/day	1.0 ± 1.2	1.1 ± 1.3	0.9 ± 1.1
Alcohol, drinks/day	1.4 ± 1.4	1.6 ± 1.5	1.2 ± 1.2
Caffeine, mg/day	171 ± 168	176 ± 172	168 ± 166
		N (%)	
History of disease			
High blood pressure	5335 (39%)	1803 (36%)	3532 (41%)
Angina	1547 (11%)	728 (15%)	819 (9.4%)
Heart attack	1396 (10%)	828 (17%)	568 (6.5%)
Stroke	670 (4.9%)	351 (7.0%)	319 (3.7%)
Cancer	1593 (12%)	467 (9.4%)	1126 (13%)
Diabetes	841 (6.2%)	414 (8.3%)	427 (4.9%)
Rheumatoid arthritis	807 (5.9%)	220 (4.4%)	587 (6.8%)
Cigarette use			
Never	6436 (47%)	1664 (33%)	4772 (55%)
Past	5724 (42%)	2900 (58%)	2824 (33%)
Current	1514 (11%)	428 (8.6%)	1086 (12%)
Total attitude			
Missing response	657 (4.8%)	207 (4.1%)	450 (5.2%)
7–20	2646 (19%)	995 (20%)	1651 (19%)
21–24	3421 (25%)	1286 (26%)	2135 (25%)
25–26	2757 (20%)	1051 (21%)	1706 (20%)
27–28	4193 (31%)	1453 (29%)	2740 (32%)
Alive at follow-up	269 (2.0%)	44 (0.9%)	225 (2.6%)

Abbreviation: SD, standard deviation. $p < 0.0001$ for all differences between men and women except caffeine ($p < 0.009$) and total attitude ($p < 0.0006$).

women. For all seven items, the HRs for the poorest mental attitude (response of "none or little of the time") were larger in men than women (about 20% or more except for "My mind is clear as it used to be"). With elimination of the first five years of follow-up, the age-adjusted HRs for women changed by less than 10% for all items except "My mind is as clear as it used to be," where the HR for the poorest mental attitude (response of "none or little of the time") was reduced from 1.43 to 1.14. The multivariable-adjusted HRs showed smaller reductions, and the HRs for the poorest mental attitude (response of "none or a little of the time") for three of the seven items ("mind is clear," "easy to make decisions," and "feel useful and needed") were no longer statistically significant. For men with the elimination of the first five years of follow-up, the age-adjusted HRs for the poorest mental attitude (response of "none or a little of the time") for all seven items were reduced 10–15% but remained statistically significant; the HRs for other response categories changed by less than 10%. The multivariable-adjusted HRs showed smaller reductions, and HRs for the poorest mental attitude remained statistically significant for all seven items.

4. Discussion

We found modest increased risks of death with poor mental attitude that persisted after adjustment for potential confounders including disease history and lifestyle practices. The observed risks, especially for the most negative attitudes, were attenuated after eliminating the first five years of follow-up suggesting that diseases leading to early death might be the cause of some of the negativity. The associations found after adjustment and elimination of the first five years of follow-up may thus be more accurate from a perspective of a causal relationship. Although mental attitude is associated with lifestyle practices and disease states which are also related with mortality, a poor attitude appears to confer additional risk of death.

Those with a positive mental attitude or psychological well-being differ from those with a more negative outlook on a number of health processes—healthier lipid profile, lower levels of inflammatory markers, higher levels of serum antioxidants, better immune responses, and healthier autonomic function [26]—and on a number of healthier behaviors—increased physical activity, nonsmoking, healthier diets, and higher quality of sleep [27]. These may partly serve as mechanisms for the association of mental attitude with mortality.

Previous prospective population-based studies have evaluated mental attitude and all-cause mortality in older population groups [10–15, 28–35]. However, follow-up has generally been less than 10 years, the cohort size less than 10,000, or the study has included only one sex. Table 5 summarizes these studies. Similar to our study, all previous studies except two [12, 28] found that persons with the most positive attitude (measured in different ways) had the lowest

Table 3: Attitude and hazard ratio of death among women: the Leisure World Cohort Study, 1981–2016.

	All subjects (N = 8682)						Excluding first five years of follow-up (N = 7828)					
	No. subjects[†]	No. deaths	Model 1[a] HR	Model 1[a] 95% CI	Model 2[b] HR	Model 2[b] 95% CI	No. subjects[†]	No. deaths	Model 1[a] HR	Model 1[a] 95% CI	Model 2[b] HR	Model 2[b] 95% CI
My mind is as clear as it used to be												
None or little of the time	124	121	1.43	1.20, 1.72	1.28	1.07, 1.54	78	75	1.14	0.91, 1.43	1.02	0.81, 1.29
Some of the time	495	491	1.39	1.27 1.52	1.27	1.16, 1.40	406	402	1.43	1.30, 1.59	1.33	1.20, 1.47
A good part of the time	1937	1901	1.09	1.03, 1.15	1.07	1.01, 1.12	1716	1680	1.09	1.03, 1.15	1.07	1.01, 1.13
Most or all of the time	6048	5866	1.00		1.00		5558	5366	1.00		1.00	
I find it easy to do the things I used to do												
None or little of the time	544	539	1.65	1.51, 1.82	1.39	1.26, 1.53	373	368	1.54	1.38, 1.72	1.30	1.16, 1.46
Some of the time	1920	1898	1.29	1.22, 1.37	1.18	1.11, 1.26	1635	1613	1.30	1.22, 1.38	1.18	1.11, 1.26
A good part of the time	3283	3214	1.03	0.98, 1.09	0.99	0.94, 1.04	3072	3003	1.05	0.99, 1.11	1.01	0.95, 1.06
Most or all of the time	2826	2697	1.00		1.00		2664	2535	1.00		1.00	
I feel hopeful about the future												
None or little of the time	331	328	1.53	1.36, 1.71	1.34	1.20, 1.50	242	239	1.46	1.28, 1.66	1.29	1.13, 1.47
Some of the time	924	911	1.25	1.16, 1.34	1.16	1.08, 1.24	785	772	1.22	1.13, 1.31	1.13	1.05, 1.22
A good part of the time	1973	1941	1.09	1.04, 1.15	1.07	1.02, 1.13	1767	1735	1.08	1.02, 1.14	1.07	1.01, 1.13
Most or all of the time	5275	5099	1.00		1.00		4885	4709	1.00		1.00	
I find it easy to make decisions												
None or little of the time	289	282	1.18	1.05, 1.33	1.10	0.97, 1.24	213	206	1.09	0.95, 1.26	1.04	0.90, 1.19
Some of the time	1101	1080	1.10	1.03, 1.17	1.05	0.99, 1.13	967	946	1.11	1.03, 1.18	1.07	0.99, 1.14
A good part of the time	2698	2642	0.96	0.92, 1.01	0.96	0.91, 1.01	2451	2395	0.97	0.92, 1.02	0.96	0.91, 1.01
Most or all of the time	4509	4370	1.00		1.00		4125	3986	1.00		1.00	
I feel that I am useful and needed												
None or little of the time	412	406	1.28	1.16, 1.42	1.14	1.03, 1.26	305	299	1.21	1.08, 1.36	1.09	0.97, 1.22
Some of the time	1038	1027	1.24	1.16, 1.33	1.16	1.09, 1.24	876	865	1.21	1.13, 1.31	1.14	1.06, 1.23
A good part of the time	1750	1705	1.03	0.97, 1.08	1.02	0.96, 1.08	1581	1536	1.02	0.96, 1.08	1.01	0.95, 1.07
Most or all of the time	5364	5203	1.00		1.00		4976	4815	1.00		1.00	
My life is pretty full												
None or little of the time	316	310	1.58	1.41, 1.78	1.33	1.19, 1.50	228	222	1.45	1.26, 1.66	1.22	1.06, 1.40
Some of the time	856	848	1.38	1.28, 1.48	1.25	1.16, 1.35	701	693	1.33	1.23, 1.44	1.21	1.12, 1.31
A good part of the time	1996	1955	1.14	1.08, 1.20	1.09	1.03, 1.14	1788	1747	1.14	1.08, 1.20	1.09	1.03, 1.15
Most or all of the time	5412	5242	1.00		1.00		5034	4864	1.00		1.00	
I still enjoy the things I used to												
None or little of the time	289	285	1.62	1.44, 1.82	1.39	1.23, 1.57	200	196	1.44	1.25, 1.67	1.27	1.10, 1.46
Some of the time	990	973	1.29	1.20, 1.38	1.18	1.10, 1.26	820	803	1.27	1.18, 1.37	1.17	1.08, 1.26
A good part of the time	2011	1978	1.07	1.02, 1.13	1.02	0.97, 1.08	1812	1779	1.07	1.01, 1.13	1.02	0.97, 1.08
Most or all of the time	5304	5133	1.00		1.00		4925	4754	1.00		1.00	
Attitude score (persons with missing items excluded)												
<21	1651	1632	1.38	1.29, 1.46	1.24	1.16, 1.32	1354	1335	1.35	1.26, 1.44	1.22	1.14, 1.31
21–24	2135	2092	1.12	1.05, 1.18	1.07	1.01, 1.13	1927	1883	1.11	1.05, 1.18	1.06	1.00, 1.13
25-26	1706	1662	1.02	0.96, 1.09	0.99	0.94, 1.06	1589	1543	1.03	0.96, 1.10	1.00	0.94, 1.07
27-28	2740	2625	1.00		1.00		2592	2472	1.00		1.00	
Attitude score (missing items given score of 1)												
<21	1925	1904	1.37	1.29, 1.45	1.23	1.16, 1.31	1561	1540	1.34	1.26, 1.43	1.22	1.14, 1.30
21–24	2289	2244	1.12	1.06, 1.19	1.06	1.00, 1.13	2067	2021	1.12	1.06, 1.19	1.07	1.01, 1.13
25-26	1728	1684	1.02	0.96, 1.09	1.00	0.94, 1.06	1608	1562	1.03	0.97, 1.10	1.00	0.94, 1.07
27-28	2740	2625	1.00		1.00		2592	2472	1.00		1.00	
Attitude score (missing items given score of 4)												
<21	1741	1721	1.38	1.30, 1.47	1.24	1.17, 1.32	1418	1397	1.34	1.26, 1.44	1.22	1.14, 1.30
21–24	2272	2227	1.12	1.06, 1.18	1.07	1.01, 1.13	2039	1994	1.11	1.05, 1.18	1.07	1.01, 1.13
25-26	1823	1779	1.04	0.98, 1.10	1.01	0.95, 1.07	1686	1642	1.04	0.97, 1.10	1.01	0.95, 1.08
27-28	2846	2730	1.00		1.00		2686	2570	1.00		1.00	

Abbreviations: CI, confidence interval; HR, hazard ratio. [†]Subjects do not always total 8682 or 7828 due to those with missing values. [a]Model 1: adjusted for age (i.e., age as time scale). [b]Model 2: adjusted for age, smoking, body mass index, exercise, alcohol intake, caffeine consumption, and histories of hypertension, angina, heart attack, stroke, diabetes, rheumatoid arthritis, and cancer.

TABLE 4: Attitude and hazard ratio of death among men: the Leisure World Cohort Study, 1981–2016.

	All subjects (N = 4992)						Excluding first five years of follow-up (N = 3980)					
	No. subjects†	No. deaths	Model 1[a] HR	Model 1[a] 95% CI	Model 2[b] HR	Model 2[b] 95% CI	No. subjects†	No. deaths	Model 1[a] HR	Model 1[a] 95% CI	Model 2[b] HR	Model 2[b] 95% CI
My mind is as clear as it used to be												
None or little of the time	109	109	1.55	1.27, 1.88	1.41	1.16, 1.71	55	55	1.38	1.06, 1.80	1.34	1.02, 1.75
Some of the time	328	327	1.47	1.31, 1.65	1.31	1.17, 1.47	203	202	1.44	1.25, 1.66	1.30	1.13, 1.50
A good part of the time	1202	1194	1.10	1.03, 1.17	1.06	0.99, 1.13	957	949	1.16	1.08, 1.25	1.13	1.05, 1.21
Most or all of the time	3327	3292	1.00		1.00		2749	2713	1.00		1.00	
I find it easy to do the things I used to do												
None or little of the time	425	425	2.02	1.81, 2.25	1.64	1.46, 1.83	205	205	1.76	1.52, 2.05	1.49	1.28, 1.73
Some of the time	1160	1157	1.32	1.22, 1.42	1.19	1.10, 1.28	848	845	1.32	1.21, 1.44	1.20	1.10, 1.32
A good part of the time	1931	1914	1.10	1.03, 1.18	1.05	0.98, 1.13	1645	1628	1.13	1.05, 1.22	1.09	1.01, 1.17
Most or all of the time	1429	1405	1.00		1.00		1250	1225	1.00		1.00	
I feel hopeful about the future												
None or little of the time	199	199	1.79	1.55, 2.07	1.51	1.31, 1.75	104	104	1.62	1.33, 1.98	1.46	1.20, 1.79
Some of the time	514	512	1.31	1.19, 1.44	1.17	1.06, 1.29	353	351	1.23	1.10, 1.38	1.11	0.99, 1.24
A good part of the time	1197	1188	1.04	0.98, 1.12	0.99	0.92, 1.06	953	944	1.04	0.96, 1.12	0.99	0.92, 1.07
Most or all of the time	2998	2966	1.00		1.00		2520	2487	1.00		1.00	
I find it easy to make decisions												
None or little of the time	155	155	1.90	1.62, 2.24	1.53	1.30, 1.80	71	71	1.83	1.44, 2.31	1.48	1.17, 1.89
Some of the time	495	494	1.17	1.07, 1.29	1.10	1.00, 1.21	354	353	1.14	1.02, 1.27	1.07	0.96, 1.20
A good part of the time	1500	1489	1.07	1.01, 1.14	1.03	0.96, 1.09	1207	1196	1.09	1.01, 1.17	1.04	0.97, 1.12
Most or all of the time	2803	2771	1.00		1.00		2317	2284	1.00		1.00	
I feel that I am useful and needed												
None or little of the time	182	181	1.83	1.57, 2.12	1.64	1.40, 1.90	88	87	1.53	1.23, 1.89	1.44	1.16, 1.78
Some of the time	535	531	1.29	1.17, 1.41	1.14	1.04, 1.25	374	370	1.20	1.07, 1.33	1.06	0.95, 1.18
A good part of the time	1145	1136	1.10	1.02, 1.17	1.08	1.01, 1.16	907	898	1.06	0.98, 1.14	1.05	0.97, 1.13
Most or all of the time	3070	3041	1.00		1.00		2575	2546	1.00		1.00	
My life is pretty full												
None or little of the time	224	223	1.89	1.64, 2.16	1.56	1.36, 1.80	111	110	1.59	1.31, 1.92	1.38	1.14, 1.68
Some of the time	465	462	1.37	1.24, 1.51	1.20	1.09, 1.33	306	303	1.25	1.11, 1.41	1.10	0.97, 1.24
A good part of the time	1290	1279	1.14	1.07, 1.22	1.06	0.99, 1.14	1022	1011	1.14	1.06, 1.23	1.07	1.00, 1.15
Most or all of the time	2958	2929	1.00		1.00		2509	2480	1.00		1.00	
I still enjoy the things I used to												
None or little of the time	225	225	2.23	1.95, 2.56	1.76	1.53, 2.03	86	86	1.86	1.50, 2.31	1.45	1.16, 1.81
Some of the time	672	668	1.36	1.25, 1.48	1.20	1.10, 1.31	455	451	1.31	1.18, 1.45	1.18	1.06, 1.31
A good part of the time	1363	1354	1.11	1.04, 1.19	1.05	0.99, 1.13	1116	1107	1.14	1.06, 1.22	1.08	1.00, 1.16
Most or all of the time	2700	2669	1.00		1.00		2305	2274	1.00		1.00	
Attitude score (persons with missing items excluded)												
<21	995	993	1.54	1.42, 1.67	1.30	1.19, 1.41	631	629	1.43	1.30, 1.58	1.24	1.12, 1.37
21–24	1286	1273	1.16	1.08, 1.25	1.09	1.01, 1.18	1056	1043	1.19	1.10, 1.29	1.13	1.04, 1.23
25-26	1051	1041	1.13	1.04, 1.22	1.06	0.98 1.15	893	883	1.17	1.08, 1.28	1.12	1.02, 1.22
27-28	1453	1435	1.00		1.00		1270	1252	1.00		1.00	
Attitude score (missing items given score of 1)												
<21	1132	1130	1.55	1.43, 1.67	1.32	1.21, 1.43	706	704	1.43	1.31, 1.57	1.25	1.14, 1.38
21–24	1344	1330	1.15	1.07, 1.24	1.08	1.00, 1.16	1103	1089	1.18	1.09, 1.28	1.12	1.03, 1.22
25-26	1063	1053	1.13	1.04, 1.23	1.06	0.98, 1.15	901	891	1.18	1.08, 1.28	1.12	1.03, 1.22
27-28	1453	1435	1.00		1.00		1270	1252	1.00		1.00	
Attitude score (missing items given score of 4)												
<21	1048	1046	1.55	1.43, 1.67	1.31	1.21, 1.42	655	653	1.43	1.30, 1.57	1.24	1.13, 1.37
21–24	1345	1332	1.17	1.09, 1.26	1.10	1.02, 1.18	1092	1079	1.20	1.10, 1.30	1.13	1.04, 1.23
25-26	1094	1084	1.13	1.04, 1.22	1.06	0.98 1.14	924	914	1.17	1.08, 1.28	1.11	1.02, 1.21
27-28	1505	1486	1.00		1.00		1309	1290	1.00		1.00	

Abbreviations: CI, confidence interval; HR, hazard ratio. †Subjects do not always total 4992 or 3980 due to those with missing values. [a]Model 1: adjusted for age (i.e., age as time scale). [b]Model 2: adjusted for age, smoking, body mass index, exercise, alcohol intake, caffeine consumption, and histories of hypertension, angina, heart attack, stroke, diabetes, rheumatoid arthritis, and cancer.

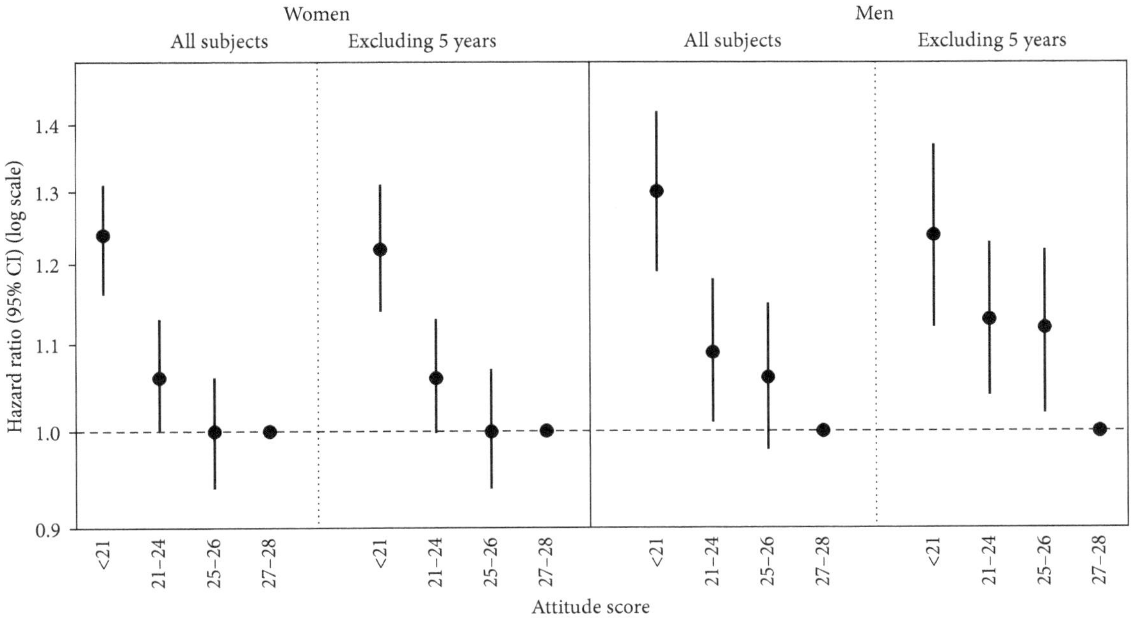

FIGURE 1: Attitude score and hazard ratios of death: the Leisure World Cohort Study, 1981–2016. Note: data shown are from analyses of total attitude score as quartile categories excluding persons with missing items. HRs and 95% confidence intervals derived from Cox regression analysis model 2, which adjusts for age (as the time scale), smoking, body mass index, exercise, alcohol intake, caffeine consumption, and histories of hypertension, angina, heart attack, stroke, diabetes, rheumatoid arthritis, and cancer.

risk of death, and that the risk was attenuated after adjustment of health conditions and lifestyle factors. An inverse dose-response relationship (decreased risk of mortality with increasing levels of positive mental attitude) was seen in both women and men and in studies conducted in diverse countries (USA, Canada, England, the Netherlands, Spain, Sweden, Finland, and China).

As in previous studies, risk of death was attenuated after adjustment of health conditions and lifestyle factors associated with both mental attitude and survival. To reduce concerns that recent changes in mental attitude may be due to underlying illness, we analyzed the data excluding participants who died within five years of study baseline. Likewise, early deaths were eliminated in the Nurses' Health Study (within two years) [11] and the Million Women Study (within five years) [12] to reduce these concerns about reverse causality. However, mental attitude may alter the time course of disease processes and influence health behaviors directly, so the possibility of overadjustment exists and we may be adjusting for the effect of intermediate factors in the causal pathway.

Although some studies have evaluated the association of the Zung self-rating depression scale with mortality [36–38], only those reporting results on the individual items can be directly compared to our study. Takeida and colleagues analyzed the Zung scale as a predictor of death in a Japanese cohort of 2,166 aged 60–74 years and followed five years [39]. Of the seven items included in our study, they found six significantly related to mortality. Those items and their relative risks (RR) were "I find it easy to do the things I used to" (RR = 3.84), "My life is pretty full" (RR = 2.39), "I find it easy to make decisions" (RR = 2.27), "My mind is as clear as it used to be" (RR = 2.05), "I feel hopeful about the future" (RR = 1.67), and "I feel that I am useful and needed" (RR = 1.44). The item "I still enjoy the things I used to do" (RR = 1.35) was not related to mortality. In our older cohort, all seven items were related to mortality. That the individual items we used had a high predictive value of risk of death indicates that refusing to answer any single question does not invalidate the use of the questionnaire nor does the use of the seven rather than the 20 items of the Zung scale.

Several strengths and limitations of this study must be considered. Our data on mental attitude were self-reported using a mailed questionnaire. The seven items included in our survey were extracted from the Zung self-rating depression scale, but we did not ask the other 13 items. Thus, we are not able to compare our results with studies reporting the full Zung scale. Similar to other studies, we previously found our mental attitude score to be related to suicide in the first five years of follow-up [40]. However, conclusions regarding attitude are limited by the crudeness of measurement. Although assessing the true level of attitude is difficult, self-reported rating is suitable for ranking of individuals.

Our large cohort size allowed us to analyze men and women separately. We did this for comparison with other studies reporting sex-specific results [11, 13, 30], because of differences between men and women on baseline characteristics and mortality rates, and due to the possibility of differential response on attitude between men and women. Chang and coworkers showed significant sex differences in reporting of psychological outcomes with more women

Table 5: Prospective cohort studies of mental attitude and mortality in the elderly.

First author, date [reference]	Study name Population	Number	Age (years)	Follow-up (years)	Sex	Mental attitude instrument	HR, 95% CI† Age- and sex-adjusted Most adjusted model
Gitlay, 2004 [30]	Arnhem Elderly Study The Netherlands	999	65–85	Mean = 9	M,F	Scale of Subjective Well-Being for Older Persons	0.55, 0.42–0.77 0.71, 0.52–0.97
Pitkala, 2004 [32]	Helsinki Aging Study Finland	491	75, 80, 85	10	M,F	6 questions on positive life orientation	0.67, 0.53–0.87‡ 0.89, 0.83–0.93
Tindle, 2009 [13]	Women's Health Initiative USA	97,253	50–79	8	F	Life Orientation Test-Revised	— 0.86, 0.79–0.93
Koopmans, 2010 [14]	Arnhem Elderly Study The Netherlands	861	65–85	15	M,F	2 "happiness" questions	0.78, 0.64–0.95 0.92, 0.75–1.14
Benito-Leon, 2010 [29]	Neurological Disorders in Central Spain	2516	65+	7	M,F	Philadelphia Geriatric Center Morale Scale	1.60, 1.29–2.21‡ 1.35, 1.00–1.81
Tilvis, 2012 [35]	National Sample Finland	2490	>75	5	M,F	6 questions on positive life orientation	0.65, 0.53–0.81 0.85, 0.67–1.08
Niklasson, 2015 [31]	GERDA Sweden and Finland	646	85+	5	M,F	Philadelphia Geriatric Center Morale Scale	1.73, 1.33–2.26 1.36, 1.03–1.80
St John, 2015 [33]	Manitoba Study of Health and Aging, Canada	1751	65+	5	M,F	Terrible-Delightful Scale	0.75, 0.66–0.86 0.90, 0.78–1.04
Steptoe, 2015 [34]	English Longitudinal Study of Aging	9050	Mean = 65	Mean = 8	M,F	Eudemonic well-being	0.42, 0.36–0.49 0.70, 0.58–0.83
Anthony, 2016 [28]	Rancho Bernardo Study USA	876	50+	<= 12 mean = 8	M,F	Life Orientation Test-Revised	0.98, 0.94–1.02 0.99, 0.94–1.03
Gong, 2016 [10]	Chinese Longitudinal Healthy Longevity Survey	18,676	80–122	16	M,F	7 items on psychological well-being	— 0.84, 0.79–0.88
Liu, 2016 [12]	Million Women Study United Kingdom	719,671	50–69	10	F	"How often do you feel happy?"	1.29, 1.25–1.33 0.98, 0.94–1.01
Kim, 2017 [11]	Nurses' Health Study USA	70,021	Mean = 70	6	F	Life Orientation Test-Revised	0.71, 0.66–0.76* 0.91, 0.85–0.97
Okely, 2018 [15]	Survey of Health Aging and Retirement in Europe	13,596	50+	~12	M,F	CASP-12	0.41, 0.38–0.43 0.57, 0.53–0.61

†HR for high vs. low category of positive mental attitude, except for Benito-Leon, Niklasson, and Liu studies which compared low vs. high category. ‡Unadjusted HR. *Adjusted for additional demographic factors as well.

reporting negative outcomes [41]. This was also seen in several of the prospective studies of attitude and mortality [29, 31], but they did not report sex-specific HRs for death. Differential reporting may help explain the lower HRs for negative attitudes we observed in women compared with men. The cohort reported here is elderly, white, and in the upper middle socioeconomic stratum. Therefore, our results may not be generalizable to other populations.

Our study has the advantages of a prospective design, large size, long and essentially complete follow-up, and the capability to control for numerous potential confounding factors. Still our investigation is an observational study, not a randomized trial. It does, however, suggest that confounders account for only a portion of the associations between mental attitude and risk of death. However, residual confounding due to suboptimal variables or to unmeasured variables remain possibilities.

5. Conclusions

Results in this large elderly cohort with long follow-up are consistent with a modest relationship between mental attitude and long-term mortality. The development of interventions to foster a positive outlook may improve the personal and public health of the elderly and prolong life.

Abbreviations

BMI: Body mass index
CI: Confidence interval
HR: Hazard ratio
PGCMS: Philadelphia Geriatric Center Morale Scale
LOT-R: Life Orientation Test-Revised
RR: Relative risk.

Conflicts of Interest

The authors declare that they have no conflicts of interest.

Acknowledgments

This work was supported by the National Institutes of Health under Grant nos. R01CA32197 and R01AG21055, Wyeth-Ayerst Laboratories, and the Earl Carrol Trust Fund.

References

[1] J. K. Boehm, C. Peterson, M. Kivimaki, and L. Kubzansky, "A prospective study of positive psychological well-being and coronary heart disease," *Health Psychology*, vol. 30, no. 3, pp. 259–267, 2011.

[2] J. K. Boehm, C. Trudel-Fitzgerald, M. Kivimaki, and L. D. Kubzansky, "The prospective association between positive psychological well-being and diabetes," *Health Psychology*, vol. 34, no. 10, pp. 1013–1021, 2015.

[3] R. A. Burns, J. Byles, P. Mitchell, and K. J. Anstey, "Positive components of mental health provide significant protection against likelihood of falling in older women over a 13-year period," *International Psychogeriatrics*, vol. 24, no. 9, pp. 1419–1428, 2012.

[4] C. R. Gale, C. Cooper, I. J. Deary, and A. Aihie Sayer, "Psychological well-being and incident frailty in men and women: the english longitudinal study of ageing," *Psychological Medicine*, vol. 44, no. 4, pp. 697–706, 2014.

[5] J. C. Huffman, S. R. Legler, and J. K. Boehm, "Positive psychological well-being and health in patients with heart disease: a brief review," *Future Cardiology*, vol. 13, no. 5, pp. 443–450, 2017.

[6] D. G. Blazer and C. F. Hybels, "What symptoms of depression predict mortality in community-dwelling elders?," *Journal of the American Geriatrics Society*, vol. 52, no. 12, pp. 2052–2056, 2004.

[7] M. T. Pankalainen, T. V. Kerola, and J. J. Hintikka, "Pessimism and the risk for coronary heart disease among middle-aged and older finnish men and women: a ten-year follow-up study," *BMC Cardiovascular Disorders*, vol. 15, no. 1, p. 113, 2015.

[8] P. Saz and M. E. Dewey, "Depression, depressive symptoms and mortality in persons aged 65 and over living in the community: a systematic review of the literature," *International Journal of Geriatric Psychiatry*, vol. 16, no. 6, pp. 622–630, 2001.

[9] M. A. Whooley, W. S. Browner, and S. O. F. R. Grp, "Association between depressive symptoms and mortality in older women," *Archives of Internal Medicine*, vol. 158, no. 19, pp. 2129–2135, 1998.

[10] E. Y. Gong, Y. C. Hua, and L. J. L. Yan, "Psychological wellbeing and all-cause mortality in the oldest old in China: a longitudinal survey-based study," *The Lancet*, vol. 388, p. S22, 2016.

[11] E. S. Kim, K. A. Hagan, F. Grodstein, D. L. DeMeo, I. De Vivo, and L. D. Kubzansky, "Optimism and cause-specific mortality: a prospective cohort study," *American Journal of Epidemiology*, vol. 185, no. 1, pp. 21–29, 2017.

[12] B. Liu, S. Floud, K. Pirie et al., "Does happiness itself directly affect mortality? the prospective UK million women study," *The Lancet*, vol. 387, no. 10021, pp. 874–881, 2016.

[13] H. A. Tindle, Y. F. Chang, L. H. Kuller et al., "Optimism, cynical hostility, and incident coronary heart disease and mortality in the Women's Health Initiative," *Circulation*, vol. 120, no. 8, pp. 656–662, 2009.

[14] T. A. Koopmans, J. M. Geleijnse, F. G. Zitman, and E. J. Giltay, "Effects of happiness on all-cause mortality during 15 Years of follow-up: the arnhem elderly study," *Journal of Happiness Studies*, vol. 11, no. 1, pp. 113–124, 2010.

[15] J. A. Okely, A. Weiss, and C. R. Gale, "The interaction between individualism and wellbeing in predicting mortality: survey of health ageing and retirement in Europe," *Journal of Behavioral Medicine*, vol. 41, no. 1, pp. 1–11, 2018.

[16] W. W. Zung, "A self-rating depression scale," *Archives of General Psychiatry*, vol. 12, no. 1, pp. 63–70, 1965.

[17] A. Paganini-Hill, A. Chao, R. K. Ross, and B. E. Henderson, "Exercise and other factors in the prevention of hip fracture: the leisure world study," *Epidemiology*, vol. 2, no. 1, pp. 16–25, 1991.

[18] A. Paganini-Hill, R. K. Ross, and B. E. Henderson, "Prevalence of chronic disease and health practices in a retirement community," *Journal of Chronic Diseases*, vol. 39, no. 9, pp. 699–707, 1986.

[19] A. Paganini-Hill and G. Hsu, "Smoking and mortality among residents of a California retirement community," *American Journal of Public Health*, vol. 84, no. 6, pp. 992–995, 1994.

[20] A. Paganini-Hill, C. H. Kawas, and M. M. Corrada, "Non-alcoholic beverage and caffeine consumption and mortality: the leisure world cohort study," *Preventive Medicine*, vol. 44, no. 4, pp. 305–310, 2007.

[21] A. Paganini-Hill, C. H. Kawas, and M. M. Corrada, "Type of alcohol consumed, changes in intake over time and mortality: the leisure world cohort study," *Age and Ageing*, vol. 36, no. 2, pp. 203–209, 2007.

[22] M. M. Corrada, C. H. Kawas, F. Mozaffar, and A. Paganini-Hill, "Association of body mass index and weight change with all-cause mortality in the elderly," *American Journal of Epidemiology*, vol. 163, no. 10, pp. 938–949, 2006.

[23] A. Paganini-Hill, C. H. Kawas, and M. M. Corrada, "Activities and mortality in the elderly: the leisure World cohort study," *Journals of Gerontology Series A: Biological Sciences and Medical Sciences*, vol. 66, no. 5, pp. 559–567, 2011.

[24] A. Paganini-Hill, "Risk factors for Parkinson's disease: the leisure world cohort study," *Neuroepidemiology*, vol. 20, no. 2, pp. 118–124, 2001.

[25] D. R. Cox, "Regression models and life-tables," *Journal of the Royal Statistical Society Series B-Statistical Methodology*, vol. 34, no. 2, pp. 187–220, 1972.

[26] A. Steptoe, P. Demakakos, C. de Oliveira, and J. Wardle, "Distinctive biological correlates of positive psychological well-being in older men and women," *Psychosomatic Medicine*, vol. 74, no. 5, pp. 501–508, 2012.

[27] L. Sapranaviciute-Zabazlajeva, D. Luksiene, D. Virviciute, M. Bobak, and A. Tamosiunas, "Link between healthy lifestyle and psychological well-being in Lithuanian adults aged 45-72: a cross-sectional study," *BMJ Open*, vol. 7, no. 4, p. e014240, 2017.

[28] E. G. Anthony, D. Kritz-Silverstein, and E. Barrett-Connor, "Optimism and mortality in older men and women: the rancho bernardo study," *Journal of Aging Research*, vol. 2016, article 5185104, 9 pages, 2016.

[29] J. Benito-Leon, E. D. Louis, J. Rivera-Navarro, M. J. Medrano, S. Vega, and F. Bermejo-Pareja, "Low morale is associated with increased risk of mortality in the elderly: a population-based prospective study (NEDICES)," *Age and Ageing*, vol. 39, no. 3, pp. 366–373, 2010.

[30] E. J. Giltay, J. M. Geleijnse, F. G. Zitman, T. Hoekstra, and E. G. Schouten, "Dispositional optimism and all-cause and cardiovascular mortality in a prospective cohort of elderly Dutch men and women," *Archives of General Psychiatry*, vol. 61, no. 11, pp. 1126–1135, 2004.

[31] J. Niklasson, C. Hornsten, M. Conradsson et al., "High morale is associated with increased survival in the very old," *Age and Ageing*, vol. 44, no. 4, pp. 630–636, 2015.

[32] K. H. Pitkala, M. L. Laakkonen, T. E. Strandberg, and R. S. Tilvis, "Positive life orientation as a predictor of 10-year outcome in an aged population," *Journal of Clinical Epidemiology*, vol. 57, no. 4, pp. 409–414, 2004.

[33] P. D. St John, C. Mackenzie, and V. Menec, "Does life satisfaction predict five-year mortality in community-living older adults?," *Aging and Mental Health*, vol. 19, no. 4, pp. 363–370, 2015.

[34] A. Steptoe, A. Deaton, and A. A. Stone, "Subjective wellbeing, health, and ageing," *The Lancet*, vol. 385, no. 9968, pp. 640–648, 2015.

[35] R. S. Tilvis, V. Laitala, P. Routasalo, T. E. Strandberg, and K. H. Pitkala, "Positive life orientation predicts good survival prognosis in old age," *Archives of Gerontology and Geriatrics*, vol. 55, no. 1, pp. 133–137, 2012.

[36] S. Arve, A. Lehtonen, and R. S. Tilvis, "Prognosis of depression with and without dementia in old age," *Archives of Gerontology and Geriatrics*, vol. 27, no. 2, pp. 141–146, 1998.

[37] M. Hiltunen, T. Nieminen, R. Kettunen et al., "Depressive symptoms and cardiovascular burden-related mortality among the aged," *European Journal of Clinical Investigation*, vol. 44, no. 5, pp. 486–492, 2014.

[38] R. S. Tilvis, T. E. Strandberg, and K. Juva, "Apolipoprotein E phenotypes, dementia and mortality in a prospective population sample," *Journal of the American Geriatrics Society*, vol. 46, no. 6, pp. 712–715, 1998.

[39] K. Takeida, M. Nishi, and H. Miyake, "Zung's depression scale as a predictor of death in elderly people: a cohort study in Hokkaido, Japan," *Journal of Epidemiology*, vol. 9, no. 4, pp. 240–244, 1999.

[40] R. K. Ross, L. Bernstein, L. Trent, B. E. Henderson, and A. Paganini-Hill, "A prospective study of risk factors for traumatic deaths in a retirement community," *Preventive Medicine*, vol. 19, no. 3, pp. 323–334, 1990.

[41] E. C. Chang, L. J. Sanna, J. M. Kim, and K. Srivastava, "Optimistic and pessimistic bias in European americans and asian americans: a preliminary look at distinguishing between predictions for physical and psychological health outcomes," *Journal of Cross-Cultural Psychology*, vol. 41, no. 3, pp. 465–470, 2010.

8

Barriers are not the Limiting Factor to Participation in Physical Activity in Canadian Seniors

Kristy L. Smith, Kelly Carr, Alexandra Wiseman, Kelly Calhoun, Nancy H. McNevin, and Patricia L. Weir

Department of Kinesiology, University of Windsor, Windsor, ON, Canada N9B 3P4

Correspondence should be addressed to Patricia L. Weir, weir1@uwindsor.ca

Academic Editor: Lynn Rochester

The identification of barriers to physical activity and exercise has been used for many decades to explain exercise behavior in older adults. Typically health concerns are the number one barrier to participation. Data from CCHS-HA dataset ($N = 20{,}875$) were used to generate a sample of Canadians, 60+ years, who did not identify a health condition limitation, illness, or injury as a barrier to participation in physical activity ($n = 4{,}900$) making this dataset unique in terms of the study of barriers to participation. While the vast majority of older adults participated in physical activity, 9.4% did not. The relationships between nonparticipation, barriers, self-reported health status, and chronic health conditions were determined using binary logistic regression. The main findings suggest that traditional barriers and self-reported health status are not responsible for nonparticipation. Nonparticipation was best predicted by chronic health conditions suggesting a disconnect between self-reported health status and underlying health conditions. The data are clear in suggesting that barriers are not the limiting factor and physical activity programming must be focused on meeting the health needs of our aging population.

1. Introduction

The world's population is aging. In 2009, 14% of Canada's 32 million people were aged 65 years or older. This proportion is expected to rise to between 23 and 25% by 2036; effectively doubling the number of seniors observed in 2009 [1], placing increased demand on the health care system and the nation's workforce. With this dramatic demographical change in the population, it has become increasingly important to find effective ways to improve health and prolong independence among older adults. Participation in regular physical activity can provide numerous physiological, cognitive, and psychological health benefits in the aging population. While some level of decline, such as reduced muscle strength and slower responding, is a normal part of the aging process [2], there is evidence that habitual exercise can minimize the physiological effects of an otherwise sedentary lifestyle and prolong active life expectancy [3]. However, despite this knowledge, many individuals do not engage in recommended levels of regular physical activity [4], and the Seniors in Canada report card [5] gave Canadian seniors a grade of C+ for participation in physical activity, with 62% of seniors being inactive.

The sizeable proportion of inactive individuals forces a critical examination of the unique challenges faced by older adults, aimed at developing the most effective health strategies to promote physical activity in this cohort [6]. Efforts to optimize health in this manner have led to numerous studies focused on identifying barriers and motivators to exercise among the older adult population, and several determinants have been consistently identified in the research literature as significant factors related to exercise behaviour among older individuals [7]. Considerations such as health concerns [6, 8, 9], lack of knowledge [6, 10], fear of falling or injury [6, 9, 11], time constraints [6, 8, 9], and lack of transportation [6] are generally reported as disincentives to participation by older adults.

Typically, issues contributing to the lack of participation are elicited through the use of focus group discussions [6, 9], interviews [11], or questionnaires [12]. These studies can be complex, such that some issues such as health problems are highly related to each other and can function both as a barrier and a motivator to exercise [6, 8]. In addition, the aging population is a diverse group [9, 13], with no one common barrier reported across all racial and ethnic groups [9]. Level of mobility [12], current exercise status [9], and past experiences [11] can all influence what respondents identify as posing a barrier or an enabler to physical activity.

The majority of older adults do, however, identify at least one of these considerations. In the cohort studied by O'Neill and Reid [14], 87% of the elderly respondents identified at least one barrier that prevents them from engaging in exercise. While the most common barriers appear to be related to health concerns, there are members of the sedentary population that do not identify any barriers to physical activity participation. For example, Cohen-Mansfield et al. [8] stated that 89 of their 324 person sample either reported no barriers at all or that they already engaged in exercise. Ironically, Connell et al. [15] reported that good health itself was a barrier to exercise because it provided the older adults with no reason to exercise.

The goal of the current study was to identify the relationship, if any, between what older adults perceived as barriers to physical activity and participation. Because previous research has suggested that health concerns pose a significant barrier to participation and would thus likely skew the data towards health-related barriers, we chose to focus on a subset of older adults who reported having no health condition limitation, illness, or injury that prevented them from participating in physical activity. We further delineated the analyses by gender as it has been well documented that older women tend to report more chronic diseases than men and this difference may impact overall participation rates [16–18]. Using data from the Canadian Communities Health Survey-Healthy Aging, an overall sample size of 4,900 seniors was identified, and, of these, 9.4% reported no participation in physical activity over the last seven days. We examined the relationship between their nonparticipation and barriers to participation, self-reported health, and chronic health conditions, and hypothesized that traditional barriers would not predict nonparticipation and there may be a dissociation between self-reported health status and reported chronic health conditions. The overarching goal of this study was to identify why Canadian seniors who do not report a health limitation do not participate in regular physical activity.

2. Methods

2.1. Canadian Communities Health Survey-Healthy Aging (CCHS-HA). Data from the Canadian Community Health Survey-Healthy Aging (CCHS-HA) (Statistics Canada, [19]) were used for the current study. This cross-sectional survey gathered self-reported data on the "factors, influences and processes that contribute to healthy aging through a multidisciplinary approach focusing on health, social and economic determinants" [19, page 1]. CCHS-HA data were derived through a standardized interview of adults aged 45 years of age and greater from the ten provinces in Canada, between December 2008 and November 2009. Using computer-assisted personal interviewing (CAPI), trained field interviewers conducted 94% of the interviews face-to-face, with the remainder being conducted over the telephone. The objectives of the survey were to (1) better understand the aging process; (2) examine how lifestyle impacts health; (3) use a multidisciplinary approach to examine relationships between healthy aging and geographical, social, demographic, and economic factors; and, (4) provide information on successful aging.

2.2. Participants. For the purposes of our study, we only used responses from the CCHS-HA dataset for people aged 60 years and older (N = 20,875). Given the interest in identifying barriers to participation, we further limited our sample to those seniors who did not identify a "health condition limitation" or "illness or injury" as barriers to participation. This ensured that we were not examining individuals who did not believe they were physically able to participate. Master weights were applied to the overall dataset such that the weights had a mean of 0. The weighting value for each respondent corresponded to the number of persons in the entire population that the respondent represented. The final weighted sample size was 4,900 participants (23.47% of total N; male: n = 2183; female: n = 2717). To estimate the average age of participants, the mid-point of each age-range was used (e.g., 60–64 years = 62.5). For the 85+ age range, we used 87.5 years, which may result in a slight underrepresentation. The overall average age of the sample was 68.39 ± 6.91 years.

2.3. Variables of Interest

2.3.1. Participation. This was determined using the derived variable for participation in leisure physical activities. This categorical variable indicated whether the respondent had participated in walking for pleasure or exercise, light sports, moderate sports, strenuous sports, and exercises to increase muscle strength and endurance over the 7 days prior to the interview. It was scored as either a "1" indicating reported participation over the last 7 days, a "2" indicating no participation over the last 7 days, or a "9" indicating at least one required activity had not been responded to (these were excluded from future analyses). To confirm differences in participation, the PASE (Physical Activity for the Elderly Scale) score was also examined [20]. The PASE score combines information on the frequency and duration of participation in leisure, household, and occupational activity over a seven-day period. While it does not differentiate frequency and duration, a higher score indicates greater levels of participation.

2.3.2. Barriers to Participation. Thirteen barriers to participation were listed in the CCHS-HA dataset: cost, transportation problem, not available in area, location not physically accessible, location is too far, health condition limitation, illness or injury, fear of injury, lack of time, lack of energy, lack of motivation, lack of skills or knowledge, other. Similar to the participation measure, these were categorical variables where respondents indicated that "yes" it prevented participation, or "no" it did not prevent participation. Of these thirteen variables, ten were used to predict participation. Health condition limitation, illness or injury were used only to identify the current sample, and "other" was not included as it was not possible to draw a conclusion about illness, or injury from this response. The total number of barriers was derived (range: 0–8 barriers; mean = 1.06 ± 0.72 barriers; median = 1.00) from the number of barriers each participant responded "yes" to.

2.3.3. Self-Reported Health Status. Respondents were asked "In general, would you say your health is" excellent, very good, good, fair, poor. This categorical variable was recoded such that excellent and very good were collapsed together, and fair and poor were collapsed together leaving three levels of self-reported health status.

2.3.4. Chronic Health Conditions. The CCHS-HA included a number of self-reported chronic condition variables that were coded categorically. The following seven were used in the current study: (1) vision function—this variable was derived from five items based on the respondent's ability and/or inability to see well enough to read newsprint and be able and/or unable to recognize a friend on the other side of the street, with and/or without glasses or contact lenses. This resulted in three vision categories: no vision problems, problems corrected by lenses, and problems not corrected by lenses. No vision problems and corrected vision were collapsed together resulting in the two categories of no vision problems and vision problems; (2) heart disease—if the respondents reported having either angina or a heart attack, they were considered to have heart disease; (3) chronic obstructive pulmonary disease (COPD)—if the respondent reported having been diagnosed with chronic bronchitis, emphysema, or COPD, which yielded a broad category used to describe limitations in lung airflow; (4) diabetes; (5) osteoporosis; (6) living with the effects of a stroke—this was used to reflect neurological damage; (7) mobility trouble—this variable was derived from five items based on the respondent's ability to walk a short distance and/or around their neighborhood, with and/or without the assistance of another person and/or walking equipment and/or a wheelchair. This resulted in four mobility categories: no mobility problems, mobility problems—no assistance required; mobility problems—requires wheelchair; mobility problems—requires help/cannot walk. The mobility problems were collapsed together resulting in two mobility categories.

2.4. Data Analyses. Logistic regression techniques were used to examine the relationships between nonparticipation and barriers to participation, self-reported health status, and the seven chronic health conditions. Data were analyzed separately for male and female respondents. Odds ratios and 95% confidence intervals were used to identify the risk of nonparticipation as a function of the predictor variables. Due to the small sample size of nonparticipants ($n = 459$), results associated with a large range in confidence intervals should be interpreted with caution as they may overestimate the practical significance. SPSS 19 was used for all data analyses, with $P < 0.05$.

3. Results

Table 1 reveals that a majority of the Canadian seniors in this sample were participants in physical activity over the last 7 days. While a small percentage of the respondents had not been physically active, this is the group of interest. Given that none of these respondents has identified barriers due to a health condition limitation, illness, or injury, the data show that approximately 10% do not participate in physical activity. Lower participation in the nonparticipants was confirmed through a lower PASE score (139.68) as compared to participants (142.99). Overall, the majority of the respondents report excellent/very good health, and a large majority do not suffer from the identified health conditions.

As can been seen in Table 2, approximately 89% of participants, regardless of participation level, did not identify a barrier. When the barriers were used to predict nonparticipation, the results of the logistic regressions suggested that older males and females have different barriers to participation (see Table 3). Males were more likely to be nonparticipants as a function of the availability of the activity (OR = 4.50, CI = 1.09, 18.68), while females were more likely to be a nonparticipants due to a lack of time (OR = 1.45, CI = 1.09, 1.92). Nonparticipation was not related to a lack of motivation in males (OR = 0.69, CI = 0.48, 0.98) and was not related to a lack of energy in females (OR = 0.54, CI = 0.39, 0.76). Overall, the data suggest that barriers do not appear to be responsible for the nonparticipation of Canadian seniors.

Given that barriers were not strong predictors of nonparticipation, we examined the influence of self-reported general health status. As seen in Table 1, the distribution of respondents across the three levels of health did vary between participants and nonparticipants. Participants more frequently reported their health as being excellent/very good (61.2% versus 49.2%), and fewer participants reported their health as fair/poor (9.1% versus 13.5%). While these differences in frequency existed, for both males and females there was no relationship between self-reported health status and nonparticipation in physical and leisure activities (see Table 4).

With regards to chronic health conditions, males and females identified a different number of predictors to nonparticipation (see Table 5). For males, who identified three predictors, the greatest likelihood of nonparticipation was predicted by vision function (OR = 3.06, CI = 1.30, 7.21), followed by mobility troubles (OR = 2.65, CI = 1.01, 6.95), and diabetes (OR = 1.66, CI = 1.12, 2.44). Women identified four significant predictors of nonparticipation; mobility troubles (OR = 2.71, CI = 1.70, 4.31), COPD (OR = 2.11, CI = 1.34, 3.32), diabetes (OR = 1.85, CI = 1.30, 2.63), and heart disease (OR = 1.54, CI = 1.19, 1.99).

4. Discussion

The purpose of this study was to examine the relationship between barriers to participation, self-reported health status, and chronic health conditions on nonparticipation in physical activity in Canadian seniors aged 60+ years who did not identify a health condition limitation, illness, or injury

Table 1: Sample descriptive statistics (weighted sample).

Variable	Category	N	%
Participation	Participant	4438	90.60
	Nonparticipant	459	9.40
PASE	Participant		142.99
	Nonparticipant		139.68
Gender	Male	2180	44.50
	Female	2717	55.50
Self-reported health status	Excellent/very good	2944	60.10
	Participant	2715	61.2
	Nonparticipant	226	49.2
	Good	1491	30.40
	Participant	1320	29.7
	Nonparticipant	171	37.3
	Fair/Poor	465	9.50
	Participant	404	9.1
	Nonparticipant	62	13.5
Chronic health conditions	Vision function		
	Yes	66	1.40
	No	4806	98.60
	Heart disease		
	Yes	2212	45.20
	No	2676	54.80
	COPD		
	Yes	231	4.70
	No	4664	95.30
	Diabetes		
	Yes	595	12.10
	No	4303	87.90
	Osteoporosis		
	Yes	641	13.10
	No	4253	86.90
	Effects of a stroke		
	Yes	63	1.30
	No	4837	98.70
	Mobility trouble		
	Yes	149	3.10
	No	4748	96.90

as a barrier to participation. Across both participants and nonparticipants, respondents on average identified 1.06 ± 0.72 barriers to participation in physical activity, with 89% of the respondents identifying no barriers to participation.

The barrier that had the highest likelihood of predicting nonparticipation differed between males and females. Males were more likely to be nonparticipants due to the activity not being available in their area, although this needs to be interpreted with some caution given the small sample size. In contrast, women were more likely to be nonparticipants due to time. Time being the most significant barrier to nonparticipation in women is supported by earlier work by Yoshida et al. [21] and Johnson et al. [22]. However, it is in contrast to the findings of O'Neill and Reid [14], where respondents ranked time as the 14th barrier to participation. The participants in O'Neill and Reid also identified "I get tired easily" as the second most frequent barrier. In the current study, a lack of energy was not related to nonparticipation in women.

Self-reported health status was not related to nonparticipation in the current sample. This may not be surprising given that this sample represented only those who did not identify a health condition, illness, or injury as barriers to participation. By limiting the sample to those who perceived their health as not posing a limiting factor, it is difficult to directly compare the results to other studies where health was consistently identified as the number one barrier to participation. What is surprising in the current study, however, is the relationship between chronic health conditions and

TABLE 2: Barriers by participation (weighted sample).

Variable	Category	N	%
Cost	Participant		
	Yes	308	6.9
	No	4130	93.1
	Nonparticipant		
	Yes	26	5.7
	No	433	94.3
Transportation	Participant		
	Yes	147	3.3
	No	4291	96.7
	Nonparticipant		
	Yes	15	3.3
	No	444	96.7
Not available in area	Participant		
	Yes	283	6.4
	No	4156	93.6
	Nonparticipant		
	Yes	14	3.1
	No	445	96.9
Not physically accessible	Participant		
	Yes	50	1.1
	No	4389	98.9
	Nonparticipant		
	Yes	4	0.9
	No	455	99.1
Location is too far	Participant		
	Yes	173	3.9
	No	4266	96.1
	Nonparticipant		
	Yes	8	1.7
	No	451	98.3
Fear of injury	Participant		
	Yes	76	1.7
	No	4363	98.3
	Nonparticipant		
	Yes	5	1.1
	No	454	98.9
Lack of time	Participant		
	Yes	1922	43.3
	No	2517	56.7
	Nonparticipant		
	Yes	184	40.1
	No	275	56.9
Lack of energy	Participant		
	Yes	456	10.3
	No	3982	89.7
	Nonparticipant		
	Yes	72	15.7
	No	387	84.3

TABLE 2: Continued.

Variable	Category	N	%
Lack of motivation	Participant		
	Yes	1281	28.9
	No	3158	71.1
	Nonparticipant		
	Yes	146	31.8
	No	313	68.2
Lack of skills or knowledge	Participant		
	Yes	34	0.8
	No	4404	99.2
	Nonparticipant		
	Yes	4	0.9
	No	454	99.1

TABLE 3: Odds of nonparticipation as a function of type of barrier.

Barrier	Males		Females	
	Odds ratios	95% CI	Odds ratios	95% CI
Cost	2.05	0.73, 5.74	1.07	0.67, 1.71
Transportation	0.89	0.16, 5.04	1.03	0.56, 1.88
Not available in area	**4.50***	**1.09, 18.68**	1.50	0.81, 2.78
Location not physically accessible	0.33	0.05, 2.31	1.53	0.39, 5.94
Location is too far	11.96	0.46, 313.09	1.70	0.76, 3.80
Fear of injury	2.29	0.25, 21.50	1.59	0.58, 4.34
Lack of time	0.79	0.56, 1.13	**1.45***	**1.09, 1.92**
Lack of energy	0.91	0.56, 1.48	**0.54***	**0.39, 0.76**
Lack of motivation	**0.69***	**0.48, 0.98**	1.18	0.88, 1.58
Lack of skills/knowledge	0.75	0.07, 8.09	0.78	0.25, 2.40

*$P < 0.05$.

TABLE 4: Odds of nonparticipation as a function of self-rated general health status.

Barrier	Males		Females	
	Odds ratios	95% CI	Odds ratios	95% CI
Excellent/very good	0.74	0.45, 1.20	0.74	0.45, 1.20
Good	0.78	0.46, 1.30	0.79	0.46, 1.30
Fair/poor	1.00	Referent	1.00	Referent

TABLE 5: Odds of nonparticipation as a function of health condition.

Barrier	Males		Females	
	Odds ratio	95% CI	Odds ratios	95% CI
Vision function	**3.06***	**1.30, 7.21**	0.25	0.37, 1.67
Heart disease	1.03	0.75, 1.41	**1.54***	**1.19, 1.99**
COPD	0.76	0.33, 1.77	**2.11***	**1.34, 3.32**
Diabetes	**1.66***	**1.12, 2.44**	**1.85***	**1.30, 2.63**
Osteoporosis	0.42	0.11, 1.63	0.94	0.69, 1.28
Effects of a stroke	1.07	0.36, 3.21	1.42	0.51, 3.98
Mobility trouble	**2.65***	**1.01, 6.95**	**2.71***	**1.70, 4.31**

*$P < 0.05$.

nonparticipation. These results suggest that while Canadian seniors have underlying chronic health conditions they do not always identify them as being associated with their self-reported general health, nor do they view them as limiting conditions to participation in physical activity. This potential disconnect between self-reported health status and chronic health conditions is interesting, as heart disease, vision, COPD, diabetes, and mobility trouble increased the likelihood of nonparticipation across males and females. It is possible that these older adults have learned to compensate for these chronic health conditions in their everyday life and therefore no longer consider them barriers to participation nor consider them impacting their self-reported general health status. It is clear, however, that there are limiting factors to participation. Although health concerns have been considered motivators to participation [23], this does not seem to be the case in the current study.

These findings have implications for physical activity programming for seniors. While only a small number of older Canadians were identified who did not participate, this sample represented those who believed they did not have limitations to participation; effectively creating a "healthy" sample of older adults. Regardless of their self-perceptions, this group of seniors was less likely to participate because of underlying health conditions. This would suggest that programming should target the specific needs of older adults; whether that takes the form of activities and classes designed specifically for those with targeted health conditions, or increased knowledge of how to integrate and attract those with health conditions into preexisting classes. What is clear is that the results identify a dissociation between self-perceptions of health and the reasons older adults are at greater risk for nonparticipation.

This study is not without limitations. The derived variable we chose from the CCHS-HA dataset captures physical activity as any one of walking for pleasure or exercise, light sports, moderate sports, strenuous sports, and exercises to increase muscle strength and endurance. While this variable is all encompassing for physical activity, it does not include activities of daily living, which may also be considered by some to contribute to their daily physical activity levels. Second, the self-reporting of general health status does not take into account the fact that many older adults learn to accommodate health concerns and to compensate for their impact on daily activities. Thus, a physical performance based measurement of health status could quite possibly have produced a different pattern of findings. Third, the chronic health conditions selected were done so to represent an overall picture of health-related issues that may impact participation. Specifically, they were chosen to represent vision, respiratory function, cardiovascular health, neurological health, diabetes, and mobility. It is by no means an exhaustive list of all chronic health conditions; any of which could impact ones' ability to participate in physical activity. The chronic health conditions were not validated in any way through performance measures, suggesting that their presence may have been under- or overrepresented in the self-reporting. Fourth, in predicting nonparticipation, the overall sample of nonparticipants represented only 9.4% of the total sample derived. Thus, the potential for type I error may be increased. Lastly, it was not possible to determine whether participants were meeting the recommended guidelines for participation in physical activity. While the PASE scores confirmed this group was more active than the nonparticipants, it was not possible to determine if this was due to frequency of participation or the duration of participation.

Overall this paper raises the issue that despite having created a "healthy" sample of older Canadians, there are still those who do not participate in regular physical activity. The 9.4% of seniors in this sample who did not participate is substantially smaller than the national average of 62%. However, it is important to note that this sample has been derived from older adults who reported no health condition or limitation preventing them from participating and thus is not representative of the general population of older adults. As such, their nonparticipation is not related to the presence of barriers such as opportunity or desire, but to specific chronic health conditions, and suggests a potential disconnect between self-perceived health and actual health status. Considering that only one-third or less of older Canadians achieve the recommended guidelines for leisure time physical activity [4], it is important to shift the focus from simply describing the barriers and motivators to physical activity to working towards designing programs that will address the health conditions facing older Canadians. With the changing age demographic, it will be important to encourage all older adults to participate in some form of physical activity on a daily basis, including a renewed focus on the role that activities of daily living can play in achieving fitness goals. One positive note to take from our findings is that 90% of the healthy older adults identified do engage in some form of physical activity, suggesting that public health messaging is reaching its mark.

Acknowledgment

This research was funded by the Social Sciences and Humanities Research Council of Canada, Grant no. 862-2010-0007 (P. L. Weir).

References

[1] Statistics Canada, "Population Projections for Canada, Provinces and Territories," http://www.statcan.gc.ca/pub/91-520-x/2010001/aftertoc-aprestdm1-eng.htm, 2010.

[2] V. A. Hughes, W. R. Frontera, M. Wood et al., "Longitudinal muscle strength changes in older adults: influence of muscle mass, physical activity, and health," *Journals of Gerontology*, vol. 56, no. 5, pp. B209–B217, 2001.

[3] W. J. Chodzko-Zajko, D. N. Proctor, M. A. Fiatarone Singh et al., "Exercise and physical activity for older adults," *Medicine and Science in Sports and Exercise*, vol. 41, no. 7, pp. 1510–1530, 2009.

[4] M. C. Ashe, W. C. Miller, J. J. Eng, and L. Noreau, "Older adults, chronic disease and leisure-time physical activity," *Gerontology*, vol. 55, no. 1, pp. 64–72, 2009.

[5] Seniors in Canada Report Card, National Advisory Council on Aging, Public Health Agency of Canada, Division of Aging and Seniors, 2006.

[6] A. E. Mathews, S. B. Laditka, J. N. Laditka et al., "Older adults' perceived physical activity enablers and barriers: a multicultural perspective," *Journal of Aging and Physical Activity*, vol. 18, no. 2, pp. 119–140, 2010.

[7] K. A. Schutzer and B. S. Graves, "Barriers and motivations to exercise in older adults," *Preventive Medicine*, vol. 39, no. 5, pp. 1056–1061, 2004.

[8] J. Cohen-Mansfield, M. S. Marx, and J. M. Guralnik, "Motivators and barriers to exercise in an older community-dwelling population," *Journal of Aging and Physical Activity*, vol. 11, no. 2, pp. 242–253, 2003.

[9] F. D. Lees, P. G. Clark, C. R. Nigg, and P. Newman, "Barriers to exercise behavior among older adults: a focus-group study," *Journal of Aging and Physical Activity*, vol. 13, no. 1, pp. 23–33, 2005.

[10] S. O'Brien Cousins, "'My heart couldn't take it': older women's beliefs about exercise benefits and risks," *Journals of Gerontology B*, vol. 55, no. 5, pp. P283–P294, 2000.

[11] M. P. Buman, L. Daphna Yasova, and P. R. Giacobbi, "Descriptive and narrative reports of barriers and motivators to physical activity in sedentary older adults," *Psychology of Sport and Exercise*, vol. 11, no. 3, pp. 223–230, 2010.

[12] M. Rasinaho, M. Hirvensalo, R. Leinonen, T. Lintunen, and T. Rantanen, "Motives for and barriers to physical activity among older adults with mobility limitations," *Journal of Aging and Physical Activity*, vol. 15, no. 1, pp. 90–102, 2007.

[13] R. N. Butler, R. Davis, C. B. Lewis, M. E. Nelson, and E. Strauss, "Physical fitness: exercise prescription for older adults," *Geriatrics*, vol. 53, no. 11, pp. 45–56, 1998.

[14] K. O'Neill and G. Reid, "Perceived barriers to physical activity by older adults," *Canadian Journal of Public Health*, vol. 82, no. 6, pp. 392–396, 1991.

[15] C. M. Connell, R. M. Davies, A. M. Rosenberg, and E. B. Fisher Jr., "Retiree's perceived incentives and barriers to participation in health promotion activities," *Health Education Research*, vol. 3, no. 3, pp. 325–330, 1988.

[16] M. Denton, S. Prus, and V. Walters, "Gender differences in health: a Canadian study of the psychosocial, structural and behavioural determinants of health," *Social Science and Medicine*, vol. 58, no. 12, pp. 2585–2600, 2004.

[17] P. McDonough and V. Walters, "Gender and health: reassessing patterns and explanations," *Social Science and Medicine*, vol. 52, no. 4, pp. 547–559, 2001.

[18] F. Orfila, M. Ferrer, R. Lamarca, C. Tebe, A. Domingo-Salvany, and J. Alonso, "Gender differences in health-related quality of life among the elderly: the role of objective functional capacity and chronic conditions," *Social Science and Medicine*, vol. 63, no. 9, pp. 2367–2380, 2006.

[19] Statistics Canada, Canadian Community Health Survey (CCHS-HA), Healthy Aging. User Guide, 1-65, 2010.

[20] R. A. Washburn, E. McAuley, J. Katula, S. L. Mihalko, and R. A. Boileau, "The physical activity scale for the elderly (PASE): evidence for validity," *Journal of Clinical Epidemiology*, vol. 52, no. 7, pp. 643–651, 1999.

[21] K. K. Yoshida, K. R. Allison, and R. W. Osborn, "Social factors influencing perceived barriers to physical exercise among women," *Canadian Journal of Public Health*, vol. 79, no. 2, pp. 104–108, 1988.

[22] C. A. Johnson, S. A. Corrigan, P. M. Dubbert, and S. E. Gramling, "Perceived barriers to exercise and weight control practices in community women," *Women and Health*, vol. 16, no. 3-4, pp. 177–191, 1990.

[23] R. S. Newson and E. B. Kemps, "Factors that promote and prevent exercise engagement in older adults," *Journal of Aging and Health*, vol. 19, no. 3, pp. 470–481, 2007.

9

Personality Traits in College Students and Caregiving for a Relative with a Chronic Health Condition

Michael A. Trujillo, Paul B. Perrin, Aaliah Elnasseh, Bradford S. Pierce, and Melody Mickens

Virginia Commonwealth University, Richmond, VA, USA

Correspondence should be addressed to Paul B. Perrin; pperrin@vcu.edu

Academic Editor: Elke Bromberg

The purpose of this study was to investigate among college students the relationship between personality traits and willingness to care for a relative with a chronic health condition. 329 undergraduate students completed an online questionnaire. Hierarchical multiple regressions found that after controlling for demographics personality traits explained 10% of the variance in willingness to provide emotional care, 7% in instrumental care, and 7% in nursing care. Within these models, greater empathy was uniquely associated with willingness to provide emotional, instrumental, and nursing care for a family member in the future. Similarly, participants with high agreeableness were more willing to provide emotional care, and participant older age was a unique predictor of instrumental care. The results can help shape research on interventions that incorporate perspective taking, motivational interviewing, and training in life skills as a means of boosting college students' willingness to provide care for a relative with a chronic health condition.

1. Introduction

By 2050, the number of people over the age of 65 is projected to increase from an estimated 524 million to nearly 1.5 billion, representing 16% of the world's population [1]. Many of these individuals and their families will experience challenges as older adults learn how to manage and cope with chronic health problems such as cancer, heart disease, and diabetes that require long-term care [1]. Over the past decade, significant increases in healthcare costs have led to greater utilization of and increased need for informal caregiving from family members who provide emotional support, assistance with activities of daily living (e.g., bathing, grooming, and feeding), and instrumental support (e.g., paying bills, shopping, and assistance with medication) for individuals with chronic illness and disabilities [2, 3].

Trends of older adults living longer with chronic illnesses have coincided with younger adults (i.e., 18–25-year-olds) assuming caregiving responsibilities for family members [2], especially since marriage and childbearing have been delayed and college enrollment overall in the young adult population has increased [4]. Young adults comprise 12–18% of adult caregivers, and the average age of a young adult caregiver is 21 years [4], suggesting that many young caregivers are college-age. Although young adult caregivers cannot be automatically equated with college students, as social selection processes may predispose certain young adults to take on a family caregiving role, the National Center for Education Statistics estimates that 40 percent of the US population between the ages of 18 and 24 is enrolled in degree-granting postsecondary institutions, representing a sizeable group of young adults who are or could become caregivers [5]. One study of young adult caregivers, for example, found 38 percent of participants caring for grandparents reported completing some college [6]. Although little is known about undergraduate students acting as family caregivers, research has found that caregiving by college students has been associated with increased burden in transitioning to college, reduced social engagement, and greater stress and depression [6, 7]. Similarly, college caregivers may experience additional stress because they may be relatively inexperienced with providing care [8], which may pose more challenges for them in fulfilling their duties.

The more general literature outside of college students has shown that factors such as caregiving history, SES, and the availability of support programs, along with mediators such as social support systems and personal coping responses, may influence an individual's ability to handle the stressors that accompany transitioning to the caregiving role [9]. There is considerable variety between families and individual members in their ability to recognize and plan for the caregiving needs of others. Individuals who anticipate and plan for the needs of older adult family members are more satisfied with the amount of family discussion and planning than those who ignore those needs [10]. Beliefs and personality characteristics play a meaningful role in an individual's anticipation of and decision to adopt a caregiving role. For example, family members with an internal locus of control tend to anticipate and prepare for the caregiving needs of their parents and grandparents [11]. Those with an avoidant attachment style perceive caregiving as a burden and are less willing to provide future care for parents [12]. In contrast, adult children who possess more filial obligation and display attachment to parents are more likely to commit to future help [13].

Despite the research examining predictors of adjustment to becoming a caregiver and the more specific research beginning to identify the widespread nature of caregiving duties among college students, no research has examined the personality characteristics that might predispose college students to assuming a caregiving role. This is unfortunate because the more general research has identified personality variables as playing a major role in shaping caregiving experiences [14, 15]. A well-established measure of personality is the Five-Factor model, which includes the dimensions extraversion, agreeableness, conscientiousness, neuroticism, and openness to experience [16]. The Big Five personality traits have been found to be related to caregiver evaluation of care tasks, use of coping strategies, and evaluation of the care recipient's impairment [17, 18].

Extraversion in particular has been associated with positive experiences in providing care and a greater ability to recognize the benefits of caregiving [19, 20]. Also, caregiver agreeableness and conscientiousness have been related to a better relationship with the care recipient [21], as well as to increased benefit finding [19]. Caregiver neuroticism, on the other hand, has been associated with more mental health problems [18], increased susceptibility to care-related stressors [19, 22], and decreased salutogenic behaviors [18]. There is also evidence suggesting extraversion and neuroticism may predict caregivers' level of optimism concerning their future health [23]. Finally, caregiver openness has been related to awareness for future care needs and more gathering of care-related information [24].

Outside of the Big Five model, caregivers with greater empathy report higher life satisfaction and less depression, as well as appraising caregiving as less threatening and stressful [25]. Broadly defined, empathy is the ability to correctly perceive another's feelings [26]. A proposed model of caregiver compassion [27] suggests personality characteristics such as empathy, level of intimacy, and attachment style moderate the level of compassion people feel in response to another's suffering, resulting in (or inhibiting) various helping behaviors [12]. As individuals develop empathy, they learn to recognize and feel what others feel before developing the capacity to maintain emotional distance from another's internal experience while retaining the ability to recognize another's feelings [25]. Caregivers in the early stages of empathy development may quickly feel overwhelmed by the emotional experience they share with the recipient [25]. In contrast, greater empathy has been associated with better provision of support by caregivers and reduced anxiety [28].

Given the aging demographic trends in the US and the increasing likelihood that today's college-age young adults will one day provide care for their relatives with a chronic health condition [2], it is extremely important to examine the factors that might predict their willingness to provide care. While previous studies have examined the relationship between a number of personality traits and different aspects of caregiving [15], including how personality traits are associated with assuming and maintaining a caregiving role [29], limited research to date has investigated the relationship between personality traits and one's willingness to provide care for a family member with a chronic health condition, especially in a young adult population that will be increasingly likely to do so.

Objective. The purpose of the current study is to examine whether the Big Five personality traits and empathy are associated with college students' willingness to provide care for a family member with a chronic condition. First, it is hypothesized that empathy, agreeableness, and conscientiousness will be positively associated with willingness to provide emotional care. Research has suggested that agreeableness and conscientiousness are both related to a better relationship with the care recipient [21], as well as to increased benefit finding [19]. Second, it is hypothesized that openness will be positively associated with willingness to provide instrumental care. Previous research has shown that openness is related to awareness of future care needs and more gathering of care-related information [24]. Third, it is hypothesized that neuroticism will be negatively associated with willingness to care more generally. Prior research indicates caregiver neuroticism is associated with more mental health problems [18], increased susceptibility to care-related stressors [19, 22], and decreased salutogenic behaviors [18]. And finally, it is hypothesized that extraversion and empathy will be positively associated with general willingness to care. Research has shown that extraversion is related to positive experiences in providing care and to recognizing the benefits of caregiving [19, 20].

2. Method

2.1. Participants. Data collection occurred from March through May of 2014. Participants were undergraduate students enrolled in psychology courses at a large urban university. All participants were over age 18 and enrolled in a psychology course at the university. Initially, 343 students completed the study. Only participants who answered at least five of seven (71%) reliability-check items correctly were included in the current study with 13 respondents omitted for this reason (see Table 1 for a description of participant

TABLE 1: Summary of participant characteristics.

Characteristics	*N*	%
Age, M (SD)	21.6 (4.29)	
Gender		
Male	95	28.9
Female	234	71.1
Race/ethnicity		
White, Caucasian	142	43.2
Black, African American	81	24.6
Asian, Asian American	55	16.7
Hispanic or Latino	21	6.4
Mixed	30	9.1
Family social class		
Lower class	12	3.6
Working class	34	10.3
Lower middle class	84	25.5
Middle class	181	55.0
Upper class	18	5.5
Employment status		
Unemployed	160	48.6
Part-time (<35 hrs/wk)	139	42.2
Full-time (36–40 hrs/wk)	30	9.1
Prior caregiving experience		
Yes	80	24.3
No	249	75.7

demographics). Additionally, one participant was excluded who was identified as intersex in order to be able to include gender as a covariate in our analyses, yielding a final sample size of 329.

2.2. Measures

2.2.1. Social Class. Participants indicated social class by answering, "What is your family's social class? Upper Class: $200,000 & up (CEOs, Politicians); Upper Middle Class: $60,000–199,999 (Professionals); Lower Middle Class: $30,000–59,999 (Professional Support & Sales); Working Class: $15,000–29,999 (Clerical, Service, & Blue Collar); Lower Class: $7,000–14,999 (Part-time & Unemployed)." Responses were coded 5, 4, 3, 2, and 1 respectively. Given that income was the primary component assessing social class, it was treated as a continuous variable in all analyses.

2.2.2. Employment Status. Participants indicated employment status by answering, "Are you currently employed? (Please select one). No. Yes, Full Time (at least 36–40 hours/week). Yes, Part-Time (no more than 35 hours/week)." Responses were coded as 1, 3, and 2 respectively.

2.2.3. Prior Caregiving Experience. Participants answered "Yes" or "No" to the following question, "In the past (but no longer), did you provide unpaid informal care to a relative or friend with a chronic health condition lasting three months or longer?" "No" responses were coded as 0 while "Yes" responses were coded as 1.

2.2.4. Gender. Participants indicated gender by answering, "What gender label best describes you (select one)? Man, Woman, Intersex, Transman, Transwoman." Responses were coded as 1, 2, 3, 4, or 5, respectively. All but one participant were identified as either man or woman and as such gender was treated as a dichotomous variable.

2.2.5. Age. Participants reported their age in response to "How old are you (in years)?"

2.2.6. Willingness to Care (WTC). The WTC scale is a 30-item measure assessing an individual's attitude toward providing instrumental, nursing, and emotional support for individuals with a chronic condition [30]. The original scale was intended to assess willingness to care for a person with HIV/AIDS; thus the directions were modified such that "person with HIV/AIDS" was replaced by "a family member that you might have to provide care for at some point because they have a chronic illness, injury, or disability." Individual caregiving items within the questionnaire are general in nature (e.g., providing encouragement, cleaning up, and paying for medicines) and not specific to persons with HIV/AIDS, so no further modifications were necessary. In order to prevent alternative explanations that may explain nonwillingness of participants to take over care responsibilities, such as an inability or financial circumstances, we instructed participants to "assume that you are able to provide the following types of care. Select the response that best shows how willing you are to do each one." Additionally, participants were told that a "chronic health condition is a disease or a disability that lasts for THREE MONTHS OR LONGER." The WTC has four scores: a global willingness-to-care score as well as three mean subscale scores including emotional care (providing emotional support such as encouraging someone who feels hopeless, e.g., to "listen to someone's concerns about death or dying"), instrumental care (assisting with everyday tasks such as preparing meals for someone, e.g., to "bring home groceries for someone"), and nursing care (measuring physical caretaking activities such as helping someone take medicine, e.g., to "clean up after someone who has lost bowel or bladder control"). Higher scores indicate greater willingness to provide care. The WTC score has high reliability for each subscale (alphas range: .84–.91) [30].

2.2.7. Big Five Inventory-10 (BFI-10). The BFI-10 is a 10-item scale with an optional 11th item derived from the Big Five Inventory-45 measuring the "Big Five" factors of personality: neuroticism, extroversion, openness, agreeableness, and conscientiousness. The 11-item version was used for the current study, producing subscales composed of two items except for agreeableness, which was composed of three items [31]. Higher scores indicate higher levels of the personality trait. The BFI-10 has shown good convergent validity [31]. In the current study, Pearson product moment correlations were calculated for the extraversion ($r = .391$), conscientiousness ($r = .362$), and neuroticism ($r = .348$) items, which were all significant ($p < .001$), as were the correlations among the three items composing the agreeableness subscale (r: .213–.256; $p < .001$). The bivariate correlation for the items assessing openness was not significant (r = .058, p = .290) suggesting a potential issue with the internal consistency for this subscale.

2.2.8. Toronto Empathy Questionnaire (TEQ). The TEQ is a 16-item scale that assesses the ability to perceive the emotional state of another person and respond sympathetically. Higher scores indicate higher empathy [26]. The TEQ has good internal consistency (Cronbach's alpha = .85) and convergent validity [26].

2.3. Procedure. Study personnel emailed psychology course instructors with information describing the study. Instructors who were willing to assist provided students with study information and a link to the survey. Interested students reviewed and completed an online consent prior to participation and completed the survey by submitting their responses using the online platform. Participants received extra credit points at the instructor's discretion, but not totaling more than 1% of their overall grade. This study received institutional review board approval by the authors' institution prior to recruitment.

2.4. Data Analysis. Preliminary analyses examined correlations within each of the WTC subscales, the BFI subscales, and the TEQ. Three hierarchical multiple regressions investigated the extent to which personality traits (neuroticism, openness, extraversion, agreeableness, and conscientiousness) and empathy were associated with each of the willingness-to-care subscales (emotional care, instrumental care, and nursing care). Prior to running primary analyses, a series of bivariate correlations between the three types of willingness to care and demographic characteristics including age, gender, family socioeconomic status, and employment status were conducted to identify important covariates to include in the models, as demographics have previously been shown to be associated with care provision [32, 33]. As prior work has found that individuals with less time available due to their employment status (e.g., families with dual earners compared to single earners) provide less care [32], we treated employment status as a continuous variable to assess if this phenomenon extended to willingness to provide care. Given that much of the prior work has not been conducted with college-age samples, only demographic characteristics that were significantly associated with outcome variables in the current sample would be included in the final analyses. Age, gender, and employment status were shown to be associated with the outcomes in the bivariate correlations and were included as covariates in all analyses (Table 2). In each of the three regressions, demographics were entered in the first step, with all of the personality variables as well as empathy entered in the second step. The three willingness-to-care subscales were entered as the dependent variable in each regression. To explore if age, gender, or employment status interacted with personality traits, a series of exploratory analyses were conducted. Interactions between each personality trait and age and each demographic characteristic were included in the third step predicting each outcome variable and are summarized following the primary results for each criterion variable.

3. Results

3.1. Normality Assumptions. Normality assumptions were assessed prior to running analyses. For all five personality subscales (neuroticism, openness, extraversion, agreeableness, and conscientiousness), empathy, and nursing care, normality assumptions were met. However, emotional and instrumental care had skewness of −3.82 and −1.46 and kurtosis of 18.62 and 2.60, respectively, and thus did not meet the assumption of normality. To address these violations, a reflection of emotional and instrumental care data was performed via log transformation and produced new skewness values of .70 and −.40 and kurtosis values of −.29 and −1.07 for emotional and instrumental care, respectively. An assessment of VIF and tolerance statistics indicated no multicollinearity was present among the variables. Additionally, an examination of bivariate correlations indicated no correlations greater than .70.

3.2. Correlation Matrix. A series of correlations were conducted to examine the bivariate relationships between all variables (Table 3). All willingness-to-care variables were positively associated with each other, as well as being positively related to empathy and personality traits of agreeableness and conscientiousness. Willingness to care was not related to extraversion, neuroticism, or openness. Extraversion was positively related to agreeableness and empathy but negatively associated with neuroticism, while agreeableness was positively related to conscientiousness and empathy. Additionally, neuroticism and conscientiousness were negatively related, while empathy was positively related, to all personality traits except for neuroticism and openness. All other bivariate relationships were not statistically significant.

3.3. Emotional Care. In the first hierarchical multiple regression (Table 4), NEO personality traits and empathy were regressed onto willingness to provide emotional care after accounting for age, gender, and employment status. Demographics were entered into the first step, for which the overall model was significant, $F(3, 325) = 3.21$, $p < .05$, and $R^2 = .03$. No demographic characteristics produced any unique effects (all $p > .053$). All personality variables as well as empathy were entered in the second step which was also significant, $F(9, 319) = 5.41$, $p < .001$, and $R^2 = .13$, with a significant increase in the amount of variance explained in emotional care, $\Delta F(6, 320) = 6.35$, $p < .001$, and $\Delta R^2 = .10$. The personality trait of agreeableness as well as empathy was uniquely and positively associated with emotional care. All other personality variables were not independently related to emotional care (all $p > .184$). This suggests that greater agreeableness and empathy are associated with greater willingness to provide emotional care.

To explore if age, gender, or employment status interacted with each personality trait, interaction terms with each of these demographic variables and the personality traits were included in step three. The overall model was significant, $F(27, 301) = 2.13$, $p < .01$, and $R^2 = .16$; however, there was no significant increase in explainable variance $\Delta F(18, 301) = 0.55$, $p = .931$, and $\Delta R^2 = .03$. There were also no significant

TABLE 2: Correlations among willingness to provide care and demographic variables.

	Age	Gender	Employment status	Social class
Emotional care	.11*	.12*	.08	.02
Instrumental care	.17**	.12*	.11*	.05
Nursing care	.13*	.09	.05	.00

Note. $^*p < .05$ and $^{**}p < .01$, two-tailed. Correlations with continuous demographics were calculated as Pearson and with dichotomous demographics as point-biserial.

TABLE 3: Correlations among willingness to provide care variables, NEO, and empathy.

	1	2	3	4	5	6	7	8
(1) Emotional Care	—							
(2) Instrumental care	.66***	—						
(3) Nursing care	.60***	.68***	—					
(4) Extraversion	.11	.05	.03	—				
(5) Agreeableness	.25***	.18**	.19**	.14*	—			
(6) Conscientiousness	.17**	.16**	.17**	.11	.19**	—		
(7) Neuroticism	.01	.01	.03	−.16**	−.10	−.11*	—	
(8) Openness	.01	.03	.05	.05	.06	.07	−.06	—
(9) Empathy	.31***	.28***	.25***	.11*	.44***	.21***	.09	.07

Note. $^*p < .05$, $^{**}p < .01$, and $^{***}p < .001$, two-tailed.

TABLE 4: Hierarchical multiple regression: association between demographics, personality traits, empathy, and willingness to provide emotional care.

Variable	Model 1			Model 2		
	B	SE *B*	*β*	*B*	SE *B*	*β*
Age	.01	.01	.11	.01	.01	.07
Gender	.10	.05	.11	.06	.05	.07
Employment	.02	.02	.05	.01	.02	.02
Extraversion				.01	.01	.06
Agreeableness				.03	.01	.14**
Conscientiousness				.02	.01	.07
Neuroticism				.00	.01	.01
Openness				.00	.01	.02
Empathy				.01	.00	.20***
R^2			.03*			.13***

Note. $N = 329$; SE = standard error.
$^*p < .05$, $^{**}p < .01$, and $^{***}p < .001$, two-tailed.

TABLE 5: Hierarchical multiple regression: association between demographics, personality traits, empathy, and willingness to provide instrumental care.

Variable	Model 1			Model 2		
	B	SE *B*	*β*	*B*	SE *B*	*β*
Age	.02	.01	.17**	.02	.01	.14*
Gender	.09	.06	.09	.05	.06	.04
Employment	.06	.03	.12*	.04	.03	.09
Extraversion				.00	.01	.02
Agreeableness				.02	.01	.07
Conscientiousness				.02	.02	.07
Neuroticism				.00	.01	.01
Openness				.00	.02	.01
Empathy				.01	.00	.19**
R^2			.05**			.12***

Note. $N = 329$; SE = standard error.
$^*p < .05$, $^{**}p < .01$, and $^{***}p < .001$, two-tailed.

interactions between personality traits by age (all $p > .257$), gender (all $p > .240$), or employment status (all $p > .186$).

3.4. Instrumental Care. In the second hierarchical multiple regression (Table 5), demographics were entered in the first step, yielding a significant test, $F(3, 325) = 6.21$, $p < .001$, and $R^2 = .05$. Both age and employment status were uniquely and positively associated with instrumental care. In the second step, empathy and all personality variables were entered, producing an overall significant model, $F(9, 319) = 4.81$, $p < .001$, and $R^2 = .12$. There was also a significant increase in the amount of variance explained in instrumental care, $\Delta F(6, 319) = 3.94$, $p < .001$, and $\Delta R^2 = .07$. After accounting for demographics, empathy was independently positively associated with instrumental care with age maintaining significance. No NEO personality traits were associated with instrumental care (all $p > .187$) and employment status dropped in significance in follow-up analyses ($p = .090$). This finding suggests that greater empathy and older age are related to greater willingness to provide instrumental care.

As part of the exploratory multiple regressions, separate interaction terms between age, gender, and employment status with personality characteristics were included in step three. The overall model was significant, $F(27, 301) = 1.990$, $p < .01$, and $R^2 = .15$; however, there was no significant increase in explainable variance $\Delta F(18, 301) = 0.631$, $p = .874$, and $\Delta R^2 = .03$. There was a significant interaction of

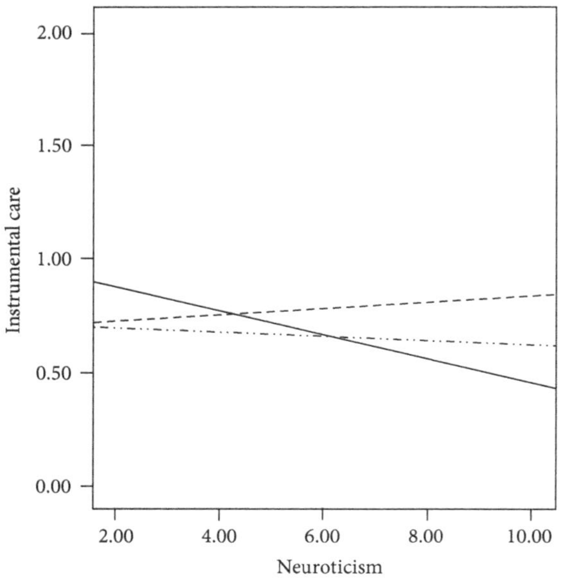

FIGURE 1: Interaction of employment status by neuroticism on willingness to provide instrumental care.

employment status by neuroticism ($\beta = .44$, $p = .030$), such that individuals who were more neurotic and were employed full-time were less likely to provide care than unemployed or part-time employed individuals (Figure 1). All other interactions with personality traits (all $p > .380$) as well as interactions between personality traits by age (all $p > .267$) and by gender (all $p > .089$) were not significant.

3.5. Nursing Care. In the third regression (Table 6), demographics were entered in the first step, which was not significant, $F(3, 325) = 2.45$, $p = .063$, and $R^2 = .02$. All personality traits and empathy were entered into the second step, which was significant, $F(9, 319) = 3.61$, $p < .001$, and $R^2 = .09$, with a significant increase in the amount of variance explained, $\Delta F(6, 319) = 4.12$, $p < .01$, and $\Delta R^2 = .07$. Only empathy was uniquely related to willingness to provide nursing care. No NEO personality traits or demographic characteristics were uniquely related to willingness to provide nursing care (all $p > .08$). This suggests that greater empathy was associated with greater willingness to provide nursing care.

Similar to the third step in the first two exploratory multiple regressions, separate interaction terms between age, gender, and employment status with personality traits were included in step three. The overall model was significant, $F(27, 301) = 1.74$, $p < .05$, and $R^2 = .14$; however, there was no significant increase in explainable variance $\Delta F(18, 301) = 0.82$, $p = .672$, and $\Delta R^2 = .04$. All interactions of personality traits by age (all $p > .366$), by gender (all $p > .100$), and by employment status (all $p > .182$) were not significant.

TABLE 6: Hierarchical multiple regression: association between demographics, personality traits, empathy, and willingness to provide nursing care.

Variable	Model 1			Model 2		
	B	SE B	β	B	SE B	β
Age	.26	.12	.12*	.20	.12	.09
Gender	1.63	1.15	.08	.73	1.19	.04
Employment	.12	.55	.01	−.13	.54	−.01
Extraversion				−.03	.27	−.01
Agreeableness				.48	.29	.10
Conscientiousness				.56	.32	.10
Neuroticism				.18	.26	.04
Openness				.21	.30	.04
Empathy				.20	.08	.16*
R^2			.02			.09***

Note. $N = 329$; SE = standard error.
$^{*}p < .05$, and $^{***}p < .001$, two-tailed.

4. Discussion

With more adults living to an older age and with chronic health conditions, younger adults are assuming greater roles as family caregivers. Though many young caregivers are in college, no studies have examined the association between personality traits and willingness to provide care in a college-age population. As such, the purpose of this study was to investigate the relationship between the Big Five personality traits and empathy and willingness to provide care for a relative with a chronic health condition in a college-aged sample. It was hypothesized that empathy, agreeableness, and conscientiousness would be positively associated with willingness to provide emotional care, that openness would be positively associated with willingness to provide instrumental care, that neuroticism would be negatively associated with willingness to care more generally, and that extraversion and empathy would be positively associated with general willingness to care. A series of hierarchal multiple regressions found that after controlling for demographics, personality traits explained 10% of the variance in willingness to provide emotional care, 7% in instrumental care, and 7% in nursing care. Within these models, greater empathy was uniquely associated with willingness to provide emotional, instrumental, and nursing care for a family member in the future. Similarly, participants with high agreeableness were more willing to provide emotional care, and older age was a unique predictor of instrumental care.

The finding that college students who exhibit a greater level of empathy are more willing to care for a family member with a chronic health condition is in line with previous research indicating empathy is a source of altruistic motivation. According to the empathy-altruism hypothesis, the motivation to help is altruistic to the degree that it is evoked by an empathic emotional response, such that empathic concern can lead to altruistic motivations to help others [34, 35]. By extension, dispositional empathy has been shown to be predictive of greater empathic concern [36]. This suggests that those who exhibit more empathic characteristics may have a greater tendency for empathic responding and subsequently are more motivated to help or care for a family member, as found in the current study. Given that empathy was uniquely predictive of all three willingness-to-care subscales, participants who were more empathic may have been more willing to help or provide care irrespective of the type of care, which is supported by numerous studies linking empathic concern to various helping behaviors [37, 38].

Agreeableness was also identified as being uniquely and positively associated with willingness to provide emotional care for a family member with a chronic health condition. Broadly, agreeableness has been argued to be representative of more humanitarian aspects of personality including nurturance and altruism [39] and has long been identified as personality disposition positively related to volunteering [40] and prosocial behaviors [41]. This suggests that people who are more agreeable may be better able to provide emotional support such as being encouraging, caring, and comforting, as well as more inclined to engage in helping behavior. This is in line with prior research outlining that nurses with greater levels of agreeableness are likely to utilize positive emotional social support [42]. Additionally, previous work indicates that those who exhibit greater levels of agreeableness are more likely to perceive the caregiving role as meaningful and positive [19]. Within the context of the previous literature, in the current study, those scoring higher on agreeableness may have been better able to find the caregiving role as important and beneficial and therefore were more willing to provide care.

Female gender, older age, and a higher level of employment were associated with more willingness to provide various types of care in the bivariate correlation matrix. Although these findings are generally in line with the previous literature [32], it is important to note that all of these effects were small-sized in the matrix, with the statistically significant correlations indexing 1.2% (e.g., age and emotional care) to a maximum of 2.9% (e.g., age and instrumental care) of shared variance. And when entered into the multiple regressions along with the personality predictors in each model's step two, none of these demographics remained significant predictors except for age predicting willingness to provide instrumental care (β = .14), which just surpassed the α = .05 threshold. As a result, these demographic effects should largely be seen as negligible and only statistically significant in the bivariate correlations because of the current study's large sample size. However, a significant interaction of employment status by neuroticism emerged, whereby college students who were more neurotic and were employed full-time were less likely to be willing to provide instrumental care than unemployed or part-time employed individuals. A potential interpretation of this effect is that college students who are working full-time, in combination with being high in neuroticism, may feel particularly overwhelmed by their employment demands and as a result may not have the personal resources necessary to be devoted to providing instrumental care for a family member with a chronic condition. However, this effect should be interpreted with caution given that 54 demographics by personality interactions were examined in an exploratory fashion as predictors (three demographics by six personality traits, for each of the three willingness-to-care criterion variables), and this was the only interaction to reach statistical significance. This exploratory approach was highly prone to familywise error, so this effect should be examined in future studies before definitive interpretations are made.

Although results did not support our hypotheses of positive relationships between willingness to care with extraversion and openness, it is possible that the substantial amount of variance accounted for by empathy eclipsed the effect these personality aspects had on willingness to care. Additionally, it is worth noting that the correlation of the two items composing the openness subscale was relatively low and not significant, calling into question the internal consistency of this subscale in the current sample. While this scale has been previously validated among a college-aged sample and the subscale intercorrelations from the current sample are in line with those from the validated study [31], it is possible that there are additional characteristics that may have impacted the potential reliability of the openness subscale in particular and prevented it from showing an effect on willingness to care.

Though individuals with higher levels of extraversion have been shown to recognize the benefits of caregiving and tend to report positive experiences in providing care [19, 20], these rewards may not be apparent or compelling enough for extraverted college students. Research indicates potential caregivers perceiving fewer gains than losses as a caregiver may be less likely to adopt a caregiving role [43]. For extraverted college students in particular (and perhaps in comparison to caregivers from other age groups or population segments), the losses to one's social life or losses to the progression in one's academic pursuits may be fairly dramatic, and as a result some extraverted college students may be less willing to make sacrifices in their social lives in order to provide care given the extremely social nature of college settings.

5. Clinical Research Implications

The results of this study suggest that research on interventions attempting to increase empathy or to make it more salient may be particularly useful in exploring how to increase college students' willingness to provide care. In an intervention aimed to improve peer counseling skills in students, Hatcher et al. [44] provided instruction in nonjudgmental and empathic listening, facilitative feedback, and self-observation through role play. College students in the intervention group showed significant increases in empathic concern and perspective taking suggesting this type of intervention that targets empathic communication may be especially helpful with college students, as they may become better able to identify as the potential family member with a chronic health condition and thus more willing to provide care.

In terms of the current study's finding that agreeableness was associated with willingness to provide emotional care, intervention research making salient for college students the values of being cooperative, kind, and considerate (all facets of agreeableness) in the context of the family system may be a helpful direction. Such research could involve interventionists designing motivational interviewing techniques [45] that attempt to help college students identify discrepancies between these aspects of their personality and their actual behaviors of providing care for their family member with a health condition. Additionally, research on training that target daily life skills such as food preparation, financial management, and home maintenance may help the field better learn how to improve college student's self-efficacy in the provision of care and perhaps resultantly willingness to do so in the future. Similarly, college students who are better equipped with the necessary skills to care for themselves may be better positioned and more willing to care given greater personal resources (e.g., energy, social support) to enact informal care.

6. Limitations and Future Directions

There are some limitations that should be considered when interpreting the findings of this study. First, participants were asked to anticipate their willingness to provide care for a relative but were not asked to identify the person, the likelihood of actually becoming a caregiver, or the quality of their relationship to this family member. The relationship of a participant to particular family members (e.g., niece/nephew, child, and cousin), the quality of that relationship, and the likelihood of actually taking on a caregiving role with that person could indeed influence one's self-reported willingness to care. Research should ask participants specifically whom they are thinking about providing care for and what the quality of that relationship is, as these variables could make one more or less apt to provide care for the family member. Additionally, data on the severity of the illness, injury, or disability imagined by the participant were not collected and may impact willingness to provide care. Related to this, participants were asked to imagine someone that they "might have to provide care for at some point because they have a chronic illness, injury, or disability." The definition of "chronic illness, injury, or disability" encompasses a wide range of issues and differing care demands and "at some point" covers a wide time-frame. As a result, responses may vary depending on what a respondent imagined based on this prompt. Future research may benefit from including more specific language regarding the potential provision of care by participants in the future. Family members with more severe injuries or illnesses, for instance, dementia, require greater care on behalf of the caregiver than others do, which may impact how much and what type of care they are willing to provide. Furthermore, issues related to familial responsibility were also not assessed. Students who have a greater sense of obligation and/or lack of choice to care for those in the family network may be more or less willing to care than those who perceive fewer obligations [43]. Finally, the sample consisted entirely of psychology students and was overrepresented by participants from middle-class families and women and thus may not generalize to all college students. Future studies should assess relationship quality between the potential caregiver and future care recipient as well as familial responsibility in an effort to better understand the effects of personality on willingness to provide care for a relative with a chronic health condition.

7. Conclusions

This study adds to the growing body of research assessing willingness to provide care for future family members by outlining specific personality traits among college students that may be influential for future care. With a growing population of older adults, young adults are primed to become caregivers in the near future. The results of this study identifying agreeableness, empathy, and age as being important for one's potential for future caregiving can help shape future interventions especially those that incorporate perspective taking and training in life skills as a means of boosting empathic concern and subsequently greater willingness to care.

Competing Interests

The authors report no competing interests related to the submission of this manuscript.

Acknowledgments

This study was supported in part by a grant from the National Science Foundation (DGE-1147383).

References

[1] World Health Organization, *Global Health and Aging (NIH publication no. 11-7737)*, National Institutes of Health, US Department of Health and Human Services, Bethesda, Md, USA, 2011.

[2] E. Brody, *Caregiving in the 1990s*, Menorah Park, Cleveland, Ohio, USA, 1995.

[3] R. L. Kane and R. A. Kane, "Transitions in long-term care," in *Aging and Health Care*, pp. 217–242, 1989.

[4] C. Levine, G. G. Hunt, D. Halper, A. Y. Hart, J. Lautz, and D. A. Gould, "Young adult caregivers: a first look at an unstudied population," *American Journal of Public Health*, vol. 95, no. 11, pp. 2071–2075, 2005.

[5] National Center for Education Statistics, "Percentage of 18- to 24-year-olds enrolled in degree-granting postsecondary institutions, by level of institution and sex and race/ethnicity of student: 1970 through 2014," http://nces.ed.gov/programs/digest/d15/tables/dt15_302.60.asp.

[6] M. Dellmann-Jenkins, M. Blankemeyer, and O. Pinkard, "Young adult children and grandchildren in primary caregiver roles to older relatives and their service needs," *Family Relations*, vol. 49, no. 2, pp. 177–186, 2000.

[7] U. Henz, "Informal caregiving at working age: effects of job characteristics and family configuration," *Journal of Marriage and Family*, vol. 68, no. 2, pp. 411–429, 2006.

[8] R. Baus, D. Dysart-Gale, and P. Haven, "Caregiving and social support: a twenty-first century challenge for college students," *Communication Quarterly*, vol. 53, no. 2, pp. 125–142, 2007.

[9] L. I. Pearlin, J. T. Mullan, S. J. Semple, and M. M. Skaff, "Caregiving and the stress process: an overview of concepts and their measures," *Gerontologist*, vol. 30, no. 5, pp. 583–594, 1990.

[10] S. Sörensen and S. H. Zarit, "Preparation for caregiving: a study of multigeneration families," *International Journal of Aging and Human Development*, vol. 42, no. 1, pp. 43–63, 1996.

[11] S. Sörensen, "Predictors of anticipating caregiving in multi-generation families: an exploratory study," *Journal of Applied Gerontology*, vol. 17, no. 4, pp. 499–520, 1998.

[12] G. C. Karantzas, L. Evans, and M. Foddy, "The role of attachment in current and future parent caregiving," *Journals of Gerontology—Series B: Psychological Sciences and Social Sciences*, vol. 65, no. 5, pp. 573–580, 2010.

[13] V. G. Cicirelli, "Adult children's helping behavior to elderly parents: the influence of divorce," *Journal of Family Issues*, vol. 5, no. 3, pp. 419–440, 1984.

[14] Y. Kim, P. R. Duberstein, S. Sörensen, and M. R. Larson, "Levels of depressive symptoms in spouses of people with lung cancer: effects of personality, social support, and caregiving burden," *Psychosomatics*, vol. 46, no. 2, pp. 123–130, 2005.

[15] C. E. Löckenhoff, P. R. Duberstein, B. Friedman, and P. T. Costa Jr., "Five-factor personality traits and subjective health among caregivers: the role of caregiver strain and self-efficacy," *Psychology and Aging*, vol. 26, no. 3, pp. 592–604, 2011.

[16] R. R. McCrae and O. P. John, "An introduction to the five-factor model and its applications," *Journal of Personality*, vol. 60, no. 2, pp. 175–215, 1992.

[17] K. Hooker, D. Monahan, K. Shifren, and C. Hutchinson, "Mental and physical health of spouse caregivers: the role of personality," *Psychology and Aging*, vol. 7, no. 3, pp. 367–375, 1992.

[18] M. P. Gallant and C. M. Connell, "Neuroticism and depressive symptoms among spouse caregivers: do health behaviors mediate this relationship?" *Psychology and Aging*, vol. 18, no. 3, pp. 587–592, 2003.

[19] S. S. Koerner, D. B. Kenyon, and Y. Shirai, "Caregiving for elder relatives: which caregivers experience personal benefits/gains?" *Archives of Gerontology and Geriatrics*, vol. 48, no. 2, pp. 238–245, 2009.

[20] Q. Zhai, M. Willis, B. O'Shea, Y. Zhai, and Y. Yang, "Big five personality traits, job satisfaction and subjective wellbeing in China," *International Journal of Psychology*, vol. 48, no. 6, pp. 1099–1108, 2013.

[21] L. A. Hollis-Sawyer, "Mother–daughter eldercare and changing relationships: a path-analytic investigation of factors underlying positive, adaptive relationships," *Journal of Adult Development*, vol. 10, no. 1, pp. 41–52, 2003.

[22] S. S. Koerner and D. B. Kenyon, "Understanding 'good days' and 'bad days': emotional and physical reactivity among caregivers for elder relatives," *Family Relations*, vol. 56, no. 1, pp. 1–11, 2007.

[23] M. Hoerger, M. Coletta, S. Sörensen et al., "Personality and perceived health in spousal caregivers of patients with lung cancer: the roles of neuroticism and extraversion," *Journal of Aging Research*, vol. 2016, Article ID 5659793, 7 pages, 2016.

[24] S. Sörensen, P. R. Duberstein, B. Chapman, J. M. Lyness, and M. Pinquart, "How are personality traits related to preparation for future care needs in older adults?" *Journals of Gerontology, Series B: Psychological Sciences and Social Sciences*, vol. 63, no. 6, pp. P328–P336, 2008.

[25] H. S. Lee, P. F. Brennan, and B. J. Daly, "Relationship of empathy to appraisal, depression, life satisfaction, and physical health in informal caregivers of older adults," *Research in Nursing and Health*, vol. 24, no. 1, pp. 44–56, 2001.

[26] R. N. Spreng, M. C. McKinnon, R. A. Mar, and B. Levine, "The Toronto empathy questionnaire: scale development and initial validation of a factor-analytic solution to multiple empathy measures," *Journal of Personality Assessment*, vol. 91, no. 1, pp. 62–71, 2009.

[27] R. Schulz, R. S. Hebert, M. A. Dew et al., "Patient suffering and caregiver compassion: new opportunities for research, practice, and policy," *The Gerontologist*, vol. 47, no. 1, pp. 4–13, 2007.

[28] L. Bramwell and A. L. Whall, "Effect of role clarity and empathy on support role performance and anxiety," *Nursing Research*, vol. 35, no. 5, pp. 282–287, 1986.

[29] M. K. Rohr, J. Wagner, and F. R. Lang, "Effects of personality on the transition into caregiving," *Psychology and Aging*, vol. 28, no. 3, pp. 692–700, 2013.

[30] N. Abell, "Assessing willingness to care for persons with AIDS: validation of a new measure," *Research on Social Work Practice*, vol. 11, no. 1, pp. 118–130, 2001.

[31] B. Rammstedt and O. P. John, "Measuring personality in one minute or less: a 10-item short version of the big five inventory in English and German," *Journal of Research in Personality*, vol. 41, no. 1, pp. 203–212, 2007.

[32] N. Chesley and K. Poppie, "Assisting parents and in-laws: gender, type of assistance, and couples' employment," *Journal of Marriage and Family*, vol. 71, no. 2, pp. 247–262, 2009.

[33] E. M. Friedman and J. A. Seltzer, *Providing for Older Parents: Is It a Family Affair*, On-Line Working Paper Series, California Center for Population Research, 2010.

[34] C. D. Batson, *The Altruism Question: Toward a Social-Psychological Answer*, Erlbaum, Hillsdale, NJ, USA, 1991.

[35] M. Toi and C. D. Batson, "More evidence that empathy is a source of altruistic motivation," *Journal of Personality and Social Psychology*, vol. 43, no. 2, pp. 281–292, 1982.

[36] M. H. Davis, "Empathic concern and the muscular dystrophy telethon: empathy as a multidimensional construct," *Personality and Social Psychology Bulletin*, vol. 9, no. 2, pp. 223–229, 1983.

[37] M. H. Davis, "The effects of dispositional empathy on emotional reactions and helping: a multidimensional approach," *Journal of Personality*, vol. 51, no. 2, pp. 167–184, 1983.

[38] J. P. Rushton, "The altruistic personality," in *Development and Maintenance of Prosocial Behavior*, E. Staub, D. Bar-Tal, J. Karylowski, and J. Reykowski, Eds., vol. 31 of *Critical Issues in Social Justice*, pp. 271–290, Springer, 1984.

[39] J. M. Digman, "Personality structure: emergence of the five-factor model," *Annual Review of Psychology*, vol. 41, no. 1, pp. 417–440, 1990.

[40] B. M. Smith and L. D. Nelson, "Personality correlates of helping behavior," *Psychological Reports*, vol. 37, no. 1, pp. 307–310, 1975.

[41] W. G. Graziano and N. H. Eisenberg, "Agreeableness: a dimension of personality," in *Handbook of Personality Psychology*, R. Hogan, J. Johnson, and S. Briggs, Eds., pp. 795–824, Academic Press, San Diego, Calif, USA, 1997.

[42] K. L. Zellars and P. L. Perrewé, "Affective personality and the content of emotional social support: coping in organizations," *Journal of Applied Psychology*, vol. 86, no. 3, pp. 459–467, 2001.

[43] M. K. Rohr and F. R. Lang, "The role of anticipated gains and losses on preferences about future caregiving," *The Journals of Gerontology Series B: Psychological Sciences and Social Sciences*, vol. 71, no. 3, pp. 405–414, 2016.

[44] S. L. Hatcher, M. S. Nadeau, L. K. Walsh, and M. Reynolds, "The teaching of empathy for high school and college students: testing rogerian methods with the interpersonal reactivity index," *Adolescence*, vol. 29, no. 116, pp. 961–974, 1994.

[45] W. R. Miller and S. Rollnick, *Motivational Interviewing: Helping People Change*, Guilford Press, 2012.

10

Age-Related Increase in Electromyography Burst Activity in Males and Females

Olga Theou,[1] Darl Edwards,[2] Gareth R. Jones,[3] and Jennifer M. Jakobi[3]

[1] *Geriatric Medicine, Dalhousie University, 5955 Veterans' Memorial Lane, Halifax, NS, Canada B3H 2E1*
[2] *Medicine, University of Toronto, Toronto, ON, Canada M5S 1A8*
[3] *Health and Exercise Sciences, University of British Columbia Okanagan, 3333 University Way, Kelowna, BC, Canada V1V 1V7*

Correspondence should be addressed to Jennifer M. Jakobi; jennifer.jakobi@ubc.ca

Academic Editor: Iris Reuter

The rapid advancement of electromyography (EMG) technology facilitates measurement of muscle activity outside the laboratory during daily life. The purpose of this study was to determine whether bursts in EMG recorded over a typical 8-hour day differed between young and old males and females. Muscle activity was recorded from biceps brachii, triceps brachii, vastus lateralis, and biceps femoris of 16 young and 15 old adults using portable surface EMG. Old muscles were active 16–27% of the time compared to 5–9% in young muscles. The number of bursts was greater in old than young adults and in females compared to males. Burst percentage and mean amplitude were greater in the flexor muscles compared with the extensor muscles. The greater burst activity in old adults coupled with the unique activity patterns across muscles in males and females provides further understanding of how changes in neuromuscular activity effects age-related functional decline between the sexes.

1. Introduction

Accelerometers, pedometers, and global position system (GPS) have become familiar tools for assessing age-related changes in mobility and physical activity during daily life [1, 2], but these devices provide no indication of muscle activity governing movement. Laboratory studies using electromyography (EMG) have provided considerable understanding of age-related changes in muscle activity for simple isometric and anisometric contractions [3–5], gait [6], and discrete tasks [7] executed under experimental constraints. With the advancement of technology, portable EMG devices now offer a means to characterize muscle activity (bursts) and quiescence (gaps) over long durations outside the laboratory, enabling discrete measurement of neuromuscular control within the environmental context of daily life [8, 9].

Quantification of gaps in EMG for a discrete task and during daily life activities, in young and old adults, suggests muscle quiescence decreases in old adults and is less in women compared with men [10]. For a discrete task when the EMG is quantified through bursts, muscle activity increases in old adults relative to young adults and is also greater in women [8, 11]. Together, measurement of bursts and gaps for a discrete task, such as carrying a bag of groceries, suggests that muscles are active more often and "rest" less in older adults and women. Age-related remodeling [12, 13], decreased muscle strength [3, 14, 15], and greater declines in performance for fast velocity relative to slow velocity movements [16, 17] likely predispose old adults to increased bursts to execute activities of daily life. Similarly, reduced muscle mass and quality have been observed in upper and lower limbs of women and may necessitate a higher level of muscle activity to execute daily life [18, 19]. Quantification of burst activity during daily life will provide insight into muscle activation required for functional movement executed within the lived environment beyond the confines of a controlled laboratory setting where factors such as stress and fatigue are not encompassed within a discrete task.

In addition to the increase in burst activity in the arm and thigh muscles of old adults for a discrete task [10, 11], prior studies suggest that the duration of burst activity was longer in females than males in the biceps brachii of young adults [20]. Muscle-dependent differences should not be surprising during daily life as laboratory-based motor unit and surface

EMG measures describe muscle specific age-related decline in motor unit activity [3, 21] and sex-specific decline in force control [22]. Thus, to better understand whether muscle activity increases with age during daily life and determine sex-specific changes in functional muscle pairs, assessment of EMG in young and old males and females needs to be undertaken during a typical day. The purpose of this study was to quantify age- and sex-related alterations in burst activity in young and old males and females in lower limb and upper limb muscles over the course of a weekday. It was hypothesized that burst activity would be greater in old adults relative to young adults due to age-related changes in neuromuscular properties. In addition, burst activity would be exacerbated in females and in flexor muscles consistent with a previous report in young adults [20].

2. Methods

Thirty-one healthy adults from the general populous of greater Windsor-Essex County of South Western Ontario participated in this study. All subjects were free of known neurological or neuromuscular conditions. Individuals were excluded if they participated in structured regular exercise training programs greater than three times per week. Volunteers were divided into four groups based upon age and sex. Age criterion for the young adults was less than 26 years whereas the minimum age for the old adults was 70 years. The local Human Research Ethics Board approved this experiment, and informed written consent was obtained prior to participation.

Subjects participated in one 8-hour recording day and visited the laboratory twice on the same day. The first session was in the morning, approximately 90 minutes after the subjects awoke. The Yale Physical Activity Survey [23] was administered to assess differences in energy expenditure and physical activities between age and sex. Subsequently, electrodes were placed on the biceps brachii (BB), triceps brachii (TB), vastus lateralis (VL), and biceps femoris (BF), and maximum voluntary exertions (MVEs) were performed for the four muscles to record maximal electromyography (EMG) for normalization of surface recordings. Following the initial MVE assessment, subjects left the laboratory and were asked to partake in normal daily activities, defined as events that were typically and regularly performed. Subjects were asked not to engage in any water activities (i.e., swimming, showering). After eight hours, subjects returned to the laboratory and the MVEs were repeated to verify the integrity of the recording off-line. Subsequently, the EMG equipment was removed and subjects were debriefed.

2.1. Electromyography. Long-term EMG was recorded using surface electrodes (20 mm interelectrode distance) placed on the long head of the BB and the lateral head of the TB as well as the VL and BF as previously described [8–11, 24, 25]. BB and TB are the principle elbow flexors and extensors, respectively, and are the primary contributors to reaching in order to execute functional upper limb movements. VL and BF are large muscle groups utilized to transport the body during upright posture and gait and exert flexion and extension force about the knee and undergo severe age-related weakening which is related to functional decline. Electrodes were attached to the skin using double-sided medical grade die cut application tape [26]. The DataLOG unit (Biometrics P3X8, Gwent, UK; 9.5 × 15.8 × 3.3 cm, 380 gram) which recorded signals was attached to a belt and worn on the hip. The electrodes and device did not impair or limit movement or activities of daily living.

2.2. Maximum Voluntary Exertions. MVEs were performed three times for each muscle (VL, BF, BB, and TB) both in the morning and afternoon, as previously described [11, 24]. Briefly, for the arm muscles the MVEs were performed with the elbow joint at 90°. The experimenter instructed and resisted a maximum pull-up (flex arm) and push-down effort (extend arm) for approximately 3 seconds to assess maximum BB and TB activities, respectively. For the two lower limb muscles, the subject was seated in a rigid chair against a wall that was adjusted to the subject's height so that the knee and hip joint could be positioned to 90° for the maximum flexion/extension efforts of the leg that were executed against experimenter resistance. A canvass strap was fixed around, the waist of the subject and the chair to support consistent positioning. All subjects were highly encouraged with verbal instruction prior to the MVE and subsequent to the attempt to exert the greatest possible effort. When aberrations in position occurred the subject was informed of the deviations and attempted the MVE effort again. The EMG value derived from the MVE was a computed rectified and integrated value recorded from the middle of the MVE contraction.

2.3. Signal Processing and Data Analysis. All EMG signals recorded during the MVE and the 8 hours testing were amplified (1000x), filtered (20–450 Hz), and stored on the 512 MB MMC flashcard at a sampling rate of 100 Hz for subsequent analysis. Data from the flashcard was transferred to the computer hard drive via USB cable and imported into the Biometrics (Gwent, UK) program. From the Biometrics (Gwent, UK) program, data was exported to Spike 2 version 5 (Cambridge Electronics Design, Cambridge, UK) for further processing in a custom analysis script. All signals were rectified, smoothed (0.01 sec), and down-sampled (100x) to 10 Hz prior to analysis. In some instances, artifacts due to electrode or device contact occurred, and these sections were time-locked and deleted across all channels simultaneously. These artifacts were limited and their occurrence was similar between age and sex groups. Data artifact was identified through visual inspection which was then confirmed by taking the root mean square (RMS) amplitude of the waveform in 0.1-second increments and identifying plateaus (square waves) in the recording. A custom script was utilized within Spike 2 for the burst analysis. An EMG burst was defined as any interval in the recording that had an amplitude >2% of the maximum EMG value and duration >0.1 seconds. The EMG data was analyzed and quantified using five burst characteristics: number of bursts, mean duration (seconds), burst percentage (% of total recording time occupied by bursts), peak amplitude (the peak amplitude of bursts averaged across all bursts, %MVE), and mean amplitude (average of the mean amplitude of all bursts, %MVE).

2.4. Statistical Analysis. The Statistical Package for the Social Sciences (SPSS, Chicago, IL, USA) for windows version 17.0 was used for statistical analysis. A 2 × 2 analysis of variance (ANOVA), with age and sex as between-subject factors, was conducted on results from the Yale Physical Activity Survey. A paired t-test was utilized to compare the morning and evening values for the maximum and average MVEs from each session. The five dependent variables of the burst characteristics were compared with a 2 × 2 × 4 multivariate ANOVA for the between-subject factors of age (young, old) and sex (male, female) and the within-subject factor of muscle (VL, BF, BB, and TB). The probability level for all statistical measures was set at 0.05.

3. Results

The eight young males were 24.0 ± 2.5 years (90.6 ± 13.1 kg, 182.0 ± 9.4 cm) and the eight young females were 22.0 ± 1.6 years (57.4 ± 8.5 kg, 162.6 ± 4.4 cm). The eight old males were 76.6 ± 2.8 years (83.9 ± 4.0 kg, 172.3 ± 4.9 cm) and the seven old females were 77.3 ± 4.5 years (74.3 ± 21.8 kg, 159.2 ± 5.9 cm). Total physical activity did not differ between age groups (young 8032 ± 2386 kcal/week; old 7532 ± 4975 kcal/week; $P = 0.72$) or sexes (male 7788 ± 4637 kcal/week; female 7792 ± 2819 kcal/week; $P = 0.99$).

The maximal and average MVE values from the morning and evening sessions did not differ; thus, the highest MVE recorded from the six attempts was utilized for normalization of the long-term EMG data and determination of burst characteristics. The three-way interaction between age, sex, and muscle was significant ($P = 0.04$). In order to identify the contribution of individual dependent variables to this significant interaction of the multivariate ANOVA, a 2 × 2 × 4 (age × sex × muscle) univariate ANOVA was utilized for each burst variable.

For the number of bursts, mean amplitude, and burst percentage, there was no three-way interaction (age × sex × muscle; $P = 0.06$). The 2 × 2 (age × sex) interactions were not significant for these variables ($P > 0.05$); however, there was a 2 × 4 (sex × muscle) interaction for burst percentage ($P = 0.01$) and a 2 × 4 (age × muscle) interaction for the number of bursts ($P = 0.04$). All three of these variables were greater ($P < 0.05$) in old adults compared with young adults (Table 1), and females had greater ($P = 0.04$) number of bursts compared with males. There was no sex effect on mean amplitude ($P = 0.77$) and burst percentage ($P > 0.05$) across muscles (Table 2).

For burst duration and peak amplitude, significant three-way interactions were observed ($P < 0.05$). These interactions were examined further by performing a 2 × 2 univariate ANOVA (age × sex) for each muscle group separately and a 2 × 4 univariate ANOVA (sex × muscle) for young and old. The 2 × 2 (age × sex) interactions were significant for burst duration in the TB ($P = 0.02$) and peak amplitude in the BF ($P = 0.01$). The 2 × 4 (sex × muscle) interactions were observed for burst duration and peak amplitude of the old adults ($P < 0.05$). Burst duration was greater in old adults compared with young adults in all muscles except the TB of males ($P = 0.92$) (Table 1). Burst duration in the BB of both young and old adults ($P = 0.01$) and in the TB of old adults ($P = 0.03$) were greater in females than males. Peak amplitude in the BF of old adults was greater ($P = 0.03$) in males (Table 2).

Significant differences were found between muscles for all burst characteristics except for burst duration in old females ($P = 0.49$). In young adults, the number of bursts and burst percentage were greater ($P < 0.01$) in the flexor muscles compared with the extensor muscles in both arm (BB > TB) and thigh muscles (BF > VL). In addition, the number of bursts and burst percentage were greater ($P = 0.01$) in BF compared with TB (Figures 1(a) and 1(b)). Burst duration in BF of young adults was longer ($P < 0.01$) than the BB and VL (Figure 1(c)), and peak burst amplitude in the thigh muscles (VL and BF) was greater compared with the arm muscles (BB and TB) ($P < 0.001$) (Figure 1(d)). In old adults, the number of bursts was less ($P < 0.01$) in the VL than the other three

TABLE 1: Age-related differences in burst characteristics for each muscle group.

	Young	Old
Number		
BB	6200 ± 3112	12935 ± 4142*
TB	3763 ± 2382	10700 ± 5167*
VL	4698 ± 2280	8048 ± 3395*
BF	6030 ± 2504	11676 ± 4391*
Duration (sec)		
BB	0.4 ± 0.1	0.6 ± 0.3*
TB†	0.4 ± 0.1	0.6 ± 0.1*
VL	0.4 ± 0.1	0.6 ± 0.2*
BF	0.5 ± 0.1	0.6 ± 0.2*
Peak amplitude (% MVE)		
BB	5.0 ± 0.8	6.0 ± 1.7
TB	4.9 ± 0.7	4.8 ± 0.6
VL	8.8 ± 2.0	9.4 ± 4.0
BF	9.3 ± 1.8	9.6 ± 3.8
Mean amplitude (% MVE)		
BB	0.6 ± 0.3	1.9 ± 1.1*
TB	0.6 ± 0.4	1.5 ± 0.8*
VL	0.8 ± 1.0	1.4 ± 0.9*
BF	1.2 ± 0.9	2.2 ± 1.4*
Percentage (% time)		
BB	8.3 ± 5.0	26.8 ± 11.8*
TB	5.4 ± 4.0	19.9 ± 12.5*
VL	5.6 ± 2.6	16.2 ± 8.0*
BF	9.3 ± 3.8	24.1 ± 7.3*

BB: biceps brachii; TB: triceps brachii; VL: vastus lateralis; BF: biceps femoris; sec: seconds; %: percentage; MVE: maximal voluntary exertion.
*Significantly different from young adults.
†Only females.

TABLE 2: Sex-related differences in burst characteristics for each muscle group.

	Male	Female
Number		
BB	8887 ± 5398	10069 ± 4541*
TB	5609 ± 4206	8731 ± 5919*
VL	5886 ± 2642	6781 ± 3922*
BF	7869 ± 4334	9713 ± 4650*
Duration (sec)		
BB	0.4 ± 0.1	0.6 ± 0.3*
TB†	0.4 ± 0.1	0.6 ± 0.1*
VL	0.5 ± 0.2	0.4 ± 0.2
BF	0.6 ± 0.2	0.6 ± 0.1
Peak amplitude (% MVE)		
BB	5.4 ± 1.5	5.6 ± 1.4
TB	4.8 ± 0.6	4.9 ± 0.8
VL	10.1 ± 3.6	8.1 ± 1.9
BF†	11.5 ± 3.7	7.5 ± 2.8*
Mean amplitude (% MVE)		
BB	1.1 ± 1.0	1.4 ± 1.1
TB	0.8 ± 0.6	1.2 ± 0.9
VL	1.2 ± 1.0	1.0 ± 1.0
BF	1.9 ± 1.4	1.5 ± 1.0
Percentage (% time)		
BB	13.6 ± 11.0	21.1 ± 13.9
TB	9.1 ± 8.7	15.9 ± 13.5
VL	11.2 ± 8.7	10.3 ± 7.2
BF	15.3 ± 9.0	17.7 ± 9.9

BB: biceps brachii; TB: triceps brachii; VL: vastus lateralis; BF: biceps femoris; sec: seconds; %: percentage; MVE: maximal voluntary exertion.
*Significantly different from males.
†Only old adults.

muscles (Figure 2(a)). Burst percentage in old adults was greater ($P < 0.05$) in flexor muscles compared with extensor muscles in both arm (BB > TB) and thigh muscles (BF > VL). In addition, burst percentage was greater ($P = 0.01$) in BB compared with VL (Figure 2(b)). In old males, burst duration and peak amplitude were greater ($P < 0.05$) in thigh muscles (VL and BF) compared with the arm muscles (BB and TB) (Figures 3(a) and 3(b)). Peak burst amplitude in old females was greater ($P < 0.05$) in the thigh muscles (VL and BF) compared with the TB (Figure 3(b)). Mean burst amplitude in both young and old adults was greater ($P < 0.05$) in BF compared with the other three muscles and in BB compared with TB.

4. Discussion

The purpose of this study was to quantify age- and sex-related differences in burst activity measured with portable EMG devices during the course of a day. The key finding in this investigation was the age-related increase in muscle activation where the number of bursts was greater in females than males and flexor muscles were more active than extensor muscles. Measuring muscle activity that governs movement during daily life with portable EMG offers an early indication of the physiological alterations in muscle that manifest prior to overt declines in activities of daily living that are required for independent living.

The most striking difference in this study was the age-related increase in burst percentage (~190–270%Δ) with young muscles being active 5–9% of the time whereas older muscles were active 16–27%. These data clearly indicate that the manner in which daily tasks are accomplished differs at the level of the muscle, and this can be captured by long-term EMG. The observed differences between young and old adults likely arise from age-related change in neuromuscular function as physical activity was similar between these groups of adults that were separated by >50 years in age. Differences in burst activity are unlikely to be related to tasks undertaken during the day. Although daily tasks were not monitored, because subjects were free to undertake normal activities without bias of an observer, our previous work has shown that burst activity is greater in old adults when the task is matched between age groups [11]. Thus, the difference in burst activity during daily life supports our prior findings from discrete tasks [11]. Muscle weakness in old adults is a contributing factor in the age-related increase in muscle activity as laboratory-based studies report greater muscle activity in weaker individuals when the relative load for isolated contractions is matched [11]. Because old adults are typically weaker than young adults [3, 27], strength might contribute to the age-related increase in muscle activity observed for a typical day; however, strength cannot be the sole factor. Burst duration was similar between males and females in the thigh muscles, yet men are stronger than women [27]. This highlights the need to acknowledge that strength occupies a role in muscle activity that necessitates success in daily activities, but it is not the singular contributor to age- and sex-related increase in muscle activity.

The decrease in motor unit number with increased age coupled with the remaining pool of motor units becoming less heterogeneous and larger in individual size (innervation ratio) may contribute to the age-related augmentation in burst activity. There is a positive relationship between the size of a motor unit and the resultant amplitude of EMG signal [28]; therefore, the older and larger motor units would likely have higher burst activity. This could be detected as greater mean burst amplitude in old adults compared with young adults during daily life. With increased age, movement times slow in old adults compared with young adults for a variety of tasks, and fast velocity movements are more affected by aging than slow velocity movements [16, 17, 29]. Increased movement time would likely augment that the amount of time force is maintained during execution of activities of daily life and in turn merge as greater total and mean burst duration. This increase in burst duration may allow for an enhanced level of force production to execute tasks of daily life. However, the increase in EMG burst activity during daily life, which likely facilitates the production of movement, could predispose older adults to an earlier onset of fatigue, and this may, over time, contribute to reduced fine motor control of everyday tasks similar to the decreased ability of

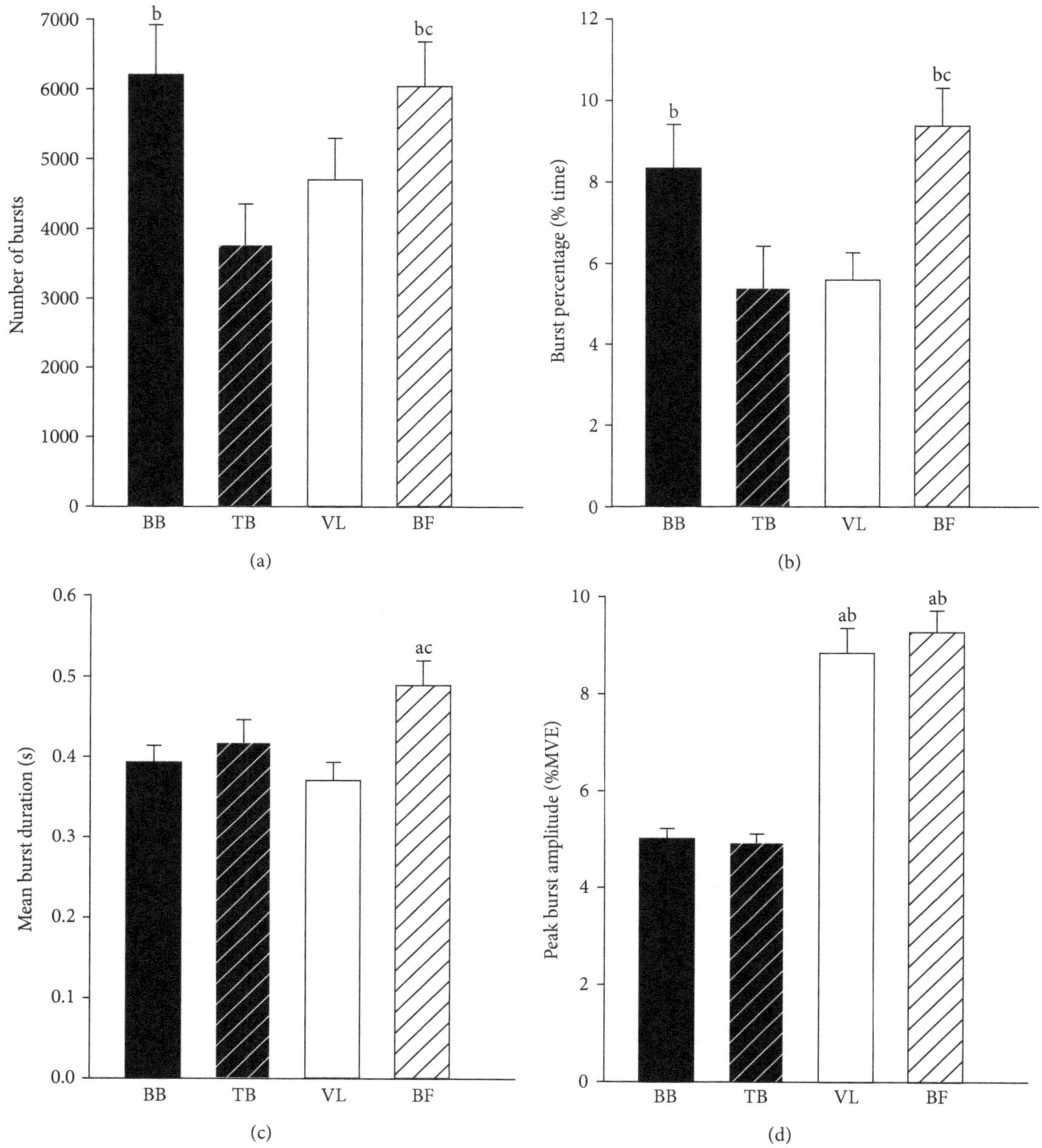

FIGURE 1: Muscle effect on burst characteristics for young adults. (a) Number of bursts; (b) burst percentage; (c) mean burst duration; (d) peak burst amplitude. BB: biceps brachii; TB: triceps brachii; VL: vastus lateralis; BF: biceps femoris; sec: seconds; %: percentage; MVE: maximal voluntary exertion. [a]Significantly different from BB; [b]significantly different from TB; [c]significantly different from VL.

older adults to produce steady contractions in controlled laboratory-based studies [4].

The number of bursts in females was 13–56% greater than males for both young and old adults. Increased bursts in females compared with males may be due to intrinsic properties of muscle. Studies suggest that fiber area, number, and force per cross-sectional area are reduced in females compared with males [19], and in animal models the innervation ratio is estimated to be greater in males compared to females [30]. These anatomical features coupled with a longer electromechanical delay [31], slower rate of force development [32], and slow reciprocal activation in triphasic EMG burst patterns in females compared with males [33] cause differential burst activity between sexes. These physiological and anatomical differences that culminate in greater burst activity in females are not unlike the age-related adaptations.

The age-related increase in burst duration of the TB was only evident in females. The sex-related differences in burst duration of the TB as well as the peak burst amplitude of the BF were only evident in old adults. In addition, muscle differences in burst duration and peak amplitude were similar between young males and females but not between old males and females. Thus, muscles of females are predisposed to

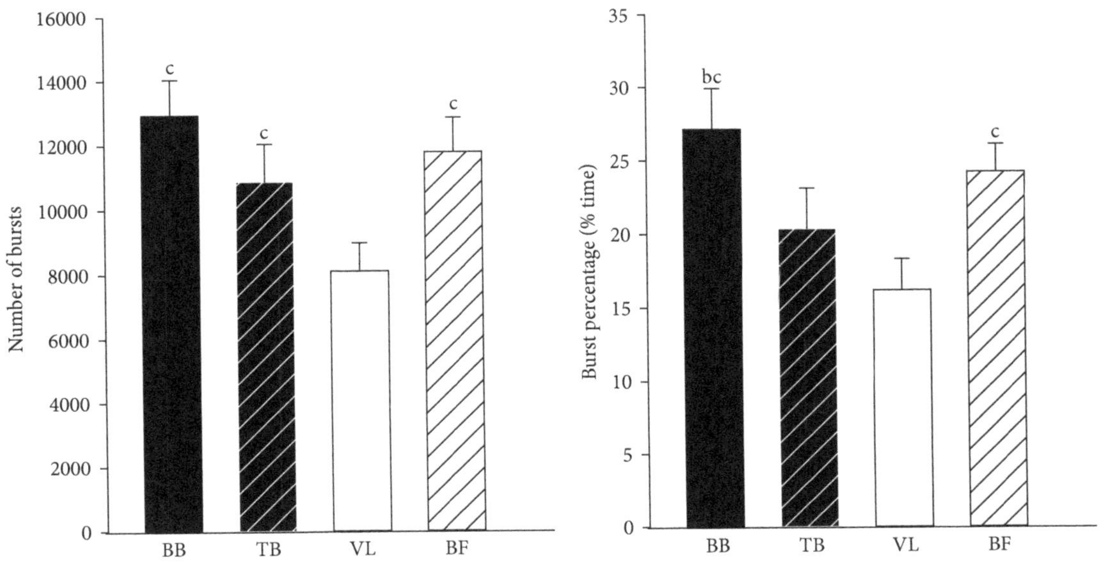

(a) (b)

FIGURE 2: Muscle effect on number of bursts and burst percentage for old adults. (a) Number of bursts; (b) burst percentage. BB: biceps brachii; TB: triceps brachii; VL: vastus lateralis; BF: biceps femoris; %: percentage. [a]Significantly different from TB; [b]significantly different from VL.

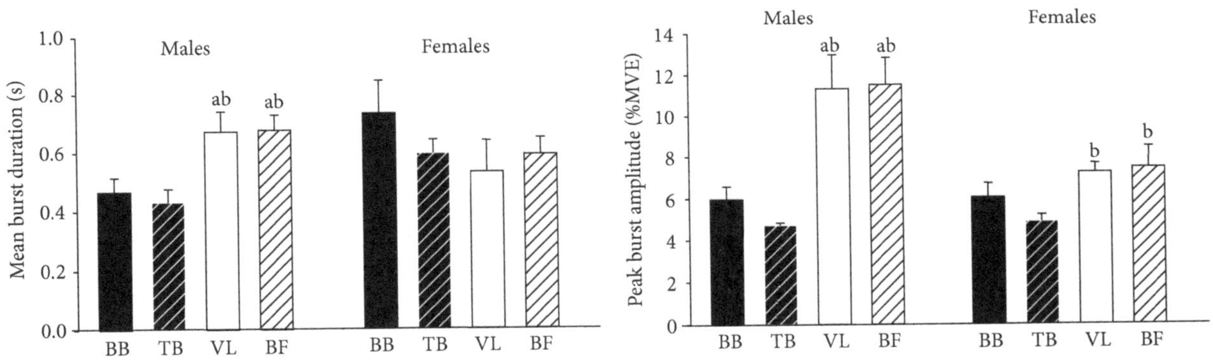

(a) (b)

FIGURE 3: Muscle effect on mean burst duration and peak burst amplitude for old adults. (a) Mean burst duration; (b) peak burst amplitude. BB: biceps brachii; TB: triceps brachii; VL: vastus lateralis; BF: biceps femoris; sec: seconds; %: percentage; MVE: maximal voluntary exertion. [a]Significantly different from BB; [b]significantly different from TB.

alterations that culminate in earlier age-related functional decline relative to males; these changes are detectable through daily EMG. This tool offers a means for sex-specific detection of altered muscle activity with age which may enable earlier identification of impending functional changes that may have a significant impact upon physical independence [24]. Females are more likely to become frail and experience functional decline and/or loss of independence [34, 35].

Differences in burst characteristics between flexor and extensor muscles were found in both the arm and thigh muscles. Flexor muscles were active for a longer duration than the extensor muscles (35–66%Δ). The greater burst characteristics of the flexor muscles compared with the extensor muscles in old adults might be related to greater age-related decline in strength and motor unit discharge rates of the flexor muscles [3, 14, 15]. Thus, the flexor muscles of the old adults need to function at a higher relative level because they have undergone greater age-related decline relative to the extensors. Therefore, this augmentation in flexor activity relative to the extensor is in part due to movements undertaken to execute daily life (self-care and feeding) which largely involve the flexors as the agonist which are reported to undergo greater age-related change [3].

5. Conclusions

In summary, there are definitive age differences with respect to burst activity over an 8-hour recording. The muscles of old adults burst more, with higher mean amplitudes and for longer duration throughout the day and muscle of females burst more and longer than males. Overall burst activity in the flexor muscles is greater than the extensor muscles. In addition, muscle differences are consistent between young males and females but not between old males and females. Differences in muscle activity for a typical day quantified as bursts in EMG highlight alterations in neuromuscular function with age that are sensitive to sex and specific to muscle. Assessment of long-term EMG, recorded with portable devices, can be an effective way to identify physiological change prior to functional loss. This offers an effective tool for diagnosing impending physical decline in older adults through earlier identification of changes in muscle activity prior to overt functional loss.

Acknowledgment

This work was supported by the Natural Science Engineering Research Council. Olga Theou receives postdoctoral funding from the University Internal Medicine Research Foundation of Dalhousie University.

References

[1] J. S. Frank and A. E. Patla, "Balance and mobility challenges in older adults: implications for preserving community mobility," *The American Journal of Preventive Medicine*, vol. 25, no. 3, pp. 157–163, 2003.

[2] O. Theou, J. M. Jakobi, A. A. Vandervoort, and G. R. Jones, "A comparison of physical activity (PA) assessment tools across levels of frailty," *Archives of Gerontology and Geriatrics*, vol. 54, no. 3, pp. e307–e314, 2012.

[3] B. H. Dalton, J. M. Jakobi, B. L. Allman, and C. L. Rice, "Differential age-related changes in motor unit properties between elbow flexors and extensors," *Acta Physiologica*, vol. 200, no. 1, pp. 45–55, 2010.

[4] R. M. Enoka, E. A. Christou, S. K. Hunter et al., "Mechanisms that contribute to differences in motor performance between young and old adults," *Journal of Electromyography and Kinesiology*, vol. 13, no. 1, pp. 1–12, 2003.

[5] B. Harwood, D. L. Edwards, and J. M. Jakobi, "Age independent and position-dependent alterations in motor unit activity of the biceps brachii," *European Journal of Applied Physiology*, vol. 110, no. 1, pp. 27–38, 2010.

[6] A. Schmitz, A. Silder, B. Heiderscheit, J. Mahoney, and D. G. Thelen, "Differences in lower-extremity muscular activation during walking between healthy older and young adults," *Journal of Electromyography and Kinesiology*, vol. 19, no. 6, pp. 1085–1091, 2009.

[7] S. Morrison and J. Sosnoff, "Age-related changes in the adaptability of neuromuscular output," *Journal of Motor Behavior*, vol. 41, no. 3, pp. 274–283, 2009.

[8] J. M. Jakobi, D. L. Edwards, and D. M. Connelly, "Utility of portable electromyography for quantifying muscle activity during daily use," *Gerontology*, vol. 54, no. 5, pp. 324–331, 2008.

[9] O. Theou, S. H. Bruce, K. Roland, G. R. Jones, and J. M. Jakobi, "Portable electromyography: application for understanding muscle function of daily life in older adults," *Gerontechnology*, vol. 10, no. 3, pp. 146–156, 2011.

[10] B. Harwood, D. L. Edwards, and J. M. Jakobi, "Age- and sex-related differences for electromyography gaps during daily activity and a discrete task," *Gait and Posture*, vol. 34, no. 1, pp. 6–12, 2011.

[11] B. Harwood, D. L. Edwards, and J. M. Jakobi, "Age- and sex-related differences in muscle activation for a discrete functional task," *European Journal of Applied Physiology*, vol. 103, no. 6, pp. 677–686, 2008.

[12] J. G. Ryall, J. D. Schertzer, and G. S. Lynch, "Cellular and molecular mechanisms underlying age-related skeletal muscle wasting and weakness," *Biogerontology*, vol. 9, no. 4, pp. 213–228, 2008.

[13] A. A. Vandervoort, "Aging of the human neuromuscular system," *Muscle and Nerve*, vol. 25, no. 1, pp. 17–25, 2002.

[14] W. R. Frontera, V. A. Hughes, R. A. Fielding, M. A. Fiatarone, W. J. Evans, and R. Roubenoff, "Aging of skeletal muscle: a 12-yr longitudinal study," *Journal of Applied Physiology*, vol. 88, no. 4, pp. 1321–1326, 2000.

[15] V. A. Hughes, W. R. Frontera, M. Wood et al., "Longitudinal muscle strength changes in older adults: influence of muscle mass, physical activity, and health," *Journals of Gerontology*, vol. 56, no. 5, pp. B209–B217, 2001.

[16] D. G. Candow and P. D. Chilibeck, "Differences in size, strength, and power of upper and lower body muscle groups in young and older men," *Journals of Gerontology*, vol. 60, no. 2, pp. 148–156, 2005.

[17] J. K. Petrella, J.-S. Kim, S. C. Tuggle, S. R. Hall, and M. M. Bamman, "Age differences in knee extension power, contractile velocity, and fatigability," *Journal of Applied Physiology*, vol. 98, no. 1, pp. 211–220, 2005.

[18] N. A. Lynch, E. J. Metter, R. S. Lindle et al., "Muscle quality. I. Age-associated differences between arm and leg muscle groups," *Journal of Applied Physiology*, vol. 86, no. 1, pp. 188–194, 1999.

[19] S. Trappe, P. Gallagher, M. Harber, J. Carrithers, J. Fluckey, and T. Trappe, "Single muscle fibre contractile properties in young and old men and women," *Journal of Physiology*, vol. 552, no. 1, pp. 47–58, 2003.

[20] D. S. Kern, J. G. Semmler, and R. M. Enoka, "Long-term activity in upper- and lower-limb muscles of humans," *Journal of Applied Physiology*, vol. 91, no. 5, pp. 2224–2232, 2001.

[21] J. G. Semmler, D. V. Kutzscher, and R. M. Enoka, "Limb immobilization alters muscle activation patterns during a fatiguing isometric contraction," *Muscle and Nerve*, vol. 23, no. 9, pp. 1381–1392, 2000.

[22] R. E. Brown, D. L. Edwards, and J. M. Jakobi, "Sex differences in force steadiness in three positions of the forearm," *European Journal of Applied Physiology*, vol. 110, no. 6, pp. 1251–1257, 2010.

[23] L. Dipietro, C. J. Caspersen, A. M. Ostfeld, and E. R. Nadel, "A survey for assessing physical activity among older adults," *Medicine and Science in Sports and Exercise*, vol. 25, no. 5, pp. 628–642, 1993.

[24] O. Theou, G. R. Jones, A. A. Vandervoort, and J. M. Jakobi, "Daily muscle activity and quiescence in non-frail, pre-frail, and frail older women," *Experimental Gerontology*, vol. 45, no. 12, pp. 909–917, 2010.

[25] O. Theou, Z. Soon, S. Filek et al., "Changing the sheets: a new system to reduce strain during patient repositioning," *Nursing Research*, vol. 60, no. 5, pp. 302–308, 2011.

[26] H. J. Hermens, G. Rau, C. Disselhorst-Klug, and B. Freriks, *Surface ElectroMyoGraphy: Application Areas and Parameters*, proceedings of the third general SENIAM workshop, Roessingh Research and Development, Aachen, Germany, 1998.

[27] W. R. Frontera, V. A. Hughes, K. J. Lutz, and W. J. Evans, "A cross-sectional study of muscle strength and mass in 45- to 78-yr-old men and women," *Journal of Applied Physiology*, vol. 71, no. 2, pp. 644–650, 1991.

[28] T. J. Doherty, D. W. Stashuk, and W. F. Brown, "Determinants of mean motor unit size: impact on estimates of motor unit number," *Muscle and Nerve*, vol. 16, no. 12, pp. 1326–1331, 1993.

[29] H. Kinoshita, P. R. Francis, T. Murase, S. Kawai, and T. Ogawa, "The mechanical properties of the heel pad in elderly adults," *European Journal of Applied Physiology and Occupational Physiology*, vol. 73, no. 5, pp. 404–409, 1996.

[30] B. Mierzejewska-Krzyzowska, H. Drzymala-Celichowska, and J. Celichowski, "Gender differences in the morphometric properties of muscle fibres and the innervation ratio of motor units in rat medial gastrocnemius muscle," *Journal of Veterinary Medicine*, vol. 40, no. 4, pp. 249–255, 2011.

[31] D. G. Bell and I. Jacobs, "Electro-mechanical response times and rate of force development in males and females," *Medicine and Science in Sports and Exercise*, vol. 18, no. 1, pp. 31–36, 1986.

[32] H. Valkeinen, J. Ylinen, E. Mälkiä, M. Alen, and K. Häkkinen, "Maximal force, force/time and activation/coactivation characteristics of the neck muscles in extension and flexion in healthy men and women at different ages," *European Journal of Applied Physiology*, vol. 88, no. 3, pp. 247–254, 2002.

[33] J. C. Ives, W. P. Kroll, and L. L. Bultman, "Rapid movement kinematic and electromyographic control characteristics in males and females," *Research Quarterly for Exercise and Sport*, vol. 64, no. 3, pp. 274–283, 1993.

[34] R. M. Andela, A. Dijkstra, J. P. J. Slaets, and R. Sanderman, "Prevalence of frailty on clinical wards: description and implications," *International Journal of Nursing Practice*, vol. 16, no. 1, pp. 14–19, 2010.

[35] R. E. Hubbard and K. Rockwood, "Frailty in older women," *Maturitas*, vol. 69, no. 3, pp. 203–207, 2011.

Gray and Green Revisited: A Multidisciplinary Perspective of Gardens, Gardening, and the Aging Process

Scott D. Wright[1] and Amy Maida Wadsworth[2]

[1] *Gerontology Interdisciplinary Program, University of Utah, Salt Lake City, UT 84112-5880, USA*
[2] *Family and Consumer Studies Department, University of Utah, Salt Lake City, UT 84112, USA*

Correspondence should be addressed to Scott D. Wright; scott.wright@hsc.utah.edu

Academic Editor: Kee L. Chou

Over fourteen years ago, the concept of "gray and green" was first introduced by Wright and Lund (2000) to represent a new awareness and a call for increased scholarship at the intersection of environmental issues and the aging process. This review paper revisits that concept with a fresh perspective on the specific role of gardens and gardening in the aging experience. As example, gardening is one of the most popular home-based leisure activities in the US and represents an important activity in the lives of older adults in a variety of residential settings. Yet, there has been a lack of any comprehensive and multidisciplinary (science and humanities) examination of the nexus between gardening and the aging experience, and in particular with research connections to stewardship and caring. In this paper, we review contemporary articles demonstrating the multidisciplinarity of gardening and the aging process. First, we will focus on the beneficial psychological effects resulting from the cultivation of caring, including personal contentment and artistic expression. Second, we will focus on stewardship and how gardening increases health, community awareness, and a connection to future generations. On the surface, this may demonstrate a separation between the humanities and science, but we will clarify a symbiotic relationship between the two disciplines in our conclusion.

1. Introduction

Over fourteen years ago, the concept of "gray and green" was first introduced by Wright and Lund [1] as representing new awareness and call for increased scholarships at the intersection of environmental issues and the aging process [2–4]. An important dimension of that original article [1] was to bring more attention to the role of the natural environment in contrast to the "built environment" in relation to successful aging [5]. This review paper revisits the concept of *gray and green* with a fresh perspective using selected examples from the literature on the specific role of gardens and gardening as it enhances the aging experience. Although the examination of the horticultural and human experience has been previously examined, especially in the context of well-being and social development [6, 7] and in the lives of the elderly [8], this review paper offers a more contemporary perspective on the increasing number of publications since the early 1990s that have addressed gardening, gardens, and aging, particularly since the emergence of the "gray and green" publication in the year 2000 [1].

Gardening is one of the most popular home-based leisure activities in the US and represents a significant and salient activity in the lives of older adults [9–15]. The National Gardening Association claimed that 80% of US households tended to plants, which represented an increase of 65% from the year 1996 [16]. The 55- to 64-year-old age group was the cohort that spent the most on horticultural products and services and this trend will most likely continue with aging baby-boomers [16, 17]. Some have proposed that there is an increased return to the small-scale farming approach as a new calling in life for many aging individuals. This trend is supported by the growing interest in the organic food movement for both environmental and health-conscious ideals [18].

However, it is proposed in this paper that gardening may represent a facet of a much deeper gerontological connection between the natural environment, well-being, legacy, sense of meaning, and interpersonal connections to community and larger social structures [12]. The functional allure of gardens and gardening in the later years is the result of multiple factors: historical, aesthetic, cultural, generational, psychological, and physiological factors. It is the premise of this paper that there is much more to the nexus of *gardening and aging* than a favorite pastime, hobby, or a task aligned with passive drudgery. For example, in the book, *Gardening for a Lifetime: How to Garden Wiser as You Grow Older*, the author Eddison [19] believes gardening can become a joy-filled activity in later life even with the onset of comorbidities and chronic conditions associated with advancing age, if the gardener considers adopting wise alternatives to high maintenance practices in the garden. Gardening and gardens represent an important facet of the *gray and green* concept where the interaction with horticulture and landscaping is a holistic experience for a "mind-body-spirit" connection [15]. This interactive connection is further highlighted by representative books such as Patricia Cassidy's [20] *The Age Proof Garden* and *The Illustrated Practical Guide to Gardening for Seniors: How to maintain your outside space with ease into retirement and beyond,* where the focus is on gardening and the aging experience, but as an adaptive process that understands and appreciates the benefits of gardening, but with adjustments in maintenance and goals in the older adult's garden.

In this paper, we review contemporary articles demonstrating the multidisciplinarity of gardening and the aging process. First, we will focus on the beneficial psychological effects resulting from the cultivation of caring, including personal contentment and artistic expression. To do this, we will reference contemporary editions of classic texts to explore the still-relevant implications of historical gardening themes and allegories. We will also discuss aging painters, writers, and filmmakers to demonstrate how the theme of gardening permeates the aging experience in various expressions of human adaptation, creativity, and existential significance even in the face of challenge and loss.

Second, we will focus on stewardship and how gardening increases health, community awareness, and represents a connection with future generations. Most importantly, we advocate the premise that gardens and gardening represent an important bridge to connect the aging experience to the natural world where stewardship, caring, and well-being are realized.

On the surface, this multidisciplinary focus may demonstrate affinity for C.P. Snow's *Two Cultures* and a separation between the humanities and science, but we will clarify a symbiotic relationship between the two disciplines in our conclusion.

2. Process and Procedure for the Selected Literature Review

The literature was systematically reviewed for relevant and peer-reviewed journals, books, and book chapters as well as contemporary annotated releases of classic and modern literature such as Thoreau's *Walden* and Virgil's *Georgics.* Relevant books were identified through published scholarly journal book reviews, published journal article references, and Google Scholar and through the Amazon.com search tool. To generate a list of selected articles (as of January 12, 2014) for the paper, searches were done in four electronic databases: PsychINFO, PubMed, ProQuest, and Scopus. The search strategy was complemented by inspecting the included articles and their reference lists. The tactical goal was to use PsychINFO, PubMed, ProQuest, and Scopus as the databases to conduct searches in the literature and establish a convergence of relevant publications from multiple database search tools. The review was primarily grounded in a Scopus query algorithm to establish corroboration of relevant publications and to generate analytics for the primary search terms (*gardening and aging*).Scopus is a large abstract and citation database of research literature and web sources representing 50 million records, 21,000 titles, and 5,000 publishers. The search using Scopus was conducted through a university system (retrieved January 12, 2014) and it is considered to have a robust index and coverage of publications. The Scopus search for (gardening AND aging) in ALL fields in journals articles published or in press and limited to a Date Range from 1990 to Present resulted in 492 document results and the analytics revealed a modest increase in the total number of documents for this query by year since 1990 to the search in January 12, 2014. When using the limiter "Article title, Abstract, Keywords" (i.e., TITLE-ABS-KEY) default in the query, the search resulted in 66 document results. A thorough examination was conducted of the 66 documents retrieved from Scopus and then articles were selected for relevancy and content affinity to the main themes of this paper.

3. How Does Your Garden Grow? Definitions, History, and Purposes

For many people, the word "garden" can evoke varied emotions and leaps of cognitive associations. According to the Oxford English Dictionary (OED), "garden" can be approached and treated as a noun and defined as, "a piece of ground adjoining a house, used for growing flowers, fruits, or vegetables," and as a modifier such that, gardens can represent "ornamental grounds laid out for public enjoyment and recreation." [21]. The OED also recognizes that one can become an active participant by working in a garden as a "gardener" (noun), by having "gardened" (verb). These distinctions serve as a basis for the reader to consider the intersection of the aging process with gardens and gardening, which can be active and passive, functional and aesthetic, and subjective and objective. For example, the term, "garden" may signify many things that have little to do with cultivating vegetables and flowers and instead, as example, focus on landscaping as gardening *with nature* [22]. Or some may immediately think of an entertainment/sports venue (e.g., Madison Square Garden); a biblical setting (e.g., The Garden of Eden) or some historical wonder of the world (e.g., The Hanging Gardens of Babylon); or pieces of literature such as *The Garden of Forking Paths* by Jorge Luis Borges or the film *The Constant Gardener* directed by Fernando Meirelles (based on the novel by John le Carre); or exotic paintings like *The Garden of Earthly Delights* by Hieronymus Bosch. For others, "garden" may represent the Butchart Gardens in Greater Victoria on Vancouver Island, Canada, or Zen rock garden of the Ryoanji Temple in Kyoto, Japan [23–25]. In the sociological domain, gardens have served as a focal point for assessing collectivist and bureaucratic cultures in context of the "urban gardening movement" [26], and more recently as a practice to engage in the illicit cultivation of someone else's land known as "guerrilla gardening" [27]. In the historical domain, there were the "Victory Gardens" in the 1940s and with contemporary television, perhaps the PBS series, "The Victory Garden." But for many people, a garden can simply be a plot of soil as close as your backyard and as modest as raised box with a few marigolds and tomato plants. Thus, as Ross [28–39] has noted, trying to pinpoint an exact definition of gardens is daunting given the kaleidoscopic variations of gardens across many cultures and geographies. For example, Pizzoni [30] has advocated that "*gardens can be thought of as a place set aside for multiple uses such associated with horticulture and the cultivation of plants for food and medicinal herbs but it can also be seen as an expression of ornamental, religious and even political purposes*"(see also [12, 31–40] for further discussion). In this paper, we will advance a similar understanding of gardens and gardening and the aging experience but broaden the horizon such that health and well-being can be derived as a benefit, and this includes the psychological expression in our main premise: *to be generative, to cultivate, to care is both utilitarian and sacred and finds its joyful expression in the reverential duty in the garden.*

3.1. Humanities Discipline: How Gardens and Gardening Cultivate Caring and a Personal Connection with Life and Nature. The word "garden" may conjure memories of warm, fertile dirt in your hands, the smell of blossoms, the sound of bees collecting pollen, or the beautiful, flourishing sight of what humans and nature can accomplish together. Gardens are experienced through the senses, and therefore, the psychological assimilation of a garden and all it may represent is highly personal. It is no wonder, then, that a deep personal understanding of life results from such communion with nature and may translate into the expression of self through art.

For example, the interrelationship between painting and the use of garden as motif or actual object for inspiration represents an important, intense, and intimate thread in the history of art and reinforces the sensory connection between human and garden. There is perhaps the most spectacular and enigmatic work of Hieronymus Bosch and his haunting imagery associated with the triptych, *Garden of Earthly Delights*. *The Garden of Earthly Delights* was painted around the years 1503 and 1504 when Bosch was about 50 years of age [41], although he lived well into the mid-sixties of life. *Garden of Earthly Delights* is the middle panel of the triptych and captures sinful pleasures in a garden-like setting where naked figures parade about and into pools of water which can bring to mind primeval fountains of youth. Compared to the panel "Paradise" which depicts a more balanced ecosystem of sorts, the middle panel is awash in people, and the garden appears to be magically self-sustaining with little human activity involved in maintenance or cultivating its rich resources for all. And indeed, there are no children to be found in this Arcadian landscape and everyone appears to be *ageless*. This is a presentation of a carefree world where the garden serves as a symbolic Utopia and humankind resides in paradise untouched by the "Fall" [41]. Of course, it is the other panel, *Hell*, which exacts the most hallucinatory experience and presentation of nightmarish figures. Perhaps, we can think of that desperate landscape, like T.S. Eliot's waste land, as a reminder of where there are repercussions for engaging *careless* activities that did not take into account the stewardship clause when residing in the Garden of Eden. We reap what we sow, but in this case the "Fall" may represent itself when all was spent in the present and little effort was taken to cultivate for the next season, or the next generation, thus leading to the hellish demise of humanity.

In direct contrast is the work of Claude Monet, who is considered as one of the founders of style of painting known as French Impressionism, lived a remarkable eighty-six years of life that spanned across two centuries (from 1840 to 1926). Monet proved to be extremely productive with creating some of his most famous paintings into his later years and along with other many other painters (e.g., Henri Matisse, Rembrandt, and Georgia O'Keefe) he has been the subject of research examining creative and artistic style and productivity into the second half of life [42–46].

Many people are certainly aware of the vast array of Monet's work and many can also readily identify the unique style and composition of his paintings, such that, for example, when examining *water lilies* with rich textures or admiring *irises* with saturated colors, we come to think that those flowering plants are virtually synonymous with *his* portfolio of art. But then again many people may *not* know that those paintings were created based on the living landscape of his own home and garden located in Giverny, France. Monet was both painter *and* gardener and he spent the last 43 years of his long life with his close-knit family by cultivating his passion for creating color with flowering plants on a one-hectare (2.5 acre) garden site and then capturing the dynamic and fluid presence of those plants onto his canvas with brushwork and oils [45]. But his garden would also be a healing and therapeutic oasis that helped him cope and adjust to the loss of his second wife and his son Jean. Monet was reported as saying, "*My most important work of art is my garden*" [47]. From 1908 and at the age of 68, Monet focused his artistic work almost entirely on depicting his garden and was then commissioned by the state to create a remarkable large format series of paintings of water-lilies (*Grandes Decorations*), his tour de force, that formed an enveloping circle that was to reside in a specially constructed pavilion in the Musée de l Orangerie, which was an extension to the Louvre [47, 48]. Around the age of 74, Monet only painted summer subjects in his garden and during the winter months he worked in his studios retouching his works and finishing his canvases [49], but he was then diagnosed with a cataract in his right eye and eventually would come to affect both eyes. Despite his visual impairments, Monet proclaimed in 1920, "*I'm extremely busy with my garden; it's such a joy to me, and on fine days like those we've had recently I am in raptures at the wonders of nature."* Monet continued to paint but his deteriorating eyesight caused him severe problems in distinguished colors for many of his final years [49]. While there have been many theoretical arguments about whether the change in Monet's paintings of his garden was due to "late style" or specifically due to limitations in his vision, Marmor used medical knowledge and computer simulation to investigate the impact of visual disabilities on perception. Marmor [50] demonstrated how Monet (and the painter Degas) had their perceptions of their preferred scenes or subjects changed due to disease, which affected their style of painting [51–53]. And for Monet, the loss of color perception due to his complications with cataracts was a major problem (see [45, 53, 54]). As Marmor [50] pointed out, Monet used his beloved garden landscape to capture the nuances of color and light, "*but his cataracts severely changed and challenged the marvelous qualities of color in his works*" (p. 1769). Even though different eye pathologies cause different visual limitations, we now know how low vision can affect both the physical and mental well-being of older adults and the ability to function in a variety of activities of daily living (ADLS) and instrumental activities of daily living (IADLS) [55, 56]. Despite these challenges, Monet stayed connected with the enchantment of his garden space, and his paintings, especially of the water lilies, were his sense of legacy to the world—that to care and cultivate the beautiful is to embrace a larger cosmic sense of nature. Another part of his legacy is his ability to engage this belief while facing physical limitations and obstacles.

The conjunction of gardening and art is substantial and includes mediums from painting to literature to film. Readers are encouraged to review the literary companion publication of Simonds [57], Marranca's [58] anthology, and Garmey's edited book [59] for an introduction and extensive review in this form of art. For a more contemporary nonfiction perspective, Arthur Hellyer's *Your Garden Week by Week* [60], Jamaica Kincaid's *My Garden (Book)* [61], Diane Ackerman's *Cultivating Delight: A Natural History of My Garden* [62], Michael Pollan's *Second Nature: A Gardener's Education* [36], Caroline Holme's *New Shoots, Old Tips* [63], Barbara Kingsolver's *Animal, Vegetable, Miracle: A Year of Food Life* [64], and Robert Fenton's [65] critical review in *The New York Review of Books* are highly recommended.

When it comes to dedication to gardening, many people will think of one of the best-selling American nonfiction classics, *Walden* by Thoreau [66, 67]. But while Thoreau had the ability to capture the art and beauty of being connected to the soil, his stay at Walden was relatively short, a two-year experiment into his late twenties, and then he left to pursue other travels. If one wanted to find a more "constant gardener," across the entire life course and *into the retirement years*, we could better discuss Thomas Jefferson, Governor of Virginia and Vice-president and President of the United States, who was also an avid gardener. We are fortunate to read of his observations and activities in gardening in a publication titled, *The Garden Book* [68], which he began in 1776 and continued until the autumn of 1824, two years before his death at the age of 83. *The Garden Book* is a remarkable account of Jefferson's meticulous note taking on his botanical interests and indicated a devotion to the "culture of the earth." At the age of 68 years old, in a letter to a Charles Willson Peale written in 1811 [68], Thomas Jefferson remarked that, "*But though an old man, I am but a young gardener.*" And the theme of gardening continues as both therapeutic activity and metaphor for life itself in the works of Hans Christian Andersen; the garden became an allegory for his lifework writing folk tales ("fairy tales"), which had more significance with the world of adulthood than for children. The folk tale, "The Gardener and the Gentry" was written *toward the end of his career* and two years before his death in 1872. The use of gardening as a metaphor and allegory continues in the works of noted writers such as Frances Hodgson Burnett's *The Secret Garden* [69], Charles Baudelaire's *Les Fleurs du mal* [70] and Eliot's imagery of the rose-garden in the *Four Quartets* [71] carries a multilayered meaning of spirituality and the loss of Paradise within the cycles of life and death [72]. The *Four Quartets* were written over a span of several years (1935–1942) and in the last quarter of Eliot's life. In "Burnt Norton" the rose-garden conveys memories and mythology of time passing with human existence (mere moments) compared to the history of humanity, civilization, and all that has gone before. We find it correlative that Carl Jung was using a similar theme to address his understanding of his own life in his book *Memories, Dreams, Reflections* (1989). In 1957, at eighty-one years of age, Jung began to work with Aniela Jaffe to complete this major work before he died in 1961. The enlightening passage is from the prologue and is both vegetative and seminal in its garden metaphor by picturing life individually and collectively as sustaining and regenerative over the ages (see also [73]).

> *When we think of the unending growth and decay of life and civilizations, we cannot escape the impression of absolute nullity. Yet I have never lost a sense of something that lives and endures underneath the eternal flux. What we see is the blossom, which passes. The rhizome remains (p. 4).*

Although Jung's use of the rhizome metaphor supports the philosophical impression of life as continuous and unending, despite the relentless seasons and centuries of time, gardens are also very much transitory and impermanent. And so while gardens can be perceived as being artistic [74], they may not necessarily represent the outcome that matches the Hippocratic dictum, "Life is short, art is long" (*Ars longa, vita brevis*) in the sense that a garden is cultivated and cared for in an effort to outlast its caretaker, while on the other hand, gardens exist to reenchant the present [75, 76]. Yet, one long-lasting medium for the expression of art is through the vehicle of film. Here we will examine the crossroads of the use of garden imagery (symbolic and realistic) in relation to the aging experience and focus on two exemplars: *Wild Strawberries and Dreams.*

Wild Strawberries is the 1957 film by Bergman [77] that depicts the story of the aged Dr. Isak Borg who is traveling in his car to receive an honorary degree. Erikson [78] has provided a comprehensive analysis, based on his own theoretical interpretation, of Bergman's film and it is here that Erikson sees the emergent virtue of *care* as a necessary strength for "*the life cycle as well as the cycle of generations*" (p. 7). For example, Erikson noted that the tensions found between Dr. Borg and Marianne (his daughter) and Borg's son Evald reflect the core issues of generativity such that it is Borg who must confront his own rejectivity and the resulting lack of care and interest in his own family and many others around him (see also [79]). The turning point for Isak Borg, and obviously the primary inspiration for the title of the film, is when Dr. Borg leaves the main highway (his journey of life) and drives down a side road to revisit an old summer home (a chance for reminiscence and remembrance out of the rigid pattern of living in rote predictability). Borg remembers a specific location that would serve as catalyst for a reawakening much like the Proustian madeleine, but in this case, it is a strawberry patch near the summer home [80]. And it is here that we find a richly layered symbolism that involves the magical transformation of the landscape surrounding the home into blooming plants and trees and lush greenery. Even though the film is in black and white, one can almost imagine that large yard as colorful as Monet's gardens at Giverny. The wild strawberries that grow along the side of the yard are the triggering mechanism to transport Borg back through time and allow him to revisit his own young adulthood in relation to Sara, his "first love." In this film, the bounty of the earth in the form of wild strawberries is richly symbolic of the decisions made and the missed opportunities at forming intimate relationships (with Sara) and the resulting isolation and aloofness that made him think of himself as a "living corpse." Erikson [78] offers his analysis of the Arcadian scene,

> *"one senses that this whole earthy scene, beyond its precious gaiety and its symbolic reference to defloration, points to something primeval, some garden, long forfeited by Isak" (p. 8).*

At least from Erikson's perspective, that small patch of botanical life, the wild strawberries, is at once symbolic of the epigenetic pathway and a crossroads through adulthood and into the commitments of *mature caring within mid and later life*. This theme shall become an important factor to consider when we examine the role of stewardship as a dimension of the "gray and green" concept for the aging experience.

Kurosawa, at the age of 80, directed and then released the film, *Dreams* [81], in 1990 (his 28th film), which featured several portrayals of Kurosawa's own dreams experienced over the course of his life. The first and last episodes of *Dreams* feature two processions that symbolize the opening and closing of the life cycle: a wedding and a funeral [82]. The film also captures luminous sequences of botanical wonderment and rural scenes of wheat fields (*crows*) with Van Gogh (who also loved gardens; see [83]) at work painting his landscapes and other segments that portrayed the ruins of ecological disasters and the break with nature. The last segment, "The Village of the Watermills" of the film is especially significant which captures a lush farm with blooming flowers, lush green grass, and crystal clear rivers that drive the watermills in a wheel-like fashion. It is a "*paradisiacal place: a village where modern technology has not invaded people's lives and they live in harmony with nature*" [83]. The Kurosawa surrogate (the younger man), while walking through the village, encounters a 103-year-old man, who is working on a smaller water wheel structure. The older man communicates the necessity of treating the land with respect and articulates the perils if it being mistreated. The symbolic depth of the old man imparting wisdom (a representation of Eriksonian "generativity") to the younger man is a critical link in the message of the segment which highlights that working in harmony with the land helps to create a natural cycle of living, and dying. The watermills turn with the river of water, which provides nourishment for the plants and the flowers, which in turn the villagers use to celebrate the wheel of life, and death. At the end of the film, we are left watching a slow moving river current with undulating clusters of long swirling stands of lush aquatic plants swaying with the flow of water that reflects multiple colors on its surface, blues, greens, and the liquid silver of indirect sunlight. Much like a Monet oil painting, *Water Lilies*, and his Japanese Bridge over his pond.

These artists demonstrate the ability to engage and connect despite challenges—an ideal for any aging adult. However, the process of disengagement seems to contradict the presence of this ability as the individual retreats into himself, and rather than being a constant gardener, he becomes isolated and trapped in his memory and his past. An example of this is Grey Gardens, a documentary so fascinating that it has been translated into a Broadway musical and an HBO film. With the title of Grey Gardens (1976) such a film would appear to be the perfect connecting point for examining aging issues ("grey") and gardens. But the film is less about gardening in the later years (per se) and more about what was once cared for in relationships with people, home, and landscape in the past has instead fallen into a state of neglect due to the disconnect with cultivating what is alive in the present. Grey Gardens is actually the name of the decaying estate that belongs to Edith Bouvier Beale ("Big Edie") age 79 and her daughter Edie (or "Little Edie") in her fifties, both frozen in time and place, in an East Hampton home that is graying along with them [84]. In the early 1970s, their 28-room mansion was found to be a health hazard and mother and daughter were threatened with eviction. The film opens up with Little Edie telling the Maysles about what used to be in terms of the beautiful and exotic gardens that once was [84]. Throughout the film, there are shots of the house surrounded by thickets of vegetation, a landscape "gone wild," that makes it appear deserted, forlorn, and enveloped in an ivy-snarled ruin. In Grey Gardens there actually is a man who is introduced as the "gardener" at the beginning of the film, but it is clear that the intruding jungle of vegetation is overwhelming to him. As the mother and daughter live in the past, the present landscape is removed from care and attention and nature encroaches and erodes the house. After years of neglect, raccoons move into the attic, ivy presses through window seals, and cats continue to reproduce and turn every room into a new wing of a sprawling litter box. The two women cook, eat, and spend most of their time in the bedroom the two of them share, warming canned goods on a hotplate near Big Edi's bed. Decay envelops what was once lush, beautiful, and a welcoming example of cooperation between nature and human interaction. Harrison [75] succinctly stated the connection between the need for constant gardening in the face of our obligations to the here and now, "If we are not able to keep our garden, if we are not able to take care of our mortal world, heaven and salvation are vain" (p. 11).

Gardening, then, is not just a hobby or a task meant to keep one physically active or to keep the mind occupied. It is effort against entropy. It is the cooperation between nature and humanity, fine-tuned through experience and nurturing. Gardening is age and wisdom.

Wisdom may be gained in the privacy of one's own mind, but it's true worth manifests as wisdom is shared. The artistic examples referenced here are not just means of self-expression, they are bridges from individual understanding to community stewardship and care. The proper starting point for this discussion of art bridging personal wisdom and community should be with Virgil's *Georgics*. Virgil (70 BCE-19 BCE) wrote the poem *Georgics* (the word *Georgics* refers to primarily to "farming") during the 30s BCE and this would put Virgil at just over 40 years of age, and relatively speaking, at the peak of his senior status in the understanding of the life course at that time but perhaps not *senectus* yet [85]. *Georgics* is a didactic and very much a template and design for interacting with the land and being attentive to what Ferry [86] noted as Virgil's ability to engage the "*ecstatic and tender celebrations of the very life in things,*" and more importantly how these "celebrations" interact with human existence (see also [87]). In the *Georgics*, one can appreciate Virgil's attentiveness to the cycles of seasons, and the cycle of birth and death, and the inevitable unfolding of sickness and aging. Virgil's *Georgics* emphasizes that through *care* of the land, we begin to care for each other, and from there follow the arts and cultural blossoming and the resulting harvesting of another kind: poetry, art, music, sculptures, law, and ethics. In the fourth Georgic, Virgil writes of an old man who is at work on his small patch of land that was at one time not fertile enough to be plowed by oxen, but with his dedicated attention it has been transformed. The lines in this vignette are less didactic and more poetic in the sheer strength of the action and sensuality by use of vivid descriptions of the labor that is needed for all the seasons [88]. Quint [89] has proposed in his review of the new translations of *Georgics* by [86] and Lembke [90] that, "*the old gardener thus carries some of the poem's political hopes as well as its ethical message. From a life of turmoil, he has settled into quiet usefulness and contentment, tamed by work and hardship, and even makes a thing of beauty in his flower garden, an analogue to the poem itself*" (p. 35).

An overarching theme throughout the *Georgics* is the didactic lesson of "as you sow, so shall you reap." The lesson is that progress towards happiness and well-being is highly dependent on the service that you have rendered to the land, kith and kin, to neighbors and to community. And it all begins in your backyard. Thus, gardening serves as the cornerstone of civilization-that is, *to care, constantly*. Harrison [75] has succinctly woven these themes together by stating, "*The true gardener is always 'the constant gardener*'" (p. 7).

3.2. Science Discipline: How Gardens and Gardening Increase Stewardship, Community Awareness, and a Connection to Future Generations and Individual Health. The constant gardener cares for and nurtures nature, community, and future generations to come. Gardens not only provide rejuvenation of plant life and the aging individual, but also inject life and vitality into the community. Here, we examine two prime examples of the "gray and green" concept where the "green" effect of gardens and gardening can instill the potential for stewardship toward not only one's backyard, but toward a much larger sphere of environmental concern and care directed "outward" in the form of legacy, community, and welfare for future generations. Gardens and gardening can also provide a direct benefit through the restorative impact of either interacting with and in the garden as a physical activity or that the presence of a garden itself as a sensory experience can enhance well-being and health.

If the lesson from the *Georgics* is that community begins in the backyard, it is no wonder that thoughts turn to residential landscaping and lawn care while thinking of communities and gardens. Lawn care has been the most prevalent form of gardening nationwide. However, this dimension has been going through its own transformation and redefinition as many more people are looking to redefine the "lawn" into a more environmental friendly and regionally appropriate recreational and social site for families, including the expansion of gardens [35, 91]. Brown and Jameton [92] have indicated that there are numerous benefits for the increase and support of gardening: food security and nutritional health (home grown produce has the potential to offset the cost of purchasing food), positive effects on physical health (as exercise), and overall community improvement (to enhance social capital; it can serve as a community organizing tool to combat poverty and provide a collective response to blighted city neighborhoods) and as a way of raising consciousness about environmental stewardship. Brown and Jameton [92] also suggest various community-based policy recommendations to encourage urban garden activities because, "*Urban gardening raises our public awareness of the need to safeguard our environment, and especially our urban soils, from future pollution, erosion, and neglect*" (p. 33). More specifically to older adults, Ashton-Shaeffer et al. [10] discovered many motivational factors for gardening in their investigation. For example, they found significant differences among older adults by marital status, education, and health status in terms of motivational categories. The two most important categories were physical fitness and creativity. Similarly, Wang and Glicksman [93] reported that low-income minority older adults expressed several motivations and benefits of community gardening. For example, Wang and Glicksman identified nine themes of why older adults chose to participate in gardening: mental health benefits, the end product (fruits and vegetables), continuation of a past life, something to do/responsibility, beauty and connection to growth, connecting with others, physical health, learning something new, and helping each other out [93].

Fänge and Ivanoff [94] also discovered mixed results with gardening in men and women aged 80–89 in Sweden.

Fänge and Ivanoff indicated that while gardens provided opportunities to go outdoors and offered a meditative space for older adults, having a garden to take care of could be a "considerable practical burden and was something that bothered the very old peoples' minds" (p. 342). In contrast, Pettigrew and Roberts [95] have proposed in their study that gardening had served as an effective way for older adults to ameliorate the experience of loneliness and feelings of emotional isolation. Gardening was also identified as a mechanism to help facilitate "self-reconstruction" through spatiotemporally establishing biographical continuity between older Chinese immigrants in their new lives in New Zealand [91].

We also know that gardening can serve as a "bridge-building" activity for enhancing intergenerational cooperation in community settings [96–100] and that it can represent a form of legacy in older adults [101] and serve as a mechanism to engage in "successful aging" [102].

The phrase "successful aging" recollects Monet and his ability to continue producing art despite his failing eyesight. The aging process requires adaptation and the ability to approach tasks in a different, more sustainable way. There are research findings to indicate gardening as an activity to enhance the physical and emotional well-being for older adults who reside in home and community-based dwellings [103]. For example, Infantino [104] found that the gardening experience had sustained older women in their cognitive and spiritual development. Heliker et al. [105] found that horticultural projects (consisting of 12 weeks of interactive gardening classes) were instrumental in increasing a sense of psychological well-being in racial and culturally diverse groups. They also found that gardening helped to instill a deeper sense of legacy and spirituality and a deeper relationship with the earth and nature in the older participants. Quandt et al. [106] explored the nutritional role of "food sharing" among a diverse set of older rural adults and also highlighted the "social meaning" in such activities as well. Similarly, Milligan et al. [107] found that older adults benefited from gardening in communal allotments as it helped to overcome social isolation and contributed to the development of social networks. An additional benefit of affective restoration from stress was found among adults (mean age 57.6) in an experimental study comparing gardening to indoor reading [108]. The authors noted that gardening may permit people to enjoy the restorative effects of nature on a regular basis. In another related study, Hawkins et al. [109] discovered that allotment gardeners appreciated "doing" gardening activity as well as "being" at the allotment landscape for affording a wide range of benefits to their health and being, specifically in stress reduction.

Gardening as an activity to improve the quality of life for older adults has generated a substantial number of publications that address gardening as a physical activity for older adults that may facilitate healthy aging [14, 15, 110–112] and as an intervention with *indoor* gardening and horticultural therapy for institutional populations [15, 113–129]. The intersection of gray and green is also reflected in the paradigmatic shift of "The Eden Alternative" in managing long-term care facilities [130, 131]. For example, Lee and Kim [132] found that indoor gardening was found to be effective for improving several dimensions of sleep patterns, decreasing agitation, and improving cognition functioning of dementia patients (see also [133]). There are also significant publications on *outdoor* gardening activities for people who live in geriatric care settings [134], specifically for persons with dementia [135], and the importance of "patient-specific gardens" for the restorative effects of nature [136]. Goto et al. concluded that organized gardens can positively affect both mood and cardiac physiology of elderly individuals [137]. Gardening has also been identified as a potential activity to incorporate into fall prevention programs as gardeners reported significantly better balance and gait speed and had fewer chronic conditions and functional limitations than nongardeners [138]. However, both Kwak et al. [139] and Larner [140] have also suggested that many cognitive abilities may be required for successful gardening and horticultural activities and that if gardening is being considered as a component for intervention and therapy for dementia patients, an individual approach that is customized to abilities and deficits and the various symptoms may be required.

In Valliant's [141] monumental study of aging and well-being, *Aging Well,* he ended with a chapter titled, "Positive Aging: A Reprise," and in that section there was the creative metaphor that captured the nuances of growing older as akin to gardening or, more precisely, the lessons learned in *being* a gardener could serve as a positive role model for finding fulfillment in later life.

Among the many positive attributes, Valliant proposed that gardening is an activity that encourages a therapeutic *slowness* [142, 143] and brings with it the additional benefit of creating opportunities for introspection and reflection (that you should stop and "smell the roses") and that it encourages and facilitates the overarching Eriksonian concept of *care*: a hallmark and defining positive attribute of the aging process [144]. We are reminded of Shakespeare's lament, "*sweet flowers are slow and weeds make haste*" which all but exudes the wisdom of living a long and cultivating the rewards of a life well-lived *and cared for*. Valliant also proclaimed that gardeners are very much in the spirit of generativity and symbolically working (i.e., being concerned and having responsibility); the soil is embedded with the meaning of rebirth and regeneration, stewardship, and the essence of cultivating for the next cycle of life [145]. And with this kind of care, there is the potential for the legacy of *caritas*, a *vita activa*, and a vocation of care transmitted through the generations. Thus, as Valliant succinctly states it, "*There is a kind of immortality about gardens, at least until next spring and the spring after that*" (p. 309).

Not only does Valliant make reference to Cicero and the ancient Roman tradition of viniculture as an honorable activity for aging, he revisits the famous line from Voltaire's *Candide* [146] where after many journeys, hardships and mishaps and a great deal of theorizing, Candide instructs Pangloss, "*We should cultivate our gardens.*" That pithy philosophical statement was crafted by Candide and inspired from an earlier encounter with an old man who was sitting outside his house "*minding his own business*" and taking in the day and enjoying the "*fruits of his labor*." This encounter sounds very familiar to a similar story of the old man previously mentioned in Virgil's *Georgics*.In Voltaire's novel, the old man knew little of worldly affairs and events but graciously offered Candide, Pangloss and Martin a sumptuous meal of exotic fruits and nuts that were grown on his farm. Candide assumed the old man must have some vast and magnificent estate, but the old man said, "*I have only twenty acres and I cultivate them with my children; and my work keeps at bay three great evils: boredom, vice and need.*" It took a while, but Candide had suddenly become a fast learner. *Gardening?* Yes, of course. Candide thought it to be a far better existence compared to anything else they had encountered as history unfolded not too kindly in all of their travels and experiences.

Perhaps it is best to summarize the findings of the importance of gardening in the lives of older adults by highlighting the work of Bhatti [11] who found that the presence of and the interaction with gardens can have a major significance in the (re)creation of "home" in later life. In addition to the benefits of physical activity [13–15, 110, 147] there is the added dimension of what the garden symbolizes psychologically as a meaningful reason for existence, or as one older adult expressed it, "*when I'm in the garden I can create my own paradise.*"

Here, we have come full circle. We began with the sensory qualities of gardens and gardening and the personal spirit-mind-body benefits to cooperation between man and nature. Personal well-being often translates into artistic expression, whether it is through painting, literature, film, or the act of gardening itself. This artistic expression benefits communities and creates a legacy for the aging adult while providing physical and mental health benefits. The give-and-take between nature and individual, individual and community, and community and nature is ongoing and rejuvenating. Science and the humanities continue in a symbiotic relationship just as nature and human beings do, and this cooperation is vital to the well-being of aging individuals and of every human being at any stage of life.

We should cultivate our gardens, but what is it exactly about gardens and gardening that would supply meaningful significance to the life course, and particularly to the aging process? What is the connection between gardening and care and well-being? The analysis of the scientific validity of the health benefits of gardening for older adults has been aptly analyzed by Wang and MacMillan [15] and they correctly conclude that there is a need for larger-scale studies using probability samples and combined methodologies to develop a more comprehensive understanding of the nuances with gardening and the aging experience. While the systematic review of Wang and MacMillan focused on the merits of gardening in the domain of connections to family and community and cultures, we would submit that the additional *connection to the natural environment*—the gray and green concept—is worthy of sustained investigation as well, especially as it relates to larger macrodynamics of legacy, sustainability, generativity, and intergenerational support and caring [148, 149].

4. Synopsis and Conclusions to the Review Paper

The purpose of this paper was to review several multidisciplinary nodes of gardening and the aging experience and to examine two specific issues: (a) gardening as a significant activity to engage the cultivation of caring across the life course, and (b) as a way to enhance the notion of stewardship in supporting environmental health in the context of home and community based settings. Based on the review of the selected literature and the examination of various multidisciplinary perspectives, we can propose that gardens and gardening represent multidimensional phenomena in the lives of many older adults and it is much more than a physical activity in a designated space where time and energy are exerted for cultivating fruits and vegetables. Gardens and gardening can also represent an intimate connection with life itself through caring and being a steward for living organisms that also reciprocate with nourishment, aesthetics, and existential meaning in the context of senescence. As Roszak [150] has noted, the added dimension of environmental connection and awareness into the experience of the aging process could serve as a template for a new "elder culture" and a sustainable future.

In addition, there are the beneficial therapeutic interactions with gardens as healing spaces, as in the example of "great-granny's garden" (Oslo, Norway), which not only is represented as a living archive for botanicals, but also serves as a "sensory garden" for persons with dementia [151]. This captures an excellent concept for both conservational activities *and* supporting the therapeutic goal of the positive attributes of a garden space for older adults with cognitive impairments.

There is much to discuss within a synopsis of these themes, but one link to appreciate is the connection back to Valliant's synthesis of his research findings that point to gardening as including, but much more than, *activity* of physical effort, and rather, it takes on the gravity of a philosophy of life, a *Weltanschauung*, a raison d'être, and much more. Valliant indicated that instead of the all-elusive high expectations of *happiness* to be sought for in later life, the concept that might instead be a better fit given the realism of the aging process in terms of challenges and promise is a *joy in life*. The experience of a joyful attention to life (and a life) that is cultivated in gardening is very much akin to a meditative practice [152] and helps to create a new kind of "homecoming" that allows one to become native to a place where there is a deeper connection to seasons of growth, and decline [153, 154]. To many, the garden exemplifies a new agrarian standard [155] that integrates the many realms of the "Great Garden" that is a seamless gateway between many realms of nature including trees, streams, pastures and it helps to instill a redirecting of *mindful care* [156].

Before you might think that the topic of gardening is exclusively an opportunity for those who are geographically located in rural areas or along the exurban fringes, and thus beyond the reach for urban and inner city dwellers, consider the following example. In the low-income residential neighborhood geographically located in the Bronx (New York) known as Tremont, there exists a community garden that recently celebrated its 37th anniversary. And it is here that the residents of Tremont find a sense of belonging even while surrounded in a world of concrete. Tina Kelley wrote a story for *The New York Times* on the Tremont Community garden and said that the "*gardens are oases, where a collective spirit and a sense of community grow from the topsoil.*" The President of the community garden is Elizabeth Butler (age 77) and she said that the garden is like a refuge, "*If I couldn't come here, it would be rough . . . I cannot stay in the house.*" Another garden member, a retired nurse, said the garden is site for celebrating birthdays and as a place for memorial services as well. "*They were like deeply part of the garden, like a soul thing,*" while another community member said of the garden, "*It's my joie de vivre. I like the way it looks. I enjoy the view. I sit here by myself.*"

Joie de vivre means joy of life.

And then there is Candide: *Il faut cultiver notre jardin*. Yes, we should cultivate our gardens. But listen to how Harrison [75] has interpreted *notre jardin* from Voltaire's story,

> *Notre jardin* is never a garden of merely private concerns into which one escapes from the real; it is that plot of soil on the earth, within the self, or amid the social collective, where the cultural, ethical, and civic virtues that save reality from its own worst impulses are cultivated. Those virtues are always *ours* (p. x).

It may be difficult to imagine this much ado about a patch of soil, some seeds, watering, and having a "strong back and a weak mind" with all the weeding and mulching [157]. But Voltaire was onto something. And that "something" has resonated with many older adults throughout history and is today still both a viable and contemplative activity that is both elemental and transcendental. That "something" is related to the core virtue of the mature and responsible adult in mid and later life: *the ethical basis of care* [144, 145]. The caring for the garden (local) is then extended into the caring of something *beyond* the home and community and outward into social and cultural levels (global) [158]. This is exactly the link that Collins [159] discovered in her study of community dwelling older adults who were transformed into "keepers of the earth" through the activities of a "gardening life" and as a result, environmental stewardship was facilitated. It is our conclusion, that the ultimate expression of why the act of cultivating is so compelling in the later years of life is connected with Stanley Kunitz who spent a lifetime (over a hundred years) reflecting on the importance of gardens through poetry. In the book, *The Wild Braid* [76], the nexus of cultivation, caring, and the life course are poignantly discovered,

> *I think of gardening as an extension of one's own being, something as deeply personal and intimate as writing a poem. The difference is that the garden is alive and it is created to endure just the way a human being comes into the world and lives, suffers, enjoys, and is mortal. The lifespan of a flowering plant can be so short, so abbreviated by the changing of the seasons, it seems a compressed parable of human existence (p. 14).*

The opportunity to consider the benefits of gardening in the aging process as including a viable connection to outcomes relating to stewardship and care and as a part of the process of older adults being engaged with natural contexts beyond the physical and built environment is also the possibility of further investigating the gray and green phenomena as an important dimension in well-being and optimal aging in mid and later life [1, 3, 4, 93, 148, 160–162]. To be generative, to cultivate, to care is both utilitarian and sacred and finds its joyful expression in the reverential duty in the garden.

References

[1] S. D. Wright and D. Lund, "Gray and green?: stewardship and sustainability in an aging society," *Journal of Aging Studies*, vol. 14, no. 3, pp. 229–249, 2000.

[2] The Gerontological Society of America, "Gray And Green Together: Older Adults Can Play Role in Creating Healthier Environment. ScienceDaily. 2008. Web. 23 Nov, Full report: Public Policy & Aging Report (PPAR):18(2)," 2013, http://www.geron.org/.

[3] K. Pillemer, N. M. Wells, L. P. Wagenet, R. H. Meador, and J. T. Parise, "Environmental sustainability in an aging society: a research agenda," *Journal of Aging and Health*, vol. 23, no. 3, pp. 433–453, 2010.

[4] K. Sykes and K. Pillemer, "The intersection of aging and the environment: introduction," *Generations*, vol. 33, no. 4, pp. 6–9, 2009.

[5] K. Carr, P. I. Weir, D. Azar, and N. R. Azar, "Universal design: a step toward successful aging," *Journal of Aging Research*, vol. 2013, Article ID 324624, 8 pages, 2013.

[6] J. Janick, "Horticulture and human culture," in *The Role of Horticulture in Human Well-Being and Social Development: A National Symposium*, D. Relf, Ed., Timber Press, Portland, Ore, USA, 1992.

[7] D. Relf, "Human Issues in Horticulture. HortTechnology," April/June: 2(2), 1992, http://www.ctahr.hawaii.edu/hih/human.asp.

[8] C. A. Browne, "The role of nature for the promotion of well-being in the elderly," in *The Role of Horticulture in Human Well-Being and Social Development: A National Symposium*, D. Relf, Ed., pp. 75–79, Timber Press, Arlington, Va, USA, 1990.

[9] M. C. Ashe, W. C. Miller, J. J. Eng, and L. Noreau, "Older adults, chronic disease and leisure-time physical activity," *Gerontology*, vol. 55, no. 1, pp. 64–72, 2009.

[10] C. Ashton-Shaeffer and A. Constant, "Why do older adults garden?" *Activities, Adaptation and Aging*, vol. 30, no. 2, pp. 1–18, 2005.

[11] M. Bhatti, "'When I'm in the garden i can create my own paradise': homes and gardens in later life," *Sociological Review*, vol. 54, no. 2, pp. 318–341, 2006.

[12] J. Carman, "Elders' lifelong connection with the natural environment," *Educational Gerontology*, vol. 37, no. 6, pp. 488–498, 2011.

[13] S.-A. Park, C. A. Shoemaker, and M. D. Haub, "Physical and psychological health conditions of older adults classified as gardeners or nongardeners," *HortScience*, vol. 44, no. 1, pp. 206–210, 2009.

[14] C. A. Shoemaker and M. Lin, "A model for healthy aging with horticulture," in *Proceedings of the 27th International Horticultural Congrss-INC2006: International Symposium on Horticultural Practices and Therapy for Human Well-Being*, pp. 978–990, 2008, http://www.actahort.org/books/775/.

[15] D. Wang and T. MacMillan, "The benefits of gardening for older adults: a systematic review of the literature," *Activities, Adaptation & Aging*, vol. 37, pp. 153–181, 2013.

[16] P. Francese, "Horticulture is hot," *American Demographics*, vol. 24, no. 5, pp. 50–51, 2002.

[17] H. Gross and N. Lane, "Landscapes of the lifespan: exploring accounts of own gardens and gardening," *Journal of Environmental Psychology*, vol. 27, no. 3, pp. 225–241, 2007.

[18] Passey, "The new gentleman farmer. Wall Street Journal Money," 2013, http://on.wsj.com/1iBPJlU.

[19] S. Eddison, *Gardening for a Lifetime: How to Garden Wiser as You Grow Older*, Timber Press, Portland, Ore, USA, 2011.

[20] P. Cassidy, *the Age Proof Garden and the Illustrated Practical Guide to Gardening for Seniors: How to Maintain Your Outside Space with Ease into Retirement and Beyond*, Arness, London, UK, 2011.

[21] "Oxford English Dictionary," 2014, http://www.oxforddictionaries.com/definition/english/garden.

[22] J. Van Sweden, *Gardening with Nature: How James Van Sweden and Wolfgang Oehme Plant Slopes, Meadows, Outdoor Rooms & Garden Screens*, Random House, New York, NY, USA, 1997.

[23] S. Harte, *Zen Gardening*, Stewart, Tabori & Chang, New York, NY, USA, 1999.

[24] J. P. Pigeat, *Gardens of the World: Two Thousand Years of Garden Design*, Flammarion, Paris, France, 2003.

[25] M. Schinz, *Visions of Gardens: Themes and Variations on the Garden*, Stewart, Tabori & Chang, New York, NY, USA, 1985.

[26] M. Jamison, "The joy of gardening: collectivist and bureaucratic cultures in conflict," *The Sociological Quarterly*, vol. 26, no. 4, pp. 473–490, 1985.

[27] R. Reynolds, *On Guerrilla Gardening*, Bloomsbury, London, UK, 2007.

[28] S. Ross, "Garden's powers," *Journal of Aesthetic Education*, vol. 33, no. 3, pp. 4–17, 1999.

[29] S. Ross, *What Gardens Mean*, University of Chicago Press, Chicago, Ill, USA, 1998.

[30] F. Pizzoni, *The Garden: A History in Landscape and Art*, Rizzoli, New York, NY, USA, 1999.

[31] W. H. Adams, *Nature Perfected: Gardens Through History*, Abbeville Press, New York, NY, USA, 1991.

[32] T. Comito, *The Idea of the Garden in the Renaissance*, Rutgers University Press, New Brunswick, NJ, USA, 1978.

[33] M. Conan and C. Whangheng, Eds., *Gardens, City Life and Culture*, Harvard University Press, Cambridge, Mass, USA, 2008.

[34] S. Constantine, "Amateur gardening and popular recreation in the 19th and 20th centuries," *Journal of Social History*, vol. 14, no. 3, pp. 387–406, 1981.

[35] C. Grampp, *From Yard to Garden: The Domestication of America's Home Grounds*, University of Chicago Press, Chicago, Ill, USA, 2008.

[36] M. Pollan, *Second Nature: A Gardener's Education*, Grove Press, New York, NY, USA, 2003.

[37] M. Pollan, "Afterword: the garden's prospects in America," in *Keeping Eden: A History of Gardening in America*, W. Punch, Ed., pp. 261–265, Brown and Company, Boston, Mass, USA, 1992.

[38] W. Punch, *Keeping Eden: A History of Gardening in America*, Little, Brown and Company, Boston, Mass, USA, 1992.

[39] P. Taylor, Ed., *The Oxford Companion to the Garden*, The Oxford University Press, New York, NY, USA, 2006.

[40] T. Turner, *Garden History: Philosophy and Design 2000BC–2000AD*, Spon Press, Taylor & Francis, New York, NY, USA, 2005.

[41] H. Belting, *Hieronymus Bosch: Garden of Earthly Delights*, Prestel, New York, NY, USA, 2002.

[42] G. Cohen, *The Creative Age: Awakening Human Potential in the Second-Half of Life*, Harper Paperbacks, New York, NY, USA, 2001.

[43] H. Kauppinen and P. McKee, "Old age, painting, and gerontology," *Journal of Aesthetic Education*, vol. 22, no. 2, pp. 87–100, 1988.

[44] M. Lindauer, *Aging, Creativity, and Art: A Positive Perspective on Late-Life Development*, Springer, New York, NY, USA, 2003.

[45] G. Ravin and C. Kenyon, "Artistic vision in old age: claude Monet and Edgar Degas," in *Creativity and Successful Aging: Theoretical and Empirical Approaches*, C. E. Adams-Price, Ed., pp. 251–268, Springer , New York, NY, USA, 1998.

[46] D. Rosand, "Style and the aging artist," *Art Journal*, vol. 46, no. 2, pp. 91–93, 1987.

[47] B. Denvir, *Impressionism: The Painters and the Paintings*, Studio Editions, London, UK, 1991.

[48] M. T. Southgate, "Water lilies," *Journal of American Medical Association*, vol. 286, no. 7, p. 764, 2001.

[49] C. Holmes, *Monet at Giverny*, A Seven Dials Book/Weidenfeld & Nicolson, London, UK, 2003.

[50] M. F. Marmor, "Ophthalmology and art: simulation of Monet's cataracts and Degas' retinal disease," *Archives of Ophthalmology*, vol. 124, no. 12, pp. 1764–1769, 2006.

[51] N. N. Bakalar, "A New Look at Impressionists'Failing Vision, New York Times," 2007, http://www.someaddress.com/full/url/http://www.nytimes.com/2007/04/17/health/17eye.html?n=Top/Reference/Times%20Topics/People/D/Degas,%20Edgar.

[52] R. R. Dotinga, "Photoshop re-creates aging impressionists' eye on the world, Wired Magazine," 2007, http://www.wired.com/science/discoveries/news/2007/05/impressionist_vision.

[53] J. G. Ravin, "Geriatrics and painting," *Art Journal*, vol. 27, no. 4, p. 397, 1968.

[54] J. Werner, "Aging through the eyes of Monet," in *Color Vision: Perspectives From Different Disciplines*, pp. 1–41, Walter de Gruyter & Company, New York, NY, USA, 1998.

[55] S. Berger and F. Porell, "The association between low vision and function," *Journal of Aging and Health*, vol. 20, no. 5, pp. 504–525, 2008.

[56] C. O'Donnell, "The greatest generation meets its greatest challenge: vision loss and depression in older adults," *Journal of Visual Impairment and Blindness*, vol. 99, no. 4, pp. 197–208, 2005.

[57] M. Simonds, Ed., *Gardens: A Literary Companion*, Greystone Books, Vancouver, Canada, 2008.

[58] B. Marranca, Ed., *American Garden Writing, Expanded Edition: An Anthology*, Taylor Trade Publishing, Lanham, Md , USA, 2003.

[59] J. Garmey, Ed., *The Writer in the Garden*, Algonquin Books, New York, NY, USA, 1999.

[60] A. Hellyer, *Your Garden Week by Week*, Collingridge, London, UK, 1936.

[61] J. Kincaid, *My Garden*, Farrar, Straus and Giroux, New York, NY, USA, 1999.

[62] D. Ackerman, *Cultivating Delight: A Natural History of my Garden*, Harper Collins Publishers, New York, NY, USA, 2001.

[63] C. Holmes, *New Shoots, Old Tips*, Frances Lincoln, London, UK, 2004.

[64] B. Kingsolver, *Animal, Vegetable, Miracle: A Year of Food Life*, Harper Collins Publishers, New York, NY, USA, 2007.

[65] J. Fenton, "Gardening with attitude. New York Review of Books," 49(13), 2002, http://www.nybooks.com/articles/15634.

[66] H. D. Thoreau and W. Harding, Eds., *Walden: An Annotated Edition*, Houghton Mifflin Company, Boston, Mass, USA, 1995.

[67] H. D. Thoreau, *Walden: One Hundred Fiftieth-Anniversary Edition*, Shambhala, Boston, Mass, USA, 2005.

[68] E. W. Betts, *Thomas Jefferson's Garden Book*, vol. 22, The American Philosophical Society, Philadelphia, Pa, USA, 1944.

[69] F. H. Burnett, *The Secret Garden*, J.B. Lippincott Company, Philadelphia, Pa, USA, 1949.

[70] C. Baudelaire and R. Howard, *Les Fleurs Du Mal*, David R. Godine, Boston, Mass, USA, 2006.

[71] T. S. Eliot, *Collected Poems: 1909–1962*, Harcourt Brace & Company, New York, NY, USA, 1991.

[72] R. Wagner, "The meaning of Eliot's rose-garden," *PMLA*, vol. 69, no. 1, pp. 22–33, 1954.

[73] M. Sabini, Ed., *The Earth Has a Soul: The Nature Writings of C.G. Jung*, North Atlantic Books, Berkeley, Calif, USA, 2002.

[74] L. Albers, "The perception of gardening as art," *Garden History*, vol. 19, no. 2, pp. 163–174, 1991.

[75] R. P. Harrison, *Gardens: An Essay and the Human Condition*, University of Chicago Press, Chicago, Ill, USA, 2008.

[76] S. Kunitz and G. Lentine, *The Wild Braid: A Poet Reflects on a Century in the Garden*, W.W. Norton & Company, New York, NY, USA, 2005.

[77] I. Bergman, *Wild Strawberries: A Film by Ingmar Bergman, Translated From the Swedish by Lars Malmstrom and David Kushner*, translated from the Swedish by Lars Malmstrom and David Kushner, Simon and Schuster, New York, NY, USA, 1960.

[78] E. Erikson, "Reflections of Dr. Borg's life cycle," in *Adulthood*, E. Erickson, Ed., pp. 1–31, W. W. Norton & Company, New York, NY, USA, 1978.

[79] S. Weiland, "Erik Erikson: ages, stages, and stories," *Generations*, vol. 1, pp. 17–22, 1993.

[80] E. Archer, "Wild strawberries, (a film review)," *Film Quarterly*, vol. 13, pp. 44–47, 1959.

[81] A. Kurosawa, *Dreams*. Film released 1990. Warner Brothers. DVD released, Warner Home Video, 2003.

[82] Z. Serper, "Kurosawa's dreams: a cinematic reflection of a traditional japanese context," *Cinema Journal*, vol. 40, no. 4, pp. 81–103, 2001.

[83] N. Reider, "Akira Kurosawa's Dreams, as seen through the principles of classical Japanese literature and performing art," *Japan Forum*, vol. 17, no. 2, pp. 257–272, 2005.

[84] A. Maysles, D. Maysles, E. Hovde, M. Meyer, and S. Froemke, (Directors). Grey Gardens [DVD]. A Maysles Films Inc. Production, [DVD, 2001, The Criterion Collection], 1976.

[85] T. Parkin, *Old Age in the Roman World: A Cultural and Social History*, The Johns Hopkins University Press, Baltimore, Md, USA, 2003.

[86] D. Ferry, *The Georgics of Virgil: A Translation*, Farrar, Straus & Giroux, New York, NY, USA, 2005.

[87] T. J. Haarhoff, "Virgil's garden of lowers and his philosophy of nature," *Greece & Rome*, vol. 5, no. 1, pp. 67–82, 1958.

[88] F. De Bruyn, "Reading Virgil's georgics as a scientific text: the eighteenth-century debate between Jethro Tull and Stephen Switzer," *English Literary History*, vol. 71, no. 3, pp. 661–689, 2004.

[89] D. Quint, *The Farmer as Hero*, vol. 20, The New Republic, 2006.

[90] J. Lembke, *Virgil's Georgics: A New Verse Translation*, Yale University Press, New London, Conn, USA, 2005.

[91] S. A. Golberg, "The glory of the garden. The Smart Set (Drexel University), October 24," 2013, http://thesmartset.com/article/article/10241301.aspx.

[92] K. H. Brown and A. L. Jameton, "Public health implications of urban agriculture," *Journal of Public Health Policy*, vol. 21, no. 1, pp. 20–39, 2000.

[93] D. Wang and A. Glicksman, "Being grounded: benefits of gardening for older adults in low-income housing," *Journal of Housing for the Elderly*, vol. 27, no. 1-2, pp. 89–104, 2013.

[94] A. Fänge and S. D. Ivanoff, "The home is the hub of health in very old age: findings from the ENABLE-AGE Project," *Archives of Gerontology and Geriatrics*, vol. 48, no. 3, pp. 340–345, 2009.

[95] S. Pettigrew and M. Roberts, "Addressing loneliness in later life," *Aging and Mental Health*, vol. 12, no. 3, pp. 302–309, 2008.

[96] A. Blake and D. Cloutier-Fisher, "Backyard bounty: exploring the benefits and challenges of backyard garden sharing projects," *Local Environment*, vol. 14, no. 9, pp. 797–807, 2009.

[97] K. Goff, "Senior to senior: living lessons," *Educational Gerontology*, vol. 30, no. 3, pp. 205–217, 2004.

[98] P. McKee, "Gardening: an equal opportunity joy," *Activities, Adaptation & Aging*, vol. 20, no. 1, pp. 71–78, 1995.

[99] J. Larson and M. Hockeberry, *Generations Gardening Together: Sourcebook for Intergenerational Therapeutic Horticulture*, Food Products Press, New York, NY, USA, 2006.

[100] M. L. Predny and D. Relf, "Horticulture therapy activities for preschool children, elderly adults and intergenerational groups," *Activities, Adaptation & Aging*, vol. 28, no. 3, pp. 1–18, 2004.

[101] V. Moller, "Attitudes to food gardening from a generational perspective: a south African case study," *Journal of Intergenerational Relationships*, vol. 3, pp. 63–80, 2005.

[102] S. Oh, "Successful aging through leisure gardening: study on constraints negotiation," *Dissertation Abstracts International*, vol. 66, no. 4, article 1497, 2005.

[103] C. A. Browne, "The role of nature for the promotion of well-being of the elderly," in *The Role of Horticulture in Human Well-Being and Social Development*, D. Relf, Ed., pp. 75–79, Timber Press, Portland, Ore, USA, 1992.

[104] M. Infantino, "Lived experience of gardening among five well older women in suburbia," *Dissertation Abstracts International*, vol. 62, no. 3, article 1319, 2001.

[105] D. Heliker, A. Chadwick, and T. O'Connell, "Meaning of gardening and the effects on perceived well being of a gardening

project on diverse populations of elders," *Activities, Adaptation and Aging*, vol. 24, no. 3, pp. 35–56, 2001.

[106] S. A. Quandt, T. A. Arcury, R. A. Bell, J. McDonald, and M. Z. Vitolins, "The social and nutritional meaning of food sharing among older rural adults," *Journal of Aging Studies*, vol. 15, no. 2, pp. 145–162, 2001.

[107] C. Milligan, A. Gatrell, and A. Bingley, "'Cultivating health': therapeutic landscapes and older people in northern England," *Social Science & Medicine*, vol. 58, no. 9, pp. 1781–1793, 2004.

[108] A. E. Van Den Berg and M. H. G. Custers, "Gardening promotes neuroendocrine and affective restoration from stress," *Journal of Health Psychology*, vol. 16, no. 1, pp. 3–11, 2011.

[109] J. L. Hawkins, J. Mercer, K. J. Thirlaway, and D. A. Clayton, "'Doing'gardening and "being"at the allotment site: exploring the benefits of Allotment gardening for stress reduction and health aging," *Ecopsychology*, vol. 5, no. 2, pp. 110–125, 2013.

[110] S.-A. Park, C. A. Shoemaker, and M. D. Haub, "A preliminary investigation on exercise intensities of gardening tasks in older adults," *Perceptual and Motor Skills*, vol. 107, no. 3, pp. 974–980, 2008.

[111] S.-A. Park and C. A. Shoemaker, "Observing body position of older adults while gardening for health benefits and risks," *Activities, Adaptation and Aging*, vol. 33, no. 1, pp. 31–38, 2009.

[112] A. J. Sommerfeld, T. M. Walicsek, and J. M. Zajicek, "Growing minds: evaluating the effect of gardening on quality of life and physical activity level of older adults," *HortTechnology*, vol. 20, no. 4, pp. 705–710, 2010.

[113] T. Barnicle and K. S. Midden, "The effects of a horticulture activity program on the psychological well-being of older people in a long-term care facility," *HortTechnology*, vol. 13, no. 1, pp. 81–85, 2003.

[114] S. Bassen and V. Baltazar, "Flowers, flowers everywhere: creative horticulture programming at the Hebrew home for the aged at riverdale: the Hebrew home for the aged at riverdale uses horticulture as a multidimensional approach in geriatric programming," *Geriatric Nursing*, vol. 18, no. 2, pp. 53–56, 1997.

[115] V. M. Brown, A. C. Allen, M. Dwozan, I. Mercer, and K. Warren, "Indoor gardening older adults: effects on socialization, activities of daily living, and loneliness," *Journal of Gerontological Nursing*, vol. 30, no. 10, pp. 34–42, 2004.

[116] C. W. Burgess, "Horticulture and its application to the institutionalized elderly," *Activities, Adapation & Aging*, vol. 14, no. 3, pp. 51–62, 1989.

[117] C. Collins and A. O'Callaghan, "Healing gardens for assisted living: an interdisciplinary approach to health education," *Journal of Extension*, vol. 45, no. 6, Article ID 6IAW7, 2007, http://www.joe.org/joe/2007december/iw7.shtml.

[118] M. B. Detweiler, T. Sharma, J. G. Detweiler, P. F. Murphy et al., "What is the evidence to support the use of therapeutic gardens for the elderly?" *Psychiatry Investigation*, vol. 9, no. 2, pp. 100–110, 2012.

[119] C. F. Grant and J. D. Wineman, "The garden-use model—an environmental tool for increasing the use of outdoor space by residents with dementia in long-term care facilities," *Journal of Housing for the Elderly*, vol. 21, no. 1-2, pp. 89–115, 2007.

[120] B. Kreidler, *Growing with Care: Using Greenery, Gardens and Nature with Aging and Special Populations*, Venture Publishers, State College, Pa, USA, 2002.

[121] M. J. Lovering, C. A. Cott, D. L. Wells, J. S. Taylor, and L. M. Wells, "A study of a secure garden in the care of people with Alzheimer's disease," *Canadian Journal on Aging*, vol. 21, no. 3, pp. 417–427, 2002.

[122] P. J. Ousset, F. Nourhashemi, J. L. Albarede, and P. M. Vellas, "Therapeutic gardens," *Archives of Gerontology and Geriatrics*, vol. 26, no. 1, pp. 369–372, 1998.

[123] H. Parr, *Mental Health and Social Space: Toward Inclusionary Geographies?* Blackwell, Malden, Mass, USA, 2008.

[124] E. Rappe and S.-L. Kivelä, "Effects of garden visits on long-term care residents as related to depression," *HortTechnology*, vol. 15, no. 2, pp. 298–303, 2005.

[125] R. Reid, "Today's healing gardens: more than shrubs and flowers," *Nursing Homes Long Term Care Management*, vol. 5, no. 3, pp. 60–63, 2006.

[126] R. J. Riordan and C. S. Williams, "Gardening therapeutics for the elderly," *Activities, Adaptation & Aging*, vol. 12, no. 1, pp. 103–111, 1988.

[127] L. K. Stein, "Horticultural therapy in residential long-term care: applications from research on health, aging, and institutional life," *Activities, Adaptation & Aging*, vol. 22, pp. 107–123, 1997.

[128] M. M. Y. Tse, "Therapeutic effects of an indoor gardening programme for older people living in nursing homes," *Journal of Clinical Nursing*, vol. 19, no. 7-8, pp. 949–958, 2010.

[129] S. Wells, *Horticulture Therapy and the Older Adult Population*, Haworth Press, Binghamton, NY, USA, 1997.

[130] W. H. Thomas and C. Johansson, "Elderhood in Eden," *Topics in Geriatric Rehabilitation*, vol. 19, no. 4, pp. 282–290, 2003.

[131] L. Weinstein, "The Eden alternative: a new paradigm for nursing homes," *Activities, Adaptation & Aging*, vol. 22, 1998.

[132] Y. Lee and S. Kim, "Effects of indoor gardening on sleep, agitation, and cognition in dementia patients—a pilot study," *International Journal of Geriatric Psychiatry*, vol. 23, no. 5, pp. 485–489, 2008.

[133] T. R. Jonveaux, M. Batt, R. Fescharek, A. Benetos et al., "Gardens and cognitive behavioral units in the management of alzheimer's disease patients: the Nancy experience," *Journal of Alzheimer's Disease*, vol. 34, no. 1, pp. 325–338, 2013.

[134] J. Ottosson and P. Grahn, "A comparison of leisure time spent in a garden with leisure time spent indoors: on measures of restoration in residents in geriatric care," *Landscape Research*, vol. 30, no. 1, pp. 23–55, 2005.

[135] S. Rodiek and B. Schwarz, *Outdoor Environments for People with Dementia*, Routledge, New York, NY, USA, 2008.

[136] G. Senes, N. Fumagalli, R. Crippa, and F. Bolchini, "Nursing homes: engaging patients and staff in healing garden design through focus group interviews," *Neuropsychological Trends*, vol. 12, no. 1, pp. 135–146, 2012.

[137] S. Goto, B. J. Park, Y. Tsunetsugu, K. Herrup, and Y. Miyazaki, "The effect of garden design on mood and heart output in older adults residing in an assisted living facility," *Health Environments Research and Design Journal*, vol. 6, no. 2, pp. 27–42, 2013.

[138] T.-Y. Chen and M. C. Janke, "Gardening as a potential activity to reduce falls in older adults," *Journal of Aging and Physical Activity*, vol. 20, no. 1, pp. 15–31, 2012.

[139] H. Kwak, P. D. Relf, and J. Rudolph, "Adapting garden activities for overcoming difficulties of individuals with dementia and physical limitations," *Activities, Adaptation & Aging*, vol. 29, no. 1, pp. 1–13, 2005.

[140] A. J. Larner, "Gardening and dementia," *International Journal of Geriatric Psychiatry*, vol. 20, no. 8, pp. 796–797, 2005.

[141] G. Valliant, *Aging Well: Surprising Guideposts to a Happier Life from the Landmark Harvard Study of Adult Development*, Little, Brown and Company, New York, NY, USA, 2003.

[142] C. Goldman, "The wisdom of elders," *Revision*, vol. 28, no. 1, pp. 46–48, 2005.

[143] C. Goldman and R. Mahler, *Tending the Earth, Mending the Spirit—the Healing Gifts of Gardening*, Hazelden, Center City, MN, USA, 2000.

[144] C. Hoare, *Erikson on Development in Adulthood: New Insights from the Unpublished Papers*, Oxford University Press, New York, NY, USA, 2002.

[145] J. Kotre, *Outliving the Self: How We Live on Future Generations*, W.W. Norton & Company, New York, NY, USA, 1996.

[146] J. F. M. Voltaire, *Candide*, The Literary Guild, New York, NY, USA, 1929.

[147] T. Vogel, P.-H. Brechat, P.-M. Leprêtre, G. Kaltenbach, M. Berthel, and J. Lonsdorfer, "Health benefits of physical activity in older patients: a review," *International Journal of Clinical Practice*, vol. 63, no. 2, pp. 303–320, 2009.

[148] "Gray is green: The national senior conservation corps," http://grayisgreen.org/home/about-us/.

[149] "The US EPA Aging Initiative. Kathy Sykes, Senior Advisor, Aging and Sustainability. Office Research and Development, U.S. EPA," http://www.ep.gov/aging.

[150] T. Roszak, *The Making of an Elder Culture: Reflections on the Future of America's Most Audacious Generation*, New Society Publishers, Philadelphia, Pa, USA, 2009.

[151] L. Borgen and A. S. Guldahl, "Great-granny's Garden: a living archive and a sensory garden," *Biodiversity and Conservation*, vol. 20, no. 2, pp. 441–449, 2011.

[152] W. Johnson, *Gardening at the Dragon's Gate: At Work in the Wild and Cultivated World*, Bantam Books, New York, NY, USA, 2008.

[153] W. Berry, *A Continuous Harmony: Essays Cultural and Agricultural*, Shoemaker & Hoard, Washington, DC, USA, 1972.

[154] W. Jackson, *Becoming Native to This Place*, University of Kentucky Press, Lexington, Ky, USA, 1994.

[155] W. Berry, *Citizenship Papers*, Shoemaker & Hoard, Washington, DC, USA, 2003.

[156] G. Logsdon, *At Nature's Pace: Farming and the American Dream*, Pantheon Books, New York, NY, USA, 1994.

[157] R. Stout, *Gardening without Work: For the Aging, the Busy, and the Indolent*, The Devin-Adair Company, Old Greenwich, Conn, USA, 1974.

[158] F. Montague, "Gardening: an ecological approach," 2010, http://www.mountainbearink.com/index.html.

[159] C. S. Collins, "Older gardeners as keepers of the earth: a phenomenological study," University of Maryland, College Park, Md, USA, 2007, http://hdl.handle.net/1903/6897.

[160] M. V. E. McCain, *GreenSpirit: Path to a New Consciousness*, Earth Books, New Alresford, UK, 2010.

[161] J. Warburton and M. Gooch, "Stewardship volunteering by older Australians: the generative response," *Local Environment*, vol. 12, no. 1, pp. 43–55, 2007.

[162] B.-S. Kweon, W. C. Sullivan, and A. R. Wiley, "Green common spaces and the social integration of inner-city older adults," *Environment and Behavior*, vol. 30, no. 6, pp. 832–858, 1998.

12

Efficacy of Wii-Fit on Static and Dynamic Balance in Community Dwelling Older Veterans

Kalpana P. Padala,[1,2] Prasad R. Padala,[1,2,3] Shelly Y. Lensing,[1,4] Richard A. Dennis,[1,2] Melinda M. Bopp,[1] Christopher M. Parkes,[1] Mark K. Garrison,[1,5] Patricia M. Dubbert,[1] Paula K. Roberson,[1,4] and Dennis H. Sullivan[1,2]

[1] *Geriatric Research Education and Clinical Center, Central Arkansas Veterans Healthcare System, Little Rock, AR, USA*
[2] *Department of Geriatrics, University of Arkansas for Medical Sciences, Little Rock, AR, USA*
[3] *Department of Psychiatry, University of Arkansas for Medical Sciences, Little Rock, AR, USA*
[4] *Department of Biostatistics, University of Arkansas for Medical Sciences, Little Rock, AR, USA*
[5] *Department of Physical Therapy, University of Central Arkansas, Conway, AR, USA*

Correspondence should be addressed to Kalpana P. Padala; kppadala@uams.edu

Academic Editor: Arshad Jahangir

Background/Objectives. Balance problems are well-established modifiable risk factors for falls, which are common in older adults. The objective of this study was to establish the efficacy of a Wii-Fit interactive video-game-led physical exercise program to improve balance in older Veterans. *Methods.* A prospective randomized controlled parallel-group trial was conducted at Veterans Affairs Medical Center. Thirty community dwelling Veterans aged 68 (±6.7) years were randomized to either the exercise or control groups. The exercise group performed Wii-Fit program while the control group performed a computer-based cognitive program for 45 minutes, three days per week for 8-weeks. The primary (Berg Balance Scale (BBS)) and secondary outcomes (fear of falling, physical activity enjoyment, and quality of life) were measured at baseline, 4 weeks, and 8 weeks. *Results.* Of 30 randomized subjects, 27 completed all aspects of the study protocol. There were no study-related adverse events. Intent-to-treat analysis showed a significantly greater improvement in BBS in the exercise group (6.0; 95% CI, 5.1–6.9) compared to the control group (0.5; 95% CI, −0.3–1.3) at 8 weeks (average intergroup difference (95% CI), 5.5 (4.3–6.7), $p < 0.001$) after adjusting for baseline. *Conclusion.* This study establishes that the Wii-Fit exercise program is efficacious in improving balance in community dwelling older Veterans. This trial is registered with ClinicalTrials.gov Identifier NCT02190045.

1. Introduction

Gait and balance problems increase with age, making older adults vulnerable to falls. Community dwelling adults, aged 65 years or older, have a 22% yearly incidence of falls [1]. Falls are associated with increased morbidity and mortality [2, 3]. For example, falls are the preeminent cause of hip fractures in older adults, which in turn are associated with decreased mobility, quality of life, and premature death. Among older adults hospitalized as a result of a fall, only 50% are alive one year later [4]. Although there are numerous intrinsic and extrinsic risk factors for falls, gait and balance problems are the most consistent predictors of future falls [5]. Balance is a complex issue with components of static and dynamic stability, sensory integration, and reactive postural control [6]. Some of these components can be improved by interventions making balance a modifiable risk factor for falls [7, 8]. The current study primarily targets static and dynamic stability.

Exercise improves gait and balance in the elderly. A Cochrane review found statistically significant improvement in balance following exercise interventions compared to usual activity [8]. Another review of 54 exercise studies in older adults concluded that interventions with challenging balance training and high dose exercise (≥2 hrs/wk) had the greatest impact on preventing falls [9]. Even low intensity exercises improve balance and gait, particularly in deconditioned elders at high risk of falling [10]. Furthermore, the benefits of exercise on reducing falls and injuries accumulate over time suggesting a need for adopting exercise as a lifestyle [11]. Despite the many proven benefits of exercise, older adults in the USA remain sedentary and show declines in moderate and vigorous physical activity with increasing age. Among adults aged 65 to 74 years, only 34% of men and 17% of women expend more than 2000 kcal per week in exercise [12]. Thus, a novel approach to increase the time engaged by older adults in exercise by making the exercises fun and safe would be valuable.

Exergames are interactive video games involving physical activity or exertion tracked as body movement [13]. The technology may enable sedentary older adults to safely add exercise to their lifestyle. The Nintendo Wii-Fit® exergame provides aerobics, strength, and balance training using a balance board that senses shifts in weight [14]. This gaming system is widely available and affordable and has the potential for self-directed home use by older adults. Even though the Wii-Fit program has been found to be safe and feasible in older adults, the efficacy of the program has not been well-established. Thus, the primary objective of the current study was to test the efficacy of an 8-week Wii-Fit program for improving balance in older Veterans with balance problems. The secondary objectives were to explore the effects of the exergames on fear of falling, exercise enjoyment, and quality of life.

2. Methods

2.1. Study Design and Participants. This pilot study was an 8-week, prospective randomized controlled parallel-group trial comparing the effects on measures of balance in the exercise group (Wii-Fit program) to that in the control group (Brain-Fitness program). The study was conducted at Department of Veterans Affairs Medical Center. The protocol was approved by the Institutional Review Board of the Central Arkansas Veterans Healthcare System. Thirty subjects were recruited to inform sample size calculations for a larger study. After responding to advertisements, recruits were prescreened by medical records review to determine eligibility. Community dwelling adults aged ≥ 60 years were included in the study. Subjects using wheel chairs or walkers for mobility, having absolute contraindications to exercise per American College of Sports Medicine guidelines, and those with medical conditions that in the opinion of the study physician were likely to compromise safe study participation were excluded [15].

2.2. Study Procedure. Subjects who cleared the prescreening were invited for the baseline visit during which they provided a written informed consent. At this visit, eligibility was further assessed with Berg Balance Scale (BBS) and Mini Mental State Exam (MMSE). Those that scored BBS ≤ 52 and MMSE ≥ 24 were included in the study. The cut-off score of 52 on BBS was selected in an effort to avoid ceiling effects and to include those with mild-to-moderate balance problems. Demographics and anthropometric data were collected at the baseline visit. Eligible subjects were trained to use Wii-Fit and Brain-Fitness programs over one to two sessions to ensure they were willing and capable of safe participation in either program. Subjects were randomized using a randomized block design to the exercise (n = 15) and control groups (n = 15) using sealed envelopes prepared by the statistician. Research assistants monitored participation in both groups for exercise fidelity, safety, and compliance. Participation time and activities performed were recorded. Subjects were allowed to choose the activities performed for Wii-Fit or Brain-Fitness though research assistants encouraged progression to higher level and inclusion of activities from each category, described below, at each session.

2.3. Exercise Group. Subjects trained for 45 minutes three days per week for 8 weeks in a well-lit exercise suite in a VA Medical Center. The room was set such that sufficient space was available for exercises free of any obstacles or fall hazards. The Wii-Fit group performed exercises from five categories: Yoga, Strength Training, Aerobics, Balance Games, and Training Plus which includes more complex exercise tasks. Balance exercises involved static and dynamic postural control (Half Moon, Torso Twist, and Deep Breathing), lateral weight shifting (Ski Slalom, Penguin Slide, and Tight Rope Walking), multidirectional balance (Table Tilt, Balance Bubble), and multidirectional balance with a cognitive component (Perfect 10). Subjects tracked their activity and progress using an individualized icon ("Mii," virtual avatar). Each session included a warm-up, exercise, and cool-down phase. During the warm-up and cool-down phases, subjects walked for five minutes at a self-selected comfortable pace using the program's "basic walk" activity. The exercise phase was designed to be patient centric. Instead of doing exactly the same exercises, subjects were encouraged to choose one or more exercises from every Wii-Fit category during each session. Research assistants were in the exercise room during the entire session maintaining visual contact and being readily available if necessary.

2.4. Control Group. Subjects performed cognitive exercises using a commercially available computer program, Brain-Fitness (HAPPYneuron Inc., Lyon, France) [16, 17] for 45 minutes three days per week for 8 weeks. The control group performed the cognitive exercises in a well-lit room at the VA Medical Center at the same frequency to ensure equal contact of all subjects with the research team. The program focused on five cognitive domains: memory (Entangled Figures, Turn Around and Around, and Money Time), language (Split Words, Right Words, Squeaky Mouse, Secret Files, and Dance with the Fireflies), attention (Split Words, Right Words, and Towers of Hanoi), executive function (American in Paris, Objects Where Are You), and visual and spatial domain (Around the World in 80 Trips).

2.5. Primary Outcomes Measures. All outcomes were measured at baseline and four and eight weeks after intervention initiation. The primary efficacy outcome was the Berg Balance Scale (BBS), which assesses balance impairments in older adults and is a good measure of static and dynamic stability [18]. It consists of 14 tasks performed in a standardized order with each task scored on a five-point scale according to quality or time ranging from "0" (lowest level of function) to "4" (highest level). The maximum score is 56. BBS has an excellent interrater reliability (0.98) [18]. A change of four points is considered the minimally detectable change for community dwelling older adults that ambulate without an assistive device [19].

2.6. Secondary Outcome Measures. The secondary outcomes included Activities-Specific Balance Confidence (ABC) scale, Physical Activity Enjoyment Scale (PACES), Modified Mini Mental State Exam (3MS), Rand Short Form 36 (SF-36), and incidence of adverse events. The ABC scale measures fear of falling and self-confidence to maintain balance [20]. Subjects rate their confidence in maintaining balance while engaging in 16 nonhazardous activities of daily living. Lower scores indicate greater fear of falling. The test-retest reliability is 0.92 with Cronbach's alpha of 0.96 [20]. PACES scale (8-item version) assesses perceived enjoyment of exercise [21, 22]. PACES score ranges from 8 to 56. Higher scores signify greater enjoyment. It has good validity and internal consistency (0.93) [21, 22].

3MS is a global screen for cognitive function that covers orientation to time and place, registration, recall, simple language, and construction. Test-retest reliability ranges from 0.91 to 0.93 [23]. The total score places the individual on a well-accepted scale of cognitive function. Different versions were used at each testing occasion to minimize practice effects. An MMSE score derived from 3MS was used in the inclusion criteria of the study. The Rand Short Form-36 is a generic measure of quality of life (QOL). The two components (mental and physical) and the physical function scores were utilized. Each component ranges from 0 to 100, with higher values indicating better QOL. It has good interrater reliability of 0.76–0.96 [24]. Adverse events (near falls, falls, dizziness, joint, muscle or chest pain, and shortness of breath) were monitored via medical records review before each session and by subject query during the sessions.

2.7. Statistical Analyses. Subject demographics and baseline characteristics were compared using t-tests or nonparametric Wilcoxon rank sum tests (continuous data) and Fisher's exact tests (categorical data). Changes from baseline at 4 and 8 weeks in primary and secondary outcomes were analyzed using repeated measures mixed model analyses of covariance. Group (exercise and control) and time (4 and 8 weeks) as well as the interaction between the two were independent variables; the dependent variable's baseline measure was included as a covariate. In post hoc analyses, groups were compared in terms of the changes from baseline at 4 and 8 weeks using t-tests derived from model-based contrasts. Additionally, comparisons were made to separately assess improvements within each group. A sensitivity analysis to investigate bias due to missing data for subjects ($n = 3$) who dropped out of the study was performed by carrying forward baseline values to conservatively impute missing data as no change; we also investigated the impact of including MMSE and SF-36 Physical and Mental summary scores as covariates in the sensitivity analysis. Two-sided p values less than 0.05 indicated statistical significance. Data were analyzed using SAS Enterprise Guide v5.1 (SAS, Cary, SC).

3. Results

Figure 1 depicts the screening, enrollment, and participation process. A total of 115 subjects were prescreened (record review) of which 79 subjects were found eligible for in-person screening. These subjects were invited to come for the baseline visit. Of the 40 subjects evaluated at the baseline visit, 30 met the full eligibility criteria and were randomized. Three subjects dropped out from the exercise group. One was withdrawn after randomization as his weight exceeded the weight limit for the Wii-Board. The other two subjects dropped out of the study due to loss of interest and difficulties traveling to the medical center, respectively. The demographic characteristics of the study sample are presented in Table 1. Twenty-six out of 30 subjects were male, which is representative of the Veteran population age ≥ 60 years. There were no significant differences between the two groups with regard to age, race, gender, medical comorbidities, and medications (Table 1). As shown in Table 2, there were no significant differences at baseline between the two groups with regard to primary or secondary outcome measures except for MMSE. All study visits were attended by the 27 subjects who completed the study (100% adherence). Subjects did not experience any study-related adverse events. At no time during the study did any subject need any physical help from the research assistants. Subjects were able to operate the video game remote and perform the exercises on their own. All subjects completed the stipulated exercise time at each session.

3.1. Program Preferences. Balance Games were the most accessed exercises in the exercise group (Ski Jump (median 11 of 24 visits), followed by Bubble Balance, Penguin Slide, and Table Tilt (median of 9, 8, and 7.5 visits, respectively)). Simple Yoga poses (Deep Breathing, Half Moon, and Warrior), Strength Training (Torso Twist, Triceps Extension), Training Plus (Perfect 10, Obstacle Course, Island Cycling, and Segway Circuit), and Balance Games (Soccer Heading, Ski Slalom, Tight Rope Walking, and Lotus Focus) were chosen at least once by at least 50% of the participants. Some of the outcomes could depend on the game preferences, the details of which are included in Table 4. Subjects in the control group accessed all the categories frequently (median ≥ 20 of 24 visits). Brain games involving attention and language (Split Words, Towers of Hanoi, and Right Word) and executive function (American in Paris) were the most accessed.

3.2. Outcome Measures. For the subjects who completed the study ($N = 27$), there was a significant group-by-time interaction for the primary outcome measure BBS ($p < 0.001$, Figure 2). Post hoc analysis showed that the change in BBS from baseline for the exercise group significantly differed from that in the control group at both 4 and 8 weeks. After adjusting for baseline BBS score, the average between-group

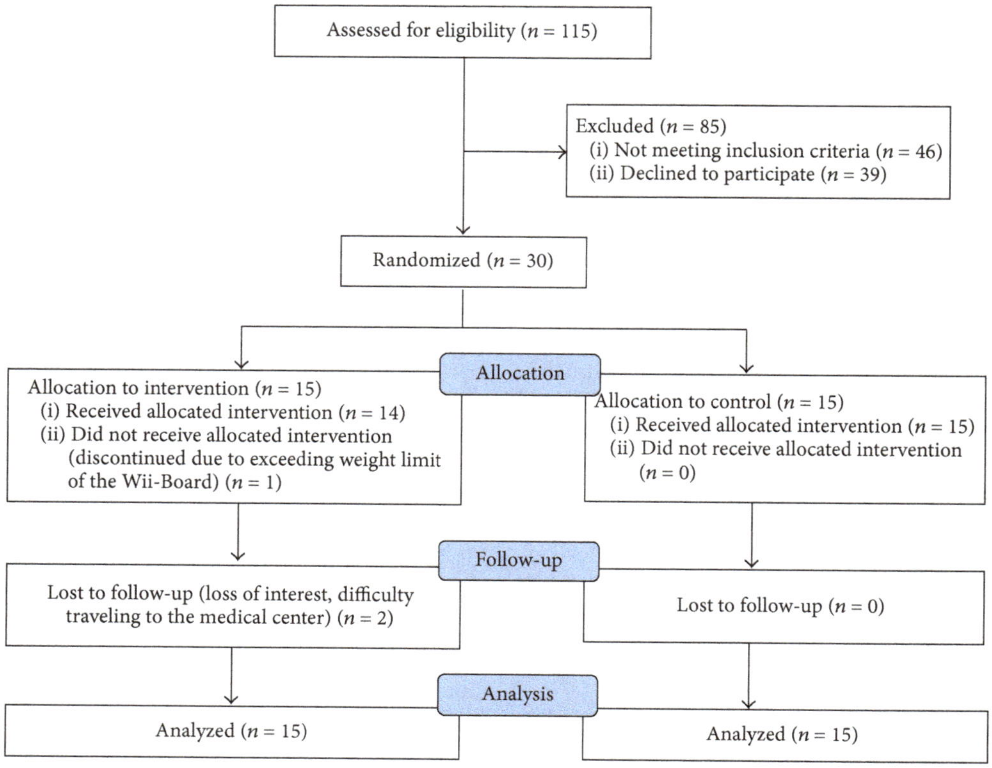

FIGURE 1: Screening, enrollment, and participation.

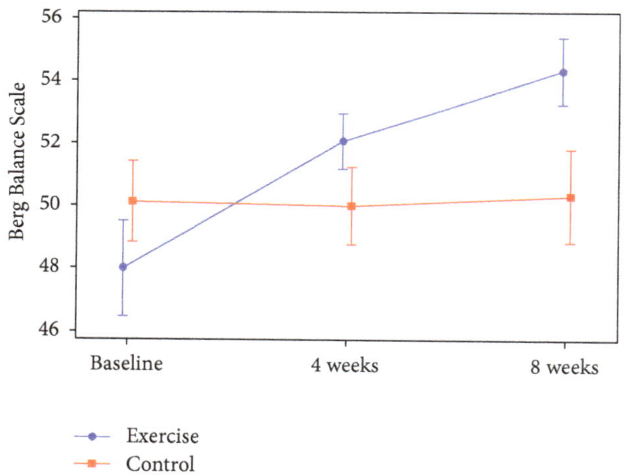

FIGURE 2: Berg Balance Scale over time in exercise and control groups (observed mean ± 2SE).

differences (95% CI) were 3.6 (2.3–4.8; $p < 0.001$) at 4 weeks and 5.5 (4.3–6.7; $p < 0.001$) at 8 weeks. Within-group analysis showed significant improvement in BBS in the exercise group at 4 weeks (3.7 [2.8–4.6], $p < 0.001$) and at 8 weeks (6.0 [5.1–6.9], $p < 0.001$) but no improvement in the control group at 4 weeks (0.2 [−0.6–0.9], $p = 0.70$) or at 8 weeks (0.5 [−0.3–1.3], $p = 0.22$). All subjects in the exercise group who completed the study demonstrated a clinically relevant change of greater than or equal to four on the BBS at 8 weeks [19]. Additionally, when the missing outcomes data for the three subjects in the exercise group were imputed as no change in a sensitivity analysis (intent-to-treat approach), the effect of exercise was decreased but still statistically significant: the average between-group differences (95% CI) were 2.7 (1.2–4.2, $p = 0.001$) at 4 weeks and 4.1 (2.6–5.7, $p < 0.001$) at 8 weeks. Adjusting for MMSE and SF-36 Physical and Mental summary scores resulted in between-group differences that were only slightly (<10%) larger, and these covariates were nonsignificant (all $p > 0.15$, results not shown).

There was a significant average improvement (95% CI) within the exercise group at 8 weeks on the secondary outcome measure, ABC scale (5.9 [0.1–11.6], $p = 0.046$) (Table 3). Analysis of exercise enjoyment at the end of 8 weeks was conducted in the Wii-Fit arm. The average score on the PACES was 49.2 (±7.4) on a 56-point scale. 83% of the subjects rated Wii-Fit to be high (6 or 7) on the measure of pleasure. A similarly high percentage rated Wii-Fit to be fun (75%), pleasant (75%), invigorating (67%), gratifying (83%), exhilarating (83%), stimulating (92%), and refreshing (92%). There were significant within-group improvements in the exercise group at 4 weeks and at 8 weeks and in control group at 4 weeks for both 3MS and MMSE ($p < 0.05$ for all comparisons, Table 3). There was a significant within-group improvement in SF-36 Physical function scale at 4 weeks in the exercise group (9.2 [0.5–17.9], $p = 0.039$) but not at 8 weeks. However, the group-by-time effect was nonsignificant for these variables. There were no significant group-by-time

TABLE 1: Descriptive characteristics of exercise and control groups.

	All participants ($N = 30$)	Exercise group ($N = 15$)	Control group ($N = 15$)	p value[a]
Age, mean (SD)	68.0 (6.7)	67.5 (8.1)	69.0 (3.8)	0.71
Male, n (%)	26 (86.7)	13 (86.7)	13 (86.7)	>0.99
Race, n (%)				0.12
Non-Hispanic Caucasian	20 (66.7)	8 (53)	12 (80)	
Non-Hispanic African American	10 (33.3)	7 (47)	3 (20)	
Anthropometry				
Height (inches), mean (SD)	69.3 (3.6)	69.3 (3.8)	69.3 (3.4)	>0.99
Weight (lbs.), median (IQR)	206 (176, 236)	198 (173–262)	208 (176–227)	0.37
BMI (kg/m^2), mean (SD)	30.6 (5.9)	32.0 (7.1)	29.3 (4.3)	0.21
Education, n (%)				>0.99
High school	6 (20.0)	3 (20.0)	3 (20.0)	
More than high school	24 (80.0)	12 (80.0)	12 (80.0)	
Number of comorbidities, median (IQR)	6.5 (4, 9)	7 (6–9)	5 (3–8)	0.27
Hypertension, n (%)	21 (70.0)	11 (73.3)	10 (66.7)	>0.99
Diabetes, n (%)	9 (30.0)	3 (20.0)	6 (40.0)	0.43
Heart disease, n (%)	3 (10.0)	1 (6.7)	2 (13.3)	>0.99
Hyperlipidemia, n (%)	21 (70.0)	11 (73.3)	10 (66.7)	>0.99
Depression, n (%)	11 (36.7)	4 (26.7)	7 (46.7)	0.45
Obesity, n (%)	14 (46.7)	8 (53.3)	6 (40)	0.72
Number of medications, median (IQR)	6.5 (4, 9)	8 (5–11)	6 (4–8)	0.32
Systolic blood pressure, mean (SD)	126.5 (9.6)	124.9 (8.9)	128.2 (10.3)	0.44
Diastolic blood pressure, mean (SD)	78.9 (4.5)	79.7 (3.6)	78.1 (5.2)	0.72
Pulse, mean (SD)	75.2 (9.3)	75.6 (9.2)	74.9 (9.7)	0.80

[a]Comparison of exercise and control groups using t-test or Wilcoxon rank sum test for continuous data or chi-square test for categorical data.

TABLE 2: Baseline outcome measures in exercise and control groups.

Variables	All Participants ($N = 30$) Mean (SD)	Exercise group ($N = 15$) Mean (SD)	Control group ($N = 15$) Mean (SD)	p value[a]
Berg Balance Scale (BBS)	49.3 (2.6)	48.5 (2.6)	50.1 (2.5)	0.08
Activities-Specific Balance Scale (ABC)	81.9 (14.6)	80.7 (12.1)	83.0 (17.1)	0.67
Modified Mini Mental State Exam (3MS)	94.5 (4.1)	94.1 (4.0)	94.9 (4.3)	0.60
Mini Mental State Exam (MMSE)	27.1 (1.7)	26.4 (1.6)	27.7 (1.7)	0.03*
Short Form-36 (Mental)	52.8 (13.2)	56.8 (9.8)	48.8 (15.2)	0.10
Short Form-36 (Physical)	44.6 (8.8)	42.2 (8.3)	47.0 (8.9)	0.14
Short Form-36 (Physical function)	65.0 (21.1)	63.3 (24.5)	66.7 (17.8)	0.67

[a]Comparison of exercise and control groups using t-test or Wilcoxon rank sum test.
*p value significant at <0.05.

interactions or between-group differences for any of the other secondary outcomes.

4. Discussion

The study sought to establish the efficacy of Wii-Fit exercise for improving balance in older adults with mild-to-moderate balance problems. As in prior studies, participants in this study experienced no adverse events, indicating that older adults with comorbidities can safely complete the program. The study also verified that Wii-Fit is feasible to use for training since the adherence rate was high and participants were able to exercise independently. Efficacy was demonstrated for the primary outcome, BBS. The average BBS change was six points and all subjects improved by at least four points at 8 weeks, a clinically relevant change observed in a similar

TABLE 3: Changes from baseline (4 or 8 weeks minus baseline) in outcomes for exercise and control groups and differences between the two groups.

	Change at 4 weeks Mean and 95% CI				Change at 8 weeks Mean and 95% CI			
	Exercise	Control	Difference[a]	p value[b]	Exercise	Control	Difference[a]	p value[b]
BBS	3.7 2.8 to 4.6	0.2 −0.6 to 0.9	3.6 2.3 to 4.8	<0.001*	6.0 5.1 to 6.9	0.5 −0.3 to 1.3	5.5 4.3 to 6.7	<0.001*
ABC	4.7 −1.0 to 10.4	−0.9 −6.1 to 4.2	5.6 −2.1 to 13.4	0.15	5.9 0.1 to 11.6	2.4 −2.8 to 7.5	3.5 −4.2 to 11.2	0.36
3MS	2.4 1.2 to 3.7	3.0 1.9 to 4.2	−0.6 −2.3 to 1.1	0.48	2.0 0.7 to 3.3	1.2 0.1 to 2.4	0.8 −0.9 to 2.5	0.36
MMSE	1.5 0.7 to 2.3	1.5 0.9 to 2.2	0.0 −1.1 to 1.0	0.95	1.1 0.3 to 1.8	0.8 0.1 to 1.5	0.3 −0.7 to 1.3	0.57
SF36:M	−0.2 −5.2 to 4.8	0.8 −3.6 to 5.3	−1.0 −7.8 to 5.7	0.75	4.2 −0.7 to 9.2	3.3 −1.2 to 7.7	1.0 −5.8 to 7.7	0.77
SF36:P	2.1 −1.8 to 5.9	1.0 −2.5 to 4.4	1.1 −4.2 to 6.4	0.67	0.9 −3.0 to 4.7	−0.1 −3.6 to 3.4	1.0 −4.3 to 6.2	0.71
SF36:PF	9.2 0.5 to 17.9	4.6 −3.2 to 12.4	4.6 −16.3 to 7.1	0.43	5.5 −3.2 to 14.2	3.3 −4.5 to 11.1	2.2 −13.9 to 9.5	0.70

[a] All means are estimates from repeated measures model of 4- and 8-week change from baseline. Difference reflects exercise group change minus control group change and is adjusted for corresponding baseline measure.

[b] p values comparing exercise and control groups are model-based.

BBS: Berg Balance Scale; 3MS: Modified Mini Mental State Exam; MMSE: Mini Mental State Exam; ABC: Activities-Specific Balance Scale; PACES: Physical Activity Enjoyment Scale; SF36:M: Short Form-36 (Mental); SF36:P: Short Form-36 (Physical); SF36:PF: Short Form-36 (Physical function).

*p value significant at <0.05.

community dwelling population [19]. Change in BBS can be influenced by baseline scores [25], but the baseline difference between groups in the current study was modest, neither statistically nor clinically significant ($p = 0.08$). Additionally, our analyses adjusted for baseline scores to further validate the effects of the program on balance. The study was not a priori powered to detect differences in secondary outcomes.

Balance-board-based exercises have been used to improve balance [26]. Wii-Fit is a balance board exercise system that has been tested as an exercise intervention using various study designs with mixed results. Noncontrolled trials have shown that Wii-Fit is safe and feasible for older adults [27–30]. Wii-Fit has been safely used in a variety of patient populations such as stroke, Parkinson's disease, and Alzheimer's disease. RCTs have never associated Wii-Fit with harm but multiple studies have failed to find differences between the intervention and control groups for multiple outcomes including balance, where balance was either a primary or secondary outcome measure [31–35].

As described in recent reviews, 35 prior studies examined the use of Wii-Fit or other balance-board-based exercise games to improve balance or motor function [26, 36]. Of these 35 articles, 21 (60%) were RCTs [26, 36] and 15 (43%) were RCT using Wii-Fit [26, 36]. Sixteen (76%) of the 21 RCTs examined balance as an outcome; six (38%) of these studies found significant between-group differences in balance [26, 36]. However, all six of these studies had important methodologic limitations [37–42]. In all but one study (83%), subjects in the intervention group had more contact with the research staff than did the control subjects who were mainly seen to complete baseline and outcome evaluations [37–40, 42]. Intent-to-treat analysis was not utilized in three of the six studies (50%) despite having dropout rates ranging from 6% to 39% [38, 39, 41]. One study (17%) did not control for baseline differences in the primary outcome measure of balance even though these differences were statistically significant [41]. Only one of the six RCTs that reported significant between-group differences used Wii-Fit as an exercise intervention [40]. In this study, Rendon et al. demonstrated significant improvement in Timed Up and Go and the ABC scale in the Wii-Fit group compared to a nonintervention control group that was only seen for assessments at baseline and six weeks after intervention [40]. Two RCTs that used Wii-Fit and had balance as outcome measures did not report between-group differences [43, 44].

Wii-Fit exercises are shown to improve motor function independent of balance. Two RCTs of Wii-Fit demonstrated statistically significant between-group differences on motor function in select populations of older adults. Saposnik et al. demonstrated significant improvement in the motor function in poststroke subjects in the Wii-Fit augmented standardized rehabilitation therapy group compared to the recreational therapy group [45]. Jorgensen et al. demonstrated significant improvement in leg muscle strength and no improvement in the secondary outcome of postural balance in physiotherapist supervised Wii-Fit group compared to the control group who were given shoe insoles to wear [46]. These two studies also had small sample sizes and had low dose of the intervention.

The current study adds to the findings of the prior studies by demonstrating that Wii-Fit produced a significantly greater effect on balance compared to the control intervention after controlling for baseline BBS scores. This is

TABLE 4: Details of Wii-Fit exercises preferentially used by subjects in this study.

Category	Exercise	Details	Balance components targeted
Balance[a]	Ski Slalom	Maneuver between virtual poles while flexing knees and shifting weight	SB, DB, Coordination
	Bubble Balance	Lean forward, backward, left, right to guide a bubble down a course, avoiding obstacles	SB, DB, Coordination, Endurance
	Penguin Slide	Move a penguin on ice to pick a fish by moving center of gravity in mediolateral plane	SB, DB, Coordination
	Table Tilt	Directing balls into holes on a tilting platform by moving the center of gravity	SB, DB, Coordination, Endurance
	Soccer Heading	Strike a virtual soccer ball coming from the TV by moving the center of gravity	SB, DB, Coordination
	Tight Rope Walking	Rhythmic lateral weight shifting with outstretched arms to walk without falling	SB, DB, Coordination, Endurance
Yoga[a]	Deep Breathing	Inhale and exhale to video cues while maintaining steady posture	SB, DB, Endurance
	Half Moon	Lean upper body sideways with outstretched arms mirroring virtual instructor	SB, DB, Endurance, Strength
	Warrior	Stretch while bending one knee and outstretched arms	SB, DB, Endurance, Strength
Strength Training	Torso Twist[a]	Twist the trunk left and right with outstretched arms mirroring virtual instructor	SB, DB, Coordination, Strength
	Triceps Extension	Extend arm mirroring trainer with the controller in the hand	SB, Coordination, Strength
Aerobic	Basic Walk/Run	Walk in place while holding the controller and follow a cat on the screen	Warm up, DB, Coordination, Endurance
Training Plus[a]	Perfect 10	Mediolateral and anteroposterior movements to add numbers to make a score of 10	SB, DB, Coordination, Endurance
	Obstacle Course	Navigate obstacles while walking on the balance board and stopping at right moments	SB, DB, Coordination, Endurance, Strength
	Island cycling	Walk on the balance board to propel a cycle on the screen to collect flags on the route	SB, DB, Endurance
	Segway Circuit	Lean forward, backward, left, right to guide a Segway at hot air balloons to collect points	SB, DB, Coordination, Endurance

[a] Uses balance board to perform exercises.
DB = Dynamic Balance, SB = Static Balance.

perhaps due to the differences in the dose of the intervention or other aspects of study design compared to previous studies. This includes analyzing the primary outcome measure of balance using intent-to-treat principles in a sensitivity analysis, adjusting for baseline, and having an attention control group. There were several other strengths of the study. First, 30% of the subjects were African Americans, which make the results more generalizable. Second, there was a high adherence to the program. In addition, none of the subjects stopped exercising before the time allotted for them to exercise; this suggests that making the program self-guided and tailored to comply with each subject's preferences and abilities was effective in keeping the subjects engaged. Third, we clearly demonstrated that subjects were able to safely participate in the Wii-Fit program with no study-related adverse events.

The current study has several limitations. Most notable one was the limited sample size. The study was a pilot investigation and was not a priori adequately powered to address all of the outcomes. The study population primarily consisted of male Veterans; although consistent with the older population enrolled within the Veterans Health Administration, this limits the generalizability. Another major limitation was the lack of blinding of the outcomes assessor. The assessor was not part of the exercise sessions; however, the assessor was aware of the group assignment. The use of Wii-Fit as an exercise modality was a limiting factor for morbidly obese subjects as the Wii balance board has an upper weight limit. Activity levels between exercise sessions were not recorded. Although there is no reason to believe that participants in either group were more active than others in between the sessions, such information could help explain the outcomes. Another limitation of the study design was the lack of postintervention follow-up to study the retention of benefits of exercise. The duration of the exercise program in our study was 8 weeks, shorter than the recommended duration of 12 weeks, which is reported to have the largest effect on balance [47]. The additional time may increase the power of the study to detect any significant differences in the secondary outcome measures. Additional studies will be needed to test the efficacy of Wii-Fit in a female population and on more sophisticated measures of balance such as center of pressure and ultimately on fall rates; a larger sample size will likely be required for such studies.

5. Conclusion

This study confirms the safety and feasibility of a Wii-Fit exercise program for community dwelling older adults with mild-to-moderate balance problems. Furthermore, it also demonstrates that Wii-Fit exergames can be used efficaciously in this population to improve balance.

Competing Interests

There is no financial conflict of interests or personal conflict of interests relevant to the submitted manuscript for any authors.

Acknowledgments

The authors thank their research assistant Allison Hunt for helping with this research study. This study (ClinicalTrials.gov Identifier: NCT02190045) was funded by SCVAHCN Network research grant program by the Department of Veterans Affairs (PI: Kalpana Padala, MD).

References

[1] A. Shumway-Cook, A. M. Ciol, J. Hoffman, J. B. Dudgeon, K. Yorkston, and L. Chan, "Falls in the medicare population: incidence, associated factors, and on health care," *Physical Therapy*, vol. 89, no. 4, pp. 324–332, 2009.

[2] J. M. Hausdorff, D. A. Rios, and H. K. Edelberg, "Gait variability and fall risk in community-living older adults: a 1-year prospective study," *Archives of Physical Medicine and Rehabilitation*, vol. 82, no. 8, pp. 1050–1056, 2001.

[3] M. E. Tinetti, "Clinical practice. Preventing falls in elderly persons," *The New England Journal of Medicine*, vol. 348, no. 1, pp. 42–49, 2003.

[4] R. Tideiksaar, *Falls in Older People*, Health Professions Press, Baltimore, Md, USA, 3rd edition, 2016.

[5] D. A. Ganz, Y. Bao, P. G. Shekelle, and L. Z. Rubenstein, "Will my patient fall?" *JAMA*, vol. 297, no. 1, pp. 77–86, 2007.

[6] K. M. Sibley, M. K. Beauchamp, K. V. Ooteghem, S. E. Straus, and S. B. Jaglal, "Using the systems framework for postural control to analyze the components of balance evaluated in standardized balance measures: a scoping review," *Archives of Physical Medicine and Rehabilitation*, vol. 96, no. 1, pp. 122.e29–132.e29, 2015.

[7] L. D. Gillespie, W. J. Gillespie, R. Cumming, S. E. Lamb, and B. H. Rowe, "Interventions for preventing falls in the elderly," *The Cochrane Database of Systematic Reviews*, no. 2, Article ID CD000340, 2000.

[8] T. E. Howe, L. Rochester, A. Jackson, P. M. Banks, and V. A. Blair, "Exercise for improving balance in older people," *Cochrane Database of Systematic Reviews*, no. 4, Article ID CD004963, 2007.

[9] C. Sherrington, A. Tiedemann, N. Fairhall, J. C. T. Close, and S. R. Lord, "Exercise to prevent falls in older adults: an updated meta-analysis and best practice recommendations," *New South Wales Public Health Bulletin*, vol. 22, no. 3-4, pp. 78–83, 2011.

[10] C. A. DeVito, R. O. Morgan, M. Duque, E. Abdel-Moty, and B. A. Virnig, "Physical performance effects of low-intensity exercise among clinically defined high-risk elders," *Gerontology*, vol. 49, no. 3, pp. 146–154, 2003.

[11] A. J. Campbell, M. C. Robertson, M. M. Gardner, R. N. Norton, and D. M. Buchner, "Falls prevention over 2 years: a randomized controlled trial in women 80 years and older," *Age and Ageing*, vol. 28, no. 6, pp. 513–518, 1999.

[12] C. J. Crespo, S. J. Keteyian, G. W. Heath, and C. T. Sempos, "Leisure-time physical activity among US adults: results from the Third National Health and Nutrition Examination Survey," *Archives of Internal Medicine*, vol. 156, no. 1, pp. 93–98, 1996.

[13] Exergaming, 2016, https://www.acsm.org/docs/brochures/exergaming.pdf?sfvrsn=6.

[14] Nintendo's New Wii Fit Makes Fitness Fun, 2017, http://www.businesswire.com/news/home/20080519005400/en/Nintendos-Wii-Fit-Fitness-Fun.

[15] American College of Sports Medicine, "American College of Sports Medicine position stand. Exercise and physical activity for older adults," *Medicine & Science in Sports & Exercise*, vol. 41, no. 7, pp. 1510–1530, 2009.

[16] Brain Fitness, 2017, http://www.happy-neuron.com/brain-games.

[17] HAPPYneuron.Inc, http://www.happy-neuron.com.

[18] S. W. Muir, K. Berg, B. Chesworth, and M. Speechley, "Use of the Berg Balance Scale for predicting multiple falls in community-dwelling elderly people: a prospective study," *Physical Therapy*, vol. 88, no. 4, pp. 449–459, 2008.

[19] D. Donoghue and E. K. Stokes, "How much change is true change? The minimum detectable change of the Berg Balance Scale in elderly people," *Journal of Rehabilitation Medicine*, vol. 41, no. 5, pp. 343–346, 2009.

[20] L. E. Powell and A. M. Myers, "The Activities-specific Balance Confidence (ABC) scale," *Journals of Gerontology—A Biological Sciences and Medical Sciences*, vol. 50A, no. 1, pp. M28–M34, 1995.

[21] D. Kendzierski and K. J. DeCarlo, "Physical activity enjoyment scale: two validation studies," *Journal of Sport and Exercise Psychology*, vol. 13, no. 1, pp. 50–64, 1991.

[22] S. P. Mullen, E. A. Olson, S. M. Phillips et al., "Measuring enjoyment of physical activity in older adults: invariance of the physical activity enjoyment scale (paces) across groups and time," *International Journal of Behavioral Nutrition and Physical Activity*, vol. 8, article 103, 2011.

[23] E. L. Teng and H. C. Chui, "The Modified Mini-Mental State (3MS) examination," *Journal of Clinical Psychiatry*, vol. 48, no. 8, pp. 314–318, 1987.

[24] J. E. Ware, K. K. Snow, and M. Kosinski, *SF-36 Health Survey: Manual and Interpretation Guide*, The Health Institute, New England Medical Center, Boston, Mass, USA, 1993.

[25] M. K. Beauchamp, S. L. Harrison, R. S. Goldstein, and D. Brooks, "Interpretability of change scores in measures of balance in people with COPD," *Chest*, vol. 149, no. 3, pp. 696–703, 2016.

[26] D. Schoene, T. Valenzuela, S. R. Lord, and E. D. de Bruin, "The effect of interactive cognitive-motor training in reducing fall risk in older people: a systematic review," *BMC Geriatrics*, vol. 14, no. 1, article 107, 2014.

[27] M. Agmon, C. K. Perry, E. Phelan, G. Demiris, and H. Q. Nguyen, "A pilot study of Wii Fit exergames to improve balance in older adults," *Journal of Geriatric Physical Therapy*, vol. 34, no. 4, pp. 161–167, 2011.

[28] Y.-Y. Chao, Y. K. Scherer, Y.-W. Wu, K. T. Lucke, and C. A. Montgomery, "The feasibility of an intervention combining self-efficacy theory and Wii Fit exergames in assisted living residents: a pilot study," *Geriatric Nursing*, vol. 34, no. 5, pp. 377–382, 2013.

[29] D. Rosenberg, C. A. Depp, I. V. Vahia et al., "Exergames for subsyndromal depression in older adults: a pilot study of a novel intervention," *American Journal of Geriatric Psychiatry*, vol. 18, no. 3, pp. 221–226, 2010.

[30] B. Williams, N. L. Doherty, A. Bender, H. Mattox, and J. R. Tibbs, "The effect of nintendo wii on balance: a pilot study supporting the use of the wii in occupational therapy for the well elderly," *Occupational Therapy in Health Care*, vol. 25, no. 2-3, pp. 131–139, 2011.

[31] J. R. Franco, K. Jacobs, C. Inzerillo, and J. Kluzik, "The effect of the Nintendo Wii Fit and exercise in improving balance and quality of life in community dwelling elders," *Technology and Health Care*, vol. 20, no. 2, pp. 95–115, 2012.

[32] V. Fung, A. Ho, J. Shaffer, E. Chung, and M. Gomez, "Use of Nintendo Wii Fit™ in the rehabilitation of outpatients following total knee replacement: a preliminary randomised controlled trial," *Physiotherapy*, vol. 98, no. 3, pp. 183–188, 2012.

[33] J. K. Hsu, R. Thibodeau, S. J. Wong, D. Zukiwsky, S. Cecile, and D. M. Walton, "A "Wii" bit of fun: the effects of adding Nintendo Wii® Bowling to a standard exercise regimen for residents of long-term care with upper extremity dysfunction," *Physiotherapy Theory and Practice*, vol. 27, no. 3, pp. 185–193, 2011.

[34] K. Laver, S. George, J. Ratcliffe et al., "Use of an interactive video gaming program compared with conventional physiotherapy for hospitalised older adults: a feasibility trial," *Disability and Rehabilitation*, vol. 34, no. 21, pp. 1802–1808, 2012.

[35] K. P. Padala, P. R. Padala, T. R. Malloy et al., "Wii-fit for improving gait and balance in an assisted living facility: a pilot study," *Journal of Aging Research*, vol. 2012, Article ID 597573, 6 pages, 2012.

[36] Y.-Y. Chao, Y. K. Scherer, and C. A. Montgomery, "Effects of using nintendo wii™ exergames in older adults: a review of the literature," *Journal of Aging and Health*, vol. 27, no. 3, pp. 379–402, 2015.

[37] G. Duque, D. Boersma, G. Loza-Diaz et al., "Effects of balance training using a virtual-reality system in older fallers," *Clinical Interventions in Aging*, vol. 8, pp. 257–263, 2013.

[38] J. Kim, J. Son, N. Ko, and B. Yoon, "Unsupervised virtual reality-based exercise program improves hip muscle strength and balance control in older adults: a pilot study," *Archives of Physical Medicine and Rehabilitation*, vol. 94, no. 5, pp. 937–943, 2013.

[39] A. Kubicki, F. Bonnetblanc, G. Petrement, and F. Mourey, "Motor-prediction improvements after virtual rehabilitation in geriatrics: frail patients reveal different learning curves for movement and postural control," *Neurophysiologie Clinique*, vol. 44, no. 1, pp. 109–118, 2014.

[40] A. A. Rendon, E. B. Lohman, D. Thorpe, E. G. Johnson, E. Medina, and B. Bradley, "The effect of virtual reality gaming on dynamic balance in older adults," *Age and Ageing*, vol. 41, no. 4, pp. 549–552, 2012.

[41] T. Szturm, A. L. Betker, Z. Moussavi, A. Desai, and V. Goodman, "Effects of an interactive computer game exercise regimen on balance impairment in frail community-dwelling older adults: a randomized controlled trial," *Physical Therapy*, vol. 91, no. 10, pp. 1449–1462, 2011.

[42] C.-Y. Yen, K.-H. Lin, M.-H. Hu, R.-M. Wu, T.-W. Lu, and C.-H. Lin, "Effects of virtual reality-augmented balance training on sensory organization and attentional demand for postural control in people with Parkinson disease: a randomized controlled trial," *Physical Therapy*, vol. 91, no. 6, pp. 862–874, 2011.

[43] K. A. Bieryla and N. M. Dold, "Feasibility of Wii Fit training to improve clinical measures of balance in older adults," *Clinical Interventions in Aging*, vol. 8, pp. 775–781, 2013.

[44] C. Toulotte, C. Toursel, and N. Olivier, "Wii Fit® training vs. Adapted Physical Activities: which one is the most appropriate to improve the balance of independent senior subjects? A randomized controlled study," *Clinical Rehabilitation*, vol. 26, no. 9, pp. 827–835, 2012.

[45] G. Saposnik, R. Teasell, M. Mamdani et al., "Effectiveness of virtual reality using Wii gaming technology in stroke rehabilitation: a pilot randomized clinical trial and proof of principle," *Stroke*, vol. 41, no. 7, pp. 1477–1484, 2010.

[46] M. G. Jorgensen, U. Laessoe, C. Hendriksen, O. B. F. Nielsen, and P. Aagaard, "Efficacy of nintendo wii training on mechanical leg muscle function and postural balance in community-dwelling older adults: a randomized controlled trial," *Journals of Gerontology —A Biological Sciences and Medical Sciences*, vol. 68, no. 7, pp. 845–852, 2013.

[47] M. Lesinski, T. Hortobágyi, T. Muehlbauer, A. Gollhofer, and U. Granacher, "Effects of balance training on balance performance in healthy older adults: a systematic review and meta-analysis," *Sports Medicine*, vol. 45, no. 12, pp. 1721–1738, 2015.

13

Flexibility of Older Adults Aged 55–86 Years and the Influence of Physical Activity

Liza Stathokostas,[1,2] Matthew W. McDonald,[2] Robert M. D. Little,[1,2] and Donald H. Paterson[1,2]

[1] *Canadian Centre for Activity and Aging, Faculty of Health Sciences, 3M Centre 2225, The University of Western Ontario, London, ON, Canada N6A 3K7*

[2] *School of Kinesiology, Faculty of Health Sciences, 3M Centre 2225, The University of Western Ontario, London, ON, Canada N6A 3K7*

Correspondence should be addressed to Liza Stathokostas; lstatho2@uwo.ca

Academic Editor: Astrid E. Fletcher

Cross-sectional age-related differences in flexibility of older adults aged 55–86 years of varying activity levels were examined. Shoulder abduction and hip flexion flexibility measurements were obtained from 436 individuals (205 men, 71 ± 9 years; 231 women, 72 ± 8 years). Total physical activity was assessed using the Minnesota Leisure-Time Physical Activity Questionnaire. Shoulder abduction showed a significant decline averaging 5 degrees/decade in men and 6 degrees/decade in women. Piecewise linear regression showed an accelerated decline in men starting at the age of 71 years of 0.80 degrees/year, whereas in women the onset of decline (0.74 degrees/year) was 63 years. Men and women showed a significant decline in hip flexion (men: 6 degrees/decade; women: 7 degrees/decade). Piecewise linear regression revealed a rate of decline of 1.16 degrees/year beginning at 71 years in men and in women a single linear decline of 0.66 degrees/year. Multiple regression analysis showed that age and physical activity accounted for only 9% of the variance in hip flexion in women and 10% in men, with age but not physical activity remaining significant. Similarly for shoulder abduction, age was significant but not physical activity, in a model that described 8% of the variance for both sexes.

1. Introduction

As indicated in a recent systematic review by our group [1], there is conflicting information regarding both the relationship between flexibility training interventions and functional outcomes and the relationship between improved flexibility and daily functioning; health benefits have not yet been established. The comparison of studies in this area to provide a prescription of the flexibility is complicated by the variety of limb ranges of motion studied, testing procedures utilized, and methods of assessing physical activity levels. Furthermore, this component of physical health has been somewhat neglected or forgotten in the current literature despite the lack of evidence for recommendations of the amount and type of flexibility needed for health in older adults. Further, despite this lack of a synthesis of the literature to support the recommendation of the inclusion of a flexibility component to older adult exercise programs, many older adult activity programs place a considerable emphasis on flexibility. The present study attempts to add additional insight to this area by presenting the relationship between declines in flexibility across age and functional outcomes in a large sample of individuals representing the older adult age range. Joint flexibility may decrease across the age span [2–4], which has the potential to affect normal daily functioning. Upper body flexibility is known to be important for activities such as getting dressed and reaching for objects, while lower body flexibility is important for maintaining normal walking patterns and for activities involving bending and reaching [5]. While the loss in flexibility with age has been attributable, in part, to decreased activity [5], the literature describing the influence of physical activity on flexibility and the aging process is surprisingly limited. The purpose of the present study was to examine the cross-sectional age-related differences in flexibility in a large sample of independently living adults aged 55–86 years with varying activity levels. The recent systematic literature review identified the lack of an established relationship between improved flexibility and daily functioning and health benefits [1]. As such, a secondary purpose of the present study was to describe any relationships of physical activity levels and of functional outcomes (specifically walking), with flexibility measures.

2. Methods

2.1. Sample Selection, Recruitment, and Participation. The municipal tax assessment list, containing names of householders and residents in the city of London, Ontario (2011, population 366,151), provided the sampling frame. Those living in institutions, defined as nursing homes or chronic care facilities, were not eligible. A stratified random sample was drawn from the population. The strata were defined by gender and six five-year age groups, starting with age of 55, and the sampling rate was set to select 35 men and women in each stratum. Those sampled were sent a letter inviting their participation, and a follow-up call to recruit and screen the respondents was made. Exclusion criteria were those who responded no to the question of their ability to walk an 80 meter course. Thus, the target population the noninstitutionalized population aged 55–85 years who self-reported the ability to walk 80 meters. The university's human research review board approved the study, and each subject signed informed consent.

2.2. Measurements

2.2.1. Anthropometric. Body height, mass, skinfold thickness (four sites: biceps, triceps, subscapular, and suprailiac), and waist and hip girth were measured. Body mass index was calculated.

2.2.2. Joint Flexibility. Hip flexion was assessed using a Leighton flexometer fastened to the hip, with the range of motion determined by bending backward as far as possible and then forward as far as possible [6]. Shoulder abduction was measured as the range of motion of the right hand from the side of the leg, upward and outward in an arc [6].

2.2.3. Physical Activity. The Minnesota Leisure-Time Physical Activity Questionnaire (MLTPAQ) was used to assess self-reported physical activity levels [7]. The questionnaire was administered with the aid of a research assistant. For the present data in older adults, the intensity codes (metabolic rate scores) for different activities, developed for middle-aged subjects, were reduced in proportion to the age-related slowing of self-paced walking speed, to acknowledge that older adults would pursue these activities at a slower absolute pace. Specifically, the codes were decreased 8.9% for males and 4.6% for females from middle age to 55 years [8]. The codes were then decreased a further 0.61% per year in males and 1.02% per year in females for each year beyond the age of 55, corresponding to the rate of decline in self-paced walking as measured in the sample of the present study (age 55 to 85 years). Thus, the "intensity codes" for the vigor with which older adults participated in a particular activity were age-adjusted. According to the MLTPAQ scoring system, physical activity was characterized by total energy expenditure (in MET/minutes/day) and also examined for energy expenditure in activities characterized as light, moderate, or heavy intensity.

2.2.4. Muscle Strength. The design of the leg dynamometer and the procedures followed for measuring plantar flexion strength have been previously reported [9]. Subjects were seated on a bench with the thigh locked in a horizontal position and knee flexed at 85 degrees in the leg dynamometer. The dominant leg was clamped down and the subject was asked to push-off, that is, to attempt to raise their heel off the ground. The force generated against the clamp bar was recorded with a strain gauge calibrated with standard weights. Three trials were done. Maximal grip strength (of three trials) of the dominant hand was measured using a handgrip dynamometer with interchangeable casings to accommodate hand size.

2.2.5. Normal and Fast Walking. As a measure of lower body function, walking speed (time/meters) and step length were assessed by having subjects walk an 80-meter course at their normal and fast self-selected speeds [8].

2.2.6. Self-Rated Health and Life Satisfaction. Self-rated health and life satisfaction were assessed using a questionnaire containing modified questions from the Nottingham Health Profile [10], as were self-reported walking difficulty and difficulty with stairs, by rating degree of difficulty on a five-point scale.

2.3. Analysis. Data analyses were performed with the Statistical Package for the Social Sciences (SPSS 19.0, Ireland, 2010). All descriptive data are presented as mean ± SD. Frequency distributions were examined for categorical variables. Ranges of motion of the hip and shoulder joints across age were analyzed by both linear regression and piecewise linear regression with a 2-segment model (Sigma Plot 12.0, Chicago, Illinois, USA); these fits produced similar R^2 values. Age and physical activity were entered into a multiple regression analysis to determine associations with shoulder and hip flexibility. Further, expanded univariate logistic regression was performed to identify other variables associated with determining flexibility. Lastly, stepwise linear regression, allowing for entry and removal at the 0.10 level of significance, was used to examine the relationship of flexibility with physical (self-rated health, self-reported arthritis, body mass index, and upper and lower body strength), functional (walking and stair climbing difficulty, step length, and walking speed), and psychosocial (self-rated health, life satisfaction) variables.

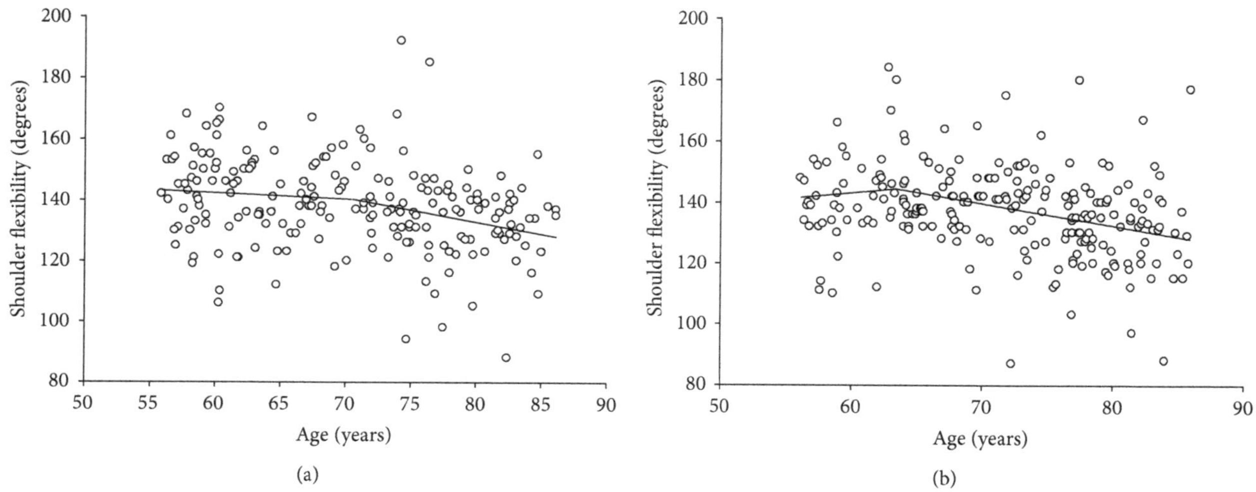

FIGURE 1: (a) Age analysis for shoulder flexibility in men. Piecewise linear regression s-segment model shows breaking at the age of 71 years. Rate of decline prior to age 71 is −0.20 degrees per year and −0.80 degrees per year after the age of 71 years. (R^2 of fit $R^2 = 0.09$). (b) Age analysis for shoulder flexibility in women. Piecewise linear regression s-segment model shows breaking at the age of 63 years. Rate of change prior to age 63 is 0.38 degrees per year and −0.74 degrees per year after the age of 63 years. (R^2 of fit $R^2 = 0.09$).

3. Results

3.1. Response Rate. The recruitment process resulted in 1451 individuals contacted; 696 were eligible, and 441 (63.4%) participated and is detailed by Koval et al. [11]. Participants were more likely to be widowed and less likely to be married, more likely to have had a white-collar job, and had some postsecondary education.

3.2. Description of the Sample. Flexibility measurements were obtained from a total of 436 community-dwelling individuals (205 men, mean age 70.4 ± 8.8 years; 231 women, mean age 71.4 ± 8.4 years). Subject characteristics are presented in Table 1. Self-rated health among the group indicated that 11% of the sample considered their health to be "excellent" and 54% rated their health as "good." Almost half of the sample was fully retired (49%) and 11% were employed full time. Seven percent of the sample reported being not "very satisfied" with life. Sixty-three reported being "quite satisfied" and 30% reported being "very satisfied." The marital status of the sample indicated that 56% were married. Based on self-reported physical activity levels, the calculated total energy expenditure in leisure time physical activity would indicate that the present sample was, on average, very active, but encompassed a wide range of activity levels.

TABLE 1: Subject characteristics.

	Total sample ($n = 436$)	Men ($n = 205$)	Women ($n = 231$)
Age (years)	71 ± 8.6	70.4 ± 8.8	71.4 ± 8.4
BMI	26 ± 3.9	26.3 ± 3.1	25.8 ± 4.4
Mass (kg)	71 ± 12.9	78.2 ± 10.5	64.5 ± 11.4
Physical activity level (MET/minutes/day)	406 ± 201	386 ± 182	423 ± 215
Shoulder abduction (degrees, $n = 431$)	138 ± 15	138 ± 15 ($n = 202$)	138 ± 16 ($n = 231$)
Hip flexion (degrees, $n = 402$)	109 ± 19	102 ± 18 ($n = 183$)	114 ± 18* ($n = 219$)

BMI: body mass index, $^*P < 0.05$.

3.3. Flexibility and Differences by Age

3.3.1. Shoulder Abduction. The mean range of motion of shoulder flexibility was 138 degrees in our sample, with no difference between men and women. Shoulder abduction showed a significant decline across age, averaging 5 degrees per decade in men and 6 degrees per decade in women. From piecewise linear regression, an accelerated decline of 0.80 degrees per year was observed in the sample of men starting with those 71 years old, whereas in women the onset of decline was 63 years and declined across age at a rate of 0.74 degrees per year (Figures 1(a) and 1(b)).

3.3.2. Hip Flexion. The women had significantly higher hip flexion of 114 degrees versus the men, with 102 degrees. However, both showed a similarly significant age-related decline in hip flexion (men: 6 degrees per decade; women: 7 degrees per decade). Piecewise linear regression revealed a rate of decline of 1.16 degrees per year, across age, beginning at 71 years in men (Figure 2(a)). In women, the decrease across the age span of the sample was a single linear decline of 0.66 degrees per year (Figure 2(b)).

3.4. Relationship of Age and Physical Activity with Flexibility. Both upper and lower body flexibility measures were normally distributed. Age was significant ($P < 0.01$), but the contribution of physical activity was not (females: $P = 0.14$; males: $P = 0.57$), when included in a regression

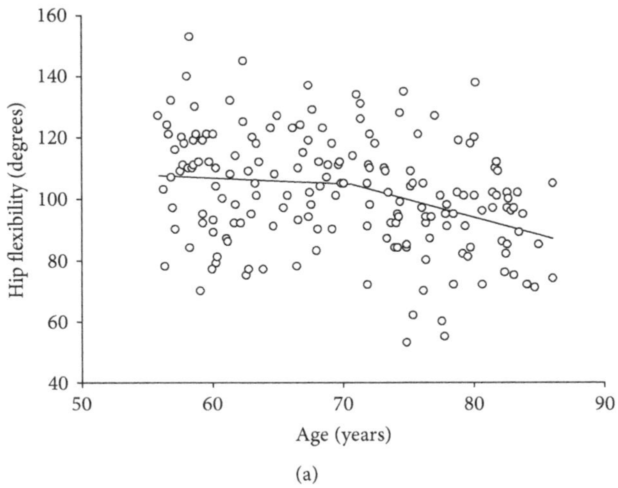

FIGURE 2: (a) Age analysis for hip flexion in men. Piecewise linear regression s-segment model shows breaking at the age of 71 years. The rate of decline prior to 71 years is −0.19 degrees per year and −1.16 degrees per year thereafter. (R^2 of fit $R^2 = 0.11$). (b) Age analysis for hip flexion in women. Piecewise linear regression s-segment model shows breaking at the age of 86 years. The rate of decline prior to 86 years is −0.66 degrees per year and −2.67 degrees per year thereafter. (R^2 of fit $R^2 = 0.08$).

model that described 9% of the variance for both males and females in the decline in shoulder abduction. The regression model accounted for only 7% of the variance (in both men and women) in the change in hip flexion. Again, age showed a significant contribution ($P < 0.01$); however, the contribution of physical activity to lower body flexibility was not significant for either males ($P = 0.71$) or females ($P = 0.42$).

3.5. Variables Associated with Flexibility. Neither total physical activity nor the components of light-, moderate-, and heavy-intensity physical activity were significantly related to flexibility of the hip or shoulder at the univariate level (Tables 2(a) and 2(b)). Age was significant and explained 8% and 7% of variance in shoulder and hip flexibility, respectively.

For upper body flexibility, age, BMI, plantar flexor strength, and handgrip strength were entered into the stepwise linear regression (Table 3(a)). Regression analysis yielded a model including age, BMI, and plantar flexion strength that resulted in 10.5% of the variance in upper body flexibility being accounted for by those variables.

Age, sex, BMI, and hand grip strength were entered into a regression model for lower body flexibility, accounting for 19.6% of the variance in hip flexibility (Table 3(b)).

3.6. Association with Function, Self-Rated Health, and Life Satisfaction. There was no association between upper body flexibility and the "functional measures" of self-reported difficulty in walking or climbing stairs. Step length was associated with upper body flexibility but not when adjustment was made for age. Normal, fast, and very fast walking speeds were associated with upper body flexibility, but only very fast walking speed ($P = 0.001$) was still associated when adjustment was made for age. Lower body flexibility was associated with all walking speeds; however, none of the associations were maintained when adjustment was made for age.

Self-rated health and life satisfaction were not associated with either upper ($P = 0.18$; $P = 0.32$) or lower body flexibility ($P = 0.09$; $P = 0.30$).

4. Discussion

This study provides descriptive data on the age-related differences (across the age range of 55–85 years) in flexibility in a large cross-sectional sample of male and female community-dwelling older adults. It also provides an examination of the role of physical activity in the changes to upper and lower body flexibility with aging and a determination of the relationship of flexibility with functional outcomes in older adults. Our sample demonstrated a mean upper body flexibility of 138 degrees and a mean lower body flexibility of 109 degrees. Bassey et al. [12] reported shoulder abduction values of 125 degrees for men and 119 for women in a similar large sample ($n = 894$) of community-dwelling adults over the age of 65 years. These values are lower than those reported for the present study's sample; however, it should be noted that the shoulder abduction measure was slightly different, and a large proportion of the sample in Bassey's study reported having a functional disability.

With respect to sex differences, the majority of the literature indicates that women have greater flexibility at all ages [4, 13–18]. Our results were in agreement for lower body flexibility, although there was no significant difference based on sex for upper body flexibility. This is in contrast to Bassey et al. [12], who reported significantly lower shoulder abduction flexibility for females in their sample. Doriot and Wang [19] did not find consistent sex differences among their 26 measures of joint range of motion. Similarly, Walker et al. [20]

TABLE 2: (a) Univariate associations with shoulder flexibility. (b) Univariate associations with hip flexibility.

(a)

	Mean (SD)	r	P value
Sex: males = 205; females = 231		−0.017	0.722
Age (years)	71 ± 8.6	−0.290	<0.001
Total physical activity	405.8 ± 201.0	0.029	0.547
Light activity	186.1 ± 82.6	0.057	0.235
Moderate activity	115.1 ± 91.1	0.030	0.530
Heavy activity	104.6 ± 141.3	−0.012	0.810
BMI	26 ± 3.9	−0.094	0.052
Sum of skinfolds	56.0 ± 20.5	0.013	0.825
Plantar flexion strength	879.5 ± 322.9	0.197	<0.001
Handgrip strength	292.1 ± 112.7	0.126	<0.001
Arthritis: no = 107; yes = 108		−0.022	0.752

BMI: body mass index; self-reported arthritis data available for 215 subjects.

(b)

	Mean (SD)	r	P value
Sex: males = 205; females = 231		0.341	<0.001
Age (years)	71 ± 8.6	−0.256	<0.001
Total physical activity	405.8 ± 201.0	0.027	0.586
Light activity	186.1 ± 82.6	0.039	0.435
Moderate activity	115.1 ± 91.1	−0.010	0.839
Heavy activity	104.6 ± 141.3	0.022	0.658
BMI	26 ± 3.9	−0.131	0.009
Sum of skinfolds	56.0 ± 20.5	0.080	0.187
Plantar flexion strength	879.5 ± 322.9	0.055	0.279
Hand grip strength	292.1 ± 112.7	−0.113	0.029
Arthritis: no = 107; yes = 108		−0.107	0.132

BMI: body mass index; self-reported arthritis data available for 215 subjects.

TABLE 3: (a) Shoulder flexibility regression model. (b) Hip flexibility regression model.

(a)

	R^2	Parameter estimate	SE	P value
Age	0.083	−0.486	0.091	<0.001*
BMI	0.009	−0.647	0.187	0.001*
Plantar flexion strength	0.039	0.006	0.002	0.045*

Cumulative R^2 = 0.117, BMI: body mass index, *significance set at = $P <$ 0.05.

(b)

	R^2	Parameter estimate	SE	P value
Age	0.066	−0.571	0.117	<0.001*
Sex—female	0.117	18.8	2.721	<0.001*
BMI	0.09	−1.014	0.265	<0.001*
Handgrip strength	0.029	0.031	0.013	0.018*

Cumulative R^2 = 0.235, BMI: body mass index, *significance set at = $P <$ 0.05, sex: male = 0; female = 1.

found no differences in ranges of motion of the shoulder, elbow, hip, or knee joints, between older men and women. These varying results are likely due to different population samples, joints studied, and customary use of the joints.

The rate of decline in flexibility with age will vary depending on the body part measured, the training status of the sample, and population being studied. In our sample of relatively healthy community-dwelling older adults, the rate of decline in our measure of upper body flexibility (shoulder abduction) was 0.5 degrees per year in males and 0.6 degrees per year in females. Declines in hip flexion of 0.6 degrees per year in males and 0.7 degrees per year in females were documented. A 1% decline per year (approximately 1.2 degrees per year, or nearly double the rate found in the present study) in shoulder abduction range of motion of older men and women was reported by Bassey et al. [12]. Comparative rates of decline are not readily available in the literature, but rates of 1.5 degrees per year have been reported for lower back flexion, and the greatest decline appears to occur with trunk extension [21].

Whereas differences in flexibility by sex may occur, the rate of change with age has been reported to be similar in both men and women [22, 23], and our results concur. In contrast, McCulloch [14] showed little decline in sit-and-reach scores in women versus men, who showed a dramatic decline in age groups of 65 to 75 years, citing differences in the decline in work activity of men over the older adult age range.

This study provides a description of potential critical periods of decline in flexibility across the older adult age range. At the age of 71 years, it appears that both upper and lower body flexibility show an accelerated decline in males, whereas in females, only upper body flexibility shows a change in the rate of decline, with lower body showing a steady rate of change. James and Parker [22] reported decreases in active and passive motion in lower limb joints during the period of 70 to 92 years, with the decline becoming more pronounced during the ninth decade. While not significant, Charkravarty and Webley [15] reported a greater decline in range of motion in a group over the age of 75 years versus a group of 65–74 years, adding support to the trend for an accelerated decline in flexibility in the oldest old. The present sample had an age range including up to 86 years, and the piecewise linear regression did suggest that an accelerated decline would occur in the oldest women.

Whereas age may be associated with a decline in flexibility, older adults still maintain the ability to improve flexibility with general exercise training programs [24–27] and with flexibility-specific training, as reviewed by Stathokostas et al. [1]. In addition, the difference in rate of change in flexibility across joints has been attributed to chronic use of those joints, for example, those used in activities of daily living. As such, one purpose of the present study was to determine if age-related losses in flexibility were associated with in physical activity levels. Our results showed no relationship between self-reported physical activity levels and upper or lower body flexibility. Walker et al. [20] also reported no differences in the ranges of motion in the shoulder, elbow, hip, or knee joints, in a sample of 60 older men and women classified into high and low physical activity categories based on self-report. Also, similar results were found by Miotto et al. [28] when comparing the hamstring flexibility in a sample of active versus sedentary adults with a mean age of 68 years; no difference was observed. Bassey et al. [12] studied the association between shoulder abduction and self-reported customary use of the shoulder and found an association; however, it should be noted that the effect was not significant in women in multiple regression (replaced by effort score), and the effect of customary use was greater in those with a disability. This finding may suggest that a more closely-matched flexibility and activity-specific measurement is more reflective of the role of physical activity in the change in flexibility with age. Nevertheless, in a smaller sample of 30 older women, Rikli and Busch [29] found a significant difference for trunk and shoulder flexibility in active versus inactive women, where active was considered as vigorous activity for at least 30 minutes, three days per week. This study reported a significant age-by-activity interaction for shoulder flexibility, but not for trunk flexion. Voorrips et al. [30], in a sample of 50 women with a mean age of 72 years, reported significantly better flexion at the hip and spine in women who self-reported high activity levels (several hours per week in aerobic-type exercises). A five-year longitudinal study by Lan et al. [31] demonstrated that baseline and follow-up thoracolumbar flexibility values were higher in older adults participating in a Chinese conditioning program of repeated motions and postures with range of motion warm-up versus a sedentary control group. Further, while both groups showed an age-related decline over the five years, the control group had a larger decline in flexibility, supporting a positive role of physical activity in attenuating the decline in flexibility with age. Thus, our results suggest that the age-related declines in flexibility of disability-free independently living older adults are not influenced by their overall level of daily physical activity (although specific stretching exercises can still alter the flexibility levels of older adults).

The present study also examined whether shoulder or hip flexibility was related to "functional" outcomes, specifically walking speeds or self-reported mobility difficulty. Normal step length and normal, fast, and very fast walking speeds were associated with shoulder abduction; however, only for very fast walking speed was the association consistently maintained when adjustments were made for age. Our results did not provide evidence that the change in lower body flexibility (hip flexion) impacted functioning with age. Normal, fast, and very fast walking speeds were associated with hip flexion, but as with shoulder abduction, the relationship was not sustained when adjustment for age was made. There was no association with self-reported difficulty in walking. A factor to consider in range-of-motion declines is the loss of compliance in connective tissue with aging. This loss can lead to decreased range of motion and therefore mobility limitations. For example, it was shown by Vandervoort et al. [32] that a loss of flexibility in the ankle joint affects walking mechanics. It might have been expected that our measure of lower body flexibility would be associated with our walking measures, as representatives of function; however this was not the case. This may be due to the lack of contribution of hip flexion to gait. Nevertheless, self-reported difficulty with stair climbing also failed to show an association in the present population. Previously, our laboratory identified shoulder flexibility as one determinant of independence when comparing a group of independently living older adults versus those in rest or nursing homes [33]. Tainaka et al. [34] showed that ankle dorsi-flexion range of motion was a significant physical fitness factor in predicting six-year incidence of disability. These studies might suggest that the roles of flexibility and function with aging are population-dependent and may not be as influential in younger or healthy subgroups of older adults, based on epidemiological data. Nevertheless, based on the reference values indicating that shoulder abduction range of motion of 120 degrees and hip flexion values of 30–50 degrees (for most hip-related functional activities) are considered lower-end thresholds associated with functional loss [35], we would consider our sample of healthy community-dwelling older adults to be high functioning. Based on the present data for shoulder abduction, using the "reference" that a value of <120 degrees was related to functional loss, the conclusion would be that, among our community-dwelling, disability-free sample the probability of the age-related decline in flexibility falling to below the reference values was very low—less than ~10 subjects beyond age 75 years fell below this "functional threshold" and the average for the 85 year old was close to 130 degrees. For the hip flexibility measure of the present study, we are not aware of data to establish a functional threshold; however from the present data where hip flexion was not related to functional outcomes, the hip flexion was above 70 degrees and the average for the 85 year old was ~100 degrees.

An individual's quality of life includes their sense of well-being, which depends on how they feel about their health and their level of satisfaction with life. In order to address the broader issue of how physical fitness attributes can contribute to health in older adults, the relationship between these health indicators and flexibility was examined. Self-rated health and life satisfaction were not associated with either upper or lower body flexibility in the present sample of independent older adults. In contrast, Bassey et al. [12] reported an association of life satisfaction and social engagement with shoulder range of motion in a large sample of older men and women. However, the difference between studies, as mentioned earlier, is that the sample of Bassey et al. [10] reported a high rate of disability, including shoulder-specific disability and arthritis. In our sample, no relationship between arthritis and flexibility was indicated. In support of the decline in flexibility playing a role in quality of life of older adults, Fabre et al. [36] reported a significant association between upper body flexibility and health-related quality of life in nonagenarians. This sample was community dwelling, with 45% of the sample reporting orthopedic conditions and 43% reporting at least one chronic condition. Thus, although further research is required to understand the role of flexibility in quality of life and successful aging, a lack of relationship is suggested from our data, and where an association of flexibility and health outcomes occurs, it is likely related to a disability, that is, a range of joint motion below some critical threshold.

4.1. Limitations. While the present study does describe a large number of men and women from a random sample, the data is cross sectional, and so reverse causality cannot be ruled out. In addition, individual trajectories of flexibility could vary due to the individuality of the aging process, which would be provided by longitudinal data. The joints measured and the functional outcomes may not be tightly matched or may not reflect functions of daily living that could potentially be limited in subgroups of the present sample, or in the older age ranges. Further to this point, based on the inclusion criteria for this study, the sample may not be representative of the "usual" aging population, but rather an independently living generally healthy one.

5. Conclusions

A decrease in flexibility of the shoulder and hip joints by approximately 6 degrees per decade was observed across ages 55 to 86 years in both men and women. Analysis of age subgroups shows that both shoulder and hip joints begin to experience significant declines after 70 years. Physical activity level did not explain a significant amount of the variance in flexibility measures, and flexibility was not associated with functional ability. While steeper gradients of flexibility with age over certain thresholds may be indicated, further analysis is warranted to discern whether the losses in flexibility impact functional outcomes and the degree of loss of range of motion that might relate to disability. In particular, a more direct matching of specific limb range of motion and meaningful functional outcome is needed, as are longitudinal studies. Additionally, the specific type of physical activity that may influence the age-related loss needs to be further elucidated. Nevertheless, overall, in community-dwelling generally healthy older adults aged 55 to 85 years, the age-related loss of flexibility appears to be small such that the normal loss of joint range of motion (i.e., in the absence of underlying clinical condition) is unlikely to neither impact significantly on daily functions nor result in disability.

References

[1] L. Stathokostas, R. M. D. Little, A. A. Vandervoort, and D. H. Paterson, "Flexibility training and functional ability in older adults: a systematic review," *Journal of Aging Research*, vol. 2012, Article ID 306818, 2012.

[2] K. E. Roach and T. P. Miles, "Normal hip and knee active range of motion: the relationship to age," *Physical Therapy*, vol. 71, no. 9, pp. 656–665, 1991.

[3] H. Nonaka, K. Mita, M. Watakabe et al., "Age-related changes in the interactive mobility of the hip and knee joints: a geometrical analysis," *Gait and Posture*, vol. 15, no. 3, pp. 236–243, 2002.

[4] M. Shields, M. S. Tremblay, M. Laviolette, C. L. Craig, I. Janssen, and S. C. Gorber, "Fitness of Canadian adults: results from the 2007–2009 Canadian health measures survey," *Health Reports*, vol. 21, no. 1, pp. 21–35, 2010.

[5] W. W. Spiriduso, K. Francis, and P. MacRae, "Physical development and decline," in *Physical Dimensions of Aging*, W. W. Spiriduso, Ed., Human Kinetics, Champaign, Ill, USA, 2nd edition, 2005.

[6] J. R. Leighton, "An instrument and technic for the measurement of range of joint motion," *Archives of physical medicine and rehabilitation*, vol. 36, no. 9, pp. 571–578, 1955.

[7] A. R. Folsom, D. R. Jacobs Jr., C. J. Caspersen, O. Gomez-Marin, and J. Knudsen, "Test-retest reliability of the Minnesota leisure time physical activity questionnaire," *Journal of Chronic Diseases*, vol. 39, no. 7, pp. 505–511, 1986.

[8] J. E. Himann, D. A. Cunningham, P. A. Rechnitzer, and D. H. Paterson, "Age-related changes in speed of walking," *Medicine and Science in Sports and Exercise*, vol. 20, no. 2, pp. 161–166, 1988.

[9] C. L. Rice, D. A. Cunningham, D. H. Paterson, and P. A. Rechnitzer, "Strength in an elderly population," *Archives of Physical Medicine and Rehabilitation*, vol. 70, no. 5, pp. 391–397, 1989.

[10] S. M. Hunt, S. P. McKenna, J. McEwen, J. Williams, and E. Papp, "The Nottingham health profile: subjective health status and medical consultations," *Social Science and Medicine A*, vol. 15, no. 3, part 1, pp. 221–229, 1981.

[11] J. J. Koval, N. A. Ecclestone, D. H. Paterson, B. Brown, D. A. Cunningham, and P. A. Rechnitzer, "Response rates in a survey of physical capacity among older persons," *Journals of Gerontology*, vol. 47, no. 3, pp. S140–S147, 1992.

[12] E. J. Bassey, K. Morgan, H. M. Dallosso, and S. B. J. Ebrahim, "Flexibility of the shoulder joint measured as range of abduction in a large representative sample of men and women over 65 years of age," *European Journal of Applied Physiology and Occupational Physiology*, vol. 58, no. 4, pp. 353–360, 1989.

[13] R. D. Bell and T. B. Hoshizaki, "Relationships of age and sex with range of motion of seventeen joint actions in humans," *Canadian Journal of Applied Sport Sciences*, vol. 6, no. 4, pp. 202–206, 1981.

[14] R. G. McCulloch, D. J. Clark, I. Pike, and Y. M. Slobodian, "Gender specific trends in fitness and anthropometric parameters in a selected Saskatchewan sample, aged 65-75 years," *Canadian Journal on Aging*, vol. 13, no. 1, pp. 30–40, 1994.

[15] K. Chakravarty and M. Webley, "Shoulder joint movement and its relationship to disability in the elderly," *Journal of Rheumatology*, vol. 20, no. 8, pp. 1359–1361, 1993.

[16] R. E. Rikli and C. J. Jones, "Functional fitness normative scores for community-residing older adults, ages 60–94," *Journal of Aging and Physical Activity*, vol. 7, no. 2, pp. 162–181, 1999.

[17] J. A. Kalscheur, P. S. Costello, and L. J. Emery, "Gender differences in range of motion in older adults," *Physical and Occupational Therapy in Geriatrics*, vol. 22, no. 1, pp. 77–89, 2003.

[18] G. van Herp, P. Rowe, P. Salter, and J. P. Paul, "Three-dimensional lumbar spinal kinematic: a study of range of movement in 100 healthy subjects aged 20 to 60+ years," *Rheumatology*, vol. 39, no. 12, pp. 1337–1340, 2000.

[19] N. Doriot and X. Wang, "Effects of age and gender on maximum voluntary range of motion of the upper body joints," *Ergonomics*, vol. 49, no. 3, pp. 269–281, 2006.

[20] J. M. Walker, D. Sue, and N. Miles-Elkousy, "Active mobility of the extremities in older subjects," *Physical Therapy*, vol. 64, no. 6, pp. 919–923, 1984.

[21] D. K. Einkauf, M. L. Gohdes, G. M. Jensen, and M. J. Jewell, "Changes in spinal mobility with increasing age in women," *Physical Therapy*, vol. 67, no. 3, pp. 370–375, 1987.

[22] B. James and A. W. Parker, "Active and passive mobility of lower limb joints in elderly men and women," *The American Journal of Physical Medicine and Rehabilitation*, vol. 68, no. 4, pp. 162–167, 1989.

[23] R. E. Rikli and C. J. Jones, "Functional fitness normative scores for community-residing older adults, ages 60–94," *Journal of Aging and Physical Activity*, vol. 7, no. 2, pp. 162–181, 1999.

[24] S. Morini, A. Bassi, C. Cerulli, A. Marinozzi, and M. Ripani, "Hip and knee joints flexibility in young and elderly people: effect of physical activity in the elderly," *Biology of Sport*, vol. 21, no. 1, pp. 25–37, 2004.

[25] J. E. Misner, B. H. Massey, M. Bemben, S. Going, and J. Patrick, "Long-term effects of exercise on the range of motion of aging women," *Journal of Orthopaedic and Sports Physical Therapy*, vol. 16, no. 1, pp. 37–42, 1992.

[26] M. C. Morey, P. A. Cowper, J. R. Feussner et al., "Two-year trends in physical performance following supervised exercise among community-dwelling older veterans," *Journal of the American Geriatrics Society*, vol. 39, no. 10, pp. 986–992, 1991.

[27] C. L. Hubley-Kozey, J. C. Wall, and D. B. Hogan, "Effects of a general exercise program on passive hip, knee, and ankle range of motion of older women," *Topics in Geriatric Rehabilitation*, vol. 10, no. 3, pp. 33–44, 1995.

[28] J. M. Miotto, W. J. Chodzko-Zajko, J. L. Reich, and M. M. Supler, "Reliability and validity of the fullerton functional fitness test: an independent replication study," *Journal of Aging and Physical Activity*, vol. 7, no. 4, pp. 339–353, 1999.

[29] R. Rikli and S. Busch, "Motor performance of women as a function of age and physical activity level," *Journals of Gerontology*, vol. 41, no. 5, pp. 645–649, 1986.

[30] L. E. Voorrips, K. A. P. M. Lemmink, M. J. G. van Heuvelen, P. Bult, and W. A. van Staveren, "The physical condition of elderly women differing in habitual physical activity," *Medicine and Science in Sports and Exercise*, vol. 25, no. 10, pp. 1152–1157, 1993.

[31] C. Lan, S. Chen, and J. Lai, "Changes of aerobic capacity, fat ratio and flexibility in older TCC practitioners: a five-year follow-up," *The American Journal of Chinese Medicine*, vol. 36, no. 6, pp. 1041–1050, 2008.

[32] A. A. Vandervoort, B. M. Chesworth, D. A. Cunningham, D. H. Paterson, P. A. Rechnitzer, and J. J. Koval, "Age and sex effects on mobility of the human ankle," *Journals of Gerontology*, vol. 47, no. 1, pp. M17–M21, 1992.

[33] D. A. Cunningham, D. H. Paterson, J. E. Himann, and P. A. Rechnitzer, "Determinants of independence in the elderly," *Canadian Journal of Applied Physiology*, vol. 18, no. 3, pp. 243–254, 1993.

[34] K. Tainaka, T. Takizawa, S. Katamoto, and J. Aoki, "Six-year prospective study of physical fitness and incidence of disability among community-dwelling Japanese elderly women," *Geriatrics and Gerontology International*, vol. 9, no. 1, pp. 21–28, 2009.

[35] E. M. Badley, S. Wagstaff, and P. H. N. Wood, "Measures of functional ability (disability) in arthritis in relation to impairment of range of joint movement," *Annals of the Rheumatic Diseases*, vol. 43, no. 4, pp. 563–569, 1984.

[36] J. M. Fabre, R. H. Wood, K. E. Cherry et al., "Age-related deterioration in flexibility is associated with health-related quality of life in nonagenarians," *Journal of Geriatric Physical Therapy*, vol. 30, no. 1, pp. 16–22, 2007.

14

Dynamic Associations of Change in Physical Activity and Change in Cognitive Function: Coordinated Analyses of Four Longitudinal Studies

Magnus Lindwall,[1] Cynthia R. Cimino,[2] Laura E. Gibbons,[3] Meghan B. Mitchell,[4] Andreana Benitez,[5] Cassandra L. Brown,[6] Robert F. Kennison,[7] Steven D. Shirk,[4] Alireza Atri,[4] Annie Robitaille,[6] Stuart W. S. MacDonald,[6] Elizabeth M. Zelinski,[8] Sherry L. Willis,[9] K. Warner Schaie,[9] Boo Johansson,[10] Marcus Praetorius,[10] Roger A. Dixon,[11] Dan M. Mungas,[12] Scott M. Hofer,[6] and Andrea M. Piccinin[6]

[1] *Department of Food and Nutrition, and Sport Science and Department of Psychology, University of Gothenburg, P.O. Box 300, 405 30 Gothenburg, Sweden*
[2] *Department of Psychology and Neurology, University of South Florida, 4202 East Fowler Avenue, Tampa, FL 33620, USA*
[3] *General Internal Medicine, Harborview Medical Center, University of Washington, 325 Ninth Avenue, P.O. Box 359780, Seattle, WA 98104, USA*
[4] *Massachusetts General Hospital, Harvard Medical School, ENRM Bedford VA Hospital, 200 Springs Road, Bedford, MA 01730, USA*
[5] *Center for Biomedical Imaging, Medical University of South Carolina, 68 President Sreet, MSC 120, Charleston, SC 29425, USA*
[6] *Department of Psychology, University of Victoria, P.O. Box 3050 STN CSC, Victoria, BC, Canada V8W 3P5*
[7] *Department of Psychology, California State University, Los Angeles, 5151 State University Drive, Los Angeles, CA 90032, USA*
[8] *Andrus Gerontology Center, Leonard Davis School of Gerontology, University of Southern California, Los Angeles, CA 90089, USA*
[9] *Department of Psychiatry and Behavioral Sciences, University of Washington, 180 Nickerson, Suite 206, Seattle, WA 98109, USA*
[10] *Department of Psychology, University of Gothenburg, P.O. Box 100, 405 30 Gothenburg, Sweden*
[11] *Department of Psychology, University of Alberta, Edmonton, AB, Canada T6G 2E9*
[12] *Davis Lawrence J. Ellison Ambulatory Care Center, University of California, 4860 Y Street, Ste 0100, Sacramento, CA 95817, USA*

Correspondence should be addressed to Magnus Lindwall, magnus.lindwall@psy.gu.se and Andrea M. Piccinin, piccinin@uvic.ca

Academic Editor: Alan J. Gow

The present study used a coordinated analyses approach to examine the association of physical activity and cognitive change in four longitudinal studies. A series of multilevel growth models with physical activity included both as a fixed (between-person) and time-varying (within-person) predictor of four domains of cognitive function (reasoning, memory, fluency, and semantic knowledge) was used. Baseline physical activity predicted fluency, reasoning and memory in two studies. However, there was a consistent pattern of positive relationships between time-specific changes in physical activity and time-specific changes in cognition, controlling for expected linear trajectories over time, across all four studies. This pattern was most evident for the domains of reasoning and fluency.

1. Introduction

Previous research has clearly demonstrated that cognitive change in old age does not occur in a homogenous manner for all individuals [1–3]. A number of predictors of cognitive change in old age have been identified, such as education, hypertension, objective indices of health and cardiovascular disease, and apolipoprotein E [4]. Regular engagement in different types of activities may also influence cognitive change. More specifically, according to the "use it or lose t" hypothesis [5], regular engagement in different activities may buffer age-related decline in cognitive functioning. A number of studies have found that general lifestyle activity engagement (often operationalized as the combination of intellectual, social, and physical activities) is associated with cognitive change [6–8] and that decline in activity in older age is associated with decline in cognitive functioning.

In addition to general activity, other studies have specifically targeted the association of physical activity with cognitive change. Indeed, a growing body of the literature highlights the potential benefits of physical activity on the structure and function of the brain [9, 10]. The first line of evidence for the relationship between physical activity and cognition comes from a number of cross-sectional studies demonstrating that physically active older adults have higher cognitive performance and functioning compared with less active older adults [11, 12].

However, the evidence derived from these cross-sectional studies is limited, as it is not. possible to draw conclusions in terms of more complex associations of change. Stronger evidence may be found in longitudinal studies. Longitudinal studies may be viewed as the second line of evidence, offering valuable information on the relationship between physical activity and cognition across time. Several prospective, longitudinal studies provide evidence for the association of physical activity with cognitive functioning [13–20]. These studies have generally shown that higher physical activity at baseline is associated with less decline in cognitive functioning over time, offering support for the notion that regular physical activity may buffer against future cognitive decline. However, results from these longitudinal studies are inconclusive [4] and several critical questions remain [21].

The longitudinal studies described above may test two different classes of hypotheses regarding the relationship of lifestyle variables, such as physical activity and cognitive change [6]. The first type of hypothesis stipulates that the level of physical activity is related to subsequent cognitive change. The majority of the abovementioned studies have targeted this first class of hypothesis, examining a stable change hypothesis by looking at how physical activity at baseline predicts change in cognitive functioning. The second class of hypothesis instead examines the relationship between concomitant change in activity and change in cognition. In contrast to the baseline effect of activity, this hypothesis deals with the concept of intraindividual change and associations among intraindividual rates of change, providing a more dynamic perspective. For example, positive changes (increases) in physical activity across time may be hypothesized to contribute to a less negative change (less decline) in cognitive functioning, whereas a negative change in activity (decreased activity) would be expected to be related to faster cognitive decline with age.

Mackinnon and colleagues [7] used a latent growth curve modeling approach to examine how change in overall activity (defined as a composite of physical activity, rest, interest and hobby related, and planned activities), rather than physical activity, was related to change in health and cognitive performance. They found substantial correlations between rates of change in activity and cognitive and health measures, and it was concluded that decline in mental and physical activity in older age is paralleled by decline in cognitive functioning and health. However, decline in cognitive functioning was still evident for participants who were stable in their level of activity across time, suggesting that maintenance of activity may not be enough to protect from cognitive decline.

Unfortunately, few previous studies have actually targeted the hypothesis of whether there are associations among rates of individual change in physical activity and cognitive functioning in long-term observational studies of aging individuals. Van Gelder and colleagues [17] found that men who decreased their physical activity duration or intensity also demonstrated a stronger decline in overall cognition (measured by the Mini Mental State Examination) compared with men who maintained their activity duration and intensity. However, several limitations should be noted in this study. First, only change in one global measure of cognitive functioning was used, rather than several different measures that may capture more diverse and complex relationships of cognitive ability with activity change. Moreover, in the study, change in physical activity was categorized in terms of quality (change/no change) rather than quantity (how much change). Finally, the analyses were based on between-group comparisons and therefore did not target relationships of within-person changes in physical activity and cognition.

Bielak and colleagues [22], however, used random effects models to examine how level and change in physical activity were related to level (within-person mean) and inconsistency (within person standard deviation across trials) of cognitive speed at baseline and change in level and inconsistency. Although physical activity at baseline was related to mean cognitive speed in some tasks, there were no associations between change in physical activity and change in cognitive speed. Moreover, a recent study [23] using bivariate dual-change-score models to analyze data from the Victoria Longitudinal Study found that changes in physical activity influenced changes in verbal speed and episodic memory. However, they also found that changes in cognition influenced changes in activity, thus supporting a dual-coupling model or a reciprocal relationship between physical activity change and change in cognition.

Although previous longitudinal studies have resulted in increased understanding of how physical activity at one point (baseline) may predict future cognitive performance, or change in cognitive performance, they have generally not helped us understand the more complex and dynamic characteristics of the longitudinal relationship between physical activity and cognition. Relevant questions remain unanswered. For example, is there an association between within-person change in physical activity and within-person changes in cognitive functioning when taking into account the change in cognition due to time? Or, put differently, do persons demonstrate lower cognitive scores (relative to their *within-person* trajectory over time) on occasions when they also report less physical activity? Relative to a cross-sectional analysis that compares individuals to other similar aged individuals, the answers to these questions afford relevant insight into the more complex and dynamic patterns of associations between changes in physical activity and cognitive functioning within individuals across time. Another question that has not been properly addressed by previous longitudinal studies is if physical activity, or change in activity, has similar effects across different cognitive domains and/or tests. From previous experimental work using randomized controlled trial designs, there is support for the notion that physical activity training has the strongest effect on executive control processes and working memory, supporting the "selective-improvement hypothesis" [24]. However, as the majority of previous longitudinal studies of the relations between physical activity and cognition have included a single measure of cognition (often MMSE) rather than different tests and domains, the theoretically, as well as practically, important question of whether changes in physical activity may relate more strongly to changes in some cognitive domains relative to others remains unresolved.

An essential step for the sound cumulative development of this body of knowledge is the reproduction and extension of research findings across independent longitudinal studies that focus on observed within-person change [25]. Although most previous longitudinal studies have found that physical activity is protective against age-related cognitive decline, the findings are disparate and far from clear [21]. Moreover, previous studies have typically used data from one population (e.g., adults ranged from 55–94 in age) and one design (e.g., 3 waves of measurements over a 6-year period), leaving the generalization of the results highly contingent on sample specific-characteristics. Differences between studies in terms of sample, design, measures, and analytical approach make it difficult to compare results across studies and to derive more general conclusions of the meaning of these results. Therefore, there is a clear need for more coordinated integrative data analyses that use data from different samples with different measures, but examine these data with the same research question and the same analytic approach [25]. Using a coordinated analysis approach for cross-study comparisons and synthesis of independent results has the potential to bring new relevant information to the field of cognitive change and physical activity [26].

The purpose of the present study is to investigate the longitudinal associations of physical activity with four domains of cognition (i.e., reasoning (executive function), episodic memory, fluency, and semantic knowledge) in older adults using a coordinated approach with data from four independent longitudinal studies: Long Beach Longitudinal Study (LBLS), the Seattle Longitudinal Study (SLS), the Victoria Longitudinal Study (VLS), and the Origins of Variance in the Oldest-Old: Octogenarian Twins Study (OCTO-Twin). More specifically, the following research questions were examined:

(i) Is physical activity at baseline associated with cognition at baseline?

(ii) Is baseline physical activity associated with the rate of change in cognition?

(iii) Are occasion-specific changes in physical activity associated with occasion-specific changes in cognition, controlling for change in cognition due to time alone?

2. Methods

2.1. Design and General Analytical Framework. This research, initiated as a partnership between the Advanced Psychometric Methods Workshop series (Mungas et al., NIA conference grant) and the Integrative Analysis of Longitudinal Studies on Aging (IALSA) network [25, 26], brought workshop participants together with researchers from four IALSA member studies. These studies were specifically selected based on their collection of cognitive, physical, and social activity data along with a range of cognitive functioning measures over multiple occasions held in common across the four studies. While the activity and cognitive functioning variables are not always identical, the subsets of variables in each study were chosen based on the rationale that they tapped similar domains at the construct level (e.g., fluid reasoning (Gf), crystallized knowledge (Gc), short-term memory (Gsm,) and long-term storage and retrieval (Glr; category fluency) [27]. In some cases the measures are the same, but more often they differ, providing opportunities for both strict and conceptual replication.

2.2. OCTO-Twin (Origins of Variance of the Oldest-Old) Sample (Sweden). The OCTO-Twin study is comprised of the oldest-cohort of the Swedish Twin Registry aged 80 and older at the time of first examination. Beginning in 1991–93, the longitudinal design included a maximum of five measurement occasions at 2-year intervals. Individuals with a dementia diagnosis at baseline ($n = 98$) were excluded from the initial sample of 702 participants. The remaining 604 individuals were included in analyses. Approximately 20% of the sample was lost to follow up at each wave (10% per year), but most of this attrition was due to death. Descriptive statistics are provided in Table 1.

2.3. OCTO-Twin Materials and Procedures

2.3.1. OCTO-Twin Cognitive Ability Measures. Reasoning was assessed using Block Design [28]. In this task, participants were presented with red and white blocks and instructed to reproduce the design shown on a card using these blocks within a predetermined time limit. *Fluency* was not assessed in the OCTO-Twin Study. *Memory* was assessed using immediate recall of the Prose Recall test, in which participants were presented with a brief, 100-word story that had a humorous element [29]. Amount of information recalled was coded in a manner similar to the scoring of story units in the Wechsler Memory Scale Logical Memory test [30]. *Semantic knowledge* was assessed using the Swedish version of the Information Task, in which participants provided responses to factual knowledge questions [31]. Raw scores were transformed into T-scores with a mean of 50

TABLE 1: OCTO-Twin participant characteristics.

Measure	Baseline (N = 574)	Year 2 (N = 471)	Year 4 (N = 363)	Year 6 (N = 275)	Year 8 (N = 201)
	Year of testing				
	M (SD)	M (SD)	M (SD)	M (SD)	M (SD)
Retention from previous testing (%)		82.0	77.1	75.8	73.1
Age	83.3 (3.0)	85.2 (2.8)	86.9 (2.5)	88.8 (2.5)	90.7 (2.4)
Education	7.3 (2.4)	7.3 (2.3)	7.3 (2.3)	7.2 (2.1)	7.2 (2.2)
Sex, female (n (%))	371 (65)	346 (65)	236 (65)	196 (71)	148 (74)
Reasoning	11.5 (7.1)	11.4 (7.2)	11.3 (7.1)	10.8 (7.2)	10.0 (7.3)
Memory	9.6 (4.0)	9.4 (4.3)	9.2 (4.4)	9.2 (4.7)	8.9 (4.5)
Semantic knowledge	28.1 (11.2)	28.6 (11.2)	27.5 (12.4)	26.7 (13.0)	26.1 (11.4)
Physical activity	0.7 (0.7)	0.9 (0.7)	0.8 (0.7)	0.7 (0.7)	0.6 (0.6)
Physical activity change[a]		0.1 (0.7)	−0.0 (0.8)	−0.1 (0.8)	−0.3 (0.9)

M: mean, SD: standard deviation. The scoring ranges for each measure with a defined upper limit are as follows: reasoning: 0–42; memory: 0–16; semantic knowledge: 0–44; physical activity: 0–2. [a]Physical activity change represents change from baseline.

and standard deviation of 10 to facilitate comparisons across measures.

2.3.2. OCTO-Twin Physical Activity Measure. Respondents were asked, at each of the five waves, the following: "*Are you presently doing or have you previously done anything special to train your body or keep your body fit?*" The possible responses were "no" (0), "yes, to some extent" (1), or "yes, to a great extent" (2). Hence, a scale from 0 to 2 was used. The participants gave one reply for their present physical activity status and one in regards to their previous status. Only the answer for the present status was used in the analyses. Physical activity change scores were computed by subtracting baseline activity from each follow-up activity measure.

2.4. Long Beach Longitudinal Study Sample (California, USA). The LBLS was initiated in 1978 when participants were recruited from the Family Health Plan Health Maintenance Organization (HMO), mainly including residents of Long Beach and Orange County. This first panel included 583 individuals aged 28–36 or 55–87. The ethnic composition of the older group (98% Caucasian) was similar to the 65+ population for the area based on the 1970 census. Panel 2, initiated in 1992, included 633 individuals from the same HMO (64 were excluded due to frank dementia or serious sensory or neurological problems).

In order to include the same measures as those in the Seattle Longitudinal Study, LBLS Panel 1 (n = 106) and Panel 2 (n = 631) data from 1994 to 2003, excluding participants younger than age 55 in 1994 (n = 541), were used in the current analysis. During this period, data were collected at 3-year intervals. Attrition was approximately 50% over each interval or 17% per year. Dementia incidence is not known. Descriptive information for the sample is presented in Table 2.

2.5. LBLS Materials and Procedures

2.5.1. LBLS Cognitive Ability Measures. *Reasoning* was based on a composite score of the Letter and Number Series tests from the Schaie-Thurstone Adult Mental Abilities Test (STAMAT; [32]. In this task, participants viewed a series of letters (e.g., a b c c b a d e f f) and were asked to identify the next letter in the series from alternate choices by extracting the rule that governed the series. Responses were made by choosing the correct alternative from an array of possible alternatives. Participants were given six minutes to complete as many of the 30 items as possible. *Fluency* was assessed using Word Fluency, in which participants wrote down as many words as possible that begin with the letter "s" during a five-minute period according to predetermined rules. These rules included no proper names and no addition of endings to words that the participant had already provided (e.g., "sit," "sitting," and "sits"). *Memory* was measured using immediate written recall of a 20-item noun list that participants had studied for 3.5 minutes. *Semantic knowledge* was assessed using the STAMAT Recognition Vocabulary test. Participants were provided with 50 target words and asked to select the synonym from four choice alternatives. Performance was based on total correct responses provided in a five-minute period.

2.5.2. LBLS Physical Activity Measure. The physical activity measure was based on selected questions from the Life Complexity Scale. A composite score was created by summing the number of physical activities (e.g., walking, outdoor hobbies, etc.) that included one or more hours of these activities per week. The range of possible scores was from 0 to 4. Activity change variables were computed by subtracting the activity measure in 1994 from activity in 1994, 1997, 2000, and 2003. This resulted in difference scores that were referent to the baseline testing in 1994.

2.6. Seattle Longitudinal Study Sample (Washington, USA). The SLS is a long-running longitudinal study initiated by K. Warner Schaie, who first recruited members of a local Health Maintenance Organization in 1956. Current analyses used up to four waves of SLS data from 1984–2005, which include an expanded set of measures that also overlapped with the Long Beach Study. Only participants 55 years and

Table 2: LBLS participant characteristics.

Measure	Year of testing			
	Baseline (N = 541)	Year 3 (N = 275)	Year 6 (N = 140)	Year 9 (N = 94)
	M (SD)	M (SD)	M (SD)	M (SD)
Retention from previous testing (%)		50.8	50.9	67.1
Age	73.6 (9.0)	75.1 (8.5)	75.1 (8.0)	75.9 (7.1)
Education	13.8 (3.0)	13.9 (2.9)	14.3 (2.7)	14.2 (2.7)
Sex, female (n (%))	258 (51)	137 (50)	71 (51)	45 (48)
Reasoning	22.5 (11.7)	24.1 (11.4)	25.4 (11.5)	25.3 (10.7)
Fluency	32.7 (11.4)	33.7 (11.2)	33.6 (12.9)	34.5 (11.8)
Memory	11.4 (4.0)	11.7 (4.3)	11.5 (4.5)	11.2 (4.8)
Semantic knowledge	38.7 (10.1)	39.6 (9.6)	40.6 (8.8)	39.7 (9.9)
Physical activity	1.7 (1.0)	1.6 (1.1)	1.5 (1.0)	1.6 (0.9)
Physical activity change	0.0 (0.0)	−0.2 (1.0)	−0.4 (1.0)	−0.4 (1.1)

M: mean, SD: standard deviation. The scoring ranges for each measure with a defined upper limit are as follows: education: 0–20, reasoning: 0–30, memory: 0–20, vocabulary: 0–36, physical activity: 0–4.

older at baseline were included in the analysis. Baseline was defined as each participant's first study visit, and time was measured in all analyses as years in study (coded as 0, 7, 14, and 21). Attrition during these 7-year intervals was approximately 50% or 7% per year. Dementia prevalence and incidence are not known. See Table 3 for SLS participant characteristics over the four waves of data analyzed here.

2.7. SLS Materials and Procedures

2.7.1. SLS Cognitive Measures. *Reasoning* was assessed with the Word Series test from the Schaie-Thurstone Adult Mental Abilities Test (STAMAT; [32]). In this task, participants were provided with a printed word series that was ordered according to an inherent rule. The participant's task was to select, from multiple-choice options, the next word in the series consistent with that rule. Total score was based on number of correct responses to the 30 trials completed in 6 minutes. As in LBLS, *Fluency* was indexed by performance on the Word Fluency Test from the Primary Mental Abilities test [33] and *Memory* by the verbal list-learning task. *Semantic knowledge* was assessed with the test of Advanced Vocabulary from the Educational Testing Service (ETS), in which participants identified synonyms for printed words from five choices [34]. The total score was derived from the number of correct responses provided within 4 minutes to the 36-itemtest.

2.7.2. SLS Physical Activity Measure. The methodology described in the LBLS method portion of this paper was used in order to generate roughly equivalent indices of physical activity. Following this methodology, a composite physical activity measure was created by summing dichotomized test responses from a modified version of the Life Complexity Scale [3], resulting in a four-item physical activity composite (playing sports, walking, fitness, and outdoor hobbies). *Activity change* was computed by subtracting baseline activity from each follow-up activity measure.

2.8. Victoria Longitudinal Study Sample (British Columbia, Canada). The Victoria Longitudinal Study began in 1986–87 with a sample of 484 community residing volunteers. Using a longitudinal sequential design, second and third independent samples began in 1992-93 (n = 530) and 2001-2002 (n = 550) [35]. Each sample is tested at three-year intervals. To date, Sample 1 has been tested on seven occasions (over 18 years), Sample 2 on five (over 12 years), and Sample 3 on two occasions (over 6 years). Participants in all three samples were recruited between the ages of 55 and 85 years.

Data from seven waves of Sample 1 and five waves of Sample 2 were included in the current investigation. Characteristics of the subsample analyzed here are provided in Table 4. Approximately 20% of the sample was lost to follow up at each wave, or 10% per year. Dementia prevalence and incidence are not known.

2.9. VLS Materials and Procedures

2.9.1. VLS Cognitive Ability Measures. *Reasoning* was indexed by Letter Series [33]. In this task, participants were presented with a series of letters and asked to identify the next letter in the sequence based on the rule that governed the sequence. *Fluency* was measured by performance on a Similarities task [34], in which participants were presented with target words and asked to write as many words as possible with the same or nearly the same meaning during a 6-minute period. *Memory* was indexed based on free recall of a 30-item noun list comprised of five semantic categories. Participants were given two minutes to study the words and then five minutes to recall them [35]. *Semantic knowledge* was assessed using a 54-item recognition vocabulary test adapted from the ETS Kit of Factor Referenced Tests [34].

2.9.2. VLS Physical Activity Measure. The physical activity measure was derived from a subset of four items from the VLS- Activity Lifestyle Questionnaire (VLS-ALQ; [6]). These items indexed the physical activities of gardening, jogging,

TABLE 3: SLS participant characteristics.

Measure	Year of testing			
	Baseline (N = 1658) M (SD)	Year 7 (N = 940) M (SD)	Year 14 (N = 447) M (SD)	Year 21 (N = 181) M (SD)
Retention from previous testing (%)		56.7	47.6	40.5
Age	67.1 (8.2)	73.0 (7.3)	78.9 (6.4)	81.9 (4.9)
Education	14.6 (2.9)	14.7 (2.8)	14.8 (2.7)	14.8 (2.8)
Sex, female (n (%))	862 (52)	507 (54)	257 (57)	108 (60)
Reasoning	15.6 (5.8)	15.2 (5.6)	14.3 (5.5)	14.0 (5.3)
Fluency	38.5 (12.8)	37.5 (13.1)	36.7 (12.7)	38.8 (14.5)
Memory	12.5 (4.0)	12.0 (4.1)	11.5 (4.2)	11.7 (3.9)
Semantic knowledge	25.0 (6.7)	25.3 (6.6)	25.8 (6.2)	25.8 (5.9)
Physical activity	1.0 (1.1)	1.8 (1.1)	1.7 (1.0)	1.6 (0.9)
Physical activity Change	—	−0.1 (1.1)	−0.2 (1.1)	−0.0 (1.1)

M: mean, SD: standard deviation. The scoring ranges for each measure with a defined upper limit are as follows: education: 0–20, reasoning: 0–30, memory: 0–20, vocabulary: 0–36, physical activity: 0–4.

TABLE 4: VLS participant characteristics.

Measure	Year of testing						
	Baseline (N = 977) M (SD)	Year 3 (N = 723) M (SD)	Year 6 (N = 571) M (SD)	Year 9 (N = 412) M (SD)	Year 12 (N = 282) M (SD)	Year 15 (N = 91) M (SD)	Year 18 (N = 52) M (SD)
Retention from Previous testing (%)[a]	—	74	79	72	68	75	57
Age	68.6 (6.7)	71.3 (6.6)	73.7 (6.4)	76.5 (5.9)	79.3 (5.2)	82.2 (4.6)	85.1 (3.6)
Years of education at baseline	14.9 (3.3)	15.4 (3.2)	15.6 (3.1)	15.8 (3.1)	15.9 (3.1)	15.2 (3.1)	14.8 (2.8)
Sex, female (n (%))	614 (63)	450 (62)	348 (61)	252 (61)	177 (63)	60 (66)	35 (67)
Reasoning[b]	11.2 (4.5)	11.7 (4.2)	10.4 (4.7)	10.4 (4.6)	9.9 (4.6)	7.5 (4.7)	6.5 (4.2)
Fluency	17.7 (4.3)	17.9 (4.4)	17.8 (4.4)	17.2 (4.8)	16.3 (4.9)	14.7 (5.8)	13.8 (5.4)
Memory[c]	13.7 (5.9)	14.6 (6.0)	14.7 (6.2)	14.9 (6.4)	11.8 (5.5)	13.0 (6.3)	—
Semantic knowledge	43.7 (7.4)	44.7 (6.2)	44.3 (6.0)	44.2 (5.8)	43.5 (5.7)	42.7 (7.1)	42.6 (6.6)
Physical activity	15.4 (5.1)	15.4 (5.1)	15.0 (4.9)	14.8 (5.2)	13.4 (5.1)	14.0 (5.2)	12.3 (5.0)
Physical activity change	0.0 (0.0)	−0.1 (4.0)	−0.8 (4.2)	−1.3 (4.6)	−2.8 (4.8)	−2.7 (5.0)	−4.4 (5.2)

M: mean, SD: standard deviation. The scoring range for each measure with a defined upper limit are as follows: Reasoning 0–20, Fluency 0-maximum number of words produced in 6 minutes, Memory 0–30, Vocabulary 0–54. Physical Activity 0–36. The physical activity change scores are on a normal metric with means of approximately 0 and SD of approximately 0.8.
[a]The 1986 cohort was followed for up to 18 years, the 1993 cohort for up to 12.
[b]The reasoning measure was not given until year 6 for the 1986 cohort.
[c]The memory measure was not given in year 18.

sailing, and tennis. For each item, participants indicated the frequency of engagement in that activity over the past two years on a scale from 0 to 9 (i.e., *never, less than once a year, about once a year, 2 or 3 times a year, about once a month, 2 or 3 times a month, about once a week, 2 or 3 times a week, and daily*).

2.10. Analytic Approach. In order to examine the effects of physical activity on cognition, a series of multilevel models was fit with time varying covariates [36] using multilevel mixed-effects regression in Stata (StataCorp, 2011), the restricted maximum likelihood estimator (REML), and an unstructured covariance matrix. Separate models were fit for each of the four cognitive measures (reasoning, fluency (except OCTO-Twin), memory, and semantic knowledge) and for each of the four studies. In order to improve ease of interpretation of our results, age, education, and activity measures were mean centered to the baseline mean of each measure in the sample so that the intercept and linear slope terms could be interpreted as the expected value for an individual at the mean age, education, and respective activity level at baseline. The reference category for sex was male. OCTO-Twin participants were modeled as nested within their twin pair and in VLS we controlled for enrolment cohort.

Our goal was to build a common model for comparisons across all outcomes for the four longitudinal studies. This common model was not necessarily the optimal model for each of the 16 cognition-physical activity combinations. An initial 19-term model included all ten two-way interactions that included activity, change in activity or time, and three 3-way interactions of time and activity with age, sex, or education. However, several terms were not significant for most of the studies and outcomes and so were trimmed to facilitate model interpretation. First, the 3-way interactions were eliminated, then the interactions with change in activity. Last, the baseline activity by sex interaction was dropped. This resulted in a final model that included 12 terms summarized in Table 5 for separate cognitive constructs of reasoning, memory, semantic knowledge, and fluency. Our significance criterion of $P < 0.05$ shaped the "familywise" alpha rate within each study, however our focus was on the repetition of results across studies, which we used to minimize the potential impact of chance associations. We did not implement formal meta-analytic techniques as they require identical measures and a larger number of studies.

3. Results

3.1. Baseline Covariates and Longitudinal Relationships. Between-person age differences are seen at the first occasion of measurement for all memory, reasoning, and fluency tests, with older adults performing less well. Semantic knowledge results are less consistent, with older adults performing less well in LBLS and OCTO-Twin, but better in VLS. At baseline, individuals with more years of education had higher cognitive performance. LBLS and SLS women scored higher than men of the same age on all measures, except for semantic knowledge. OCTO-Twin and VLS women had higher memory scores than did the men. OCTO-Twin women had lower scores on semantic knowledge.

For the reference individuals (men with sample average baseline age and years of education), within-person declines were seen over time in all cognitive abilities and all samples except SLS (the youngest), where the relationship, as in LBLS and VLS, depended on age. Older individuals declined faster on all VLS, SLS, and LBLS measures except LBLS immediate memory. No clear pattern was identified in regards to differential decline related to sex or education.

3.2. Physical Activity. Higher physical activity at baseline was associated with higher scores on reasoning and memory in OCTO-Twin and VLS and fluency in SLS. The association between physical activity score at baseline and cognitive score did not differ by age. However, there was some indication that the relation between physical activity and cognition differed by education. For semantic knowledge in LBLS and SLS the association with physical activity at baseline was stronger for people with less education. In terms of associations with cognitive decline, higher physical activity score at baseline was related only to less decline on fluency in VLS and SLS.

However, we found a consistent pattern of positive relationships between time-specific changes in physical activity and time-specific changes in cognition beyond those expected by the estimated linear trajectories in the four studies. This pattern was most evident for the domains of reasoning and fluency. More specifically, after controlling for the trend in cognitive functioning over time, time-specific changes in physical activity change were related to cognitive fluctuations in the following cognitive domains: (a) reasoning in all four studies; (b) fluency in two (VLS and SLS) of three studies; (c) memory in two studies (OCTO-Twin and VLS); (d) semantic knowledge in one study (OCTO-Twin).

4. Discussion

Using data from four longitudinal studies of aging, the present study examined the relationship between physical activity and cognitive functioning at three different levels: (a) cross-sectionally; (b) longitudinally using physical activity as predictor of cognitive change; (c) longitudinally using change in physical activity as a time-varying covariate to predict change in cognition, adjusting for the normative development (effect of time) in cognition. On the cross-sectional level, higher physical activity at baseline was associated primarily with higher scores on reasoning and fluency, generally supporting previous studies demonstrating that physically active older adults have higher cognitive performance and functioning compared with less active older adults [11, 12]. Although relevant, these well-known and well-documented findings contribute little to a deeper understanding of the likely very complex relationship between activity and cognition.

The second level of analysis addressed more theoretically relevant and interesting longitudinal associations and the question of whether physical activity at baseline is associated with cognitive change. From a broader perspective, this research question is also linked to the "use it or lose it" hypothesis [5, 21], generally proposing that physical activity may buffer against future cognitive decline. A number of prospective studies have found support for this notion [13–20], offering preliminary support for the longitudinally beneficial and buffering effect of physical activity on cognitive decline. A general limitation in many of these previous prospective studies, however, is that they have examined the association between physical activity and a broad global measure of cognition (typically MMSE), thereby proving an incomplete picture of the potentially diverse longitudinal associations between different cognitive domains and physical activity. As a consequence, these previous studies generally have not answered the theoretically and practically relevant question "what cognitive domains most benefit from physical activity?" [21].

In the present study four different domains were examined, representing a broader spectrum of cognitive abilities,

TABLE 5: Mixed effects model summaries across four studies with baseline physical activity and activity change predicting four cognitive outcomes.

	OCTO-Twin			LBLS			SLS			VLS		
	b	SE	*P*	*b*	SE	*P*	*b*	SE	*P*	*b*	SE	*P*
Reasoning												
Intercept	10.66	0.56	<.001	21.53	0.56	<.001	37.88	1.02	<.001	9.53	0.59	<.001
Age	–0.37	0.12	0.002	–0.62	0.05	<.001	–0.35	0.01	<.001	–0.25	0.02	<.001
Sex	0.90	0.68	0.186	2.12	0.81	0.009	1.67	0.24	<.001	–0.01	0.31	0.969
Education	0.57	0.13	<.001	1.30	0.14	<.001	0.52	0.04	<.001	0.33	0.05	<.001
Activity	1.19	0.40	0.003	–0.50	0.40	0.209	–0.57	0.89	0.519	0.01	0.03	0.827
Age × activity	0.06	0.14	0.699	0.03	0.04	0.502	0.01	0.01	0.398	0.00	0.00	0.587
Education × activity	–0.09	0.13	0.479	–0.12	0.14	0.372	0.00	0.04	0.983	0.00	0.01	0.840
Time	–0.51	0.09	<.001	–0.46	0.09	<.001	0.15	0.10	0.141	–0.24	0.03	<.001
Age × time	–0.02	0.02	0.296	–0.02	0.01	0.001	–0.01	0.00	<.001	–0.01	0.00	<.001
Sex × time	0.13	0.10	0.206	0.09	0.11	0.445	0.02	0.03	0.318	0.00	0.03	0.968
Education × time	0.02	0.02	0.258	–0.06	0.02	0.007	–0.01	0.00	0.090	–0.01	0.00	0.065
Activity × time	0.06	0.07	0.354	0.04	0.06	0.506	0.01	0.01	0.183	0.00	0.00	0.332
Activity change	0.85	0.21	<.001	0.54	0.24	0.028	0.18	0.09	0.045	0.05	0.02	0.013
Fluency												
Intercept				31.19	0.62	<.001	58.66	2.55	<.001	11.73	0.56	<.001
Age				–0.25	0.05	<.001	–0.34	0.04	<.001	–0.10	0.03	<.001
Sex				4.25	0.90	<.001	3.54	0.59	<.001	0.46	0.36	0.200
Education				1.04	0.16	<.001	1.29	0.11	<.001	0.64	0.05	<.001
Activity				0.45	0.45	0.314	4.45	22.4	0.047	–0.06	0.03	0.098
Age × activity				0.07	0.05	0.159	–0.06	0.03	0.070	0.00	0.00	0.952
Education × activity				–0.29	0.15	0.059	–0.02	0.09	0.844	–0.01	0.01	0.159
Time				–0.27	0.11	0.013	0.78	0.23	0.001	–0.13	0.03	<.001
Age × Time				–0.03	0.01	0.001	–0.02	0.00	<.001	–0.01	0.00	0.002
Sex × Time				–0.22	0.15	0.132	0.13	0.05	0.007	0.07	0.04	0.070
Education × Time				0.00	0.03	0.983	–0.01	0.01	0.106	0.00	0.01	0.950
Activity × Time				0.03	0.08	0.680	0.05	0.02	0.048	0.01	0.00	0.045
Activity Change				0.05	0.35	0.894	0.41	0.20	0.043	0/07	0.03	0.003
Memory												
Intercept	8.59	0.31	<.001	10.78	0.20	<.001	23.50	0.74	<.001	17.36	0.42	<.001
Age	–0.22	0.06	<.001	–0.19	0.02	<.001	–0.18	0.01	<.001	–0.19	0.02	<.001
Sex	1.14	0.38	<.002	1.55	0.30	<.001	1.65	0.17	<.001	1.65	0.27	<.001
Education	0.39	0.07	<.001	0.29	0.05	<.001	0.32	0.03	<.001	0.32	0.04	<.001
Activity	0.48	0.22	0.003	0.15	0.15	0.312	–0.17	0.65	0.789	0.05	0.03	0.042
Age × Activity	–0.09	0.08	0.232	0.00	0.02	0.817	0.00	0.01	0.671	0.00	0.00	0.223
Education × Activity	0.02	0.07	0.837	–0.05	0.05	0.346	–0.03	0.03	0.215	0.00	0.01	0.607
Time	–0.32	0.07	0.001	–0.17	0.05	0.001	0.33	0.08	<.001	–0.27	0.03	<.001
Age × Time	–0.01	0.01	0.700	0.00	0.00	0.578	–0.01	0.00	<.001	–0.01	0.00	<.001
Sex × Time	0.08	0.08	0.319	–0.04	0.07	0.601	0.03	0.02	0.077	–0.02	0.03	0.469
Education × Time	0.01	0.02	0.972	0.01	0.01	0.379	0.00	0.00	0.449	–0.01	0.00	0.232
Activity × Time	–0.02	0.05	0.660	–0.02	0.04	0.531	0.02	0.01	0.078	0.00	0.00	0.202
Activity Change	0.44	0.15	0.004	–0.08	0.15	0.593	0.08	0.08	0.309	0.06	0.02	0.001
Semantic knowledge												
Intercept	30.21	0.85	<.001	38.36	0.56	<.001	23.41	1.29	<.001	43.86	0.71	<.001
Age	–0.60	0.17	<.001	–0.26	0.05	<.001	0.01	0.02	0.531	0.08	0.03	0.013
Sex	–3.88	1.04	<.001	1.47	0.81	0.069	0.56	0.30	0.069	0.02	0.47	0.971
Education	1.60	0.21	<.001	1.11	0.14	<.001	1.11	0.05	<.001	0.77	0.07	<.001
Activity	0.85	0.57	0.134	–0.54	0.40	0.174	1.61	1.14	–0.160	–0.02	0.04	0.716
Age × Activity	0.02	0.20	0.914	–0.02	0.04	0.672	–0.02	0.02	0.174	0.01	0.01	0.331
Education × Activity	–0.22	0.21	0.307	–0.31	0.14	0.023	–0.11	0.05	0.020	–0.01	0.01	0.588
Time	–0.93	0.12	<.001	–0.44	0.09	<.001	0.45	0.08	<.001	–0.14	0.03	<.001

Table 5: Continued.

	OCTO-Twin			LBLS			SLS			VLS		
	b	SE	*P*	*b*	SE	*P*	*b*	SE	*P*	*b*	SE	*P*
Age × Time	−0.05	0.03	0.056	−0.04	0.01	<.001	−0.01	0.00	<.001	−0.01	0.00	<.001
Sex × Time	0.27	0.14	0.054	0.08	0.12	0.486	0.07	0.02	<.001	0.01	0.04	0.736
Education × Time	0.03	0.03	0.279	−0.03	0.02	0.134	0.00	0.00	0.792	−0.01	0.01	0.152
Activity × Time	−0.02	0.09	0.804	0.10	0.07	0.147	0.01	0.01	0.087	0.00	0.00	0.319
Activity Change	1.06	0.26	<.001	−0.04	0.25	0.881	0.11	0.08	0.148	0.02	0.02	0.258

Values represent model coefficients and their standard error. Across all studies, time was measured in years since baseline visit, and activity change was entered as a time-varying covariate. All other variables represent baseline measurements alone, in interaction with one another, or in interaction with time.

ranging from the more crystallized knowledge-based domain of semantic knowledge to more fluid or process-based factors of reasoning, fluency, and memory. Higher baseline physical activity was associated with less fluency decline in two of three studies. Thus, the preliminary answer to the question what cognitive domain benefits most from physical activity, based on the results of the present study, is fluency, which is one of the more process-based/fluid domains. However, it should be mentioned that for most cognitive domains across the four studies, we did not find support for the protective effect of baseline levels of physical activity on cognitive decline.

Aside from the more stationary change relationships typically investigated in previous studies (how level of physical activity at baseline relates to change in cognition), we also targeted more dynamic associations between changes in physical activity and changes in cognitive functioning by using change in physical activity from baseline as a time-varying covariate in longitudinal multilevel models. The time-varying covariate model used in this study examined occasion-specific intraindividual relations between physical activity and cognition, after controlling for individual rates of change over time. Such time-specific associations between fluctuations in activity and cognition have rarely been examined and may be highly relevant to understanding how to prescribe exercise and how to design and implement interventions including physical activity to optimize effects on cognition [37]. As associations of change and time-specific fluctuations are of key importance in the analyses and interpretation of intervention studies, the results of studies like the present one may offer new relevant information both from a scientific as well as from an applied perspective.

The results from these analyses were surprisingly consistent across studies and domains. Variation in physical activity was associated with variation in reasoning in all four studies and in fluency in two of three studies. Hence, although evidence for the association of between-person differences in baseline physical activity with subsequent cognitive change was generally weak across domains, aside from fluency, support for the notion that change in physical activity covaries with fluctuations in cognition is much more robust across studies. These results are inline with previous work [16], indicating that physical activity may specifically moderate the decline in cognitive domains that is typically associated with aging. Moreover, from a broader perspective, the stronger associations across time of physical activity with more fluid cognition may be linked to the hypothesis that exercise and aerobic fitness training results in selective improvement in executive control processes and working memory [24]. Although the cognitive tests used in the present study to measure reasoning and fluency were derived from a psychometric tradition of psychological testing and do not map well onto more recent conceptualizations of executive processing, they do share some of these features, being a more fluid measure of cognition.

An obvious limitation of the current study is the observational nature of the longitudinal designs, making inferences in terms of cause and effect irresolvable. The notion that decline in cognition leads to decline in physical activity is equal in validity to the interpretation that a decline in physical activity leads to a decline in cognition, that the relationship is reciprocal, or that both are a result of some third variable. Recent studies provide evidence for not only the reciprocal relationship across time between physical activity and mental health in older adults [38], but also for the reciprocal relationship between physical activity and cognition [23].

Another limitation is the problem associated with using different tests in different studies to tap the same cognitive domains. As noted earlier, the studies were selected because they shared similar measures of activity and cognition. Moreover, single cognitive tests are always imperfect markers of a cognitive domain. Therefore, a general feature of the integrated analytical approach in the present study, where data and tests from four different studies are used to answer the same research question, is the risk of heterogeneity in terms of how well the different tests indicate the higher order construct they should measure. As a result, when patterns of results are not consistent across studies, additional questions, testable in future research, are raised with respect to the source of these differences. It is, for example, interesting to note that for OCTO-Twin, in which physical activity was operationalized as the extent to which persons saw themselves as purposefully "keeping their body fit," baseline activity was associated with cognitive functions more consistently than were the physical activity measures in the other studies. The apparent importance of physical activity, however, may also be due to the more advanced age of this sample. In situations where the studies with identical measures agree with each other, but not the remaining studies, for example, where neither SLS nor LBLS shows associations between memory performance and either baseline or change in activity, but OCTO-Twin and VLS do, we may draw conclusions that something about the measurement is important. In contrast, LBLS and SLS fluency results do not agree, suggesting instead that some detail relevant to the sampling, retest interval, or other study characteristic may be relevant.

On the other hand, when patterns of results do show consistency across studies that have used different measures to tap the same underlying construct, such as the association of change in activity with change in reasoning and fluency, these differences become a major strength, as the reliability of the conclusions drawn is considerably strengthened compared with traditional analysis of a single dataset.

Moreover, in contrast with the more specific measurement of cognition, the physical activity variables used in the current analyses were broad and self-reported and did not differentiate aerobic from strength or resistance training. Combining objective measures of physical activity with more specific multi-item, self-report instruments would likely provide future studies with a more robust base for the analysis of the association of change in activity with change in cognition.

The dynamic associations between physical activity and cognitive functioning underscore the broader question of associations between biological and cognitive aging [39]. Also, the effect of intraindividual change in physical activity on cognitive functioning (adjusting for the trend in cognition) raises the question of what drives, or causes, these relationships across time? These dynamic associations with the more fluid cognitive domains may be mediated, or explained, by a number of factors [40], such as physical resources (sleep, energy/fatigue, appetite, pain, or drug/medication use), disease states (hypertension, diabetes, and CVD), and mental resources (chronic stress, depression, and self-efficacy). More specifically, a number of physiological mediators, such as aerobic fitness, hormones, lipid profiles, cerebral blood flow, blood pressure, neurotransmitters, and neurotrophins have all been identified as potential mediators in physical activity-cognition relationships [41]. Although intuitively appealing and quite frequently investigated, the hypothesis of physical activity leading to improved cognition via increased aerobic fitness (the cardiovascular fitness hypothesis) is not, however, supported by meta-analyses [24, 42]. Thus, although single mediation models are theoretically attractive, and may fit data to some extent, the more complete pathways explaining why physical activity and cognition seem to change together more likely include multiple mediators and complex micromediational chains [41], that also may vary in strength and validity across individuals and groups. Nevertheless, increasing knowledge about what precise mechanisms are active ingredients in the effects of physical activity on cognition constitutes a vital step towards the development of appropriate physical activity intervention designs to test these specific models of mediation and the effects of physical activity and exercise on cognition in experimentally controlled trials.

The major strength of the present study is the ability to elucidate consistent patterns of complex associations across time through coordinated analyses of data from four longitudinal studies. Contrary to previous research based on analyses of single samples, which are limited by the specific characteristics of the sample and data, we instead used a coordinated and integrated analytical approach and framework [25, 26] to examine the same research question in data from four longitudinal studies, thereby making the conclusions less vulnerable to study specific characteristics. As such, the present study is unique (in particular considering the choice of analytical approach) and may pave the way for similar collaborative projects where the same research question and analytical approaches are used to answer relevant questions simultaneously across different studies linked to the association of lifestyle, physical activity, and cognitive functioning.

The four studies included afford considerable heterogeneity in terms of age (ranging from mean age of 67 in SLS to 83 in OCTO-Twin), number of available waves of measurement (four in SLS and LBLS to seven in VLS), years of followup (8 years in OCTO-Twin to 21 years in SLS), years between measurements (every 2 years in OCTO-Twin to every 7 year in SLS), and cultural background (Scandinavia to North-America). Yet, as discussed above, a surprisingly clear pattern emerged across studies in the relation of change in activity to fluctuations in cognition. Thus, in terms of capacity to identify patterns of associations from a larger and broader perspective and to be able to generalize results and conclusions, the present study brings reproduced evidence to the field as well as to practitioners working with health related behavior, lifestyle, and cognition in elderly. Based on the results in the present study, the main message is that change in activity, and not only previous or current level of activity, seems to matter and may play a significant role in the pursuit of maintaining benign nondecreasing trajectories of cognition along the path of cognitive aging.

Acknowledgments

The research was supported by the Integrative Analysis of Longitudinal Studies of Aging (IALSA) research network (NIA AG026453, S. M. Hofer and A. M. Piccinin, PIs) and the *Conference on Advanced Psychometric Methods in Cognitive Aging Research* (NIA R13AG030995, D. M. Mungas, PI). M. Lindwall was supported by the Swedish National Centre for Research in Sports (CIF). L. E. Gibbons was supported by a grant from the NIH (AG05136, Murray Raskind, PI). A. Atri, S. D. Shirk, and M. B. Mitchell were supported by NIA Grant AG027171 (A. Atri, PI). M. Praetorius was supported by the EpiLife-FAS center at University of Gothenburg. The LBLS was funded by NIA Grants AG10569 and AG00037 (E. M. Zelinski, PI). The OCTO-Twin Study was funded by NIA AG08861 (B. Johansson, PI). SLS was funded by the National Institute of Child Health and Human Development (HD00367, 1963–1965; HD04476, 1970–1973) and the National Institute of Aging (AG00480, 1973–1979; AG03544, 1982–1986; AG04470, 1984–1989; AG08055, 1980–2006; AG027759, 2006–2008; currently AG024102, 2005–2015; S. L. Willis, PI). The VLS is currently funded by NIA Grant AG008235 (R. A. Dixon, PI). Tina L. Huang and Nadar Fallah participated in early work on the VLS portion of the paper. Finally, and most importantly, the authors express their deep gratitude for the commitment of the study participants across all four studies.The content of this study is solely the responsibility of the authors and does not necessarily represent the views of the National Institutes of Health or the United States Government. The authors report no conflict of interests with the present study.

References

[1] H. Christensen, A. J. Mackinnon, A. E. Korten et al., "An analysis of diversity in the cognitive performance of elderly community dwellers: individual differences in change scores as a function of age," *Psychology and Aging*, vol. 14, no. 3, pp. 365–379, 1999.

[2] S. M. Hofer, H. Christensen, A. J. Mackinnon et al., "Change in cognitive functioning associated with ApoE genotype in a community sample of older adults," *Psychology and Aging*, vol. 17, no. 2, pp. 194–208, 2002.

[3] K. W. Schaie, *Intellectual Development in Adulthood*, Cambridge University Press, Cambridge, UK, 1996.

[4] K. Anstey and H. Christensen, "Education, activity, health, blood pressure and apolipoprotein E as predictors of cognitive change in old age: a review," *Gerontology*, vol. 46, no. 3, pp. 163–177, 2000.

[5] T. A. Salthouse, *Theoretical Perspectives on Cognitive Aging*, Lawrence Erlbaum Associates, Hillsdale, NJ, USA, 1991.

[6] D. F. Hultsch, C. Hertzog, B. J. Small, and R. A. Dixon, "Use it or lose it: engaged lifestyle as a buffer of cognitive decline in aging?" *Psychology and Aging*, vol. 14, no. 2, pp. 245–263, 1999.

[7] A. Mackinnon, H. Christensen, S. M. Hofer, A. E. Korten, and A. F. Jorm, "Use it and still lose it? The association between activity and cognitive performance established using latent growth techniques in a community sample," *Aging, Neuropsychology, and Cognition*, vol. 10, no. 3, pp. 215–229, 2003.

[8] R. S. Newson and E. B. Kemps, "General lifestyle activities as a predictor of current cognition and cognitive change in older adults: a cross-sectional and longitudinal examination," *Journals of Gerontology*, vol. 60, no. 3, pp. P113–P120, 2005.

[9] A. F. Kramer and K. I. Erickson, "Capitalizing on cortical plasticity: influence of physical activity on cognition and brain function," *Trends in Cognitive Sciences*, vol. 11, no. 8, pp. 342–348, 2007.

[10] J. J. Ratey and J. E. Loehr, "The positive impact of physical activity on cognition during adulthood: a review of underlying mechanisms, evidence and recommendations," *Reviews in the Neurosciences*, vol. 22, no. 2, pp. 171–185, 2011.

[11] M. Lindwall, M. Rennemark, and T. Berggren, "Movement in mind: the relationship of exercise with cognitive status for older adults in the Swedish National Study on Aging and Care (SNAC)," *Aging and Mental Health*, vol. 12, no. 2, pp. 212–220, 2008.

[12] P. D. Tomporowki, "Physical activity, cognition, and aging: a review of reviews," in *Active Living, Cognitive Functioning, and Aging*, L. Poon, W. Chodzjo-Zajko, and P. D. Tomporowski, Eds., pp. 15–32, Human Kinetics, Champagne, Ill, USA, 2006.

[13] H. Bosma, M. P. J. Van Boxtel, R. W. H. M. Ponds et al., "Engaged lifestyle and cognitive function in middle and old-aged, non-demented persons: a reciprocal association?" *Zeitschrift fur Gerontologie und Geriatrie*, vol. 35, no. 6, pp 575–581, 2002.

[14] L. E. Middleton, D. E. Barnes, L. Y. Lui, and K. Yaffe, "Physica activity over the life course and its association with cognitiv performance and impairment in old age," *Journal of th American Geriatrics Society*, vol. 58, no. 7, pp. 1322–1326 2010.

[15] M. Richards, R. Hardy, and M. E. J. Wadsworth, "Does activ leisure protect cognition? Evidence from a national birt cohort," *Social Science and Medicine*, vol. 56, no. 4, pp. 785–792, 2003.

[16] A. Singh-Manoux, M. Hillsdon, E. Brunner, and M. Marmot "Effects of physical activity on cognitive functioning in middl age: evidence from the whitehall II prospective cohort study," *American Journal of Public Health*, vol. 95, no. 12, pp. 2252–2258, 2005.

[17] B. M. Van Gelder, M. A. R. Tijhuis, S. Kalmijn, S. Giampaoli, A. Nissinen, and D. Kromhout, "Physical activity in relation to cognitive decline in elderly men: the FINE study," *Neurology*, vol. 63, no. 12, pp. 2316–2321, 2004.

[18] J. Weuve, J. H. Kang, J. E. Manson, M. M. B. Breteler, J. H. Ware, and F. Grodstein, "Physical activity, including walking, and cognitive function in older women," *Journal of the American Medical Association*, vol. 292, no. 12, pp. 1454–1461, 2004.

[19] K. Yaffe, D. Barnes, M. Nevitt, L. Y. Lui, and K. Covinsky, "A prospective study of physical activity and cognitive decline in elderly women women who walk," *Archives of Internal Medicine*, vol. 161, no. 14, pp. 1703–1708, 2001.

[20] K. Yaffe, A. J. Fiocco, K. Lindquist et al., "Predictors of maintaining cognitive function in older adults: the Health ABC Study," *Neurology*, vol. 72, no. 23, pp. 2029–2035, 2009.

[21] A. A. M. Bielak, "How can we not 'lose it' if we still don't understand how to 'use it'? unanswered questions about the influence of activity participation on cognitive performance in older age—a mini-review," *Gerontology*, vol. 56, no. 5, pp. 507–519, 2010.

[22] A. A. M. Bielak, T. F. Hughes, B. J. Small, and R. A. Dixon, "It's never too late to engage in lifestyle activities: significant concurrent but not change relationships between lifestyle activities and cognitive speed," *Journals of Gerontology*, vol. 62, no. 6, pp. P331–P339, 2007.

[23] B. J. Small, R. A. Dixon, J. J. McArdle, and K. J. Grimm, "Do changes in lifestyle engagement moderate cognitive decline in normal aging? Evidence from the Victoria Longitudinal Study," *Neuropsychology*, vol. 25, pp. 144–155, 2012.

[24] S. Colcombe and A. F. Kramer, "Fitness effects on the cognitive function of older adults: a meta-analytic study," *Psychological Science*, vol. 14, no. 2, pp. 125–130, 2003.

[25] S. M. Hofer and A. M. Piccinin, "Integrative data analysis through coordination of measurement and analysis protocol across independent longitudinal studies," *Psychological Methods*, vol. 14, no. 2, pp. 150–164, 2009.

[26] S. M. Hofer and A. M. Piccinin, "Toward an integrative science of life-span development and aging," *Journals of Gerontology*, vol. 65, no. 3, pp. 269–278, 2010.

[27] J. L. Horn and S. M. Hofer, "Major abilities and development in the adult period," in *Intellectual Development*, R. J. Sternberg and C. A. Berg, Eds., pp. 44–99, Cambridge University Press, New York, NY, USA, 1992.

[28] I. Dureman and H. Sällde, *Psykometriska och Experimentalpsykologiska Metoder för Klinisk Tillämpning*, Almqvist & Wiksell, Uppsala, Sweden, 1959.

[29] B. Johansson, S. H. Zarit, and S. Berg, "Changes in cognitive functioning of the oldest old," *Journals of Gerontology*, vol. 47, no. 2, pp. P75–P80, 1992.
[30] D. Wechsler, *Wechsler Memory Scale-Revised*, Psychological Corporation, San Antonio, Tex, USA, 1987.
[31] C. O. Jonsson and L. Molander, *Manual Till CVB-Skalen*, Psykologi Forlaget, Stockholm, Sweden, 1964.
[32] K. W. Schaie, *Adult Mental Abilities Test*, Consulting Psychologists Press, Palo Alto, Calif, USA, 1985.
[33] L. Thurstone and T. Thurstone, *Examiner Manual For the SRA Primary Mental Abilities Test*, Science Research Associates, Chicago, Ill, USA, 1949.
[34] R. B. Ekstrom, J. W. French, H. H. Harman, and D. Dermen, *Kit of Factor-Referenced Cognitive Tests*, Educational Testing Service, Princeton, NJ, USA, 1976.
[35] D. F. Hultsch, C. Hertzog, and R. A. Dixon, "Ability correlates of memory performance in adulthood and aging," *Psychology and Aging*, vol. 5, no. 3, pp. 356–368, 1990.
[36] D. Hedeker and R. D. Gibbons, "Application of random-effects pattern-mixture models for missing data in longitudinal studies," *Psychological Methods*, vol. 2, no. 1, pp. 64–78, 1997.
[37] J. L. Etnier, "Physical activity programming to promote cognitive function: are we ready for prescription?" in *Aging, Exercise, and Cognition Series Vol 3 Enhancing Cognitive Functioning and Brain Plasticity*, W. W. Spirduso, W. Chodzko-Zajko, and L. W. Poon, Eds., pp. 159–176, Human Kinetics, Urbana-Champaign, Ill, USA, 2009.
[38] M. Lindwall, P. Larsman, and M. S. Hagger, "The reciprocal relationship between physical activity and depression in older european adults: a prospective cross-lagged panel design using SHARE data," *Health Psychology*, vol. 30, no. 4, pp. 453–462, 2011.
[39] S. W. MacDonald, C. A. DeCarlo, and R. A. Dixon, "Linking biological and cognitive aging: toward improving characterizations of developmental time," *The Journals of Gerontology*, vol. 66, supplement 1, pp. i59–i70, 2011.
[40] W. Spirduso, L. W. Poon, and W. Chodzko-Zaiko, "Using resources and reserves in an exercise-cognition model," in *Exercise and Its Mediating Effect on Cognition*, W. Spirduso, L. W. Poon, and W. Chodzko-Zaiko, Eds., Human Kinetics, Champaign, Ill, USA, 2008.
[41] J. L. Etnier, "Interrelationships of exercise, mediator variables, and cognition," in *Aging, Exercise and Cognition Series: Vol 2 Exercise and Its Mediating Effects on Cognition*, W. W. Spirduso, W. Chodzko-Zajko, and L. W. Poon, Eds., pp. 13–32, Human Kinetics, Urbana-Champaign, Ill, USA, 2008.
[42] J. L. Etnier, P. M. Nowell, D. M. Landers, and B. A. Sibley, "A meta-regression to examine the relationship between aerobic fitness and cognitive performance," *Brain Research Reviews*, vol. 52, no. 1, pp. 119–130, 2006.

15

Relationship between Serum and Brain Carotenoids, α-Tocopherol, and Retinol Concentrations and Cognitive Performance in the Oldest Old from the Georgia Centenarian Study

Elizabeth J. Johnson, Rohini Vishwanathan,[1] Mary Ann Johnson,[2] Dorothy B. Hausman,[2] Adam Davey,[3] Tammy M. Scott,[1] Robert C. Green,[4] L. Stephen Miller,[2] Marla Gearing,[5] John Woodard,[6] Peter T. Nelson,[7] Hae-Yun Chung,[8] Wolfgang Schalch,[9] Jonas Wittwer,[9] and Leonard W. Poon[2]

[1] *Jean Mayer US Department of Agriculture Human Nutrition Research Center on Aging at Tufts University, Boston, MA 02111, USA*
[2] *University of Georgia-Athens, Athens, GA 30602, USA*
[3] *Temple University, Philadelphia, PA 19122, USA*
[4] *Harvard University, Boston, MA 02115, USA*
[5] *Emory University, Atlanta, GA 30322, USA*
[6] *Wayne State University, Detroit, MI 48202, USA*
[7] *University of Kentucky, Lexington, KY 40536, USA*
[8] *Yonsei University, Seoul 120-749, Republic of Korea*
[9] *DSM Nutritional Products, CH-4002 Basel, Switzerland*

Correspondence should be addressed to Elizabeth J. Johnson; elizabeth.johnson@tufts.edu

Academic Editor: Paula Bickford

Oxidative stress is involved in age-related cognitive decline. The dietary antioxidants, carotenoids, tocopherols, and vitamin A may play a role in the prevention or delay in cognitive decline. In this study, sera were obtained from 78 octogenarians and 220 centenarians from the Georgia Centenarian Study. Brain tissues were obtained from 47 centenarian decedents. Samples were analyzed for carotenoids, α-tocopherol, and retinol using HPLC. Analyte concentrations were compared with cognitive tests designed to evaluate global cognition, dementia, depression and cognitive domains (memory, processing speed, attention, and executive functioning). Serum lutein, zeaxanthin, and β-carotene concentrations were most consistently related to better cognition ($P < 0.05$) in the whole population and in the centenarians. Only serum lutein was significantly related to better cognition in the octogenarians. In brain, lutein and β-carotene were related to cognition with lutein being consistently associated with a range of measures. There were fewer significant relationships for α-tocopherol and a negative relationship between brain retinol concentrations and delayed recognition. These findings suggest that the status of certain carotenoids in the old may reflect their cognitive function. The protective effect may not be related to an antioxidant effect given that α-tocopherol was less related to cognition than these carotenoids.

1. Introduction

Cognitive decline in the elderly is a significant public health issue. It has been estimated that the incidence of mild cognitive impairment (MCI) is approximately 19% in those younger than 75 years and 29% in those older than 85 years [1]. Further, 13% of people aged 65 years and older are afflicted with Alzheimer's disease. Studies in centenarians have reported considerable dementia, ranging from 42 to 100% [2, 3]. The number of individuals so affected is likely to increase given that the number of people over 65 years is rising. As with most age-related diseases, the most cost effective way to combat disease is through prevention. One possible strategy is nutrition intervention [4].

Fruit and vegetable intake has been associated with cognitive function [5–7]. For example, in a study of 13,388 women, it was found that total vegetable intake was significantly associated with reduced cognitive decline [8]. The strongest association was with greater intake of green leafy and cruciferous vegetables. Fruits and vegetables are major dietary sources of carotenoids. Carotenoids are a class of naturally occurring pigments that are synthesized by plants and produce the red, orange, and yellow colors of fruits and vegetables. Carotenoids are comprised of two subclasses: xanthophylls (lutein, zeaxanthin, and β-cryptoxanthin) and carotenes (α-carotene, β-carotene, and lycopene). In the Nurses' Health Study, among nonsupplement users, women in the highest quartile of plasma carotenoids had better cognitive performance than those in the lowest quartile [9]. Research has shown that patients with MCI had decreased plasma levels of antioxidants, including carotenoids [10]. Given that dietary carotenoids function as both antioxidants and anti-inflammatory agents and that oxidative stress and inflammation are believed to be involved in the pathogenesis of cognitive decline [11–20], intake of these dietary components may hold promise in cognitive health for the elderly.

The first objective of this study was to evaluate the relationship between serum concentrations of carotenoids and cognitive function in subjects from the Georgian Centenarian Study, a population-based multidisciplinary study of octogenarians and centenarians conducted in Georgia (USA) [21].

Given that an intervention with lutein was reported to improve cognitive function in the elderly [22] and that compared to carotenes, xanthophylls are preferentially taken up into brain tissue [23], a second objective of this research was to evaluate the cross-sectional relationship between brain carotenoids and premortem measures of cognitive function in a subgroup of the centenarian participants. For both serum and brain tissues, α-tocopherol was measured for comparison since it crosses the blood brain barrier and has antioxidant properties. Serum and brain retinol concentrations were measured because of the provitamin A activity of certain carotenoids.

This study provides a unique advantage of being able to assess the relationship between serum and brain carotenoids. If indeed serum concentrations of individual carotenoids reflect their levels in the brain and these brain carotenoids are related to better cognitive performance, serum carotenoid measures could be a useful tool for evaluating the benefits of dietary carotenoids to age-related cognitive health.

2. Materials and Methods

2.1. Study Population. The Georgia Centenarian Study (GCS) [21], a population-based multidisciplinary study conducted in 44 counties in northern Georgia (USA) from 2001 to 2009, was designed to identify and isolate longevity genes, neuropathology, functional capacity, and adaptational characteristics of centenarians [17]. Living status was classified as community dwelling or institutionalized where community dwelling included those living in private residences and institutionalized included individuals living in a skilled nursing facility or personal care home. The study involving serum analyses included 244 centenarians (defined in this study as age 98 yrs and older) and 80 octogenarians. The study involving brain tissue analyses included 47 centenarians who volunteered to donate their brain upon death. Subjects were recruited from the community, personal care homes, and skilled nursing facilities. The sample procedures and data collection methods have been described elsewhere [21].

In the analyses of serum, we excluded 2 octogenarians and 7 centenarians from whom we were unable to obtain sufficient serum for analysis. The final number of subjects with a complete dataset for serum analytes and cognitive function was 220 subjects in the centenarian group and 78 subjects in the octogenarian group.

Brain tissue was obtained from four regions of the brain: right cerebellum, right temporal cortex, and right and left frontal and occipital cortices from the subset of centenarians. Serum and tissues were stored at −80°C until analysis.

2.2. Serum and Brain Carotenoids, α-Tocopherols, and Retinoids Extraction. Serum was as described previously [24]. The brain extraction procedure was adapted from Park et al. [25] and has been described in detail by our laboratory [26].

2.3. HPLC Analysis for Carotenoid, Tocopherols, and Retinol. Serum and brain extracts were analyzed by HPLC (Alliance 2695l Waters, Milford, MA, USA) as previously described [24]. Using this method, *cis* lutein, all-*trans* lutein, *cis* zeaxanthin, all-*trans* zeaxanthin, cryptoxanthin, α-carotene, 13-*cis* β-carotene, all-*trans* β-carotene, 9-*cis* β-carotene, *cis* lycopene, and *trans* lycopene were separated and detected at 455 nm. α-Tocopherol, and retinol were detected at 292 and 340 nm, respectively. Using this method, the lower limit of detection was 0.2 pmol for carotenoids, 2.7 pmol for α-tocopherol and 2.0 pmol for retinol.

The analysis of serum and brain tissues was conducted without knowledge of values for the associated measures of cognition.

2.4. Measures of Cognitive Performance. Subjects underwent a battery of cognitive tests designed to evaluate global cognitive function, dementia, and depression as well as several cognitive domains including memory, processing speed, or attention and executive functioning (see Table S1 in the Supplementary Material available online at http://dx.doi.org/10.1155/2013/951786). The Geriatric Depression Scale-short form was administered to screen for depressive symptoms in the subjects [27]. Cognitive measures included the Mini-Mental State Examination (MMSE) [28], Global Deterioration Rating Scale (GDRS) [29], Severe Impairment Battery (SIB) [30], Fuld Object Memory Evaluation (FOME) [31], Wechsler Adult Intelligence Scale-III

(WAIS-III) Similarities Subtest [32], Behavioral Dyscontrol Scale [33], and Controlled Oral Word Association Test (COWAT) [34].

For participants in the separate brain donation component, additional cognitive tests were administered every six months until mortality. These tests included the Consortium to Establish a Registry for Alzheimer's Disease (CERAD) neuropsychological battery, which is composed of five subtests derived from previously established cognitive tests (verbal fluency, Boston Naming Test, MMSE, Constructional Praxis, and Word List Memory) [35, 36]. These subtests have been found to be valid and reliable measures of cognition in normal aging and in Alzheimer's disease [37]. Further, no differences were found between participants in the brain donation component of the GCS and the rest of the centenarian participants [38]. All of these tests or versions of them have been used and validated in aging research settings or have demonstrated sensitivity to health variables in epidemiological studies [39–42].

2.5. Covariates and Predictors. In the analyses involving serum, covariates and predictors included age (80–89 or ≥98 y), gender, and race (white or African American, by design). The proportion of participants from each age group recruited from skilled nursing facilities was based on estimates of the "institutionalized" population of the study area according to the 2000 US Census figures [21]. Residence status was not considered as a covariate because it was a potential suppressor variable. Fifteen percent of the octogenarians and 62% of the centenarians resided in skilled nursing facilities. The remaining "community dwelling" participants resided in private residences and personal care homes. In the analyses involving brain tissue, which involved centenarian decedents, 31% of the decedents had resided in skilled nursing facilities.

2.6. Statistical Analyses. Results are expressed as geometric means ± SDs. Relationships between trans and cis isomers of individual carotenoids and cognition did not differ appreciably. Therefore, the total (*trans* + *cis*) was used in the analysis. Given that the purpose of our analyses was to increase the precision with which an association could be estimated following adjustment for variables associated with our criterion, but not our predictor, we chose to analyze relationships between carotenoids, α-tocopherol, and retinol with cognitive measures using partial correlations. Thus, the partial correlation can provide an estimate of substantive interest but has the added advantage in that it does so in a standardized and easily interpretable metric. Statistical significance was set at $P < 0.05$. All statistical analyses were performed using SAS version 9.0 (serum) and SPSS version 19.0 (brain).

2.6.1. Serum Analyses. Data were verified for normality (Shapiro-Wilk test) and, when necessary, were log-transformed for normal distribution before further statistical analysis. Chi-square test and Student's t-test were used to compare subject characteristics, serum carotenoid levels, and cognitive values between groups. Pearson's correlations were performed to identify associations between cognitive indices with age, sex, anthropometric variables, and other possible confounders. The associations between cognitive indices and serum carotenoids were determined by calculating partial Pearson's correlation coefficients adjusted for age, sex, body mass index (BMI), smoking, alcohol, diagnosed hypertension, and diabetes. For the centenarians, diagnosis of hypertension and diabetes was drawn from proxy, family, staff, or charts.

2.6.2. Brain Analyses. Data were analyzed for all 47 decedents together and also separately for decedents based on their premortem GDRS scores. The purpose was to determine differences between decedents who had intact cognitive function (GDRS = 1), mild memory loss (GDRS = 2), mild cognitive impairment (GDRS = 3), and dementia (GDRS > 3) before death. One-way ANOVA was used to determine differences in age, education, BMI and brain carotenoid, α-tocopherol, and retinol concentrations between the GDRS groups. Chi-square tests were used for categorical variables, which included sex, race, living arrangement, smoking status, alcohol use, hypertension, and diabetes. Repeated measures ANOVA was used to determine differences in carotenoids, tocopherol, and retinol concentrations between the four regions of the brain. For frontal and occipital cortices, tissue from both the left and right lobes of the brain was obtained. For cerebellum and temporal cortices, tissue from only the right side of the brain was obtained. No differences were observed in carotenoid, tocopherol and retinol concentrations between the right and left lobes for ten decedents (data not shown). In order to maintain consistency, only the right lobe of the brain was analyzed for all decedents. Mean brain carotenoid, α-tocopherol, and retinol concentrations were calculated for each decedent based on measures from the four regions of the brain (cerebellum frontal, occipital, and temporal cortices). These means were used for comparison of carotenoid, α-tocopherol, and retinol profiles between the brain and serum and also to evaluate differences between brain concentrations of individual micronutrients. Partial correlation coefficients were determined in order to evaluate the relationship of carotenoids, α-tocopherol, and retinol with different measures of cognitive function. Age, sex, education, diabetes, and hypertension were used as covariates since these variables have the strongest influence on cognitive function measures. Concentration of *trans* lutein and zeaxanthin in the cerebellum was significantly greater than the three cortical regions of the brain. In order to determine associations with cognitive indices, concentration of carotenoids in the temporal, frontal, and occipital cortices was averaged, and associations were evaluated with and without cerebellum carotenoids.

3. Results

3.1. Serum Analytes and Cognition

3.1.1. Subject Characteristics. The characteristics of the octogenarians and centenarians who provided serum are given in Table 1. A significantly greater proportion of the centenarians

TABLE 1: Subject characteristics.

	≥80 to ≤89 y (n = 78)	≥98 y (n = 220)	P value*	Community dwelling (n = 150)	Institutionalized (n = 148)	P value*	Total (n = 298)
Age, yrs (mean ± SD)	84.2 ± 2.7	100.4 ± 1.9		93.3 ± 8.3	99.7 ± 4.6	<0.0001	96.6 ± 7.4
Male : female	27 : 51	36 : 184	0.0007	40 : 110	23 : 125	0.0187	63 : 235
Community dwelling (n) : institutionalized (n)	66 : 12	84 : 136	<0.0001	—	—		150 : 148
Education, yrs (mean ± SD)	13.0 ± 3.5	10.6 ± 3.8	<0.0001	12.1 ± 3.7	10.3 ± 3.7	<0.0001	11.2 ± 3.8
Body mass index (kg/m^2) (mean ± SD)	25.5 ± 4.8	22.6 ± 4.7	<0.0001	24.2 ± 4.7	22.5 ± 4.8	0.0059	23.3 ± 4.8
Smoking (n)			<0.0001			0.035	
None	33	156		88	101		189
Ex-smoker	40	54		53	41		94
Current	5	7		9	3		12
No information	0	3		0	3		3
Alcohol use (n)			<0.0001			<0.0001	
None	22	134		67	89		156
Ex-drinker	27	45		32	40		72
Current	29	39		51	17		68
No information	0	2		0	2		2
Hypertension (n)			0.394			0.306	
Yes	32	108		66	74		140
No	45	109		83	71		154
No information	1	3		1	3		4

*Significant difference between groups. Means were compared using Student's t-test. Fisher's exact test was applied for categorical variables.

were women, institutionalized, and nonsmokers compared to the octogenarians ($P < 0.001$). Furthermore, the centenarians had significantly less education years, alcohol use, and BMI ($P < 0.001$). There was no difference in the prevalence of hypertension in these two age groups.

A greater proportion of the institutionalized subjects were women and nonsmokers compared to the community dwelling subjects ($P < 0.02$ and 0.035, resp., Table 1). They were also significantly older than the community dwelling subjects ($P < 0.001$). The institutionalized subjects had significantly less education years, alcohol use, and BMI ($P < 0.001$). There was no difference in the prevalence of hypertension in these two groups.

3.1.2. Serum Carotenoids, α-Tocopherol, and Retinol Concentrations. Serum concentrations of individual carotenoids, α-tocopherol and retinol are given in Table 2. Compared to the octogenarians, the centenarians had lower mean values for all carotenoids and α-tocopherol, which was significantly different ($P < 0.05$) for all analytes except *cis* zeaxanthin and marginally significant for *trans* lutein ($P < 0.075$) and β-carotene ($P < 0.084$). Similarly, the institutionalized subjects had lower mean values for all carotenoids and α-tocopherol which was significantly different ($P < 0.05$) for all analytes except for cryptoxanthin, α-carotene, and β-carotene and marginally significant for *trans* zeaxanthin ($P < 0.052$). Serum retinol values were neither significantly different between octogenarians and centenarians nor between community dwelling and institutionalized subjects.

3.1.3. Cognitive Function in Octogenarians and Centenarians. The cognitive function status of subjects from the Georgia Centenarian Study is found in Table S2 of the Supplementary Material. For all measures of cognitive function, mean values were significantly lower in the centenarians than in octogenarians ($P < 0.0001$) except for delayed recognition which was not different between the two groups. For all measures of cognitive function, the institutionalized subjects had significantly lower values than the community dwelling subjects ($P < 0.0005$).

3.1.4. Relationships between Serum Carotenoids, α-Tocopherol, and Retinol and Cognitive Performance. In the total study population, serum lutein and zeaxanthin concentrations were most consistently related to better cognitive performance, with a significant correlation observed ($P < 0.05$) (Table 3) for all cognitive measures except delayed recognition. It should be noted that none of the serum analytes were correlated with delayed recognition. Serum concentrations of β-carotene were also significantly correlated to most measures of cognitive function ($P < 0.05$) with the exception

TABLE 2: Serum carotenoid, α-tocopherol, and retinol concentrations in subjects from the Georgian Centenarian Study (mean ± SD).

nmol/L (carotenoids) μmol/L (α-tocopherol, retinol)	≥80 to ≤89 y (*n* = 78)	≥98 y (*n* = 220)	*P* value*	Community dwelling (*n* = 150)	Institutionalized (*n* = 148)	*P* value*	Total (*n* = 298)
Lutein, *trans*	213 ± 162	199 ± 177	0.0753	223 ± 199	181 ± 141	0.0072	204 ± 174
Lutein, *cis*	58 ± 58	53 ± 65	0.0006	63 ± 77	46 ± 46	0.0162	56 ± 63
Lutein, total	316 ± 255	293 ± 285	0.0156	334 ± 329	265 ± 207	0.0116	300 ± 276
Zeaxanthin, *trans*	47 ± 23	44 ± 28	0.0194	49 ± 30	42 ± 23	0.0516	46 ± 26
Zeaxanthin, *cis*	5 ± 16	5 ± 11	0.6388	7 ± 14	4 ± 9	0.0764	5 ± 12
Zeaxanthin, total	53 ± 32	49 ± 37	0.0355	56 ± 40	46 ± 28	0.0195	51 ± 35
Cryptoxanthin	159 ± 105	148 ± 125	0.0362	166 ± 137	134 ± 96	0.3174	150 ± 119
α-Carotene	80 ± 110	63 ± 61	0.0122	71 ± 93	63 ± 54	0.6972	67 ± 76
β-Carotene, *trans*	547 ± 836	443 ± 419	0.2200	542 ± 670	398 ± 406	0.0056	471 ± 558
β-Carotene, *cis*	20 ± 26	17 ± 22	0.6538	19 ± 26	17 ± 20	0.5322	19 ± 22
β-Carotene, total	568 ± 855	460 ± 432	0.0839	560 ± 69	415 ± 419	0.0039	488 ± 573
Lycopene, *trans*	240 ± 181	138 ± 119	<0.0001	199 ± 166	130 ± 112	<0.0001	164 ± 145
Lycopene, *cis*	389 ± 277	231 ± 227	<0.0001	324 ± 276	220 ± 212	0.0003	272 ± 251
Lycopene, total	629 ± 443	369 ± 337	<0.0001	523 ± 430	348 ± 309	0.0003	436 ± 384
α-Tocopherol	31.9 ± 16.8	25.5 ± 12.9	0.0011	29.6 ± 15.0	24.8 ± 13.2	0.0016	29.2 ± 14.3
Retinol	2.14 ± 0.07	1.84 ± 0.62	0.449	2.00 ± 0.64	1.83 ± 0.59	0.247	1.92 ± 0.62

*Significant difference between groups. Means were compared using Student's *t*-test. Chi-square analysis was applied for categorical variables.

TABLE 3: Partial correlation coefficients between cognition indices and serum carotenoids, α-tocopherol, and retinol in octogenarians and centenarians from the Georgia Centenarian Study (adjusted w/age, sex, education years, BMI, smoking, alcohol, hypertension, and diabetes, *n* = 298).

	Mini-Mental State Exam	Global Deterioration Rating Scale	FOME[1] delayed recall	FOME delayed recognition	FOME delayed retention	Controlled Oral Word Association Test	WAIS-III Similarities Subtest[2]	Behavioral Dyscontrol Scale Total Score
Lutein, (*trans* + *cis*)	0.114	−0.350[a]	0.177[b]	0.009	0.114	0.148[c]	0.244[a]	0.180[b]
Zeaxanthin, (*trans* + *cis*)	0.128[c]	−0.236[a]	0.134[c]	0.069	0.146[c]	0.169[b]	0.184[b]	0.196[b]
Cryptoxanthin	0.026	−0.096	0.054	0.002	0.035	0.031	0.129[c]	0.045
α-Carotene	−0.014	−0.068	0.017	−0.029	0.009	0.015	0.074	0.029
β-Carotene, (*trans* + *cis*)	0.072	−0.244[a]	0.173[b]	0.082	0.168[b]	0.186[b]	0.144[c]	0.227[a]
Lycopene, (*trans* + *cis*)	−0.014	−0.142[c]	−0.017	−0.033	0.014	0.017	0.108	0.044
α-Tocopherol	0.118	−0.194[b]	0.097	0.097	0.145[c]	0.106	0.121[c]	0.200[b]
Retinol	0.089	−0.078	0.113	0.022	0.105	0.006	0.045	0.116

[1]FOME: Fuld Object Memory Evaluation; [2]WAIS-III Similarities Subtest: Wechsler Adult Intelligence Scale-III Similarities Subtest.
Significantly related (*P* <): [a]0.001; [b]0.01, [c]0.05.

of the MMSE and delayed recognition (Table 3). Serum α-tocopherol concentrations were inversely related to dementia severity (Geriatric Deterioration Scale) ($P < 0.01$) and positively related to delayed retention, abstract reasoning, and the Behavioral Dyscontrol Scale ($P < 0.05$). Higher serum lycopene concentrations were only related to a lower dementia severity ($P < 0.01$). Serum cryptoxanthin was only related to the WAIS-III test ($P < 0.05$, Table 5). Serum retinol concentrations were not related to any of the cognitive function measures.

In the octogenarians, serum lutein concentrations were significantly related to measures of global cognition, lower dementia severity, and executive function ($P < 0.05$) (Table S3 of the Supplementary Material). In this age group, serum cryptoxanthin was inversely related to delayed recall ($P < 0.05$). There were no other significant relationships. In the centenarians, none of the serum carotenoids or α-tocopherol were related to global cognition or delayed recognition. Higher concentrations of lutein, zeaxanthin, β-carotene, and α-tocopherol were significantly related to lower dementia severity ($P < 0.05$). Additional significant relationships were found between lutein and abstract reasoning, between β-carotene and verbal fluency (Controlled Oral Word Association Test), WAIS-III and executive function, between α-tocopherol and executive function, and between retinol and delayed recall ($P < 0.05$).

TABLE 4: Mean (±SEM) concentrations of carotenoids, α-tocopherol, and retinol in the cerebellum, frontal, occipital, and temporal cortices ($n = 47$).

Analyte (pmol/g)	Cerebellum	Frontal cortex	Occipital cortex	Temporal cortex
Lutein, *cis*	6.5 ± 1.4^{a}	$4.0 \pm 1.6^{a,b}$	2.8 ± 0.7^{b}	3.1 ± 0.8^{b}
Lutein, *trans*	169.8 ± 15.5^{a}	78.7 ± 7.6^{b}	91.8 ± 9.1^{b}	81.7 ± 7.8^{b}
Total Lutein (*cis* + *trans*)	176.4 ± 16.6^{a}	82.7 ± 8.0^{b}	94.6 ± 9.6^{c}	$84.8 \pm 8.4^{b,c}$
Zeaxanthin, *trans*	52.9 ± 4.3^{a}	25.9 ± 1.9^{b}	30.0 ± 2.0^{c}	$27.8 \pm 2.0^{b,c}$
Cryptoxanthin ($\alpha + \beta$)	$75.8 \pm 13.7^{a,b}$	63.4 ± 10.2^{a}	93.4 ± 15.6^{b}	60.7 ± 9.4^{a}
β-Carotene, *trans*	59.8 ± 5.7^{a}	60.8 ± 6.4^{a}	70.2 ± 6.9^{b}	51.8 ± 4.3^{a}
β-Carotene, 9-*cis*	12.0 ± 1.5^{a}	13.5 ± 1.8^{a}	16.9 ± 2.0^{b}	$13.1 \pm 1.9^{a,b}$
Lycopene, *trans*	26.3 ± 4.4	21.0 ± 3.7	21.9 ± 3.6	19.9 ± 3.2
α-Tocopherol	43475 ± 1877^{a}	$67027 \pm 2992^{b,c}$	72971 ± 2442^{c}	65521 ± 1940^{b}
Retinol	472 ± 24^{a}	615 ± 42^{b}	$676 \pm 43^{b,c}$	768 ± 54^{c}

Means not sharing a common superscript in the same row are significantly different at $P < 0.05$ (repeated measures ANOVA with Bonferroni adjustment for multiple comparisons).

TABLE 5: Mean (±SEM) concentrations of carotenoids, α-tocopherol, and retinol in the brain (average of cerebellum, frontal, occipital, and temporal cortices) based on premortem GDRS scores in decedents with normal cognitive function (GDRS = 1), subjective mild memory loss (GDRS = 2), and mild cognitive impairment (GDRS = 3).

pmol/g	Global deterioration scale (GDRS)[a]		
	1 ($n = 5$)	2 ($n = 7$)	3 ($n = 11$)
Lutein, *trans*	133 ± 21^{b}	$124 \pm 17^{b,c}$	67 ± 14^{c}
Total lutein (*cis* + *trans*)	145 ± 22^{b}	$127 \pm 18^{b,c}$	68 ± 15^{c}
Zeaxanthin, *trans*	45.0 ± 7.5	43.1 ± 6.3	25.9 ± 5.0
Cryptoxanthin	90.1 ± 22.4	63.2 ± 19.0	57.2 ± 15.1
β-Carotene, *trans*	77.6 ± 10.5^{b}	$48.0 \pm 8.9^{b,c}$	39.5 ± 7.1^{c}
Lycopene, *trans*	37.0 ± 9.0	26.1 ± 7.6	16.4 ± 6.1
γ-Tocopherol	1609 ± 370	2129 ± 313	1518 ± 249
α-Tocopherol	67408 ± 5295	63205 ± 4475	60028 ± 3570
Retinol	572 ± 109	530 ± 92	691 ± 74

[a] GDRS = 1: no subjective complaints or objective evidence of memory deficits; GDRS = 2: subject complaints, but no objective evidence of memory deficits; GDRS = 3: mild cognitive impairment.
Means not sharing a common superscript in the same row are significantly different at $P < 0.05$ (univariate ANOVA with Bonferroni adjustment for multiple comparisons).

In the community dwelling subjects, serum zeaxanthin had significant relationships with most measures of cognitive function (Supplementary Material, Table S4), with higher concentrations being significantly related to global cognitive performance, lower dementia severity, delayed recall and retention, verbal fluency, and concept formation/abstraction ($P < 0.05$). Higher serum lutein was significantly related to global cognitive function, lower dementia severity, and delayed recall and retention ($P < 0.05$). Other significant relationships were found between higher β-carotene concentrations and lower dementia, delayed recall and retention, and verbal fluency and executive function ($P < 0.05$). In the community dwelling subjects, α-tocopherol was only significantly related to executive function ($P < 0.05$). There were no significant relationships found between cryptoxanthin, α-carotene and retinol and cognitive measures.

Fewer significant relationships were found between serum analytes and cognitive measures in the institutionalized subjects. In this group, significant relationships were found between lower dementia severity and serum concentrations of lutein, zeaxanthin, β-carotene, and α-tocopherol. Serum lutein, zeaxanthin, cryptoxanthin, and α-carotene were significantly related to concept formation/abstraction ($P < 0.05$). Lutein, zeaxanthin, β-carotene, α-tocopherol and retinol were significantly related to executive function ($P < 0.05$).

3.2. Brain Analytes and Cognition

3.2.1. Subject Characteristics. The characteristics of the centenarian population for which brain tissues were available are described in Table S5 of the Supplementary Material. Of the 47 decedents, five had normal cognitive function (GDRS = 1), seven had subjective mild memory loss (GDRS = 2), and eleven had MCI (GDRS = 3). There were 24 decedents who had different stages of dementia (GDRS 4 to 7). Subjects with dementia were slightly older than those with intact cognitive function. However, the differences were not significant. Eighty-nine percent of the decedents were females, and 89% were Caucasians. Race/ethnicity, sex, education, BMI, smoking status, and alcohol use did not differ by GDRS status. A greater proportion of the

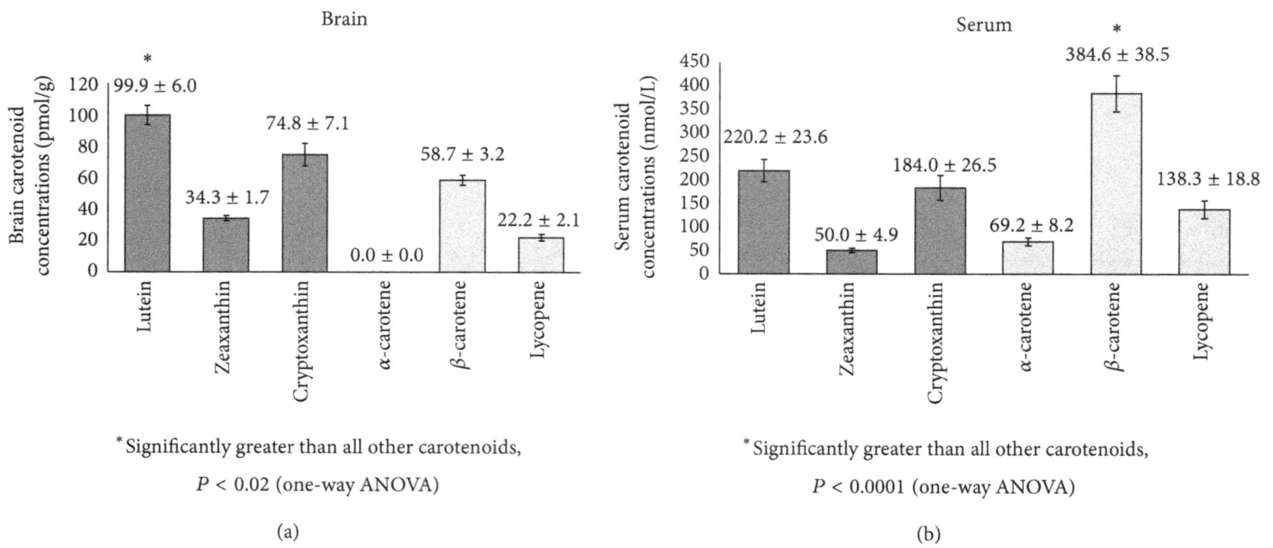

FIGURE 1: Mean (± SEM) concentrations of carotenoids (*trans* isomers) in the brain (average of cerebellum frontal serum, occipital, and temporal cortices) of decedents from the Georgia Centenarian Study ($n = 42$). Dark gray bars indicate xanthophyll carotenoids. Light gray bars indicate carotenes.

decedents were institutionalized; however, the differences between institutionalized and community dwelling subjects were not statistically significant. The prevalence of diabetes and hypertension did not differ between these two groups.

3.2.2. Brain Carotenoid, α-Tocopherol, and Retinol Concentrations. The mean concentration of individual carotenoids, α-tocopherol, and retinol in the cerebellum, frontal, occipital, and temporal cortices from the 47 decedents is shown in Table 4. The range of values for carotenoids was 0–661 pmol/g. For α-tocopherol, the range was 22,979–137,576 pmol/g and for retinol 202–2,233 pmol/g. Mean lutein and zeaxanthin concentrations were significantly greater in the cerebellum compared to the frontal, occipital, and temporal cortices. Concentrations of cryptoxanthin and β-carotene the were highest in the occipital cortex and were significantly different from the frontal and temporal cortices. α-Carotene was not detected in these brain tissues. Contrary to lutein and zeaxanthin, concentrations of α-tocopherol and retinol were the lowest in the cerebellum and significantly different from all three cortical regions.

The proportion of *cis* to *trans* isomers was much lower in the brain than in the serum. The ratio of *cis* to *trans* lutein and β-carotene was ~0.25 in the serum while in the brain it was only ~0.04. Although present in the serum, *cis* isomers of zeaxanthin and lycopene were not detected in any of the brain regions analyzed. Of note is that brain carotenoids were significantly related to their concentrations in serum ($P < 0.01$ for all, except *cis* lutein: $P < 0.05$). α-Tocopherol concentrations in the cortices were also significantly related to serum concentrations ($P < 0.01$). However, α-tocopherol in the cerebellum was not. Retinol concentrations in all brain regions were not related to serum retinol concentrations.

Figure 1 shows the mean carotenoid (*trans* isomers) concentrations in the brain and matched serum for the decedents that had both serum and brain tissue. In the brain, xanthophylls (lutein, zeaxanthin, and cryptoxanthin) accounted for 72% of total carotenoids, of which lutein accounted for 34% of the total and was significantly greater than all other carotenoids ($P < 0.02$). The proportion of carotenes (α-carotene, β-carotene, and lycopene) was higher than xanthophylls in serum, accounting for 57% of the total carotenoids of which β-carotene accounted for 37% of the total and was significantly greater than all other carotenoids ($P < 0.0001$).

3.2.3. Brain Carotenoids, α-Tocopherol, and Retinol Concentrations in Decedents with Intact Cognitive Function, Mild Memory Loss, and MCI. The mean brain concentrations of carotenoids, α-tocopherol, and retinol for decedents with GDRS ≤ 3 and GDRS > 3 were not significantly different (data not shown) with the exception of 9 *cis* β-carotene which was significantly higher in dementia (17 ± 3.1 versus 9,8 ± 1.7 pmol/g).

Table 5 shows brain carotenoids, α-tocopherol, and retinol concentrations in decedents with normal cognitive function, mild memory loss, and MCI. Due to the advanced pathological changes in brain and significant reduction in brain volume associated with dementia, decedents with dementia were not included in this analysis [43]. Additionally, the neuropathological and neurobiological brain changes associated with MCI are quantitatively less than those associated with dementia [44]. Mean concentrations of all carotenoids were found to progressively decrease with increasing GDRS scores from 1 to 3. However, only the differences in lutein and β-carotene concentrations between subjects with normal cognitive function and MCI were statistically significant ($P < 0.05$). When data were adjusted for age, sex, education, diabetes, and hypertension, only the differences observed in lutein concentrations between the

TABLE 6: Cross-sectional relationship between concentrations of carotenoids, α-tocopherol, and retinol in the cortex (average concentrations of the frontal, occipital, and temporal cortices) and premortem measures of cognitive function in subjects with normal cognitive function, mild memory loss, and MCI who completed the cognitive function tests a year prior their death ($n = 21$).

	MMSE	FOME recognition	SIB	COWAT	BDS	CERAD verbal fluency	CERAD Boston naming test
Lutein (*trans* + *cis*)	0.494[a]	−0.297	0.076	0.142	0.459	0.455	0.572[a]
Zeaxanthin	0.439	−0.281	0.139	0.177	0.286	0.461[a]	0.207
Cryptoxanthin	−0.056	0.325	−0.021	0.152	0.046	0.302	0.084
β-Carotene, *trans*	0.265	−0.010	−0.014	0.269	0.137	0.265	0.008
Lycopene, *trans*	0.124	−0.003	0.132	0.067	−0.085	0.065	0.275
α-Tocopherol	0.393	−0.295	0.568[a]	0.637[a]	0.434	0.328	0.165
Retinol	0.161	−0.456	0.168	0.400	0.067	0.108	−0.307

Values are partial correlation coefficients adjusted for sex, education, diabetes, and hypertension.
[a] $P \le 0.05$.
MMSE: Mini-Mental State Examination; FOME: Fuld Object Memory Evaluation; SIB: Severe Impairment Battery; COWAT: Controlled Oral Word Association Test; BDS: Behavioral Dyscontrol Scale; CERAD: Consortium to Establish a Registry for Alzheimer's Disease.

two groups remained significant ($P < 0.05$). Mean brain retinol concentration was not significantly different between individuals with MCI and normal cognitive function. Similar results were obtained when concentrations of carotenoids, α-tocopherol, and retinol in the cerebellum and cortex (average of frontal, temporal, and occipital) were analyzed separately. Data corrected for covariates are not reported due to the small sample size in each GDRS subgroup.

3.2.4. Relationship between Brain Carotenoids, α-Tocopherol, and Retinol and Cognitive Function Measures. Of the 23 decedents with normal cognitive function, mild memory loss, and MCI, data for 21 subjects whose cognitive function tests were performed within one year (4.3 ± 2.8 mo, range: 0.3–10.5 mo) prior to their death were analyzed for associations with cognition. A significant positive correlation was observed between lutein concentrations in the cortex and the MMSE (global measure of cognitive function) and the Boston Naming Test (CERAD battery, a measure of language), while a negative correlation was observed with Geriatric Depression Scale ($P < 0.05$) (Table 6). The positive association of zeaxanthin in the cortex and verbal fluency was statistically significant ($P < 0.05$). α-Tocopherol was positively associated with SIB (a global measure of cognitive function) and COWAT (a measure of executive function) ($P < 0.05$). In the case of retinol, there was a negative relation with FOME-delayed recognition ($P < 0.05$). No associations were observed with the other listed measures of cognitive function.

Carotenoids in the cerebellum were not associated with any of the cognitive function measures with the exception of a negative association between lutein and the Geriatric Depression Scale ($r = -0.63$, $P = 0.005$). α-tocopherol in the cerebellum was positively associated with MMSE ($r = 0.535$, $P = 0.027$) and SIB ($r = 0.602$, $P = 0.01$), both of which are measures of global cognition.

4. Discussion

In this cross-sectional study involving octogenarians and centenarians, we found significant relationships between serum and brain concentrations of dietary carotenoids and various measures of cognitive function. No specific domain of the cognitive performance showed the strongest relationship with either serum or brain concentrations of carotenoids since significant relationships were observed with memory, executive function, and language. The fact that specific carotenoids were associated with more than one cognitive function and that these associations remained statistically significant after controlling for potential confounding factors supports a possible role for these phytonutrients in age-related cognitive health. The present study is the first report on serum and brain carotenoids, α-tocopherol, and retinol concentrations and their relationship to cognitive function in the oldest of the old. This is of importance given the dramatic increase in the number of Americans surviving into their 80s and 90s and the increased prevalence of age-related cognitive diseases such as Alzheimer's disease [4].

Others have also found relationships with dietary carotenoids and age-related cognitive function. In cross-sectional and longitudinal analysis of 442 subjects aged 65–94 years, Perrig et al. [45] reported that a higher β-carotene plasma level was associated with better memory performances (free recall, recognition, and vocabulary). In the Rotterdam Study of 5182 community participants aged 55–95 yrs, cross-sectional analysis found that a lower intake of β-carotene was associated with impaired cognitive function as measured by the MMSE [46]. In both of these studies, there were no significant relationships with vitamin E. Also, no other carotenoids were evaluated. Two studies have reported that supplementation with antioxidants including β-carotene [47, 48] reduces the risk of cognitive decline. However, given that both studies involved multivitamin/mineral supplementation, a specific effect of β-carotene is difficult to determine. In the EVA, a cross-sectional study using a variety of cognitive measures in 589 subjects (68–79 yrs), it was found that those with the lowest cognitive functioning (<25th percentile) had a higher probability of having low plasma levels of lycopene and zeaxanthin, but not lutein or β-carotene [49]. However, in a prospective study of older adults (mean age 73 y), Morris and colleagues found no association between β-carotene intake and risk of

Alzheimer's disease [50]. Additionally, the Age-Related Eye Diseases Study Research Group [51] found no effect of a multivitamin/mineral supplementation which included β-carotene on MMSE score and a battery of cognitive measures in a population with a median age of 69 yrs. Rinaldi et al. found that plasma levels of lutein, zeaxanthin, and α-carotene were lower in MCI and Alzheimer's disease subjects compared to controls but no difference for lycopene and β-carotene [10]. β-Cryptoxanthin was also significantly lower than controls in subjects with Alzheimer's disease but not in subjects with MCI. Others have reported lower levels of zeaxanthin, β-cryptoxanthin, lycopene, and β-carotene but not lutein and α-carotene in Alzheimer's patients than in controls [52]. Inconsistencies among studies may be due to limited sample size, cognitive tests used, method of carotenoid assessment, or characteristics of the subject population. The major difference between our present study and previous research is the age of the population. In our population, the average age was 97 yrs compared to averages of 67–77 yrs for the studies discussed above.

Whether a possible protective effect of carotenoids differs between the old and the oldest of the old remains to be tested. However, in our study, the most consistent relationships with cognition were observed for serum lutein, zeaxanthin, and β-carotene, reflecting diets rich in green leafy vegetables and orange and yellow vegetables such as carrots, sweet potatoes, and winter squash [53]. This remained to be true for the centenarians and with respect to living status, but only lutein remained significantly related to better measures of cognitive performance in the octogenarians. Furthermore, in brain tissue only concentrations of lutein and β-carotene were significantly lower in the cortex and cerebellum of subjects with MCI compared to those with normal cognitive function. Lutein and β-carotene may thus be important carotenoids for maintaining normal cognitive function in older adults. Consumption of vegetables, particularly the green leafy varieties that are rich sources of lutein and β-carotene, was associated with slower rates of cognitive decline in two large cohort studies [5, 8]. Other evidence suggests that lutein supplementation, alone or in combination with docosahexaenoic acid, may be able to improve certain aspects of cognitive performance in healthy older women [22].

Although much recent work has focused on lutein and its role in ocular health [54], lutein was also the dominant carotenoid in various regions of the centenarian brains. On the contrary, carotenes (α-carotene, β-carotene, and lycopene) were predominant in serum, which more closely reflects dietary intake. These findings suggest that although not predominant in the diet, there seems to be a preferential uptake of lutein from the circulation into the brain. Craft et al. reported similar preferential uptake of xanthophylls in brain [23]. *Trans* isomers of lutein, zeaxanthin, cryptoxanthin and β-carotene, α-tocopherol, and retinol were detected in all the brain tissues analyzed in this study. Only three *cis* isomers, two of lutein and one of β-carotene, were detected in the centenarian brain, which were not reported in the elderly brain tissues analyzed by Craft et al. [23]. Also, the ratios of *cis* to *trans* isomers in the brain were much lower than in serum, indicating a preferential uptake of *trans* isomers in the brain of these centenarians.

The majority of our findings find an association between lutein concentrations in serum or brain with age-related cognitive performance. However, there were significant associations for zeaxanthin and β-carotene as well. Therefore, the protective effect of carotenoids does not appear to be limited to the provitamin A carotenoids (β-cryptoxanthin, α-carotene, and β-carotene) nor to a class of carotenoids (xanthophylls versus carotenes). In addition, brain retinol levels were positively related to very few of the measures of cognition and negatively related to delayed recognition.

A protective effect of carotenoids may, in part, to be related to an antioxidant effect given that an antioxidant function is common to all carotenoids [55–58]. Furthermore, α-tocopherol, a major dietary antioxidant, was found to be related to several measures of cognitive. Cortical carotenoids may be protective in nature and may also influence interneuronal communication and function via multiple mechanisms. Other mechanisms by which certain carotenoids may function include modulation of functional properties of synaptic membranes along with changes in their physicochemical and structural features [59]. Carotenoids have also been shown to enhance gap junctional communication [60] which in the retina is important for light processing and may be important for the development of neural circuitry in the visual system. Lutein and zeaxanthin, as macular pigments in the retina, have been related to increased visual processing speed and to reduced scotopic noise (noise associated with vision under dim light conditions) [61–63]. Lutein may also have anti-inflammatory action in the brain, lowering inflammatory markers, and preventing cognitive decline [64, 65]. Neuroinflammation is also one of the factors that contribute to the pathogenesis of MCI and AD with increased levels of inflammatory markers being correlated with cognitive impairment [66].

The significant progressive decline in brain lutein and β-carotene with increased impairment from normal to MCI indicates that these carotenoids may play a role in preventing cognitive decline. MCI is thought to be the transitional stage between normal aging and the earliest symptoms of AD. There may be as much as a 50% likelihood of individuals with MCI developing AD within five years [67]. Our finding of a significant decrease in lutein and β-carotene in subjects with MCI indicates that these carotenoids may play a role in maintenance of cognitive health prior to a decline to MCI. Future clinical studies should focus on nutritional interventions with lutein and β-carotene in subjects with MCI. Thus, far supplementation studies with β-carotene have yielded mixed results; the Physician Health Study II showed a long-term beneficial effect [68], while some studies showed no effect on cognitive function with β-carotene or antioxidant supplementation [69, 70]. Effects of lutein supplementation on subjects with MCI have not been studied to date.

The strength of this study is that we were able to evaluate cognitive function in the elderly using a battery of cognitive tests that included the MMSE. This approach is more powerful than using only the less sensitive measure of MMSE. With the other tests, the scores ranges are wider, allowing for a better ability to study cognitive impairment. We were also able to evaluate cognitive relationships with a variety of dietary carotenoids using measures of serum concentrations. Carotenoid assessment using serum concentrations may be preferred to food frequency questionnaires because the high interindividual variation in intestinal bioavailability of carotenoids [71] does not need to be considered. Whether such variability exists for, uptake of carotenoids into brain tissue is not known. What is known is that the macular pigment response to supplementation of lutein from diet or supplements varies widely among individuals [72, 73]. A variable response of uptake into the brain may also exist given the significant relationship between concentrations of xanthophylls in the retina and brain [26].

Thus, another strength of this study is the measures in brain tissue that are associated with premortem measures of cognition. Additionally, the strength of these cross-sectional relationships lies in the high interindividual variability in brain carotenoid concentrations, similar to that observed in the serum of these centenarians. Another strength of the study is that associations with cognitive function were evaluated with carotenoids, α-tocopherol, and retinol actually embedded in brain tissue. However, the significant correlations between carotenoid concentrations in serum and brain tissue suggest that serum carotenoid measures could be a useful tool for evaluating the benefits of dietary carotenoids to age-related cognitive health.

One limitation to this study is that, in cross-sectional analysis, it is not possible to affirm whether these low levels of carotenoids preceded or were the consequence of cognitive impairment. Low carotenoid status, that is, poor food choices, may be a reflection of poor cognitive status. The significant relationships observed may not be due to specific effects of the individual carotenoids but, indication of overall healthier diets and lifestyles. Another limitation is that our analyses were performed in a sample drawn from a relatively small population. Therefore, we were unable to perform multivariate regression analysis that would have provided additional information regarding the independent contributions of the individual nutrient components.

5. Conclusions

In conclusion, this is the first study to evaluate the role of carotenoids, α-tocopherol, and retinol in cognitive function in the oldest of the old. To date, previous studies evaluated older populations with average ages of 20–30 years younger than those of this study. Evaluations of the role of diet to health in this age group are becoming increasingly important given the rise in both life expectancy and the segment of the population who are >80 years. While far from conclusive, the idea that certain carotenoids can influence cognitive function is certainly feasible. The significance of our findings requires further research using biological studies, longitudinal epidemiological studies, and clinical trials with carotenoid supplementation.

Abbreviations

BMI: Body mass index
BDS: Behavioral Dyscontrol Scale
CERAD: Consortium to Establish a Registry for Alzheimer's Disease
COWAT: Controlled Oral Word Association Test
FOME: Fuld Object Memory Evaluation
GCS: Georgia Centenarian Study
GDRS: Global deterioration rating scale
HPLC: High-performance liquid chromatography
MTBE: Methyl tert-butyl ether
MCI: Mild cognitive impairment
MMSE: Mini-Mental State Examination
MP: Macular pigment
SIB: Severe Impairment Battery
WAIS-III: Wechsler Adult Intelligence Scale-III.

Acknowledgments

The authors acknowledge the valuable recruitment and data acquisition effort from M. Burgess, K. Grier, E. McCarthy, L. Strong, and S. Reynolds, data acquisition team managers; S. Anderson, M. Janke, and T. Savla, data management; M. Poon, project fiscal management. Additional investigators in the Georgia Centenarian Study include Jonathan Arnold (University of Georgia), S. Michal Jazwinski (Tulane University Health Sciences Center), Peter Martin (Iowa State University), William R. Markesbery (deceased), Willard L. Rodgers (University of Michigan), Ilene C. Siegler (Duke University), and J. Lisa Tenover (Palo Alto VA Health Care System). The authors' responsibilities were as follows: M. A. Johnson, L. W. Poon, designed the study; E. J. Johnson, A. Davey, L. S. Miller, J. L. Woodward, conducted and supervised the clinical research; R. C. Green, M. Gearing, P. T. Nelson, supervised brain donation, processing and storage; D. B. Hausman, coordinated inter-institutional agreements and sample transfer; R. Vishwanathan, L. T. M. Scott, H. Y. Chung, analyzed the data; R. Vishwanathan, E. J. Johnson and wrote the manuscript; R. Vishwanathan, E. J. Johnson interpreted data paper. All authors reviewed the paper; E. J. Johnson supervised the serum and brain analyses. R. Vishwanathan conducted the brain analysis. E. J. Johnson and R. Vishwanathan had equal contribution to the paper. None of the authors had a conflict of interests. This research was supported by USDA 58-1950-7-707, DSM Nutritional Products, and NIH 1P01-AG17553. Any opinions, findings, conclusions, or recommendations expressed in this are those of the author and do not necessarily reflect the view of the US Department of Agriculture.

References

[1] O. L. Lopez, W. J. Jagust, S. T. DeKosky et al., "Prevalence and classification of mild cognitive impairment in the cardiovascular health study cognition study," *Archives of Neurology*, vol. 60, no. 10, pp. 1385–1389, 2003.

[2] Y. Gondo and L. W. Poon, "Cognitive function of Centenarians and its influence on longevity," *Annual Review of Gerontology and Geriatrics*, vol. 27, pp. 129–149, 2007.

[3] L. S. Miller, M. B. Mitchell, J. L. Woodard, A. Davey, P. Martin, and L. W. Poon, "Cognitive performance in centenarians and the oldest old: norms from the georgia centenarian study," *Aging, Neuropsychology, and Cognition*, vol. 17, no. 5, pp. 575–590, 2010.

[4] *Alzheimer's Association 2010 Alzheimer's Disease Facts and Figures*, Alzheimer's Associaton National Office, Chicago, Ill, USA, 2010.

[5] M. C. Morris, D. A. Evans, C. C. Tangney, J. L. Bienias, and R. S. Wilson, "Associations of vegetable and fruit consumption with age-related cognitive change," *Neurology*, vol. 67, no. 8, pp. 1370–1376, 2006.

[6] L. Lee, S. A. Kang, H. O. Lee et al., "Relationships between dietary intake and cognitive function level in Korean elderly people," *Public Health*, vol. 115, no. 2, pp. 133–138, 2001.

[7] R. M. Ortega, A. M. Requejo, P. Andrés et al., "Dietary intake and cognitive function in a group of elderly people," *American Journal of Clinical Nutrition*, vol. 66, no. 4, pp. 803–809, 1997.

[8] J. H. Kang, A. Ascherio, and F. Grodstein, "Fruit and vegetable consumption and cognitive decline in aging women," *Annals of Neurology*, vol. 57, no. 5, pp. 713–720, 2005.

[9] J. H. Kang and F. Grodstein, "Plasma carotenoids and tocopherols and cognitive function: a prospective study," *Neurobiology of Aging*, vol. 29, no. 9, pp. 1394–1403, 2008.

[10] P. Rinaldi, M. C. Polidori, A. Metastasio et al., "Plasma antioxidants are similarly depleted in mild cognitive impairment and in Alzheimer's disease," *Neurobiology of Aging*, vol. 24, no. 7, pp. 915–919, 2003.

[11] J. N. Keller, F. A. Schmitt, S. W. Scheff et al., "Evidence of increased oxidative damage in subjects with mild cognitive impairment," *Neurology*, vol. 64, no. 7, pp. 1152–1156, 2005.

[12] E. Tarkowski, N. Andreasen, A. Tarkowski, and K. Blennow, "Intrathecal inflammation precedes development of Alzheimer's disease," *Journal of Neurology, Neurosurgery and Psychiatry*, vol. 74, no. 9, pp. 1200–1205, 2003.

[13] C. E. Teunissen, M. P. J. Van Boxtel, H. Bosma et al., "Inflammation markers in relation to cognition in a healthy aging population," *Journal of Neuroimmunology*, vol. 134, no. 1-2, pp. 142–150, 2003.

[14] M. J. Engelhart, M. I. Geerlings, J. Meijer et al., "Inflammatory proteins in plasma and the risk of dementia: the Rotterdam Study," *Archives of Neurology*, vol. 61, no. 5, pp. 668–672, 2004.

[15] M. A. Pappolla, M. A. Smith, T. Bryant-Thomas et al., "Cholesterol, oxidative stress, and Alzheimer's disease: expanding the horizons of pathogenesis," *Free Radical Biology and Medicine*, vol. 33, no. 2, pp. 173–181, 2002.

[16] T. Wyss-Coray, "Inflammation in Alzheimer disease: driving force, bystander or beneficial response?" *Nature Medicine*, vol. 12, no. 9, pp. 1005–1015, 2006.

[17] D. Praticò, "Alzheimer's disease and oxygen radicals: new insights," *Biochemical Pharmacology*, vol. 63, no. 4, pp. 563–567, 2002.

[18] D. Praticò and J. Q. Trojanowski, "Inflammatory hypotheses: novel mechanisms of Alzheimer's neurodegeneration and new therapeutic targets?" *Neurobiology of Aging*, vol. 21, no. 3, pp. 441–445, 2000.

[19] P. L. McGeer, E. G. McGeer, and K. Yasojima, "Alzheimer disease and neuroinflammation," *Journal of Neural Transmission, Supplement*, no. 59, pp. 53–57, 2000.

[20] G. Ravaglia, P. Forti, F. Maioli et al., "Homocysteine and folate as risk factors for dementia and Alzheimer disease," *American Journal of Clinical Nutrition*, vol. 82, no. 3, pp. 636–643, 2005.

[21] L. W. Poon, M. Jazwinski, R. Green et al., "Methodological consideration in studying centenarians: lessons learned from the Georgia Centenarian Studies," in *Annual Review of Gerontology and Geriatrics*, L. W. Poon and T. T. Perls, Eds., pp. 231–264, Springer, New York, NY, USA, 2007.

[22] E. J. Johnson, K. McDonald, S. M. Caldarella, H. Y. Chung, A. M. Troen, and D. M. Snodderly, "Cognitive findings of an exploratory trial of docosahexaenoic acid and lutein supplementation in older women," *Nutritional Neuroscience*, vol. 11, no. 2, pp. 75–83, 2008.

[23] N. E. Craft, T. B. Haitema, K. M. Garnett, K. A. Fitch, and C. K. Dorey, "Carotenoid, tocopherol, and retinol concentrations in elderly human brain," *Journal of Nutrition, Health and Aging*, vol. 8, no. 3, pp. 156–162, 2004.

[24] E. J. Johnson, H. Y. Chung, S. M. Caldarella, and D. Max Snodderly, "The influence of supplemental lutein and docosahexaenoic acid on serum, lipoproteins, and macular pigmentation," *American Journal of Clinical Nutrition*, vol. 87, no. 5, pp. 1521–1529, 2008.

[25] J. H. Park, H. J. Hwang, M. K. Kim, and Y. C. Lee-Kim, "Con antioxidant vitamin status of the second generation rat brain sections," *Korean Journal of Nutrition*, vol. 34, pp. 754–761, 2001.

[26] R. Vishwanathan, M. Neuringer, D. M. Snodderly, W. Schalch, and E. J. Johnson, "Macular lutein and zeaxanthin are related to brain lutein and zeaxanthin in primates," *Nutritional Neuroscience*, vol. 16, no. 1, pp. 21–29, 2013.

[27] J. I. Sheikh and J. A. Yesavage, "Geriatric Depression Scale (GDS): recent evidence and development of a shorter version," *Clinical Gerontologist*, vol. 5, no. 1-2, pp. 165–173, 1986.

[28] M. F. Folstein, S. E. Folstein, and P. R. McHugh, "'Mini mental state'. A practical method for grading the cognitive state of patients for the clinician," *Journal of Psychiatric Research*, vol. 12, no. 3, pp. 189–198, 1975.

[29] B. Reisberg, S. H. Ferris, M. J. De Leon, and T. Crook, "The global deterioration scale for assessment of primary degenerative dementia," *American Journal of Psychiatry*, vol. 139, no. 9, pp. 1136–1139, 1982.

[30] J. Saxton, K. L. McGonigle-Gibson, A. A. Swihart, V. J. Miller, and F. Boller, "Assessment of the severly impaired patient: description and validation of a new neuropsychological test battery," *Psychological Assessment*, vol. 2, no. 3, pp. 298–303, 1990.

[31] P. A. Fuld, *Fuld Object Memory Evaluation Instruction Manual*, Stoetling, Wood Dale, Ill, USA, 1981.

[32] D. Wechsler, *Wechsler Adult Intelligence Scale-III*, The Psychological Corporation, San Antonio, Tex, USA, 1997.

[33] J. Grigsby, K. Kaye, and L. J. Robbins, "Reliabilities, norms and factor structure of the Behavioral Dyscontrol Scale," *Perceptual and Motor Skills*, vol. 74, no. 3, pp. 883–892, 1992.

[34] A. Benton and K. Hamsler, *Multilingual Aphasia Examination*, University of Iowa, Iowa City, Iowa, USA, 1997.

[35] R. C. Atkinson and R. M. Shiffrin, "The control of short-term memory," *Scientific American*, vol. 225, no. 2, pp. 82–90, 1971.

[36] M. J. Chandler, L. H. Lacritz, L. S. Hynan et al., "A total score for the CERAD neuropsychological battery," *Neurology*, vol. 65, no. 1, pp. 102–106, 2005.

[37] K. A. Welsh-Bohmer and R. C. Mohs, "Neuropsychological assessment of Alzheimer's disease," *Neurology*, vol. 49, no. 3, pp. S11–S13, 1997.

[38] K. Shaw, M. Gearing, A. Davey et al., "Successful recruitment of centenarians for post-mortem brain donation: results from the Georgia Centenarian Study," *Journal of Bioscience and Medicine*, vol. 2, no. 1, pp. 1–6, 2012.

[39] S. H. Ferris, T. Crook, C. Flicker, B. Reisberg, and R. T. Bartus, "Assessing cognitive impairment and evaluating treatment effects: psychometric performance test," in *Handbook For Clinical Memory Assessment of Older Adults*, L. S. Poon, Ed., pp. 139–148, American Psychological Association, Washington, DC, USA, 1986.

[40] R. Letz, *NES2 User's Manual (version 4.4)*, Neurobehavioral Systems, Winchester, Mass, USA, 1991.

[41] B. Johansson and S. H. Sarit, "Early cognitive markers of the incidence of dementia and mortality: a longitudinal population based study of the oldest old," *International Journal of Geriatric Psychiatry*, vol. 12, pp. 53–59, 1997.

[42] M. Payton, K. M. Riggs, A. Spiro, S. T. Weiss, and H. Hu, "Relations of bone and blood lead to cognitive function: the VA normative aging study," *Neurotoxicology and Teratology*, vol. 20, no. 1, pp. 19–27, 1998.

[43] E. D. Bigler and D. F. Tate, "Brain volume, intracranial volume, and dementia," *Investigative Radiology*, vol. 36, no. 9, pp. 539–546, 2001.

[44] V. Haroutunian, L. B. Hoffman, and M. S. Beeri, "Is there a neuropathology difference between mild cognitive impairment and dementia?" *Dialogues in Clinical Neuroscience*, vol. 11, no. 2, pp. 171–179, 2009.

[45] W. J. Perrig, P. Perrig, and H. B. Stähelin, "The relation between antioxidants and memory performance in the old and very old," *Journal of the American Geriatrics Society*, vol. 45, no. 6, pp. 718–724, 1997.

[46] J. Warsama Jama, L. J. Launer, J. C. M. Witteman et al., "Dietary antioxidants and cognitive function in a population-based sample of older persons: the Rotterdam study," *American Journal of Epidemiology*, vol. 144, no. 3, pp. 275–280, 1996.

[47] S. L. Gray, J. T. Hanlon, L. R. Landerman, M. Artz, K. E. Schmader, and G. G. Fillenbaum, "Is antioxidant use protective of cognitive function in the community-dwelling elderly?" *American Journal Geriatric Pharmacotherapy*, vol. 1, no. 1, pp. 3–10, 2003.

[48] A. Smith, R. Clark, D. Nutt, J. Haller, S. Hayward, and K. Perry, "Anti-oxidant vitamins and mental performance of the elderly," *Human Psychopharmacology*, vol. 14, pp. 459–471, 1999.

[49] N. T. Akbaraly, H. Faure, V. Gourlet, A. Favier, and C. Berr, "Plasma carotenoid levels and cognitive performance in an elderly population: results of the EVA Study," *Journals of Gerontology A*, vol. 62, no. 3, pp. 308–316, 2007.

[50] M. C. Morris, D. A. Evans, J. L. Bienias et al., "Dietary intake of antioxidant nutrients and the risk of incident Alzheimer disease in a biracial community study," *Journal of the American Medical Association*, vol. 287, no. 24, pp. 3230–3237, 2002.

[51] K. Yaffe, T. E. Clemons, W. L. McBee, and A. S. Lindblad, "Impact of antioxidants, zinc, and copper on cognition in the elderly: a randomized, controlled trial," *Neurology*, vol. 63, no. 9, pp. 1705–1707, 2004.

[52] P. Mecocci, M. Cristina Polidori, A. Cherubini et al., "Lymphocyte oxidative DNA damage and plasma antioxidants in Alzheimer disease," *Archives of Neurology*, vol. 59, no. 5, pp. 794–798, 2002.

[53] http://fnic.nal.usda.gov/.

[54] D. M. Snodderly, "Evidence for protection against age-related macular degeneration by carotenoids and antioxidant vitamins," *American Journal of Clinical Nutrition*, vol. 62, no. 6, pp. 1448S–1461S, 1995.

[55] A. A. Woodall, G. Britton, and M. J. Jackson, "Carotenoids and protection of phospholipids in solution or in liposomes against oxidation by peroxyl radicals: relationship between carotenoid structure and protective ability," *Biochimica et Biophysica Acta*, vol. 1336, no. 3, pp. 575–586, 1997.

[56] A. A. Woodall, S. W. M. Lee, R. J. Weesie, M. J. Jackson, and G. Britton, "Oxidation of carotenoids by free radicals: relationship between structure and reactivity," *Biochimica et Biophysica Acta*, vol. 1336, no. 1, pp. 33–42, 1997.

[57] W. Stahl, A. Junghans, B. De Boer, E. S. Driomina, K. Briviba, and H. Sies, "Carotenoid mixtures protect multilamellar liposomes against oxidative damage: synergistic effects of lycopene and lutein," *FEBS Letters*, vol. 427, no. 2, pp. 305–308, 1998.

[58] W. Stahl and H. Sies, "Antioxidant activity of carotenoids," *Molecular Aspects of Medicine*, vol. 24, no. 6, pp. 345–351, 2003.

[59] W. I. Gruszecki, "Carotenoid orientation: role in membrane stabilization," in *Carotenoids in Health and Disease*, N. I. Krinsky, S. T. Mayne, and H. Sies, Eds., pp. 151–163, Marcel Dekker, New York, NY, USA, 2004.

[60] W. Stahl and H. Sies, "Effects of carotenoids and retinoids on gap junctional communication," *BioFactors*, vol. 15, no. 2-4, pp. 95–98, 2001.

[61] B. R. Hammond and B. R. Wooten, "CFF thresholds: relation to macular pigment optical density," *Ophthalmic and Physiological Optics*, vol. 25, no. 4, pp. 315–319, 2005.

[62] L. M. Renzi and B. R. Hammond, "The relation between the macular carotenoids, lutein and zeaxanthin, and temporal vision," *Ophthalmic and Physiological Optics*, vol. 30, no. 4, pp. 351–357, 2010.

[63] L. M. Renzi and B. R. Hammond, "The effect of macular pigment on heterochromatic luminance contrast," *Experimental Eye Research*, vol. 91, no. 6, pp. 896–900, 2010.

[64] S. B. Kritchevsky, A. J. Bush, M. Pahor, and M. D. Gross, "Serum carotenoids and markers of inflammation in nonsmokers," *American Journal of Epidemiology*, vol. 152, no. 11, pp. 1065–1071, 2000.

[65] E. J. Johnson, "Obesity, lutein metabolism, and age-related macular degeneration: a web of connections," *Nutrition Reviews*, vol. 63, no. 1, pp. 9–15, 2005.

[66] A. Schuitemaker, M. G. Dik, R. Veerhuis et al., "Inflammatory markers in AD and MCI patients with different biomarker profiles," *Neurobiology of Aging*, vol. 30, no. 11, pp. 1885–1889, 2009.

[67] *Alzheimer's Association 2010 Alzheimer's Disease Facts and Figures*, Alzheimer's Association National Office, Chicago, Ill, USA, 2010.

[68] F. Grodstein, J. H. Kang, R. J. Glynn, N. R. Cook, and J. M. Gaziano, "A randomized trial of beta carotene supplementation and cognitive function in men: the physicians' health study II," *Archives of Internal Medicine*, vol. 167, no. 20, pp. 2184–2190, 2007.

[69] J. H. Kang, N. R. Cook, J. E. Manson, J. E. Buring, C. M. Albert, and F. Grodstein, "Vitamin E, Vitamin C, Beta carotene, and cognitive function among women with or at risk of cardiovascular disease: the women's antioxidant and cardiovascular study," *Circulation*, vol. 119, no. 21, pp. 2772–2780, 2009.

[70] A. B. Mendelsohn, S. H. Belle, G. P. Stoehr, and M. Ganguli, "Use of antioxidant supplements and its association with cognitive function in a rural elderly cohort: the movies project," *American Journal of Epidemiology*, vol. 148, no. 1, pp. 38–44, 1998.

[71] E. J. Johnson, "Human studies on bioavailability and serum response of carotenoids," in *CRC Handbook of Antioxidants*, E. Cadenas and L. Packer, Eds., pp. 265–277, Marcel Dekker, New York, NY, USA, 2nd edition, 2001.

[72] B. R. Hammond, E. J. Johnson, R. M. Russell et al., "Dietary modification of human macular pigment density," *Investigative Ophthalmology & Visual Science*, vol. 38, pp. 1795–1801, 1997.

[73] E. J. Johnson, B. R. Hammond, K. J. Yeum et al., "Relation among serum and tissue concentrations of lutein and zeaxanthin and macular pigment density," *American Journal of Clinical Nutrition*, vol. 71, no. 6, pp. 1555–1562, 2000.

16

A Review of the Effects of Physical Activity and Exercise on Cognitive and Brain Functions in Older Adults

Louis Bherer,[1,2] **Kirk I. Erickson,**[3] **and Teresa Liu-Ambrose**[4,5]

[1] *PERFORM Centre, Concordia University, Montreal, QC, Canada*
[2] *Research Center, Institut Universitaire de Gériatrie de Montréal, Montreal, QC, Canada*
[3] *Department of Psychology, University of Pittsburgh, Pittsburgh, PA, USA*
[4] *Department of Physical Therapy, University of British Columbia, Vancouver, BC, Canada*
[5] *Brain Research Centre, University of British Columbia, Vancouver Coastal Health Research Institute, Vancouver, BC, Canada*

Correspondence should be addressed to Louis Bherer; louis.bherer@concordia.ca

Academic Editor: Karl Rosengren

Studies supporting the notion that physical activity and exercise can help alleviate the negative impact of age on the body and the mind abound. This literature review provides an overview of important findings in this fast growing research domain. Results from cross-sectional, longitudinal, and intervention studies with healthy older adults, frail patients, and persons suffering from mild cognitive impairment and dementia are reviewed and discussed. Together these finding suggest that physical exercise is a promising nonpharmaceutical intervention to prevent age-related cognitive decline and neurodegenerative diseases.

1. Introduction

Chronological aging, or senescence, is associated with an increased risk of chronic conditions and diseases such as cognitive impairment, cardiovascular disease, and metabolic syndrome. Due to prolonged life expectancy, age-related diseases have increased in alarming proportions in recent decades [1]. An increasing body of studies have suggested that lifestyle factors have a significant impact on how well people age. For example, Fratiglioni et al. [2] reported that three lifestyle factors can play a significant role in slowing the rate of cognitive decline and preventing dementia: a socially integrated network, cognitive leisure activity, and regular physical activity. In this review and others [3, 4], it is argued that out of these lifestyle factors, physical activity has the most support as protective against the deleterious effects of age on health and cognition. Broadly defined, physical activity refers to activity that is part of one's daily life involving bodily movements and the use of skeletal muscles. Physical exercise is a subcategory of physical activity that is planned, structured, and purposive to improve specific physical skills or physical fitness. Evidence suggests that physical activity and exercise can to some extent lower the risk of adverse outcomes associated with advancing age.

Physical activity maintained throughout life is associated with lower incidence and prevalence of chronic diseases such as cancer, diabetes and cardiovascular and coronary heart diseases [5, 6]. Recent studies suggest that physical exercise also protects against dementia [7]. Yet, despite this promise, the ways in which physical activity impacts the rate and prevalence of cognitive decline is still under investigation. Furthermore, several open issues call for further research, such as the dose-response relationship, the level of change or protection provided by physical activity, the biological and/or psychological mechanisms by which these effects occur and whether physical activity can be beneficial despite chronic medical conditions, neurological syndromes such as dementia, and the physical limitations observed in frail patients. Although recent advancements in neuroimaging techniques and genetics have opened new research avenues, more studies are required to provide definitive answers to these important questions. This literature review aims to provide an overview of studies that have attempted to assess whether and how physical activity and exercise positively impact older adults at any age and with various physical and psychological conditions.

2. Aging and Neurocognitive Functions

It is generally assumed that age brings with it declines in performance in a multitude of cognitive tasks that require a variety of perceptual and cognitive processes (for extensive reviews of the literature see [3, 8, 9]). More specifically, processing speed declines early in the course of aging, which has recently been associated with loss of white matter integrity [10]. Working memory, or the ability to maintain and consciously manipulate information, is also highly age-sensitive. The age-related difference in working memory tends to be greater if executive control processes such as inhibition, updating, and manipulation are required, and even greater if the memory load (i.e., the number of items to be maintained) is high. These deficits have sometimes been associated with reduced task-related activation in older compared to younger adults in frontal regions of the cerebral cortex. Other studies also reported higher task-related activation in older adults, a phenomenon possibly associated with compensation for age-related changes in brain structure and functions [9]. Older adults also tend to show reduced inhibition compared to younger adults. As a result, they are more distracted by irrelevant information and more affected by proactive interference (i.e., interference induced by current learning on further encoding of new information). Furthermore, episodic memory declines in late adulthood, likely due to poor encoding strategies, less use of environmental support, and deficits in binding new information with existing knowledge during encoding.

Structural and functional brain imaging studies have provided insights into potential brain mechanisms of cognitive aging. For instance, changes in brain volume occur faster in adults after 50 years of age, with an annual decline of 0.35% compared to 0.12% in young adults (see [11, 12] for reviews). Ventricle dilatation can approximate 4.25% per year at 70 years of age compared to 0.43% in young adults. The volume of the hippocampus, a cerebral structure that plays a major role in memory formation, is also sensitive to age, with an annual decline of 0.86% per year (from 26 to 82 years), 1.18% per year after 50 years, and 1.85% per year after 70 years. Yet, rate of change is difficult to appreciate due to the lack of longitudinal studies. In a recent study, Raz et al. [13] followed participants over 30 months and observed that the hippocampus, the entorhinal cortex, the orbital-frontal cortex, and the cerebellum showed volumetric changes after only 15 months, while other brain structures showed shrinkage after 30 months, including the caudate nucleus, the prefrontal subcortical white matter, and the corpus callosum. However, some brain structures showed almost no change (the primary visual cortices, the putamen, and the pons). In addition, aging is associated with overall changes in white matter integrity (e.g., leukoaraiosis), with greater changes occurring after the seventh decade, and localized preferentially in the frontal and prefrontal regions [11]. These changes are more pronounced in patients with vascular diseases such as hypertension and type-2 diabetes.

Cerebral metabolism is also altered by age, with a reduction in regional cerebral metabolic rate for glucose, oxygen, and blood flow. Although it is frequently assumed that structural changes are associated with a decline in brain metabolism, recent evidence suggests otherwise. For example, Chen et al. [14] observed that, in some brain regions, age-associated reductions in cerebral blood flow could occur independently of regional atrophy [14].

3. Physical Activity and Cognition in Healthy Seniors

Several studies support the notion that physical activity is a significant moderator of age-related cognitive decline. In cross-sectional studies, age-related differences in cognitive performance observed when older adults are compared to younger participants are reduced if the comparisons involved higher-fit individuals rather than sedentary older adults [15–19]. As a whole, these cross-sectional studies suggest that cardiorespiratory fitness is associated with more efficient cognitive functions.

In longitudinal studies, older adults that participate in physical activity show less cognitive decline over two- to 10-year follow-up periods. For instance, in a study by Barnes et al. [20] cardiorespiratory fitness assessed at baseline predicted cognitive performance six years later in a variety of cognitive domains (working memory, processing speed, attention, and general mental functioning). In nationally representative samples of noninstitutionalized persons aged 50 years and older and across 11 European countries (Austria, Germany, Sweden, Denmark, Switzerland, the Netherlands, Belgium, France, Spain, Italy, and Greece) Aichberger et al. [21] reported that individuals who participated in any type of regular physical activity showed less cognitive decline after 2.5 years, especially when they engaged in vigorous activities more than once a week.

The impact of physical activity on cognition in older adults is more strongly supported by results from intervention studies, which generally show that older adults who have completed a physical activity program that produces significant increases in cardiorespiratory fitness (indexed by direct measures or estimation of $VO_{2\,max}$) often show enhanced cognitive performance. Dustman et al. [22] compared middle-aged and older individuals who completed a four-month aerobic training program to age-matched controls who participated in strength and flexibility exercises and controls who did not exercise. Only the aerobic training group showed improved cardiorespiratory function, along with improvements on a simple RT task. Similar results were obtained in women aged 57 to 85 years old following a three-year physical training program [23]. Hawkins et al. [24] reported that, in older adults, a 10-week aquatic fitness program led to greater improvement in task conditions that tap dual-task and switching abilities compared to conditions that do not require executive or attentional control processes. In Kramer et al.'s [25] study, older adults who completed a six-month aerobic training program (walking) showed a significant improvement in cognitive performance, unlike those who completed a stretching program. Cognitive improvement was greater in tasks that tapped attentional control or executive control functions and was correlated with improvement in $VO_{2\,max}$. In another study, Albinet et al. [26] reported that 12 weeks of aerobic training lead to enhanced performance in executive control and increased heart rate variability in older men and women aged 65–78. These results suggest that aerobic exercise may be an important cardiac and brain protective factor as people age. The greater improvement induced by aerobic training in executive control compared to other cognitive domains has also been confirmed by several meta-analyses (see [27] but see [28] for different conclusions).

The selective benefit of aerobic exercise for tasks that tap executive control was also observed in another recent study [29], where 57 older adults completed a 10-month training program (aerobic versus strength and flexibility). The positive effect on executive control was observed after aerobic training only. In another study, Renaud et al. [30] observed that only 12 weeks of aerobic training induced a significant improvement in cardiorespiratory capacity (estimated $VO_{2\,max}$) along with enhanced motor response preparation, such that participants maintained response preparation over time more efficiently after the training program. These results provide additional support for the notion that improving aerobic fitness may enhance attentional control mechanisms in older adults. In a meta-analytic review of randomized-control trials of aerobic exercise on neurocognitive functions, Smith et al. [31] examined 29 studies conducted between 1966 and 2009 (including more than 2,000 participants and 234 effect sizes). They found that individuals who were randomly assigned to aerobic exercise training showed modest improvements in attention, processing speed, executive function, and memory, with less convincing effects on working memory. These results, along with those from Colcombe and Kramer [27], suggest a selective effect of aerobic exercise on neurocognitive functions. However, not all studies reported a significant correlation between improvement in cardiorespiratory fitness outcomes and cognitive improvement (see [28, 32] meta-analysis), which suggests that physiological mechanisms supporting cognitive enhancement remain to be fully understood.

Studies reported above highlight that aerobic exercise enhances cognitive function. However, recent evidence now suggests that other types of exercise training, such as resistance training, may also benefit cognition. Cassilhas and colleagues [33] demonstrated that six months of either thrice-weekly moderate or high intensity resistance training improved memory performance and verbal concept formation among 62 community-dwelling senior men aged 65 to 75 years. Liu-Ambrose and colleagues [34] demonstrated that an individualized home-based program of balance and strength retraining significantly improved selective attention and conflict resolution as measured by the Stroop Test after six months among seniors aged 70 years and older with a recent history of falls. The finding of this study is notable given that many have hypothesized that the cognitive and neural benefits of exercise must occur within the context of social engagement for it to be effective [35]. Liu-Ambrose and colleagues [36] also demonstrated that 12 months of either once-weekly or twice-weekly progressive resistance training improved Stroop Test performance among 155 community-dwelling senior women aged 65 to 75 years. Enhanced selective attention and conflict resolution were also associated with increased gait speed. Clinically, improved gait speed predicts a substantial reduction in both morbidity [37] and mortality [38, 39]. These results illustrate the clinical significance of cognitive gains induced by resistance training. Therefore, it seems that in addition to endurance training, resistance training should be seriously considered as a potential modifier of cognitive functions in older adults. Recent studies also suggest that motor learning and coordinative exercise could also be used to enhance cognitive function in this population (see [40]).

4. Physical Activity and Brain Structures and Functions in Older Adults

The biological mechanisms by which cognition is enhanced through physical exercise training remain to be completely elucidated, although the number of studies that have tried to identify these mechanisms has increased in the last 10 years. For the most part, the studies that support the notion that physical exercise has an impact on brain functions have focused on direct biological effects of exercise using both animal and human models. However, as suggested by Spirduso et al. [41] exercise may enhance cognition indirectly by improving health conditions (stress, sleep) and reducing chronic diseases (coronary heart diseases) that impact neurocognitive functions.

The evidence for the direct effects of exercise on the brain first came from animal studies. In a comprehensive literature review, Lista and Sorrentino [42] suggest that the basic neurobiological mechanisms associated with exercise can occur at two levels, supramolecular and molecular. At the supramolecular level, physical activity has been found to induce angiogenesis or the physiological process by which new blood vessels grow from preexisting vessels [43, 44]. Physical activity has also been associated with neurogenesis, or neural cell proliferation, in the hippocampus in elderly rats [45]. Although the functional significance of this effect remains unclear, there is evidence that newly formed neurons can integrate into a neural network and become functional [46]. Exercise-induced synaptogenesis has also been reported [47, 48].

The molecular mechanisms by which exercise induces angiogenesis, neurogenesis, and synaptogenesis have received growing attention in the last few years. Again, the evidence comes mainly from animal studies that showed exercise-associated changes in molecular growth factors such as brain-derived neurotrophic factor (BDNF), which plays a crucial role in neuroplasticity and neuroprotection, and increased production of insulin-like growth factor 1 (IGF-1), which is involved in both neurogenesis and angiogenesis. Moreover, neurotransmitter systems also seem to be modulated through exercise (see [42]). Until very recently, evidence for the molecular and supramolecular effects of exercise came exclusively from animal studies.

However, a very innovative study [49] recently showed that greater exercise-related increases in BDNF were associated with increased hippocampal volume. If reproduced, these results would confirm that physical exercise induces genuine neurotrophic effects on brain structures and functions at the molecular, supramolecular, and structural levels.

In humans, several studies using structural and functional brain imaging, or electrophysiological measures of brain activity, suggest that physical exercise induces transient and permanent changes at the structural and functional levels in the aging brain [50–54]. Using voxel-based morphometry (VBM), or detailed image segmentation of high-resolution brain scans, Colcombe et al. [55] reported that a higher cardiorespiratory fitness level ($VO_{2\,max}$) was associated with a reduced loss of grey and white matter in the frontal, prefrontal, and temporal regions in older adults. In another study, Erickson et al. [56] performed a region-of-interest analysis on magnetic resonance images in 165 nondemented older adults and found that higher fitness levels were associated with larger left and right hippocampi that further correlated with better spatial memory performance. These findings suggest that aerobic fitness is associated with changes in brain structures that translate into better cognitive function in older adults (see also [49, 57]).

Even more striking evidence of the benefit of fitness on brain functions comes from functional brain imaging studies (fMRI). It has been shown that enhanced cardiovascular functions after aerobic training are associated with greater task-relevant activity in brain areas recruited in an attentional control task [58]. Similarly, 12 months of resistance training in community-dwelling senior women led to functional changes in two regions of the cortex previously associated with response inhibition processes, the anterior portion of the left middle temporal gyrus, and the left anterior insula extending into lateral orbital frontal cortex [36]. These hemodynamic effects cooccurred with improved task performance. Moreover, Voss et al. [59] found changes in functional connectivity after aerobic exercise training in older adults. They observed that 12 months of training leads to increased connectivity in regional connections that support both the default-mode network and the frontal executive network, suggesting that physical exercise has a restorative effect on large-scale brain circuitry. Changes in these large-scale brain networks have received increasing attention in aging neuroscience, as they indicate massive changes in brain systems.

A complete understanding of the potential for physical activity to protect the brain from the effects of age would require investigating the indirect influences of exercise on cognition. There is growing evidence that exercise has indirect beneficial effects on cognition through its impact on factors that are known to alter neurocognitive integrity [60]. Spirduso et al. [60] suggest three groups of potential mediators in the relationship between exercise and cognition: physical resources, chronic diseases or states, and mental resources. It has been shown that physical exercise enhances mental resources by reducing depression [61], anxiety, and chronic stress and improving self-efficacy [62]. The effect of physical activity on cognitive function might also be mediated by physical resources such as diet [63] and sleep [64, 65]. It remains to be seen whether these factors in fact mediate the positive effects that exercise has on cognitive and brain health.

5. Physical Activity and Cognition in Frail Older Adults

With increasing age, and specifically with advanced age (i.e., over 75 years), many individuals eventually develop one or more of a group of related medical problems referred to as geriatric syndromes. Perceptual limitations (vision and hearing problems), urinary incontinence, falls, delirium, and dementia are examples of geriatric syndromes. These syndromes are characterized by having more than one cause and by involving several different body systems. An emerging symptom that appears particularly relevant to our purpose is frailty, as it apparently limits physical activity and exercise. Frailty is defined as a complex health state of increased vulnerability to stressors due to impairments in multiple systems. It has been associated with adverse outcomes such as disability, falls, hospitalization, and death [66]. With aging, the prevalence of frailty increases from 7% in older adults aged between 65 and 74 years to 18% between 75 and 84 years and 37% at age 85 years and older [67]. Physical inactivity is a major risk factor for frailty [66]. It is important to note that frailty is not a contraindication for physical activity. On the contrary, it may be one of the most compelling reasons to prescribe physical exercise [68].

Results from longitudinal studies show that physical activity and exercise can prevent frailty in older adults. In a recent study, 2,964 older adults were followed for five years to determine the relationship between physical activity and the risk of becoming frail [69]. Results showed that individuals who regularly exercised at baseline were less likely to develop frailty within a five-year period than sedentary individuals, even after adjusting for baseline health conditions and demographic characteristics.

Intervention studies also suggest that physical activity can improve several frailty syndrome components, especially sarcopenia (reduction in skeletal muscle mass) and functional impairment [68]. Moreover, in a recent randomized controlled trial that assessed the impact of a three-month physical training intervention on quality of life in 77 physically frail persons aged 75 years and older [70], it was observed that functional exercises twice a day to improve balance and lower extremity muscle strength, in addition to strength training twice a week, helped to improve psychological well-being associated with physical functioning, emotion, and mental health. To our knowledge, only one study has shown that physical exercise training can help improve cognition in frail older adults. Langlois et al. [71] recently observed that three months of training in frail older adults resulted in significant improvement in both physical capacity and cognitive performance (executive functions, processing speed, and working memory) as well as quality of life associated with leisure activities and satisfaction with physical capacity.

6. Physical Activity and Cognition in Older Adults with Mild Cognitive Impairment and Dementia

According to the Alzheimer's Association [72], one in eight people aged 65 and older (13%) and 43% of people 85 and older have Alzheimer's disease. Currently, there is no cure for Alzheimer's disease. However, research has suggested that physical activity and exercise can significantly reduce the risk of developing it. In a recent cross-sectional study that compared 198 subjects with mild cognitive impairment (MCI) to 1,126 with normal cognition, Geda et al. [73] observed that moderate activity during midlife was associated with a 39% lower risk of having mild cognitive impairment in later life. Late-life moderate exercise was associated with a 32% lower risk for MCI. Burns et al. [74] explored the effect of exercise on cognitively impaired individuals and found an association between direct measures of cardiorespiratory fitness (VO_2 peak) and cognition (neuropsychological test battery) in normal older participants and patients in the early stage of Alzheimer's dementia (AD). Results showed that cardiorespiratory fitness was modestly reduced in patients with AD compared to participants without dementia. Although no significant association was found between cardiorespiratory fitness and cognition in participants without dementia, higher fitness levels in early AD participants were associated with larger brain volume (less brain atrophy), even when controlling for age, sex, dementia severity, and physical frailty.

In a longitudinal study exploring the association between midlife physical activity and late-life cognitive function and dementia, Chang et al. [75] observed that being active (around 5 hours per week) was associated with higher scores in processing speed, memory, and executive functions, even after controlling for demographic and cardiovascular factors. Moreover, participants who reported being active were significantly less likely to have dementia in later life. In a prospective study following 1,740 persons older than 65 years without cognitive impairment for a period of 6.2 years, Larson et al. [7] reported reduced dementia incidence for individuals who exercised three or more times a week (13 per 1,000 person-years) compared to those who exercised fewer than three times a week (19.7 per 1,000 person-years), demonstrating a 32% reduced risk for dementia.

Interestingly, correlations have also been reported between muscle strength and a lower risk of AD and a slower rate of cognitive decline. Having followed 900 community-based older persons without dementia at baseline, Boyle et al. [76] showed a lower rate of global cognitive decline, MCI and AD in older adults with higher muscle strength. The protective effects remained after adjustment for several covariates, including body mass index, physical activity, pulmonary function, vascular risk factors, vascular diseases, and apolipoprotein E4 status. Furthermore, in a recent meta-analysis of prospective studies that covered 15 prospective studies (12 cohorts) and 33,816 nondemented individuals, 3,210 of which showed cognitive decline during the one- to 12-year followup, Sofi et al. [77] observed that physical activity significantly and consistently prevented cognitive decline. Individuals who were highly physically active showed 38% less risk of cognitive decline, and those who did low-to-moderate level exercise also showed a significantly 35% reduced risk.

Results from intervention studies are scarce. A meta-analysis of randomized controlled trials (2,020 participants; 30 trials) [78] reported beneficial effects of physical activity on physical fitness (effect size = 0.69) and cognitive function (effect size = 0.57) in adults with cognitive impairment (MCI and dementia). However, other studies have reported modest benefits [79] or no appreciable effect [80] of physical activity on cognition in patients with cognitive impairment. A recent randomized clinical study evaluated the impact of a six-month aerobic exercise intervention in individuals with mild cognitive impairment [81]. Thirty-three older adults (17 women) with amnestic mild cognitive impairment ranging in age from 55 to 85 years were randomized to either a highintensity aerobic exercise (75–85% of heart rate capacity) or a stretching control group. Results showed beneficial effects of aerobic exercise, especially in speed of processing and executive functioning, although in some tests, gender differences in cognitive improvement were observed, despite comparable gains in cardiorespiratory fitness in men and women. In a randomized controlled study, Kemoun et al. [82] examined the benefits of a 15-week physical activity program in 31 subjects (mean age of 82 years). They reported that a physical activity program can slow cognitive decline and improve quality of walking in elderly persons with dementia. A more recent study assessed the cognitive impact of a Tai-Chi intervention group (n = 171) compared to a stretching and toning group (n = 218) in older adults with cognitive impairment [83]. Results showed that both groups improved in global cognitive function, delayed recall, and subjective cognitive complaints. However, improvements in balance, visual span, and Clinical Dementia Rating scores were observed in the intervention group only. Future studies are needed to specify whether interventions should involve aerobic or strength training exercises or both to improve cognition in MCI patients. Nagamatsu et al. [84] recently reported that patients who completed six months of aerobic or strength training exercise showed improved spatial memory performance, but only the aerobic group showed a correlation between physical capacity after intervention and spatial memory performance. The mechanisms by which exercise impacts cognition in this population thus deserve further study.

7. Conclusions

In recent decades, an increasing number of studies have suggested that people should adopt physical activity and exercise as part of their lifestyle to alleviate the negative impact of aging on the body and the mind. However, we still do not understand how physical activity impacts the rate of cognitive decline. One major issue is whether physical activity broadly defined (i.e., activity that is part of one's daily life involving bodily movements and the use of skeletal muscles) or structured exercise (i.e., physical activity that is planned, structured, and purposive to improve physical fitness) leads to the same benefits in preventing age-related cognitive decline. Physical exercise often differs from physical activity by being more controlled in terms of intensity and duration, while physical activity studies tend to incorporate a large variety of unspecified activities. Future studies are required to understand the intensity, duration, and types of exercise that better enhance cognitive functions in older adults. Although recent advancements in brain imaging techniques and genetics have opened new research avenues, more studies are required to find definitive answers to these questions. Further research is needed to better document the impact of other forms of exercise, as well as the dose-response relationship that governs the positive impact of exercise on brain functions. Hopefully, ongoing randomized trials such as the AIBL Active Trial [85] and the brain-in-motion trial [86] designed to address the relationship between physical exercise intervention and brain function in at risk individuals will help answer these questions.

Acknowledgments

The authors wish to thank Francis Langlois for editing and helpful comments. Louis Bherer and Teresa Liu-Ambrose are supported by the Canadian research chair program.

References

[1] C. Y. Wang, W. L. Haskell, S. W. Farrell et al., "Cardiorespiratory fitness levels among us adults 20–49 years of age: findings from the 1999–2004 national health and nutrition examination survey," *The American Journal of Epidemiology*, vol. 171, no. 4, pp. 426–435, 2010.

[2] L. Fratiglioni, S. Paillard-Borg, and B. Winblad, "An active and socially integrated lifestyle in late life might protect against dementia," *The Lancet Neurology*, vol. 3, no. 6, pp. 343–353, 2004.

[3] C. Hertzog, A. F. Kramer, R. S. Wilson, and U. Lindenberger, "Enrichment effects on adult cognitive development: can the functional capacity of older adults be preserved and enhanced?" *Psychological Science in the Public Interest*, vol. 9, no. 1, pp. 1–65, 2008.

[4] A. F. Kramer, L. Bherer, S. J. Colcombe, W. Dong, and W. T. Greenough, "Environmental influences on cognitive and brain plasticity during aging," *Journals of Gerontology A*, vol. 59, no. 9, pp. 940–957, 2004.

[5] F. W. Booth, S. E. Gordon, C. J. Carlson, and M. T. Hamilton, "Waging war on modern chronic diseases: primary prevention through exercise biology," *Journal of Applied Physiology*, vol. 88, no. 2, pp. 774–787, 2000.

[6] J. Myers, M. Prakash, V. Froelicher, D. Do, S. Partington, and J. E. Atwood, "Exercise capacity and mortality among men referred for exercise testing," *The New England Journal of Medicine*, vol. 346, no. 11, pp. 793–801, 2002.

[7] E. B. Larson, L. Wang, J. D. Bowen et al., "Exercise is associated with reduced risk for incident dementia among persons 65 years of age and older," *Annals of Internal Medicine*, vol. 144, no. 2, pp. 73–81, 2006.

[8] F. Craik and T. Salthouse, *Handbook of Aging and Cognition*, Psychology Press, New York, NY, USA, 3rd edition, 2008.

[9] P. A. Reuter-Lorenz and D. C. Park, "Human neuroscience and the aging mind: a new look at old problems," *Journals of Gerontology B*, vol. 65, no. 4, pp. 405–415, 2010.

[10] L. Penke, S. M. Maniega, C. Murray et al., "A general facto of brain white matter integrity predicts information processin speed in healthy older people," *Journal of Neuroscience*, vol. 30 no. 22, pp. 7569–7574, 2010.

[11] N. A. Dennis and R. Cabeza, "Neuroimaging of healthy cogni tive aging," in *Handbook of Aging and Cognition*, F. I. M. Crail and T. A. Salthouse, Eds., pp. 1–54, Psychology Press, New York NY, USA, 3rd edition, 2008.

[12] N. Raz, "The aging brain observed in vivo: differential change and there modifiers," in *Cognitive Neuroscience of Aging*, R Cabeza, L. Nyberg, and D. C. Park, Eds., pp. 19–57, Oxford University Press, New York, NY, USA, 2005.

[13] N. Raz, P. Ghisletta, K. M. Rodrigue, K. M. Kennedy, and U Lindenberger, "Trajectories of brain aging in middle-aged and older adults: regional and individual differences," *NeuroImage* vol. 51, no. 2, pp. 501–511, 2010.

[14] J. J. Chen, H. D. Rosas, and D. H. Salat, "Age-associated reductions in cerebral blood flow are independent from regional atrophy," *NeuroImage*, vol. 55, no. 2, pp. 468–478, 2011.

[15] T. Abourezk and T. Toole, "Effect of task complexity on the relationship between physical fitness and reaction time in older women," *Journal of Aging and Physical Activity*, vol. 3, pp. 251–260, 1995.

[16] L. Clarkson-Smith and A. A. Hartley, "Relationships between physical exercise and cognitive abilities in older adults," *Psychology and Aging*, vol. 4, no. 2, pp. 183–189, 1989.

[17] C. H. Hillman, E. P. Weiss, J. M. Hagberg, and B. D. Hatfield, "The relationship of age and cardiovascular fitness to cognitive and motor processes," *Psychophysiology*, vol. 39, no. 3, pp. 303–312, 2002.

[18] M. Renaud, L. Bherer, and F. Maquestiaux, "A high level of physical fitness is associated with more efficient response preparation in older adults," *Journals of Gerontology B*, vol. 65, no. 3, pp. 317–322, 2010.

[19] W. W. Spirduso, "Reaction and movement time as a function of age and physical activity level," *Journals of Gerontology*, vol. 30, no. 4, pp. 435–440, 1975.

[20] D. E. Barnes, K. Yaffe, W. A. Satariano, and I. B. Tager, "A longitudinal study of cardiorespiratory fitness and cognitive function in healthy older adults," *Journal of the American Geriatrics Society*, vol. 51, no. 4, pp. 459–465, 2003.

[21] M. C. Aichberger, M. A. Busch, F. M. Reischies, A. Ströhle, A. Heinz, and M. A. Rapp, "Effect of physical inactivity on cognitive performance after 2.5 years of follow-up: longitudinal results from the survey of health, ageing, and retirement (SHARE)," *GeroPsych*, vol. 23, no. 1, pp. 7–15, 2010.

[22] R. E. Dustman, R. O. Ruhling, E. M. Russell et al., "Aerobic exercise training and improved neuropsychological function of older individuals," *Neurobiology of Aging*, vol. 5, no. 1, pp. 35–42, 1984.

[23] R. E. Rikli and D. J. Edwards, "Effects of a three-year exercise program on motor function and cognitive processing speed in older women," *Research Quarterly for Exercise and Sport*, vol. 62, no. 1, pp. 61–67, 1991.

[24] H. L. Hawkins, A. F. Kramer, and D. Capaldi, "Aging, exercise, and attention," *Psychology and Aging*, vol. 7, no. 4, pp. 643–653, 1992.

[25] A. F. Kramer, S. Hahn, N. J. Cohen et al., "Ageing, fitness and neurocognitive function," *Nature*, vol. 400, no. 6743, pp. 418–419, 1999.

[26] C. T. Albinet, G. Boucard, C. A. Bouquet, and M. Audiffren, "Increased heart rate variability and executive performance after aerobic training in the elderly," *European Journal of Applied Physiology*, vol. 109, no. 4, pp. 617–624, 2010.

[27] S. Colcombe and A. F. Kramer, "Fitness effects on the cognitive function of older adults: a meta-analytic study," *Psychological Science*, vol. 14, no. 2, pp. 125–130, 2003.

[28] J. L. Etnier, P. M. Nowell, D. M. Landers, and B. A. Sibley, "A meta-regression to examine the relationship between aerobic fitness and cognitive performance," *Brain Research Reviews*, vol. 52, no. 1, pp. 119–130, 2006.

[29] A. L. Smiley-Oyen, K. A. Lowry, S. J. Francois, M. L. Kohut, and P. Ekkekakis, "Exercise, fitness, and neurocognitive function in older adults: the "selective improvement" and "cardiovascular fitness" hypotheses," *Annals of Behavioral Medicine*, vol. 36, no. 3, pp. 280–291, 2008.

[30] M. Renaud, F. Maquestiaux, S. Joncas, M. J. Kergoat, and L. Bherer, "The effect of three months of aerobic training on response preparation in older adults," *Frontiers in Aging Neuroscience*, vol. 2, article 148, 2010.

[31] P. J. Smith, J. A. Blumenthal, B. M. Hoffman et al., "Aerobic exercise and neurocognitive performance: a meta-analytic review of randomized controlled trials," *Psychosomatic Medicine*, vol. 72, no. 3, pp. 239–252, 2010.

[32] M. Angevaren, G. Aufdemkampe, H. J. Verhaar, A. Aleman, and L. Vanhees, "Physical activity and enhanced fitness to improve cognitive function in older people without known cognitive impairment," *Cochrane Database of Systematic Reviews*, no. 2, Article ID CD005381, 2008.

[33] R. C. Cassilhas, V. A. R. Viana, V. Grassmann et al., "The impact of resistance exercise on the cognitive function of the elderly," *Medicine and Science in Sports and Exercise*, vol. 39, no. 8, pp. 1401–1407, 2007.

[34] T. Liu-Ambrose, M. G. Donaldson, Y. Ahamed et al., "Otago home-based strength and balance retraining improves executive functioning in older fallers: a randomized controlled trial," *Journal of the American Geriatrics Society*, vol. 56, no. 10, pp. 1821–1830, 2008.

[35] K. Fabel and G. Kempermann, "Physical activity and the regulation of neurogenesis in the adult and aging brain," *NeuroMolecular Medicine*, vol. 10, no. 2, pp. 59–66, 2008.

[36] T. Liu-Ambrose, L. S. Nagamatsu, P. Graf, B. L. Beattie, M. C. Ashe, and T. C. Handy, "Resistance training and executive functions: a 12-month randomized controlled trial," *Archives of Internal Medicine*, vol. 170, no. 2, pp. 170–178, 2010.

[37] C. Rosano, A. B. Newman, R. Katz, C. H. Hirsch, and L. H. Kuller, "Association between lower digit symbol substitution test score and slower gait and greater risk of mortality and of developing incident disability in well-functioning older adults," *Journal of the American Geriatrics Society*, vol. 56, no. 9, pp. 1618–1625, 2008.

[38] J. Dumurgier, A. Elbaz, P. Ducimetière, B. Tavernier, A. Alpérovitch, and C. Tzourio, "Slow walking speed and cardiovascular death in well functioning older adults: prospective cohort study," *The British Medical Journal*, vol. 339, Article ID b4460, 2009.

[39] S. E. Hardy, S. Perera, Y. F. Roumani, J. M. Chandler, and S. A. Studenski, "Improvement in usual gait speed predicts better survival in older adults," *Journal of the American Geriatrics Society*, vol. 55, no. 11, pp. 1727–1734, 2007.

[40] C. Voelcker-Rehage and C. Nieman, "Structural and functional brain changes related to different types of physical activity across the life span," *Neuroscience and Biobehavioral Reviews*, 2013.

[41] W. Spirduso, K. Francis, and P. MacRae, *Physical Dimensions of Aging*, Human Kinetics, Champaign, Ill, USA, 2nd edition, 2005.

[42] I. Lista and G. Sorrentino, "Biological mechanisms of physical activity in preventing cognitive decline," *Cellular and Molecular Neurobiology*, vol. 30, no. 4, pp. 493–503, 2010.

[43] J. E. Black, K. R. Isaacs, B. J. Anderson, A. A. Alcantara, and W. T. Greenough, "Learning causes synaptogenesis, whereas motor activity causes angiogenesis, in cerebellar cortex of adult rats," *Proceedings of the National Academy of Sciences of the United States of America*, vol. 87, no. 14, pp. 5568–5572, 1990.

[44] K. R. Isaacs, B. J. Anderson, A. A. Alcantara, J. E. Black, and W. T. Greenough, "Exercise and the brain: angiogenesis in the adult rat cerebellum after vigorous physical activity and motor skill learning," *Journal of Cerebral Blood Flow and Metabolism*, vol. 12, no. 1, pp. 110–119, 1992.

[45] H. van Praag, T. Shubert, C. Zhao, and F. H. Gage, "Exercise enhances learning and hippocampal neurogenesis in aged mice," *Journal of Neuroscience*, vol. 25, no. 38, pp. 8680–8685, 2005.

[46] P. Lledo, M. Alonso, and M. S. Grubb, "Adult neurogenesis and functional plasticity in neuronal circuits," *Nature Reviews Neuroscience*, vol. 7, no. 3, pp. 179–193, 2006.

[47] B. D. Eadie, V. A. Redila, and B. R. Christie, "Voluntary exercise alters the cytoarchitecture of the adult dentate gyrus by increasing cellular proliferation, dendritic complexity, and spine density," *Journal of Comparative Neurology*, vol. 486, no. 1, pp. 39–47, 2005.

[48] S. Hu, Z. Ying, F. Gomez-Pinilla, and S. A. Frautschy, "Exercise can increase small heat shock proteins (sHSP) and pre- and post-synaptic proteins in the hippocampus," *Brain Research*, vol. 1249, pp. 191–201, 2009.

[49] K. I. Erickson, M. W. Voss, R. S. Prakash et al., "Exercise training increases size of hippocampus and improves memory," *Proceedings of the National Academy of Sciences of the United States of America*, vol. 108, no. 7, pp. 3017–3022, 2011.

[50] K. I. Erickson and A. F. Kramer, "Aerobic exercise effects on cognitive and neural plasticity in older adults," *The British Journal of Sports Medicine*, vol. 43, no. 1, pp. 22–24, 2009.

[51] C. H. Hillman, K. I. Erickson, and A. F. Kramer, "Be smart, exercise your heart: exercise effects on brain and cognition," *Nature Reviews Neuroscience*, vol. 9, no. 1, pp. 58–65, 2008.

[52] A. F. Kramer, K. I. Erickson, and S. J. Colcombe, "Exercise, cognition, and the aging brain," *Journal of Applied Physiology*, vol. 101, no. 4, pp. 1237–1242, 2006.

[53] T. Liu-Ambrose, L. S. Nagamatsu, M. W. Voss, K. M. Khan, and T. C. Handy, "Resistance training and functional plasticity of the aging brain: a 12-month randomized controlled trial," *Neurobiology of Aging*, vol. 33, no. 8, pp. 1690–1698, 2012.

[54] C. Voelcker-Rehage, B. Godde, and U. M. Staudinger, "Physical and motor fitness are both related to cognition in old age," *European Journal of Neuroscience*, vol. 31, no. 1, pp. 167–176, 2010.

[55] S. J. Colcombe, K. I. Erickson, N. Raz et al., "Aerobic fitness reduces brain tissue loss in aging humans," *Journals of Gerontology A*, vol. 58, no. 2, pp. 176–180, 2003.

[56] K. I. Erickson, R. S. Prakash, M. W. Voss et al., "Aerobic fitness is associated with hippocampal volume in elderly humans," *Hippocampus*, vol. 19, no. 10, pp. 1030–1039, 2009.

[57] R. Ruscheweyh, C. Willemer, K. Krüger et al., "Physical activity and memory functions: an interventional study," *Neurobiology of Aging*, vol. 32, no. 7, pp. 1304–1319, 2011.

[58] S. J. Colcombe, A. F. Kramer, K. I. Erickson et al., "Cardiovascular fitness, cortical plasticity, and aging," *Proceedings of the National Academy of Sciences of the United States of America*, vol. 101, no. 9, pp. 3316–3321, 2004.

[59] M. W. Voss, R. S. Prakash, K. I. Erickson et al., "Plasticity of brain networks in a randomized intervention trial of exercise training in older adults," *Frontiers in Aging Neuroscience*, vol. 2, article 32, 2010.

[60] W. Spirduso, L. Poon, and W. Chodzo-Zajko, "Using resources and reserves in an exercise-cognition model," in *Exercise and Its Mediating Effects on Cognition*, W. Spirduso, L. Poon, and W. Chodzo-Zajko, Eds., pp. 3–11, Human Kinetics, Champaign, Ill, USA, 2008.

[61] J. Bartholomew and J. Ciccolo, "Exercise, depression, and cognition," in *Exercise and Its Mediating Effects on Cognition*, W. Spirduso, L. Poon, and W. Chodzo-Zajko, Eds., pp. 33–46, Human Kinetics, Champaign, Ill, USA, 2008.

[62] E. McAuley and S. Elavsky, "Self-efficacy, physical activity, and cognitive function," in *Exercise and Its Mediating Effects on Cognition*, W. Spirduso, L. Poon, and W. Chodzo-Zajko, Eds., pp. 69–84, Human Kinetics, Champaign, Ill, USA, 2008.

[63] J. Joseph, "Diet, motor behavior, and cognition," in *Exercise and Its Mediating Effects on Cognition*, W. Spirduso, L. Poon, and W. Chodzo-Zajko, Eds., pp. 119–129, Human Kinetics, Champaign, Ill, USA, 2008.

[64] M. Lopez, "Exercise and sleep quality," in *Exercise and Its Mediating Effects on Cognition*, W. Spirduso, L. Poon, and W. Chodzo-Zajko, Eds., pp. 131–146, Human Kinetics, Champaign, Ill, USA, 2008.

[65] M. V. Vitiello, "Exercise, sleep, and cognition: interactions in aging," in *Exercise and Its Mediating Effects on Cognition*, W. Spirduso, L. Poon, and W. Chodzo-Zajko, Eds., pp. 146–165, Human Kinetics, Champaign, Ill, USA, 2008.

[66] L. P. Fried, C. M. Tangen, J. Walston et al., "Frailty in older adults: evidence for a phenotype," *Journals of Gerontology A*, vol. 56, no. 3, pp. M146–M156, 2001.

[67] K. Rockwood, S. E. Howlett, C. MacKnight et al., "Prevalence, attributes, and outcomes of fi tness and frailty in community-dwelling older adults: report from the Canadian study of health and aging," *Journals of Gerontology A*, vol. 59, no. 12, pp. 1310–1317, 2004.

[68] F. Landi, A. M. Abbatecola, M. Provinciali et al., "Moving against frailty: does physical activity matter?" *Biogerontology*, vol. 11, no. 5, pp. 537–545, 2010.

[69] M. J. Peterson, C. Giuliani, M. C. Morey et al., "Physical activity as a preventative factor for frailty: the health, aging, and body composition study," *Journals of Gerontology A*, vol. 64, no. 1, pp. 61–68, 2009.

[70] J. L. Helbostad, O. Sletvold, and R. Moe-Nilssen, "Home training with and without additional group training in physically frail old people living at home: effect on health-related quality of life and ambulation," *Clinical Rehabilitation*, vol. 18, no. 5, pp. 498–508, 2004.

[71] F. Langlois, T. T. M. Vu, K. Chassé, G. Dupuis, M. J. Kergoat, and L. Bherer, "Benefits of physical exercise training on cognition and quality of life in frail older adults," *Journals of Gerontology B*, vol. 68, no. 3, pp. 400–404, 2013.

[72] Alzheimer's Association, "Alzheimer's disease facts and figures," *Alzheimer's & Dementia*, vol. 7, no. 2, 2011.

[73] Y. E. Geda, R. O. Roberts, D. S. Knopman et al., "Physical exercise, aging, and mild cognitive impairment a population-based study," *Archives of Neurology*, vol. 67, no. 1, pp. 80–86, 2010.

[74] J. M. Burns, B. B. Cronk, H. S. Anderson et al., "Cardiorespiratory fitness and brain atrophy in early Alzheimer disease," *Neurology*, vol. 71, no. 3, pp. 210–216, 2008.

[75] M. Chang, P. V. Jonsson, J. Snaedal et al., "The effect of midlife physical activity on cognitive function among older adults: AGES—Reykjavik study," *Journals of Gerontology A*, vol. 65, no. 12, pp. 1369–1374, 2010.

[76] P. A. Boyle, A. S. Buchman, R. S. Wilson, S. E. Leurgans, and D. A. Bennett, "Physical frailty is associated with incident mild cognitive impairment in community-based older persons," *Journal of the American Geriatrics Society*, vol. 58, no. 2, pp. 248–255, 2010.

[77] F. Sofi, D. Valecchi, D. Bacci et al., "Physical activity and risk of cognitive decline: a meta-analysis of prospective studies," *Journal of Internal Medicine*, vol. 269, no. 1, pp. 107–117, 2011.

[78] P. Heyn, B. C. Abreu, and K. J. Ottenbacher, "The effects of exercise training on elderly persons with cognitive impairment and dementia: a meta-analysis," *Archives of Physical Medicine and Rehabilitation*, vol. 85, no. 10, pp. 1694–1704, 2004.

[79] N. T. Lautenschlager, K. L. Cox, L. Flicker et al., "Effect of physical activity on cognitive function in older adults at risk for Alzheimer disease: a randomized trial," *The Journal of the American Medical Association*, vol. 300, no. 9, pp. 1027–1037, 2008.

[80] L. H. P. Eggermont, D. F. Swaab, E. M. Hol, and E. J. A. Scherder, "Walking the line: a randomised trial on the effects of a short term walking programme on cognition in dementia," *Journal of Neurology, Neurosurgery and Psychiatry*, vol. 80, no. 7, pp. 802–804, 2009.

[81] L. D. Baker, L. L. Frank, K. Foster-Schubert et al., "Effects of aerobic exercise on mild cognitive impairment: a controlled trial," *Archives of Neurology*, vol. 67, no. 1, pp. 71–79, 2010.

[82] G. Kemoun, M. Thibaud, N. Roumagne et al., "Effects of a physical training programme on cognitive function and walking efficiency in elderly persons with dementia," *Dementia and Geriatric Cognitive Disorders*, vol. 29, no. 2, pp. 109–114, 2010.

[83] L. C. W. Lam, R. C. M. Chau, B. M. L. Wong et al., "Interim follow-up of a randomized controlled trial comparing Chinese style mind body (Tai Chi) and stretching exercises on cognitive function in subjects at risk of progressive cognitive decline," *International Journal of Geriatric Psychiatry*, vol. 26, no. 7, pp. 733–740, 2011.

[84] L. S. Nagamatsu, A. Chan, J. C. Davis et al., "Physical activity improves verbal and spatial memory in older adults with probable mild cognitive impairment: a 6-month randomized controlled trial," *Journal of Aging Research*, vol. 2013, Article ID 861893, 10 pages, 2013.

[85] E. V. Cyarto, N. T. Lautenschlager, P. M. Desmond et al., "Protocol for a randomized controlled trial evaluating the effect of physical activity on delaying the progression of white matter changes on MRI in older adults with memory complaints and mild cognitive impairment: the AIBL active trial," *BMC Psychiatry*, vol. 12, article 167, 2012.

[86] A. V. Tyndall, M. H. Davenport, B. J. Wilson et al., "The brain-in-motion study: effect of a 6-month aerobic exercise intervention on cerebrovascular regulation and cognitive function in older adults," *BMC Geriatrics*, vol. 13, article 21, 2013.

17

Gender, Success, and Drop-Out during a Resistance Exercise Program in Community Dwelling Old Adults

O. G. Geirsdottir,[1,2] M. Chang,[1,3] K. Briem,[4] P. V. Jonsson,[1,5] I. Thorsdottir,[6] and A. Ramel[1,2]

[1] *The Icelandic Gerontological Research Center, Reykjavik, Iceland*
[2] *Faculty of Food Science and Nutrition, University of Iceland, Reykjavik, Iceland*
[3] *Department of Sport Science, School of Science and Engineering, Reykjavik University, Reykjavik, Iceland*
[4] *Department of Physiotherapy, University of Iceland, Reykjavik, Iceland*
[5] *Department of Geriatrics, National University Hospital of Iceland, Reykjavik, Iceland*
[6] *School of Health Sciences, University of Iceland, Reykjavik, Iceland*

Correspondence should be addressed to A. Ramel; alfonsra@hi.is

Academic Editor: Arshad Jahangir

Background. Resistance exercise training can be effective against sarcopenia. We identified predictors of drop-out and compared physical outcomes between men and women after such training. *Methods.* Subjects ($N = 236$, 73.7 ± 5.7 years) participated in a 12-week resistance exercise program. Outcome variables were measured at baseline and endpoint. *Results.* Drop-out was 11.9% and not significantly different between genders. Drop-outs were significantly older and had poorer strength and physical function in comparison to completers. Anthropometrics, QoL, and cognitive function were not related to drop-out. According to multivariate analysis, gait speed and physical activity were the strongest predictors of drop-out. After the training, gains in lean mass or appendicular muscle were significantly higher in men than women; however relative gains in appendicular muscle as well as absolute improvements in strength and function were similar in men and women, respectively. *Conclusions.* Participants who drop out are older, have poorer physical function, and are less physically active. Old women do not drop out more frequently than men and show meaningful improvements in relevant outcomes similar to men after such a training program. The trial is registered at the US National Library of Medicine (NCT01074879).

1. Introduction

Sarcopenia, the age related loss of muscle mass and strength, is frequently observed in older populations [1]. It is an unfavorable condition, because it is related to functional decline and adverse health outcomes [1]. Thus, it is important to establish therapies that prevent sarcopenia or delay its onset. Regular resistance training has been shown to be an effective intervention [2].

However, a resistance exercise program can be demanding for participants, because often high intensity resistance exercise is prescribed for old adults [2]. The rationale for this is that gains in muscle strength and size are thought to be larger following resistance training with higher intensities, although the degree of training-induced muscle hypertrophy is generally small in old adults [2].

During a high intensity training program, participants typically attend two to three sessions per week and a weekly increase in load is implemented in order to keep the intensity of around 80% (relative to the one-repetition-maximum) constant due to gains in strength that occur during a resistance exercise program [2, 3].

Drop-out during resistance exercise programs has been reported to be 22–38% [4–6] and increases with the length of the program [7]. In this context, it is important to identify participants at higher risk for drop-out beforehand, in order to provide these individuals with better supervision and attention during a resistance exercise program with the aim of preventing drop-out.

When it comes to compliance with resistance exercise, women might need particular attention. In general, women have been reported to have lower levels of physical activity than men [8] and this is also true for resistance exercise [9]. It has been suggested that women increase muscle mass less than men with the same amount of training [10]. A recently published study reported sex differences in the response to resistance exercise training also in old people with lesser improvement of maximal torque and muscle quality in women compared to men [10]. In addition to biological differences in muscular adaptation to physical training, one might also speculate that the gym environment itself could be a deterrent for some female participants [7].

In order to gain knowledge on drop-out and success after a resistance exercise program, we conducted this secondary data analysis based on results from a previously published randomized, controlled trial, designed to examine the effect of postexercise protein ingestion on the efficacy of strength training in old adults [3]. The aim of the present work was (1) to identify baseline predictors of drop-out with particular focus on physical function and (2) to compare changes in physical outcomes after the resistance exercise program between men and women.

2. Methods

Several papers have been published from this study and in the present paper we followed the methods of Geirsdottir et al. 2012 [11], Arnarson et al. 2013 [3], Arnarson et al. 2014 [12], and Ramel et al. 2015 [13]. The similarity found between the present paper and the above-mentioned articles is restricted to Methods. The present paper contains novel scientific content with focus on drop-out, success, and gender not presented previously.

2.1. Subjects. Participants ($N = 236$, range 65–92 years) were recruited within the Capital Area in Iceland. Exclusion criteria were major orthopedic disease, pharmacological interventions known to affect muscle mass, and low cognitive function according to Mini-Mental State Examination (MMSE) ≤ 19 points [12, 14]. Subjects had also to be free from disorders that could significantly affect their body composition. Some of the participants had hypertension, hyperlipidemia, or type 2 diabetes [15], although the enrolled subjects looked apparently healthy. The study received permission from the Icelandic National Bioethics Committee (VSNb2008060007/03-15) and has therefore been performed in accordance with the ethical standards as described by the Declaration of Helsinki 1964 and its later amendments. The subjects gave their written informed consent before participation in the study.

2.2. Resistance Training. The aim of the resistance exercise program was to increase strength and mass of all major muscle groups. In order to assess physiological changes, measurements were conducted at baseline and the end of the study. The training was conducted in a local fitness study where participants trained three days per week for 12 weeks in supervised groups of 26–44 individuals. Each training started with a 10–15 minute warm up. The correct exercise and lifting techniques were taught at lower loads (60% of 1 repetition maximum (1-RM)) during the first week. In the following weeks resistance training was done in three sets where each exercise was repeated six to eight times, at 75–80% of 1-RM. After each exercise the participants rested shortly until they felt ready for the next exercise. In order to keep the number of repetitions per exercise unchanged during the 12 weeks of training, training loads were increased by 5–10% each week. Stretching exercises were performed at the end of each session. The training was supervised by staff members, by fitness trainers, and occasionally by a physiotherapist. After each training, participants received a protein and carbohydrate containing drink, which was part of the original aim of this trial [3]. As the supplementation was not related to outcomes of the present analysis, it is not considered further in this paper.

2.3. Body Composition. Body weight (BW) was measured in light underwear (Seca scale model number 708, Seca, Hamburg, Germany) and height was measured with a calibrated stadiometer (model number 206; Seca, Hamburg, Germany). Body mass index (BMI) was calculated as kg/m^2. Waist circumference was measured halfway between the top of the lateral iliac crest and the lowest rib. Body composition (lean body mass = LBM, fat mass = FM, and appendicular skeletal muscle = ASM) was assessed at the Icelandic Heart Association, Kopavogur, Iceland, using dual energy X-ray absorptiometer (DXA, Hologic QDR-2000 plus®, Hologic Inc., Waltham, MA, USA).

2.4. Physical Function

2.4.1. Six-Minute Walk for Distance (6MWD). The 6MWD was conducted in a gym hall according to the guidelines from the American Thoracic Society [16]. In healthy subjects, the 6MWD usually ranges from 400 to 700 m [17–19]. For some of the statistical analyses, subjects were categorized into *below 400 m* and in *at least 400 m* (see Figure 2).

2.4.2. Quadriceps Strength. Quadriceps strength (maximum voluntary isometric contraction (MVIC)) was tested using an isokinetic dynamometer (Kin-Com® 500H Chattanooga). The participants performed three submaximal trials and then four MVIC tests for five seconds each, with a 50-second rest between tests. The greatest output was recorded as the peak torque expressed in Newton (N).

2.4.3. Timed Up and Go (TUG) Test. The participants were instructed to stand up from a chair (seat height = 43 cm), to walk 3 m, then to turn around, to return, and to sit down again. Time (sec) was taken during this procedure. The participants wore shoes during this test and used walking aids when necessary [20].

TABLE 1: Characteristics of male and female participants.

	Male ($n = 98$) Mean ± SD	Female ($n = 138$) Mean ± SD	P value*
Age (years)	74.6 ± 5.9	72.8 ± 5.5	0.018
BMI (kg/m^2)	29.7 ± 4.6	28.1 ± 4.9	0.012
Waist (cm)	108 ± 12	94 ± 13	<0.001
Body fat (%)	33.9 ± 5.9	41.3 ± 6.5	<0.001
Body fat (kg)	32.3 ± 10.4	31.4 ± 9.5	0.515
Lean body mass (kg)	57.4 ± 7.2	41.1 ± 4.7	<0.001
Appendicular skeletal muscle (kg)	29.6 ± 3.9	20.9 ± 2.6	<0.001
Appendicular skeletal muscle (%)	31.9 ± 3.2	28.3 ± 2.9	<0.001
Quadriceps strength (N)	538 ± 124	409 ± 90	<0.001
Quadriceps strength** (N/kg)	5.9 ± 1.5	5.6 ± 1.3	0.100
Grip strength (lb.)	79 ± 15	49 ± 9	<0.001
6MWD (m)	456 ± 86	452 ± 76	0.708
TUG (sec)	8.0 ± 2.1	7.9 ± 2.3	0.595
MMSE (score)	27.1 ± 2.1	27.8 ± 2.0	0.021
QoL (score)	54.9 ± 6.2	55.0 ± 6.1	0.907
Number of drugs	2.3 ± 1.4	1.9 ± 1.6	0.067
Exercise/week (min)	323 ± 341	356 ± 343	0.472
Drop-out (%)	8.2	14.5	0.138

*Differences between genders according to independent samples t-test (normally distributed variables) and Mann–Whitney U test (not normally distributed variables). **Corrected for body weight.

2.4.4. Grip Strength. Hand grip strength (lbs) was measured using a hydraulic hand dynamometer (Baseline® Baseline Evaluations Corporation). The maximal achieved grip strength from three attempts was recorded as the subject's grip strength.

2.5. Questionnaires. Questionnaires were used to receive information on demographic characteristics and medication count.

2.6. Leisure-Time Physical Activity (LTPA). LTPA during the last year was estimated using a questionnaire [21] based on the Compendium of Physical Activities [22] and Paffenberger's questionnaire [23]. It contains questions on the subjects' participation in sports, exercises, or other physical activities. In statistical analysis LTPA is used as min/week.

2.7. Health Related Quality of Life (HRQL). The HRQL questionnaire involves 12 domains that cover a range of psychological and physical functions, for example, functional status, vitality, social function, physical pain, emotions, general health, and mental health. The domains were summarized into a single score and converted into a T-score corrected for age and gender (T-score norm is 50 ± 10) [24, 25].

2.8. Statistical Analysis. Statistical analysis was conducted using SPSS for Windows version 22.0 (SPSS, Chicago, IL, USA). The Kolmogorov-Smirnov test was used to investigate the distribution of the data. In Tables 1–3, data are shown as mean ± standard deviation (SD). Comparison between groups, for example, men and women, was done using independent samples' t-test (normally distributed variables) or Mann–Whitney U test (not normally distributed variables). Correlations between variables were calculated using Pearson's correlation coefficient r. Logistic regression models with various degrees of statistical correction were used to find out whether physical function can predictor drop-out. Model 1 is crude analysis; model 2 corrected for age; model 3 additionally corrected for gender. Risk of drop-out for categories of gait speed and five-year age groups was calculated using cross tabs including chi-square statistics. The level of significance was set at $P < 0.05$.

3. Results

Baseline data and differences between genders can be seen in Table 1. There were differences between men and women in body composition and muscular strength. However, physical function (6MWD, TUG) did not differ between men and women. Drop-out rate was insignificantly higher in women. In comparison to completers, participants who dropped out were older and had poorer strength and physical function. They exercised less; however, neither body composition nor QoL nor MMSE was related to drop-out (Table 2).

In general, the intervention resulted in favorable changes in body composition (FM −0.44 kg, LBM +0.75 kg, and ASM +0.53 kg, all $P < 0.001$), muscular strength (quadriceps +53 N; grip strength +3 lb, both $P < 0.001$), and physical function (6MWD +34 m; TUG −0.7 sec, both $P < 0.001$).

TABLE 2: Characteristics of participants that dropped out or completed the program.

	Completers ($n = 208$) Mean ± SD	Drop-out ($n = 28$) Mean ± SD	P value*
Age (years)	73.0 ± 5.5	77.5 ± 5.9	<0.001
BMI (kg/m2)	28.8 ± 4.8	29.0 ± 4.9	0.853
Waist (cm)	99.7 ± 14.4	100.4 ± 14.5	0.815
Body fat (%)	37.9 ± 7.3	40.8 ± 6.8	0.073
Body fat (kg)	31.5 ± 9.6	33.6 ± 12.0	0.325
Lean body mass (kg)	48.2 ± 9.8	45.3 ± 11.1	0.175
Appendicular muscle mass (kg)	24.7 ± 5.2	22.4 ± 6.0	0.052
Appendicular skeletal muscle (%)	30.0 ± 3.5	28.2 ± 2.6	0.022
Quadriceps strength (N)	471 ± 122	386 ± 117	0.005
Quadriceps strength** (N/kg)	5.8 ± 1.4	4.9 ± 1.5	0.021
Grip strength (lb)	63 ± 19	53 ± 18	0.045
6MWD (m)	461 ± 74	394 ± 102	<0.001
TUG (sec)	7.7 ± 1.9	9.8 ± 3.7	<0.001
MMSE (score)	27.6 ± 2.0	27.0 ± 2.4	0.175
QoL (score)	55.1 ± 6.2	53.5 ± 5.1	0.199
Number of drugs for different conditions	2.0 ± 1.5	2.6 ± 1.6	0.058
Exercise/week (min)	364 ± 350	181 ± 210	<0.001

*Differences between genders according to independent samples t-test (normally distributed variables) and Mann–Whitney U test (not normally distributed variables). **Corrected for body weight.

TABLE 3: Changes in anthropometric, physical, and functional outcomes in male and female participants after the 12-week intervention.

	Male ($n = 91$) Mean ± SD	Female ($n = 119$) Mean ± SD	P value*
BMI (kg/m^2)	0.21 ± 0.58	0.09 ± 0.52	0.097
Waist (cm)	−0.90 ± 3.32	−0.50 ± 4.15	0.493
Body fat (%)	−0.65 ± 1.16	−0.93 ± 4.17	0.529
Body fat (kg)	−0.34 ± 1.34	−0.52 ± 2.72	0.573
Lean body mass (kg)	1.09 ± 1.31	0.61 ± 1.24	0.008
Lean body mass (%)	1.93 ± 2.30	1.59 ± 2.99	0.380
App. skeletal muscle (kg)	0.67 ± 0.81	0.42 ± 0.62	0.016
App. skeletal muscle (%)	2.28 ± 2.76	2.07 ± 3.05	0.619
Quadriceps strength (N)	55 ± 57	52 ± 49	0.717
Quadriceps strength (%)	11 ± 14	14 ± 13	0.179
Grip strength (lb.)	3.2 ± 6.2	3.0 ± 5.4	0.784
Grip strength (%)	4.2 ± 8.5	6.7 ± 13.0	0.017
6MWD (m)	31 ± 38	35 ± 32	0.397
TUG (sec)	0.55 ± 0.98	0.71 ± 1.22	0.296
QoL (score)	0.64 ± 3.28	1.57 ± 3.85	0.077
MMSE (score)	0.41 ± 1.91	0.48 ± 1.83	0.817

*Differences between genders according to independent samples t-test (normally distributed variables) and Mann–Whitney U test (not normally distributed variables).

Attendance rate was 91% and similar in both genders. Gains in LBM and ASM were not related to improvements in physical function; however, increases in quadriceps strength correlated with improvements in TUG ($r = 0.151$, $P = 0.032$) and 6MWD ($r = 0.137$, $P = 0.052$).

Changes after the intervention stratified by gender can be seen in Table 3. Although absolute gains in LBM or ASM were higher in men than women, relative gains in muscle as well as improvements in strength und function were similar between genders.

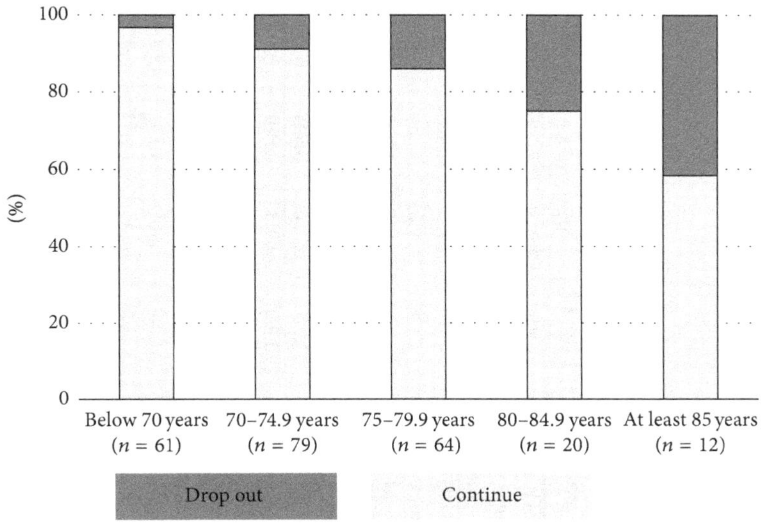

FIGURE 1: Associations between age categories and risk of drop-out (chi-square statistics, $P < 0.001$).

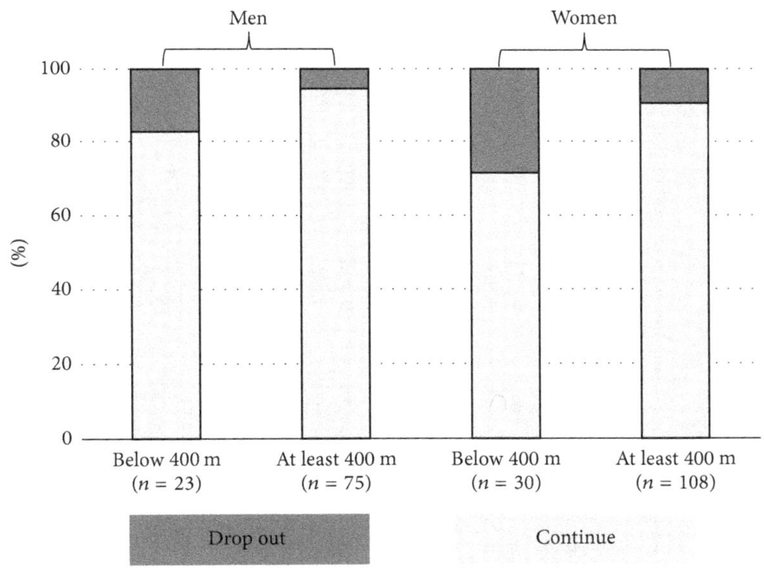

FIGURE 2: Associations between gait speed categories and risk of drop-out (chi-square statistics, $P = 0.065$ for men and 0.008 for women; $P < 0.001$ for men and women combined).

Logistic regression models in Table 4 show the prediction of drop-out by variables of physical function and physical activity. In the crude models without any statistical correction (model 1) most of the variables describing physical function and physical activity were associated with the risk of drop-out in a negative way (i.e., better function-lower risk of drop-out). However, some of these associations were partly explained by age and gender. In models 2 and 3 in which we included statistical correction for age and gender, the associations between function and drop-out got weaker and are partly no longer significant. According to models 3 physical activity per week and gait speed (borderline significant) were the strongest predictors for drop-out from all the physical function variables.

Figures 1 and 2 show the risk for drop-out depending on age groups and 6MWD, respectively. Both higher age and lower distance were associated with higher drop-out (chi-square statistics).

4. Discussion

The present study investigated drop-out and success of community dwelling old adults after a 12-week resistance exercise program with particular consideration of potential gender differences. In our study drop-out of 11.9% was low compared to previously reported studies [4–6] and not significantly different between genders. There are several potential reasons

TABLE 4: Logistic regression models showing the association between physical outcomes and the risk of drop-out.

Variable	Model 1				Model 2					Model 3				
	Exp (*B*)	95% CI for EXP (*B*)		*P* value	Variables	Exp (*B*)	95% CI for EXP (*B*)		*P* value	Variables	Exp (*B*)	95% CI for EXP (*B*)		*P* value
6MWD (m)	0.991	0.986	0.995	<0.001	6MWD (m)	0.994	0.988	1.000	0.048	6MWD (m)	0.994	0.988	1.000	0.063
					Age (years)	1.102	1.013	1.198	0.024	Age (years)	1.121	1.026	1.224	0.011
										Male	0.418	0.159	1.098	0.077
TUG (sec)	1.318	1.129	1.538	<0.001	TUG (sec)	1.185	0.995	1.412	0.057	TUG (sec)	1.174	0.983	1.403	0.076
					Age (years)	1.107	1.016	1.205	0.020	Age (years)	1.128	1.032	1.234	0.008
										Male	0.394	0.141	1.095	0.074
Quad. strength (N)	0.993	0.988	0.998	0.006	Quad. strength (N)	0.996	0.990	1.001	0.083	Quad. strength (N)	0.995	0.989	1.002	0.143
					Age (years)	1.125	1.031	1.228	0.008	Age (years)	1.123	1.018	1.239	0.021
										Male	1.062	0.286	3.949	0.928
Grip strength (lb.)	0.968	0.938	1.000	0.051	Grip strength (lb.)	0.975	0.943	1.007	0.122	Grip strength (lb.)	0.960	0.913	1.010	0.116
					Age (years)	1.141	1.049	1.242	0.002	Age (years)	1.120	1.018	1.233	0.020
										Male	1.934	0.357	10.465	0.444
Exercise (min/week)	0.997	0.996	0.999	0.011	Exercise (min/week)	0.998	0.996	1.000	0.032	Exercise (min/week)	0.998	0.995	1.000	0.029
					Age (years)	1.126	1.048	1.210	0.001	Age (years)	1.143	1.061	1.233	<0.001
										Male	0.349	0.137	0.891	0.028

Model 1 includes constant and physical measurement; model 2 includes additionally age; model 3: includes additionally gender; Exp (*B*) = hazard ratio.

why drop-out was low: (1) our study population consisted of rather healthy volunteers who did neither represent the general population at this age nor a clinical sample of patients. It can be assumed that volunteers show higher motivation and compliance towards physical training. (2) Further, the study was conducted during the lively opening hours in (at that time) one of the most modern fitness studios in the Reykjavik area as opposed to a physiotherapy facility at a hospital. (3) Training was conducted in groups of 26–44 individuals with several dedicated instructors and study staff assisting and being available for help. Although not measured, we found that there was a pleasant and kind atmosphere and that participants liked to attend the training sessions which is reflected by the high attendance rate of 91%.

Drop-out was related to baseline strength, physical function, medical drug use, and physical activity but unexpectedly not to body composition, MMSE, or QoL. According to multivariate analysis age and gait speed were the strongest baseline predictors. It is a matter of definition at what percentage drop-out is still acceptable or not. However, as shown in Figures 1 and 2, age older than 80 years and 6MWD below 400 m were both related to a drop-out risk of >20%. Consequently, these cut-off values for age and gait speed can be easily used to identify participants at higher risk for drop-out. Future studies are needed to determine whether, for example, better supervision in smaller groups might help to prevent attrition from a study program in such vulnerable participants.

Considering that the oldest and weakest individuals had the highest risk of drop-out, it can be speculated that the program was too demanding for them. Although it is widely accepted that resistance exercise with high intensity (heavy loads) is efficient [26], a controversy has arisen during recent years whether strength and muscle mass gains would also be achievable with lighter load resistance exercise programs [27, 28]. There is evidence that, when matched for mechanical work, resistance exercise provokes substantial gains in muscle mass and strength, irrespective of whether heavy or rather lighter loads were used [29].

According to a recently published meta-analysis [2] on this topic, both high and moderate resistance exercise provoke significant gains in muscle strength compared with nontraining control. However, differences between high and moderate intensities are less clear, partly due to methodological issues of the included studies. An analysis of the subset of studies to report data on the training-related changes in muscle size revealed that neither the higher nor lower load resistance training programs performed were effective in inducing significant muscle hypertrophy [2]. However, this result is most likely a consequence of short intervention periods and/or lack of an appropriate surplus of calories and protein necessary for muscle gain. As long-term adherence to resistance exercise is a general problem [30], we think that minimum effective thresholds should be determined in order to increase long-term success.

It has been proposed that a short-term increase in testosterone after heavy resistance exercise promotes muscle protein synthesis, which finally leads to protein accretion and hypertrophy [31]. Women have much lower testosterone concentrations than men and do not experience postexercise increases in testosterone compared with men [32, 33]. This sex specific response has been used to explain why women have an attenuated potential for resistance exercise-induced hypertrophy [34]. In accordance with this, women gained significantly less LBM and ASM than men in our study. However, we also found that both relative gains in LBM and ASM and clinically relevant improvements in muscle strength and physical function after a resistance exercise program were similar between genders. In order to put the improvements of TUG (−0.7 sec) and 6MWD (+34 m) in perspective, it is worth considering that age related changes have been reported +1 sec/decade for TUG [35] and −30 m/decade [36] for 6MWD. Our study also indicates that gains in muscle strength seem to be more important than gains in muscle mass in order to maintain or improve physical function. Strength gains without associated alterations in body composition but better functional status as seen in the present study possibly reflect enhanced neural adaptation in the early stages of training [37].

5. Limitations

The participants in our study were apparently healthy and motivated community dwelling volunteers. Thus, the reported drop-out rate most likely underestimates drop-out experienced in a population representative for this age or in a clinical sample. Further, our resistance exercise intervention was twelve weeks. A longer program would have increased drop-out rate as studies have shown increased drop-out with increased study length [38, 39]. Further, our study failed to establish the reasons why subjects finally decided to drop out, as correlation does not reflect necessarily causality. This could be related to a number of factors not assessed in the present study, including greater perceived exertion during exercise, pain, or social considerations. In future studies, qualitative interviews with subjects after drop-out can help to elucidate the reason.

6. Conclusion

Our study shows that participants who drop out are older, have poorer physical function and poorer health, and are less physically active. Great care has to be taken of such individuals in order to help them to participate in resistance exercise. Age > 80 years and 6MWD < 400 m might be useful screening parameters to identify participants at higher risk for drop-out.

Although there a theoretical rationale that old women improve less than old men after a resistance exercise program, we found that changes in strength and function were similar between genders and reflect improvements equal to 7–11 years of younger age.

Conflicts of Interest

The authors declare no conflicts of interest.

Acknowledgments

This study was part of the IceProQualita project, which was funded by the Icelandic Technology Development Fund (no. 071323008), Research Fund of the University of Iceland, a grant from Landspitali University Hospital Research Fund, and the Helga Jonsdottir and Sigurlidi Kristjansson Geriatric Research Fund.

References

[1] R. J. Dhillon and S. Hasni, "Pathogenesis and management of sarcopenia," *Clinics in Geriatric Medicine*, vol. 33, no. 1, pp. 17–26, 2017.

[2] R. Csapo and L. M. Alegre, "Effects of resistance training with moderate vs heavy loads on muscle mass and strength in the elderly: a meta-analysis," *Scandinavian Journal of Medicine and Science in Sports*, vol. 26, no. 9, pp. 995–1006, 2016.

[3] A. Arnarson, O. Gudny Geirsdottir, A. Ramel, K. Briem, P. V. Jonsson, and I. Thorsdottir, "Effects of whey proteins and carbohydrates on the efficacy of resistance training in elderly people: Double blind, randomised controlled trial," *European Journal of Clinical Nutrition*, vol. 67, no. 8, pp. 821–826, 2013.

[4] A. Ericsson, T. Bremell, Å. Cider, and K. Mannerkorpi, "Effects of exercise on fatigue and physical capacity in men with chronic widespread pain - a pilot study," *BMC Sports Science, Medicine and Rehabilitation*, vol. 8, no. 1, 2016.

[5] V. Almadana Pacheco, M. Pavón Masa, A. P. Gómez-Bastero Fernández, A. M. Muñiz Rodríguez, R. Tallón Moreno, and T. Montemayor Rubio, "Patient profile of drop-outs from a pulmonary rehabilitation program," *Archivos de Bronconeumologia*, 2016.

[6] A. Zech, M. Drey, E. Freiberger et al., "Residual effects of muscle strength and muscle power training and detraining on physical function in community-dwelling prefrail older adults: a randomized controlled trial," *BMC Geriatrics*, vol. 12, article 68, 2012.

[7] A. Y. Arikawa, M. O'Dougherty, and K. H. Schmitz, "Adherence to a strength training intervention in adult women," *Journal of Physical Activity and Health*, vol. 8, no. 1, pp. 111–118, 2011.

[8] U.S. Centers for Disease Control and Prevention and The Merck Company Foundation. Whitehouse Station, NJ: Merck Company Foundation; 2007. [Accessed Sep 2; 2008]. The state of aging and health in America 2007.

[9] J. W. Vezina, C. A. Der Ananian, E. Greenberg, and J. Kurka, "Sociodemographic correlates of meeting US department of health and human services muscle strengthening recommendations in middle-aged and older adults," *Preventing Chronic Disease*, vol. 11, no. 9, article E162, 2014.

[10] M. Da Boit, R. Sibson, J. R. Meakin et al., "Sex differences in the response to resistance exercise training in older people," *Physiological Reports*, vol. 4, no. 12, article e12834, 2016.

[11] O. G. Geirsdottir, A. Arnarson, K. Briem et al., "Physical function predicts improvement in quality of life in elderly icelanders after 12 weeks of resistance exercise," *Journal of Nutrition, Health and Aging*, vol. 16, no. 1, pp. 62–66, 2012.

[12] A. Arnarson, A. Ramel, O. G. Geirsdottir, P. V. Jonsson, and I. Thorsdottir, "Changes in body composition and use of blood cholesterol lowering drugs predict changes in blood lipids during 12 weeks of resistance exercise training in old adults," *Aging Clinical and Experimental Research*, vol. 26, no. 3, pp. 287–292, 2014.

[13] A. Ramel, O. G. Geirsdottir, P. V. Jonsson, and I. Thorsdottiri, "C-reactive protein and resistance exercise in community dwelling old adults," *Journal of Nutrition, Health and Aging*, vol 19, no. 7, pp. 792–796, 2015.

[14] M. F. Folstein, S. E. Folstein, and P. R. McHugh, ""Mini mental state". A practical method for grading the cognitive state of patients for the clinician," *Journal of Psychiatric Research*, vol 12, no. 3, pp. 189–198, 1975.

[15] O. G. Geirsdottir, A. Arnarson, K. Briem, A. Ramel, P. V. Jonsson, and I. Thorsdottir, "Effect of 12-week resistance exercise program on body composition, muscle strength, physical function, and glucose metabolism in healthy, insulin-resistant, and diabetic elderly icelanders," *Journals of Gerontology - Series A Biological Sciences and Medical Sciences*, vol. 67, no. 11, pp. 1259–1265, 2012.

[16] R. O. Crapo, R. Casaburi, A. L. Coates et al., "ATS statement: guidelines for the six-minute walk test," *American Journal of Respiratory and Critical Care Medicine*, vol. 166, no. 1, pp. 111–117, 2002.

[17] T. Troosters, R. Gosselink, and M. Decramer, "Six minute walking distance in healthy elderly subjects," *European Respiratory Journal*, vol. 14, no. 2, pp. 270–274, 1999.

[18] P. L. Enright and D. L. Sherrill, "Reference equations for the six-minute walk in healthy adults," *The American Journal of Respiratory and Critical Care Medicine*, vol. 158, no. 5, part 1, pp. 1384–1387, 1998.

[19] W. J. Gibbons, N. Fruchter, S. Sloan, and R. D. Levy, "Reference values for a multiple repetition 6-minute walk test in healthy adults older than 20 years," *Journal of Cardiopulmonary Rehabilitation*, vol. 21, no. 2, pp. 87–93, 2001.

[20] D. Podsiadlo and S. Richardson, "The timed "Up and Go": a test of basic functional mobility for frail elderly persons," *Journal of the American Geriatrics Society*, vol. 39, no. 2, pp. 142–148, 1991.

[21] M. A. Martínez-González, J. J. Varo, J. L. Santos et al., "Prevalence of physical activity during leisure time in the European Union," *Medicine and Science in Sports and Exercise*, vol. 33, no. 7, pp. 1142–1146, 2001.

[22] B. E. Ainsworth, W. L. Haskell, M. C. Whitt et al., "Compendium of physical activities: an update of activity codes and MET intensities," *Medicine and Science in Sports and Exercise*, vol. 32, no. 9, pp. S498–S504, 2000.

[23] R. S. Paffenbarger Jr., A. L. Wing, and R. T. Hyde, "Physical activity as an index of heart attack risk in college alumni," *American Journal of Epidemiology*, vol. 108, no. 3, pp. 161–175, 1978.

[24] T. Helgason, J. K. Bjornsson, K. Tomasson, and S. Ingimarsson, "Health related quality of life," *Laeknabladid*, vol. 83, pp. 492–502, 1997.

[25] T. Helgason, J. K. Bjornsson, K. Tomasson, and E. Gretarsdottir, "Health-related quality of life among Icelanders," *Laeknabladid*, vol. 86, pp. 251–257, 2000.

[26] ACSM. American College of Sports Medicine Position Stand, "Progression models in resistance training for healthy adults," *Medicine & Science in Sports & Exercise*, vol. 41, no. 3, pp. 687–708, 2009.

[27] B. J. Schoenfeld, "Is there a minimum intensity threshold for resistance training-induced hypertrophic adaptations?" *Sports Medicine*, vol. 43, no. 12, pp. 1279–1288, 2013.

[28] M. D. Schuenke, J. Herman, and R. S. Staron, "Preponderance of evidence proves "big" weights optimize hypertrophic and strength adaptations," *European Journal of Applied Physiology*, vol. 113, no. 1, pp. 269–271, 2013.

[29] L. M. Alegre, X. Aguado, D. Rojas-Martín, M. Martín-García, I. Ara, and R. Csapo, "Load-controlled moderate and high-intensity resistance training programs provoke similar strength gains in young women," *Muscle and Nerve*, vol. 51, no. 1, pp. 92–101, 2015.

[30] O. G. Geirsdottir, A. Arnarson, A. Ramel, I. Thorsdottir, K. Briem, and P. V. Jonsson, "Muscular strength and physical function in elderly adults 6–18 months after a 12-week resistance exercise program," *Scandinavian Journal of Public Health*, vol. 43, no. 1, pp. 76–82, 2015.

[31] W. J. Kraemer and N. A. Ratamess, "Hormonal responses and adaptations to resistance exercise and training," *Sports Medicine*, vol. 35, no. 4, pp. 339–361, 2005.

[32] W. J. Kraemer, S. J. Fleck, J. E. Dziados et al., "Changes in hormonal concentrations after different heavy-resistance exercise protocols in women," *Journal of Applied Physiology*, vol. 75, no. 2, pp. 594–604, 1993.

[33] W. J. Kraemer, S. E. Gordon, S. J. Fleck et al., "Endogenous anabolic hormonal and growth factor responses to heavy resistance exercise in males and females," *International Journal of Sports Medicine*, vol. 12, no. 2, pp. 228–235, 1991.

[34] B. J. Schoenfeld, "The mechanisms of muscle hypertrophy and their application to resistance training," *Journal of Strength & Conditioning Research*, vol. 24, no. 10, pp. 2857–2872, 2010.

[35] R. W. Bohannon, "Reference values for the timed up and go test: a descriptive meta-analysis," *Journal of Geriatric Physical Therapy*, vol. 29, no. 2, pp. 64–68, 2006.

[36] C. Casanova, B. R. Celli, P. Barria et al., "The 6-min walk distance in healthy subjects: reference standards from seven countries," *European Respiratory Journal*, vol. 37, no. 1, pp. 150–156, 2011.

[37] D. A. Gabriel, G. Kamen, and G. Frost, "Neural adaptations to resistive exercise: mechanisms and recommendations for training practices," *Sports Medicine*, vol. 36, no. 2, pp. 133–149, 2006.

[38] J. Adams and M. White, "Are activity promotion interventions based on the transtheoretical model effective? A critical review," *British Journal of Sports Medicine*, vol. 37, no. 2, pp. 106–114, 2003.

[39] A. K. Van Der Bij, M. G. H. Laurant, and M. Wensing, "Effectiveness of physical activity interventions for older adults: a review," *American Journal of Preventive Medicine*, vol. 22, no. 2, pp. 120–133, 2002.

18

Cognitive Strategies and Physical Activity in Older Adults

Nathalie André[1,2] **Claude Ferrand,**[3] **Cédric Albinet**[1,4] **and Michel Audiffren**[1,2]

[1]*Centre de Recherches sur la Cognition et l'Apprentissage, UMR CNRS 7295, Université de Poitiers, Poitiers, France*
[2]*Maison des Sciences de l'Homme et de la Société, USR CNRS 3565, Université de Poitiers, Poitiers, France*
[3]*EA 2114, Psychologie des âges de la vie, Université François Rabelais, Tours, France*
[4]*Laboratoire Sciences de la Cognition, Technologie, Ergonomie (SCoTE), Université de Toulouse, INU Champollion, Albi, France*

Correspondence should be addressed to Nathalie André; nathalie.andre@univ-poitiers.fr

Academic Editor: Barbara Shukitt-Hale

Background. Although a number of studies have examined sociodemographic, psychosocial, and environmental determinants of the level of physical activity (PA) for older people, little attention has been paid to the predictive power of cognitive strategies for independently living older adults. However, cognitive strategies have recently been considered to be critical in the management of day-to-day living. *Methods.* Data were collected from 243 men and women aged 55 years and older living in France using face-to-face interviews between 2011 and 2013. *Results.* A stepwise discriminant analysis selected five predictor variables (age, perceived health status, barriers' self-efficacy, internal memory, and attentional control strategies) of the level of PA. The function showed that the rate of correct prediction was 73% for the level of PA. The calculated discriminant function based on the five predictor variables is useful for detecting individuals at high risk of lapses once engaged in regular PA. *Conclusions.* This study highlighted the need to consider cognitive functions as a determinant of the level of PA and, more specifically, those cognitive functions related to executive functions (internal memory and attentional control), to facilitate the maintenance of regular PA. These results are discussed in relation to successful aging.

1. Introduction

Generally, physical activity adherence is examined by social psychologists and health psychologists to prevent sedentariness. Reviews of the gerontological literature on this topic reveal a number of socioeconomic, demographic, psychological, attitudinal, and accessibility correlates and/or determinants of physical activity (PA) [1–5]. For instance, when focusing on independently living elderly people, van Stralen et al. [2] and Koeneman et al. [3] reported several moderate to strong determinants of regular PA such as age, gender, education, perceived health and depression, baseline PA behavior, barriers' self-efficacy, benefits of regular PA, and social support. However, adherence also requires continuous effort and strategies underpinned by executive functions to maintain the behaviors involved in the healthy management of day-to-day living such as PA [6], diet regimen, and medication [7].

It is now well known that cognitive functions undergo a decline during aging [8], and this decline is often associated with the use of compensatory cognitive strategies that could help aging people cope with their diminished cognitive performances. For instance, some elderly people use external memory strategies, such as writing a shopping list on a piece of paper to compensate for a decline in episodic memory. In some cases, these strategies can be considered counterproductive in a long-term perspective because external memory aids could stimulate negative stereotype related to aging by reducing perceived efficacy and perceived control on memory [9]. These strategies could lead the individual to reduce the cognitive resources used to initiate behaviors and, consequently, not to stimulate or maintain their self-regulation ability. Thus, each time an elderly person chooses to write his/her shopping list on a piece of paper to avoid forgetting an item during shopping, he/she does not stimulate his/her encoding and retrieval memory systems and consequently undermines his/her episodic memory in the long term. Fortunately, not all compensatory cognitive strategies reduce the cognitive resources invested to cope with a problem but rather use alternate or vicarious cognitive systems, for instance, internal memory strategies [10]. In another respect, Lachman and Andreoletti [11] reported that when metacognitive beliefs were lacking, older adults were less strategic in solving problems, and this lack of mastery experiences reduced self-efficacy and resulted in less autonomy and more dependency.

The relationship between cognitive functioning and adherence has been studied either by examining populations with cognitive impairments [12, 13] or by training populations in cognitive processes [14–18]. These studies have been principally carried out in the context of medication adherence. For instance, studies have reported that older people with cognitive dysfunctions show poor medication adherence compared to healthy older people [12] and that working memory ability or habitual prospective memory facilitated recall of medication instructions [19, 20]. In their systematic review on the efficacy of interventions to increase medication adherence among community-dwelling seniors with cognitive impairments, Kröger et al. [13] have shown that reminder strategies are promising to improve adherence. Finally, Karr et al. [21] have shown that regardless of the population and executive functions targeted, cognitive training (specific or through physical activity) has positive effects on adherence. To our knowledge, very few studies have investigated the links between cognitive functioning and adherence to physical activity with healthy older adults [22–24]. As highlighted by McDonald-Miszczak et al. [25], despite a lack of clear identification of the cognitive functions implied in the adherence process, the research literature has identified several cognitive processes that can be considered to be responsible for psychological disturbances and nonadherence when they are impaired. Recently, Olson et al. [26] reported that cognitive functions such as working memory, controlled inhibition, attention, and task switching predicted PA adherence 6 months after the end of a PA program in older adults with metabolic diseases. Other studies have identified prospective memory [14, 27], metamemory [8, 28], and attentional control [22, 29, 30] as determinants of high levels of cognitive functioning. It can be reasonably hypothesized that remembering planned sessions during the week (prospective memory) and inhibiting the desire to stop exercise when it is difficult (controlled inhibition) are two high-level cognitive functions required to maintain the regular practice of a moderate to vigorous level of PA over weeks, months, or years. On one hand, prospective memory is related to long-term memory and declarative memory, and it describes the ability to plan and successfully execute delayed intentions in the future [31]. People in general, and more particularly aging people, use strategies to facilitate and/or solve a prospective memory task. Studies on prospective memory have demonstrated that this cognitive process facilitates medication adherence [27]. Metamemory can be defined as the control and regulation of strategies necessary to address such memory tasks [32]. More precisely, metamemory refers to two categories of strategies: (1) internal strategies, such as using mental imagery, recalling contextual cues, associating cues, or listing events; and (2) external strategies, such as making shopping lists or writing down appointments on a calendar. Gould et al. [27] have reported that older adults preferentially use internal memory strategies—although this relationship is mediated by depression and concerns about memory efficacy—to remember their medication but external memory strategies for everyday situations. On the other hand, attentional control can be conceptualized as the ability to filter information by focusing on pertinent cues and inhibiting nonpertinent cues [33]. Controlled inhibition can be considered a component of attentional control and concerns the ability to repress actions, thoughts, emotions, or impulses. Attentional control was greatly examined by Hillman et al. [22, 23] in relation to physical activity, and the authors reported that PA activates the attentional system and mobilizes attentional resources.

Many epidemiological studies have examined the benefits of PA on cognition and have shown a positive relationship between higher levels of PA and a reduced risk of cognitive impairment (for a review, see [34, 35]). For instance, some studies based on large sample sizes and long follow-up periods have shown that older adults who had previously engaged in higher levels of PA were likely to perform better on cognitive tasks when compared with participants with previously lower PA levels [36, 37]. Consequently, PA is hypothesized to have a protective effect on cognitive decline in older adults. The brain structures most negatively affected by aging are also those that benefit the most from physical activity (e.g., Colcombe et al. [38]). For instance, the prefrontal cortex and the hippocampus, which underlie executive functions and encoding of information in episodic memory, respectively, are more severely affected by aging than brain structures involved in procedural memory [39]. Because of this positive effect of PA on cognitive functions, it can be expected that active older adults will show better cognitive functioning and use better cognitive strategies than inactive ones. Reciprocally, better functioning in executive functions may facilitate the maintenance of new healthy behaviors such as a physically active lifestyle [40], and consequently, it could be expected that aging people who use more effective cognitive strategies maintain a higher level of regular physical activity.

The purpose of this study was to identify predictors of the level of PA among a sample of independent-living older healthy people from the PRAUSE project. We are particularly interested in the perception of use of cognitive strategies rather than the effectiveness of these strategies. It can be expected that because PA reduces the decline of cognitive functions and because the efficient functioning of cognitive functions facilitates the use of functional strategies, we should observe differences between active and inactive older adults in the use of cognitive strategies. As suggested by West et al. [41], cognitive functions meaningfully influence thought and actions and determine adaptive coping to challenges in everyday life. The main objective of the present study was to examine whether cognitive strategies related to executive functions and prospective memory would predict the level of engagement in physical activity in older persons.

2. Methods

2.1. Description of Sample. The present study is a part of a French regional survey, a multidisciplinary research project entitled Seniors' Autonomy Preservation in Poitou-Charentes (PRAUSE). The inclusion criteria to be eligible for the recruitment into PRAUSE were the following: (1) living in Poitou-Charentes; (2) being aged 55 years or over; and (3) not being institutionalized and not under guardianship or trusteeship. Participants were invited to take part in the study by mail and phone. Project feasibility was tested with a pilot study, and three waves of data collection were necessary to include a total of 466 participants. Each participant included in the study performed one to three sessions of data collection according to his/her motivation. For the purposes of this study, only 243 participants out of 466 completed all the data required to test our hypotheses. This sample of participants included 41.57% males and had a mean age of 74.02 (SD = 9.61) years.

2.2. Compliance with Ethical Standards. All participants signed an informed consent form. The three data collection waves occurred between 2011 and 2013. All participants were visited at home, and all face-to-face questionnaires were administered by investigators who received individual training for all data collection. The protocol of PRAUSE was approved by two national ethics committees: (1) the "general interest and statistical quality" label from the French National Council of Statistical Information (CNIS, visa no. 2012X907RG) and (2) the French National Commission on Informatics and Liberty (authorization no. 1593815).

2.3. Demographic and Health Variables. Questionnaires were completed with data including age, gender, perceived health status, education, depression, decisional balance, and BMI. Perceived health status was evaluated with a visual analogue scale from EuroQol-5D and consisted of assessing his/her perception of health from "best known health status" to "worse known health status." The *Decisional Balance* questionnaire was based on Marcus' version and adapted to physical activity. It consisted of two constructs that underlie cognitive and motivational aspects of human decision making. These constructs have been labeled the pros and cons of exercising, and they were each measured with 8 items. Participants responded to each item on a 5-point Likert-type scale ranging from totally agree (1) to totally disagree (5). Based on Bandura's guidelines [42] and the identification of main barriers in old age reported in the literature [43, 44], six barriers' self-efficacy were included based on health aspects (pain and fatigue), motivational determinants (too busy and nobody to practice with), and environmental factors (weather and accessibility). Participants rated answers on a 5-point scale ranging from 1 (not confident to overcome) to 5 (extremely confident to overcome). Cronbach's alpha values were .76 for pros, .83 for cons, and .68 for barriers' self-efficacy. Depression GDS, Depressive symptoms were assessed using the 30-item Geriatric Depression Scale validated in French by Bourque et al. [45]. A score of 0–9 is normal, a score of 10–19 indicates slight depression, and a score of 20–30 corresponds to severe depression.

2.4. Physical Activity Measure. The level of current PA was evaluated with the Historical Leisure Activity Questionnaire (HLAQ) [46]. This questionnaire was used to assess the history of PA weighted by relative intensity, and as suggested by Kriska et al. [46], the list of activities was adapted to the population. The HLAQ was previously used in French studies that demonstrated relationships between executive functions and level of physical activity [47, 48]. Participants were asked to report the frequency, type, intensity, and hours of PA performed during the present year. Using the Compendium of Physical Activities Tracking Guide 2011 [49], we obtained a specific metabolic equivalent (MET) for each PA. According to the HLAQ data and the compendium, we calculated the average energy expenditure (METs-h/week) for each participant. According to the WHO recommendations, we classified the participants above 7.5 METs-h/week in the active group and those below 7.5 METs-h/week in the inactive group.

2.5. Cognitive Variables. Cognitive strategies were measured using a questionnaire adapted from three scales: (1) the Metamemory in Adulthood scale [50], (2) the Thought Control Questionnaire [51], and (3) the Attentional Control Scale [52] (Table 1). Metamemory concerns knowledge of memory functioning, beliefs and affects about memory, as well as monitoring and autoregulation during memory activity [50]. The metamemory in adulthood scale contains eight subscales, from which two were selected and adapted for the study: the external strategy subscales (e.g., memos and calendar) and the internal strategy subscales (e.g., mental imagery and word associations). These scales evaluate the means used by people to more easily find information stored in prospective and episodic memory. The external strategy subscales include 6 items and the internal subscale 9 items. Cronbach's alphas for these two cognitive strategies were 0.66 and 0.70, respectively. The thought control questionnaire contains five subscales designed to assess people's tendency to use a variety of thought control strategies in everyday life. Two subscales were selected and adapted for the needs of the study: the reappraisal subscale (e.g., I try to reinterpret the thought) and the distraction subscale (e.g., I occupy myself with work instead). The reappraisal subscale includes 5 items and the distraction subscale 6 items. Cronbach's alphas for these two cognitive strategies were 0.83 and 0.75, respectively. The short-form Attentional Control Scale consisted of a 12-item self-report [52] measure combining attentional focusing that requires voluntary control over behaviors and attentional shifting that is related to performance on switching tasks. Only the attentional focusing strategy was evaluated in the study because of the link we posited with PA. This scale includes 6 items. Participants rated answers on a 5-point scale ranging from 1 (never used) to 5 (always used) for the five strategy subscales. Cronbach's alpha for this scale was 0.66.

Table 1: Cognitive strategy questionnaires used in the study.

External memory strategies
I keep a list or otherwise note important dates, such as birthdays and anniversaries
I write shopping list to help me remember
I write appointments on a calendar to help me remember them
I routinely keep things (keys or glasses) in a familiar spot, so I will not forget them when I need to locate them
I post reminders of things I need to do in a prominent place, such as on bulletin boards or note boards
When I want to take something with me, I leave it in an obvious, prominent place, such as putting my suitcase in front of the door
Internal memory strategies
When I am looking for something I have recently misplaced, I try to retrace my steps in order to locate it
When I want to remember something, I concentrate hard on it
When I try to remember a telephone number, I mentally repeat it to myself
I think about the day's activities at the beginning of the day, so I can remember what I am supposed to do
I make mental images or pictures to help me remember an event or an individual
I try to relate something I want to remember to something else hoping that this will increase the likelihood of my remembering later
When I have trouble remembering something, I try to remember something similar in order to help me remember
Reappraisal
When I experience an unpleasant/unwanted thought, I challenge the thought's validity
When I experience an unpleasant/unwanted thought, I analyze the thought rationally
When I experience an unpleasant/unwanted thought, I try to reinterpret the thought
When I experience an unpleasant/unwanted thought, I try a different way of thinking about it
When I experience an unpleasant/unwanted thought, I question the reasons for having the thought
Distraction
When I experience an unpleasant/unwanted thought, I call to mind positive images instead
When I experience an unpleasant/unwanted thought, I occupy myself with work instead
When I experience an unpleasant/unwanted thought, I think pleasant thoughts instead
When I experience an unpleasant/unwanted thought, I do something that I enjoy
When I experience an unpleasant/unwanted thought, I think about something else
When I experience an unpleasant/unwanted thought, I keep myself busy
Attentional control
When concentrating on something and there are noises around me, I ask for silence
When I read, I look for a calm area where I will not be distracted by people around me
When I am working hard on something and I am distracted by events around me, I try to isolate myself
When trying to focus my attention on something and thoughts distracting me, I chase them out of my mind
When concentrating on something and hunger or thirst distracts me, I satisfy my need so that it does not worry me anymore
When concentrating on something, I turn off TV or radio

2.6. Data Analysis. Descriptive statistics were examined to characterize the study population. Correlation analyses and *t*-tests were used to obtain additional descriptive information and to identify a preliminary set of predictor variables to be included in the discriminant analysis. Variables with a significant difference of $p < 0.05$ as determined by the above tests were entered into stepwise discriminant analysis. Then, a stepwise discriminant analysis was performed to determine if active and inactive participants could be discriminated based on the following variables: age, gender, body mass index (BMI), perceived health status, depression, barriers' self-efficacy, and cognitive strategies (internal memory and attentional control).

3. Results

Table 2 shows distributions of sociodemographic characteristics and other covariates. Participants who were active had a mean age of 71.45 (SD = 8.65), had a mean BMI of 26.88 (SD = 4.94), perceived themselves on average in better health (75.46, SD = 14.27), perceived themselves on average as capable of overcoming barriers (38.51, SD = 9.83), were not depressed (6.48, SD = 4.80), used on average more internal memory strategies (30.28, SD = 5.21), and were not easily distracted (19.41, SD = 4.37). Participants who were inactive had a mean age of 77.66 (SD = 9.75), had a mean BMI of 28.70 (SD = 4.70), perceived themselves in worse health (66.37, SD = 18.01), perceived themselves as less capable of overcoming barriers (31.85, SD = 10.06), used on average less internal memory (28.76, SD = 6.61), and had difficulties in concentrating (20.46, SD = 5.04).

The emphasis of this analysis was on understanding how these variables were related to each other to determine the level of physical activity. We used discriminant analysis to determine the linear combination of predictor variables that best classified the cases into the two groups. The stepwise discriminant analysis (Table 3) showed that Wilks' lambda, as a test of discriminant function, was significant (lambda = 0.736; $\chi^2 = 72.051$, df = 8, $p < 0.001$) and selected the five following variables as determinants of physical inactivity (based on structure matrix loading): older (−0.626), perceived poor health (0.442), less use of internal memory strategies (0.213), attentional control (−0.196), and poor confidence to overcome barriers to PA practice (0.555).

Table 2: Sociodemographic, health, motivational, and cognitive strategies for active versus inactive participants. The last column shows th correlations between the variable and the level of physical activity for the population sample examined in this study ($n = 243$).

Variables	Active ($n = 139$) mean (SD)	Inactive ($n = 104$) mean (SD)	p	Correlation coefficien
✓*Age (years)	71.45 (8.65)	77.66 (9.75)	†	−0.35†
✓*Gender (M/F)	71/68	29/75	†	0.23†
✓Education	10.52 (3.66)	10.20 (3.80)	ns	0.05
✓*BMI	26.88 (4.94)	28.70 (4.70)	†	−0.18†
✓*Perceived health status	75.46 (14.27)	66.37 (18.01)	†	0.26†
✓*Depression	6.48 (4.80)	9.067 (5.05)	†	−0.14†
Decisional variables				
✓Pros	15.84 (6.14)	17.27 (6.10)	ns	−0.11
✓*Barriers' self-efficacy	38.51 (9.83)	31.85 (10.06)	†	0.36†
Cognitive strategies				
EMS (from 6 to 30)	23.86 (4.02)	24.30 (4.42)	ns	−0.06
*IMS (from 9 to 45)	30.28 (5.16)	28.76 (6.61)	†	0.12
*ACS (from 6 to 30)	19.43 (3.68)	20.46 (5.04)	†	−0.11
DS (from 6 to 30)	20.60 (4.94)	20.21 (5.40)	ns	0.04
RS (from 5 to 25)	14.58 (4.05)	13.62 (4.56)	ns	0.11

✓Variables reported as moderately to strongly significant in the literature. *Variables entered in the current discriminant analysis. † = $p < 0.05$ ns = nonsignificant ($p > 0.05$). EMS: external memory strategies, IMS: internal memory strategies, ACS: attentional control strategies, DS: distraction strategies, and RS: reappraisal strategies.

Table 3: Summary of interpretive measures for stepwise discriminant analysis.

Predictor	Standardized coefficient loadings	F ratio	Rank
Age	−0.626	15.239**	1
Gender	0.413	1.469	
BMI	−0.307	3.824	
Perceived health status	0.442	4.230*	4
Depression	−0.434	0.739	
Internal memory	0.213	10.684*	2
Attentional control	−0.196	9.761*	3
Barriers' self-efficacy	0.555	3.948*	5
Canonical correlation	0.513		
Eigenvalue	0.358		
Wilks' lambda	0.736		
χ^2	72.051; df = 8		

*$p < 0.01$, **$p < 0.001$.

Wilks' lambda, which describes the proportion of total variance in the discriminant score not explained by differences between groups, was significant, indicating that it is unlikely that participants who were inactive and those who were active had the same means on the discriminant functions generated from the prediction equation.

Table 4 summarizes the group membership results of the classification routine. Of the 104 participants who were inactive, 63 (60.6%) were correctly classified as inactive, and of the 139 participants who were active, 113 (81.3%) were correctly classified as active based on the selected variables. The overall percentage of the level of PA classifications was 73%, reflecting a 23% improvement over chance alone. Of the variables investigated, age was the most discriminating and barriers' self-efficacy the least.

4. Discussion

Sedentariness and inactivity are legitimate problems in older adults because these behaviors lead to several health problems such as more pronounced cognitive decline, sarcopenia, or social isolation. Most studies that have examined the factors associated with sedentariness or inactivity have focused on psychosocial predictors. However, cognitive functions have recently been considered in adherence to treatment medication [12, 13], but to our knowledge, no study has examined the predictive value of cognitive strategies in adherence to PA in healthy older adults. The aim of the present study was to identify cognitive and psychosocial determinants of the level of PA in independently living healthy older adults in France.

First, no difference was observed between active and inactive healthy older adults when considering level of education, knowledge concerning the benefits of regular PA, the use of external memory strategies, cognitive and behavioral distractions, or reappraisal. These results are partially consistent with previous literature reviews examining the relationships between sociodemographic and psychosocial determinants and the level of PA [2, 3, 53]. The results concerning knowledge about the benefits of regular PA suggest that information provided by the campaigns of prevention are well retained by individuals in general,

Table 4: Classification results of the discriminant analysis.

Group	Number of cases	Predicted group inactive n (%)	Membership active, n (%)
Inactive	104	63 (60.6%)	41 (39.4%)
Active	139	24 (17.2%)	113 (81.3%)

73.03% of grouped cases were correctly classified and 26.97% of grouped cases were incorrectly classified.

regardless of their level of engagement in regular PA. As suggested by Gross and Rebok [53], however some demographic predictors such as gender, pros of exercising, and level of education could be used in high-risk populations, these predictors are not necessarily significant in healthy populations. It is interesting to note that, in the present study, active older adults scored lower on the pros scale than inactive ones. This result could indicate that inactive older adults overestimate pros but are not interested or concerned by these potential benefits. Three out of five cognitive strategies showed no significant differences between active and inactive older adults, with external strategies being more used than the other strategies by older adults in general ($M = 4.82$; close to "always used"), followed by distraction ($M = 3.43$; close to "sometimes used") and reappraisal strategies ($M = 2.36$; close to "rarely used"), the latter being the least used and referring to problem solving. These results could be interpreted in two ways: (1) maintaining a high level of PA involves specific cognitive functions and strategies and (2) practicing a high level of PA facilitates the use of higher cognitive functions and strategies.

This study also revealed some interesting results concerning predictors of the level of PA that could contribute to reinforce interventions intended to help older people adhere to long-term PA practice. The discriminant analysis revealed that among the variables that emerged as significantly predictive of the level of PA, age, perceived health, barriers' self-efficacy, internal memory strategies, and attentional control strategies predominantly discriminated between active and inactive older participants in successfully classifying 73% of participants. Concerning sociodemographic and psychosocial variables, these results are congruent with previous studies. First, several studies [2, 3] moderately suggested that males are generally more active than females. Unlike these studies, gender was not a predictor of the level of PA in the present study. In a recent systematic review [54], it appears that gender differences in walking is attenuated for old adults (>70 years). Second, perceived health status was presently identified as a determinant of engagement in PA but not depression. However, McHugh and Lawlor [55] have reported an overadditive interaction of these two variables on hours of exercise per week such that high perceived health status combined with low levels of depression resulted in the highest levels of exercise. In the present study, even if depression was correlated to the level of PA, this variable did not discriminate between active and inactive older adults. Consequently, it could be suggested that (1) perceived health status and depression share a common variance, certainly because global perceived health status includes a component of mental health status such as depression ($r = -0.365$ for this study) or (2) perceived health status is a better predictor of PA than depression. Third, and finally, barriers' self-efficacy, which appeared as a predictor of the level of PA in the present study, were already reported as predictive of adherence to PA [56], more precisely, in elderly women in a 6-month strength training program. In this last study, barriers' self-efficacy were a good predictor of the first three months of exercise adherence and remained a significant predictor after six months. In the present study, barriers' self-efficacy were a good predictor of regular and habitual physical activity. Both studies suggest that barriers' self-efficacy are a good predictor of exercise adherence from a long-term perspective, possibly because this variable positively influences motivation to practice by increasing effort and persistence as well as enhancing attention paid to tasks.

The important contribution of this study is the discriminant power of cognitive strategies, indicating that active older people perceive themselves as using more internal memory strategies—assessing prospective and episodic memory—and as more able of using controlled inhibition than inactive ones. In other words, these perceptions would favor engagement in physical activity because they would reinforce positive perception of one's own efficacy to interact with environment. Another explanation could be that practicing moderate to high level of physical activity improves episodic memory and consequently facilitates the use of internal memory by older adults and their perception of using these strategies. Because this study was cross-sectional, we cannot define a causal relationship between these variables. Notwithstanding, a first assumption would be that older adults who have better memory abilities and/or better attentional control engage themselves more easily in active behaviors. This explanation is reinforced by previous research that has reported that the use of memory strategies facilitates the management of daily living activities [7], medication adherence [19, 26], and PA [15]. To our knowledge, only the study carried out by Olson et al. [26] reporteda relationship between attention and adherence to PA and postulated that controlled inhibition is critical to successful behavior changes. In other words, attentional control ability is important for switching between goal-directed plans and environment-based responses. According to the temporal self-regulation model proposed by Hall and Fong [6], executive functions are involved in PA behavior. However, these authors did not provide any details concerning the specific executive functions involved in adherence, such as planning, cognitive flexibility, or controlled inhibition. The present results clearly show that specific cognitive functions are associated with PA behavior: presumably, prospective memory related to internal memory strategies and controlled inhibition related to attentional control strategies. A second assumption would be that by being active, older adults increase their memory abilities and their attentional control. For instance, Winnecke et al. [30]

reported that individuals with higher levels of PA showed better attentional control capabilities than those who are less active. This result confirms the proposition made by Hillman et al. [23] that PA can activate the attentional system and mobilize attentional resources. From that perspective, other studies showed that controlled inhibition seems to benefit more selectively from PA than from other executive functions [57, 58]. Studies on memory training programs reported that memory strategies are needed to maintain regular activity with a low investment of cognitive resources [59]. For instance, Wolff et al. [59] reported that action planning, defined by the authors as being strongly related to memory strategies, facilitates the enactment of health behavior in daily life. What is interesting to note here is that memory strategies are not necessarily associated with high prospective memory ability. In other words, physically active older adults might compensate for cognitive deficits by recruiting larger frontal areas relevant for memory and/or attentional control strategies. This compensatory mechanism would not necessarily consist of an increase of the efficiency of these functions but in a better use of the cognitive strategies. These strategies could, in turn, facilitate the day-to-day management of life and perceived health. There is now substantial literature demonstrating this reciprocal effect, and our results confirm and specify the theoretical position taken by Hall and Fong [6] on the mutual reinforcement of executive functions and PA over time. Our results argue in the direction of this model, and particular attention should be paid to the cognitive strategies involved according to the targeted behavior. The present study has certain limitations. First, the study employed cross-sectional data, precluding any assumptions concerning causality between the five variables selected as predictors and the level of PA. Moreover, those variables and the level of PA might have changed over time. Further analysis of longitudinal data is warranted to clarify the relationship between changes in the five predictors obtained and PA. Another limitation to this study is its reliance on self-reported data on the five selected variables and PA.

5. Conclusion

Rather than seeing older people as lacking motivation for physical activities, this study identified cognitive and psychosocial predictors of the level of PA to evaluate the likelihood of relapses or quitting and to reduce the risk factors through interventions among older people at increased risk of inactivity. Regardless of whether age is an irreversible process, this study raises awareness of the need to consider cognitive strategies as facilitators to engage in durable PA. The development of specific cognitive strategies related to cognitive functions seems a relevant element to facilitate the management of daily life and preservation from sedentariness.

Conflicts of Interest

The authors declare that there are no conflicts of interest regarding the publication of this article.

Authors' Contributions

All authors have contributed significantly to the research concept, literature review, objectives, and design of the study. They all are in agreement with the content of the manuscript. All authors approved the manuscript and this submission.

References

[1] S. G. Trost, N. Owen, A. E. Bauman, J. F. Sallis, and W. Brown, "Correlates of adults' participation in physical activity: review and update," *Medicine and Sciences in Sports and Exercise*, vol. 34, no. 12, pp. 1996–2001, 2002.

[2] M. M. van Stralen, H. De Vries, A. N. Mudde, C. Bolman, and L. Lechner, "Determinants of initiation and maintenance of physical activity among older adults: a literature review," *Health Psychology Review*, vol. 3, no. 2, pp. 147–207, 2009.

[3] M. A. Koeneman, M. W. Verheijden, M. J. M. Chinapaw, and M. Hopman-Rock, "Determinants of physical activity and exercise in healthy older adults: a systematic review," *International Journal of Behavioral Nutrition and Physical Activity*, vol. 8, no. 1, p. 142, 2011.

[4] A. E. Bauman, R. S. Reis, J. F. Sallis, J. C. Wells, R. J. Loos, and B. W. Martin, "Correlates of physical activity: why are some people physically active and others not?," *The Lancet*, vol. 38, no. 9838, pp. 258–271, 2012.

[5] B. Guinn and V. Vincent, "Select physical activity determinants in independent-living elderly," *Activities, Adaptation & Aging*, vol. 26, no. 4, pp. 17–26, 2002.

[6] P. A. Hall and G. T. Fong, "Temporal self-regulation theory: a neurobiologically informed model for physical activity behaviour," *Frontiers in Human Neuroscience*, vol. 9, p. 117, 2015.

[7] R. L. West, D. K. Bagwell, and A. Dark-Freudeman, "Self-efficacy and memory aging: the impact of a memory intervention based on self-efficacy," *Aging, Neuropsychology, and Cognition*, vol. 15, no. 3, pp. 302–329, 2008.

[8] S. Colcombe and A. F. Kramer, "Fitness effects on the cognitive function of older adults: a meta-analytic study," *Psychological Science*, vol. 14, no. 2, pp. 125–130, 2003.

[9] B. Levy, "Stereotype embodiment: a psychological approach to aging," *Current Directions in Physical Science*, vol. 18, no. 6, pp. 332–336, 2009.

[10] B. Bouazzaoui, M. Isingrini, S. Fay et al., "Aging and self-reported internal and external memory strategy uses: the role of executive functioning," *Acta Psychologica*, vol. 135, no. 1, pp. 59–66, 2010.

[11] M. E. Lachman and C. Andreoletti, "Strategy use mediates the relationship between control beliefs and memory performance for middle-aged and older adults," *Journal of Gerontology: Psychological Sciences*, vol. 61, no. 2, pp. P88–P94, 2006.

[12] F. Misokami, M. Hiroki, T. Kinoshita, T. Kumagai, K. Futura, and I. Kazuhiro, "Adherence to medication regimens is an effective indicator of cognitive dysfunction in elderly individuals," *American Journal of Alzheimer's Disease and Other Dementias*, vol. 31, no. 2, pp. 132–136, 2016.

[13] E. Kröger, O. Tatar, I. Vedel et al., "Improving medication adherence among community-dwelling seniors with cognitive impairment: a systematic review of interventions," *International Journal of Clinical Pharmacy*, vol. 39, no. 4, pp. 641–656, 2017.

[14] A. Hering, P. G. Rendell, N. S. Rose, K. M. Schnitzspahn, and M. Kliegel, "Prospective memory training in older adults and its relevance for successful aging," *Psychological Research*, vol. 78, no. 6, pp. 892–904, 2014.
[15] J. R. Best, L. S. Nagamatsu, and T. Liu-Ambrose, "Improvements to executive functions during exercise training predict maintenance of physical activity over the following year," *Frontiers in Human Neuroscience*, vol. 8, p. 353, 2014.
[16] M. A. Wiegand, A. K. Troyer, C. Gojmerac, and K. J. Murphy, "Facilitating change in health-related behaviors and intentions: a randomized controlled trial of a multidimensional memory program for older adults," *Aging and Mental Health*, vol. 17, no. 7, pp. 806–815, 2013.
[17] N. L. Campbell, J. Zhan, W. Tu et al., "Self-reported medication adherence barriers among ambulatory older adults with mild cognitive impairment," *Pharmacotherapy*, vol. 36, no. 2, pp. 196–202, 2016.
[18] A. Hernandez-Galiot and I. Goni, "Adherence to the Mediterranean diet pattern, cognitive status and depressive symptoms in an elderly non-institutionalized population," *Nutricion Hospitalaria*, vol. 34, no. 2, pp. 338–344, 2017.
[19] S. D. Neupert and L. McDonald-Miszczak, "Younger and older adults' delayed recall of medication instructions: the role of cognitive and metacognitive predictors," *Aging, Neuropsychology, and Cognition*, vol. 11, no. 4, pp. 428–442, 2004.
[20] K. Vedhara, E. Wadsworth, P. Norman et al., "Habitual prospective memory in elderly patient with type 2 diabetes: implications for medication adherence," *Psychology, Health & Medicine*, vol. 9, no. 1, pp. 17–27, 2004.
[21] J. E. Karr, C. N. Areshenkoff, P. Rast, and M. A. Garcia-Barrera, "An empirical comparison of the therapeutic benefits of physical exercise and cognitive training on the executive functions of older adults: a meta-analysis of controlled trials," *Neuropsychology*, vol. 28, no. 6, pp. 829–845, 2014.
[22] C. H. Hillman, A. F. Kramer, A. V. Belopolsky, and D. P. Smith, "A cross-sectional examination of age and physical activity on performance and event-related brain potentials in a task switching paradigm," *International Journal of Psychophysiology*, vol. 59, no. 1, pp. 30–39, 2006.
[23] C. H. Hillman, K. I. Erickson, and A. F. Kramer, "Be smart, exercise your heart: exercise effects on brain and cognition," *Nature Reviews*, vol. 9, no. 1, pp. 58–65, 2008.
[24] C. B. Phillips, J. D. Edwards, R. Andel, and M. Kilpatrick, "Daily physical activity and cognitive function variability in older adults," *Journal of Aging and Physical Activity*, vol. 24, no. 2, pp. 256–267, 2016.
[25] L. McDonald-Miszczak, S. D. Neupert, and G. Gutman, "Does cognitive ability explain inaccuracy in older adults' self-reported medication adherence?," *Journal of Applied Gerontology*, vol. 28, no. 5, pp. 560–581, 2009.
[26] E. A. Olson, S. P. Mullen, L. B. Raine, A. F. Kramer, C. H. Hillman, and E. McAuley, "Integrated social and neurocognitive model of physical activity behavior in older adults with metabolic disease," *Annals of Behavioral Medicine*, vol. 51, no. 2, pp. 272–281, 2017.
[27] O. N. Gould, L. McDonald-Miszczak, and B. King, "Metacognition and medication adherence: how do older adults remember?," *Experimental Aging Research*, vol. 23, no. 4, pp. 315–342, 1997.
[28] L. Taconnat and P. Lemaire, "Fonctions exécutives, vieillissement cognitif et variations stratégiques," *Psychologie Française*, vol. 59, no. 1, pp. 89–100, 2014.
[29] C. Lustig, L. Hasher, and S. T. Tonev, "Distraction as a determinant of processing speed," *Psychonomic Bulletin & Review*, vol. 13, no. 4, pp. 619–625, 2006.
[30] A. H. Winnecke, B. Godde, E.-M. Reuter, S. Vieluf, and C. Voelcker-Rehage, "The association between physical activity and attentional control in younger and older middle-aged adults: an ERP study," *GeroPsychology*, vol. 25, no. 4, pp. 207–221, 2012.
[31] M. Kliegel, M. A. McDaniel, and G. O. Einstein, *Prospective Memory: Cognitive, Neuroscience, Developmental, and Applied Perspectives*, Erlbaum, Mahwah, NJ, USA, 2008.
[32] A.-P. Le Berre, F. Eustache, and H. Beaunieux, "La métamémoire: théorie et clinique," *Revue de Neuropsychologie*, vol. 1, no. 4, pp. 312–320, 2009.
[33] D. Derryberry and M. A. Reed, "Anxiety-related attentional biases and their regulation by attentional control," *Journal of Abnormal Psychology*, vol. 111, no. 2, pp. 225–236, 2002.
[34] M. Audiffren, N. André, and C. Albinet, "Effets positifs de l'exercice physique chronique sur les fonctions cognitives des seniors: bilan et perspective," *Revue de Neuropsychologie*, vol. 3, no. 4, pp. 207–225, 2011.
[35] L. Bherer, K. I. Erickson, and T. Liu-Ambrose, "A review of the effects of physical activity and exercise on cognitive and brain functions in older adults," *Journal of Aging Research*, vol. 2013, Article ID 197326, 2 pages, 2013.
[36] F. Sofi, D. Valecchi, D. Bacci, R. Abbate, G. F. Gensini, and C. Macchi, "Physical activity and risk of cognitive decline: a meta-analysis of prospective studies," *Journal of Internal Medicine*, vol. 269, no. 1, pp. 107–117, 2011.
[37] K. Yaffe, D. Barnes, M. Nevitt, L. Y. Lui, and K. Covinsky, "A prospective study of physical activity and cognitive decline in elderly women: women who walk," *Archives of Internal Medicine*, vol. 161, no. 14, pp. 1703–1708, 2001.
[38] S. J. Colcombe, K. I. Erickson, N. Raz et al., "Aerobic fitness reduces brain tissue loss in aging humans," *Journal of Gerontology*, vol. 58, no. 2, pp. 176–180, 2003.
[39] D. B. Mitchell, "How many memory system? Evidence from aging," *Journal of Experimental Psychology: Learning, Memory, and Cognition*, vol. 15, no. 1, pp. 31–49, 1989.
[40] J. L. Allan, D. McMinn, and M. Daly, "A bidirectional relationship between executive function and health behavior: evidence, implications, and future directions," *Frontiers in Neurosciences*, vol. 10, p. 386, 2016.
[41] R. West, M. S. Beeri, J. Schmeidler et al., "Better memory functioning associated with higher total and low-density lipoprotein cholesterol levels in very elderly subjects without the apolipoprotein e4 allele," *American Journal of Geriatric Psychiatry*, vol. 16, no. 9, pp. 781–785, 2008.
[42] A. Bandura, "Guide for constructing self-efficacy scales," in *Self-Efficacy Beliefs of Adolescents*, F. Pajares and T. Urdan, Eds., pp. 307–337, Information Age Publishing, Greenwich, CT, USA, 2006.
[43] C. Thogersen-Ntoumani, "An ecological model of predictors of stages of change for physical activity in Greek older adults," *Scandinavian Journal of Medicine and Sciences in Sports*, vol. 19, no. 2, pp. 286–296, 2009.
[44] K. L. Smith, K. Carr, A. Wiseman, K. Calhoun, N. H. McNevin, and P. L. Weir, "Barriers are not the limiting factor to participation in physical activity in Canadian seniors," *Journal of Aging Research*, vol. 2012, Article ID 890679, 8 pages, 2012.
[45] P. Bourque, L. Blanchard, and J. Vezina, "Etude psychométrique de l'échelle de dépression gériatrique," *Canadian Journal of Aging*, vol. 9, no. 4, pp. 348–355, 1990.
[46] A. M. Kriska, R. B. Sandler, J. A. Cauley, R. E. Laporte, D. L. Hom, and G. Pambianco, "The assessment of historical physical-activity and its relation to adult bone parameters,"

American Journal of Epidemiology, vol. 127, no. 5, pp. 1053–1063, 1988.

[47] G. K. Boucard, C. T. Albinet, A. Bugaïska, C. A. Bouquet, D. Clarys, and M. Audiffren, "Impact of chronic exercise on executive functions in aging: a selective effect to inhibition performance among middle-old adults," *Journal of Sport and Exercise Psychology*, vol. 34, no. 6, pp. 808–827, 2012.

[48] A. Canivet, C. T. Albinet, N. André et al., "Effects of BDNF polymorphism and physical activity on episodic memory in the elderly: a cross sectional study," *European Review of Aging and Physical Activity*, vol. 12, p. 15, 2015.

[49] B. E. Ainsworth, W. L. Haskell, S. D. Herrmann et al., "Compendium of physical activities: a second update of codes and MET values," *Medicine and Sciences in Sports and Exercise*, vol. 43, no. 8, pp. 1575–1581, 2011.

[50] R. A. Dixon, D. F. Hultsch, and C. Hertzog, "The metamemory in adulthood (MIA) questionnaire," *Psychopharmacology Bulletin*, vol. 24, no. 4, pp. 671–688, 1988.

[51] A. Wells and M. I. Davies, "The thought control questionnaire: a measure of individual differences in the control of unwanted thoughts," *Behaviour Research and Therapy*, vol. 32, no. 8, pp. 871–878, 1994.

[52] M. T. Judah, D. M. Grant, A. C. Mills, and W. V. Lechner, "Factor structure and validation of the attentional control scale," *Cognition and Emotion*, vol. 28, no. 3, pp. 433–451, 2014.

[53] A. L. Gross and G. W. Rebok, "Memory training and strategy use in older adults: results from the ACTIVE study," *Psychology and Aging*, vol. 26, no. 3, pp. 503–517, 2011.

[54] T. M. Pollard and J. M. Wagnild, "Gender differences in walking (for leisure, transport and in total) across adult life: a systematic review," *BMC Public Health*, vol. 17, no. 1, p. 341, 2017.

[55] J. E. McHugh and B. A. Lawlor, "Perceived health status is associated with hours of exercise per week in older adults independent of physical health," *Journal of Physical Activity and Health*, vol. 10, no. 8, pp. 1102–1108, 2013.

[56] R. E. Rhodes, A. D. Martin, and J. E. Taunton, "Temporal relationships of self-efficacy and social support as predictors of adherence in a 6-month strength-training program for older women," *Perceptual and Motor Skills*, vol. 93, no. 7, pp. 693–703, 2001.

[57] G. K. Boucard, C. T. Albinet, A. Bugaiska, C. A. Bouquet, D. Clarys, and M. Audiffren, "Impact of physical activity on executive functions in aging: a selective effect on inhibition among old adults," *Journal of Sport and Exercise Psychology*, vol. 34, no. 6, pp. 808–827, 2012.

[58] A. L. Smiley-Oyen, K. A. Lowry, S. J. Francois, M. L. Kohut, and P. Ekkekakis, "Exercise, fitness, and neurocognitive function in older adults: the selective improvement and cardiovascular fitness hypotheses," *Annals of Behavioral Medicine*, vol. 36, no. 3, pp. 280–291, 2008.

[59] J. K. Wolff, L. M. Warner, J. P. Ziegelmann, S. Wurm, and M. Kliegel, "Translating good intentions into physical activity: older adults with low prospective memory ability profit from planning," *Journal of Behavioral Medicine*, vol. 39, no. 3, pp. 472–482, 2016.

19

Decline in Memory, Visuospatial Ability, and Crystalized Cognitive Abilities in Older Adults: Normative Aging or Terminal Decline?

R. Bendayan,[1] A. M. Piccinin,[2] S. M. Hofer,[2] D. Cadar,[1] B. Johansson,[3] and G. Muniz-Terrera[1]

[1] *MRC Unit for Lifelong Health and Ageing, University College of London, Faculty of Population Health Sciences, London, UK*
[2] *Department of Psychology, University of Victoria, Victoria, BC, Canada*
[3] *Department of Psychology, University of Göteborg, Göteborg, Sweden*

Correspondence should be addressed to R. Bendayan; r.bendayan@ucl.ac.uk

Academic Editor: F. R. Ferraro

The aim of this study is to explore the pattern of change in multiple measures of cognitive abilities in a sample of oldest-old adults, comparing two different time metrics (chronological age and time to death) and therefore examining both underlying conceptual assumptions (age-related change and terminal decline). Moreover, the association with individual characteristics as sex, education, and dementia diagnosis was also examined. Measures of cognitive status (Mini-Mental State Examination and the Swedish Clock Test) and tests of crystallized (knowledge and synonyms), memory (verbal memory, nonverbal long-term memory, recognition and correspondence, and short-term memory), and visuospatial ability were included. The sample consisted of 671 older Swedish adult participants of the OCTO Twin Study. Linear mixed models with random coefficients were used to analyse change patterns and BIC indexes were used to compare models. Results showed that the time to death model was the best option in analyses of change in all the cognitive measures considered (except for the Information Test). A significant cognitive decline over time was found for all variables. Individuals diagnosed with dementia had lower scores at the study entrance and a faster decline. More educated individuals performed better in all the measures of cognition at study entry than those with poorer education, but no differences were found in the rate of change. Differences were found in age, sex, or time to death at baseline across the different measures. These results support the terminal decline hypothesis when compared to models assuming that cognitive changes are driven by normative aging processes.

1. Introduction

Increasing levels of population aging turns research about aging related cognitive decline into a worldwide priority. Although it is well known that cognitive abilities decline with age, a better understanding of the underlying processes and individual differences in cognitive aging remains a main objective in current cognitive aging research [1].

Cognitive decline in aging studies is often explored using linear mixed models [2]. These models consist of two levels of analysis that allow researchers to explore how individuals change over time and how these changes vary across individuals [3, 4]. Depending on the context, time can represent any appropriate scale, ranging from milliseconds to millennia, and can be centered for all individuals to represent distance from any event: birth (i.e., age), time since baseline measurement, time to diagnosis, or time to death. While time is a generic concept that passes (within a person) in the same way, regardless of how it is specified [5], different time metric specifications imply a specific alignment of the individuals' scores relative to other people in the sample. From a methodological perspective, it has been shown that if scores are aligned according to a time metric that does not reflect the progression of the processes driving change, the measurement model is misidentified and estimation of the parameters of change is distorted [6].

Moreover, choosing the most appropriate time metric to model cognitive change is not only a statistical issue, but also a theoretical one. Different time metrics assume that the changes are driven by different underlying processes. For example, selecting age as time metric assumes that all the individuals at each age are in the same stage of the causal process (aging) that is driving the cognitive changes. Therefore, when changes are modelled using chronological age, these changes are considered as age-related changes, which are often conceptualized as normative aging changes [7]. However, cognitive changes in older adults may not be driven by age-related changes but by their proximity to death, proposed by the terminal decline hypothesis. This hypothesis was first described by Kleemeier [8] and extended by K. F. Riegel and R. M. Riegel [9] who hypothesized that approximately 5 years prior to death there is an acceleration in cognitive decline. Since then, a great body of research has examined this hypothesis in older adults (for a review see [10, 11]) and several studies have modelled change in cognitive abilities assuming time to death as time metric [12–14]. On the other hand, a number of reports which have modelled change in cognitive abilities in older adults assumed this change as a function of chronological age (e.g., [15, 16]).

Most of the studies explored measures of cognitive abilities using only one time metric making an a priori assumption to conceptualize the change in these abilities (e.g., [12, 17]). Johansson et al. [12] explored cognitive change in older adults using only the time to death model and found that proximity to death is predictive of decline in indicators of crystallized knowledge and verbal abilities. Laukka et al. [17] compared different cognitive measures assuming a terminal decline model and also found that some tasks are more sensitive to terminal decline than others. Moreover, they highlighted the need of further research to distinguish whether there is a differential effect for tasks measuring crystallized cognitive abilities compared to other tasks measuring, for example, fluid abilities. Few studies compared models with different time metrics [18–21]. Gerstorf et al. [18] explored change in cognitive function (using a Digit Letter test) and compared models using chronological age and time to death as time metrics. They found that the time to death metric explained better the variability of this cognitive measure than the chronological age metric, suggesting that changes in performance-based variables, as cognition, were primarily driven by mortality-related processes. Sliwinski et al. [20] focused on memory loss and compared different time metrics as chronological age, time to dropout, and time to dementia diagnosis. These authors considered that one possible explanation of the attrition effects is that individuals tended to drop out from the study as a result of death, and therefore they included time to death as time metric when studying individuals free of dementia. They concluded that chronological age may not be the best time metric to describe change in cognitive abilities in older adults and that time to an event (e.g., death or dementia diagnosis) models may be more useful to describe the pattern of change in cognition in older adults. Similar results were found by Ram et al. [19] who examined memory changes across models that aligned scores according to different time metrics, as chronological age, time to disability, and time to death, in a sample of deceased and disabled individuals. Thorvaldsson et al. [21] explored change in perceptual speed as a function of age and time to death finding time to death as the best metric. In sum, evidence about differential patterns of change in multiple measures according to contrasting metrics of time is scarce.

The aim of this study is to explore the pattern of change in measures of cognitive status and specific measures of cognitive abilities in a sample of oldest-old adults, comparing two different time metrics (chronological age and time to death) and therefore examining both underlying conceptual assumptions (age-related changes and terminal decline). Two brief and well-known measures of cognitive status (Mini-Mental State Examination and the Swedish Clock Test), memory (verbal memory, nonverbal long-term memory, recognition and correspondence, short-term memory), two tests of crystallized cognitive abilities (knowledge and synonyms), and visuospatial ability are included. In addition, the association with individual characteristics as sex, education, and dementia diagnosis is also examined.

2. Method

2.1. Sample. The sample consisted of 671 older Swedish adults (229 women and 442 men) that were participants of the Origins of Variance in the Old-Old (OCTO Twin Study). Further details about Swedish Twin Studies can be found in Pedersen et al. [22]. Participants were assessed on five measurement occasions at two-year intervals. At the first measurement occasion, respondents were 83.65 years old in average (SD = 3.19) and had a mean of 7.12 years of education (SD = 2.28). From this sample, 447 were never diagnosed with dementia while 224 were diagnosed with dementia at some point of the study. During and after the five waves of measurement, date of death was recorded for each participant. The same sample of deceased individuals was used in all the considered models. Only deceased individuals were included as comparing level of cognitive performance or rate of change in deceased and surviving individuals represents a comparison across individuals, rather than a focus within individuals, which is required given the conceptualization of terminal decline as a within-individual process [14, 23].

2.2. Measures. The OCTO Twin Study includes a number of cognitive and behavioural measures including two general measures of cognitive status, four measures of memory, two of crystallized abilities, and one of visuospatial abilities. We included standard measures to screen dementia in clinical settings [24], for example, the MMSE, based on their relevance and extended use to identify individuals in studies examining the association between cognitive impairment and mortality. Memory tasks, in general, and verbal memory tasks, in particular, were included as these have shown to be one of the strongest predictors of dementia risk in older adults [25, 26]. In addition, research has highlighted the importance of examining measures of visuospatial and crystallized cognitive abilities not yet included in previous studies with similar aims [11, 17].

2.3. Cognitive Status. Cognitive status was measured using the Mini-Mental State Examination (MMSE [27]) and the Swedish Clock Test [28]. The MMSE consists of 21 questions on orientation, immediate and delayed recall, naming, spelling, and simple arithmetic and constructional praxis. The Swedish Clock Test, which is similar to the Clock Drawing Test, includes three subtasks: clock drawing and setting hands to a certain time; setting the hands of a wooden clock with no numbers on the face to certain standard times; and reading the clock. Greater values indicate a better cognitive status.

2.4. Memory. Verbal memory was assessed by a Prose Recall Test [29]. This test is a Swedish language Prose Recall task similar to those from the Wechsler Memory Test [30]. Respondents were asked for immediate free recall of a brief story. Higher scores are indicative of a greater level of verbal memory.

Nonverbal long-term memory was assessed with the Thurstone Picture Memory Test [31]. Respondents were shown 28 pictures and asked for recognition of these among three lures. Higher scores indicate greater levels of nonverbal memory.

Memory recognition and memory correspondence were assessed by the two subtests of the Memory in Reality Test (Johansson, 1988/89). This test was developed as an alternative to standard list-learning tasks and asked the participants to place real-life objects at the same location as they were previously placed. Higher scores are indicative of better memory.

Short-term memory was assessed by the Digit Span Forward and Backward Test (WAIS [32]). The participants were asked to recall orally presented digits in the same and reverse order as they were presented. Higher scores represent higher levels of short-term memory.

2.5. Visuospatial Ability. Visuospatial ability was assessed with the Kohs Block Design Test [33]. Respondents were asked to reproduce with blocks a pattern shown in cards. Higher scores are indicative of a greater level of visuospatial ability.

2.6. Crystallized Abilities. These abilities can be described as the knowledge and skills acquired through education and other cultural experiences over the life span [34, 35]. In the OCTO Twin Study, two tests from the Swedish version of the Wechsler Adult Intelligence Scale (WAIS [32, 36]) were used to assess crystallized knowledge: the Swedish version of the Information Task and the Synonyms Test. The Information Task includes questions of general knowledge, which requires participants to provide answers to questions assessing acquired semantic knowledge of facts. The Synonyms Test is a verbal meaning test where the respondent has to find a synonym that matches a target word among five alternatives. Higher scores represent higher levels of knowledge.

2.7. Statistical Analyses. Linear mixed models, with random intercepts and slopes, were estimated using SAS Proc Mixed [3, 37], as these models allow capturing between- and within-individual variability. Conditional models for chronological age and time to death were fitted to each cognitive measure, adjusted for baseline age, sex, education, dementia diagnosis at any time point across the five measurement occasions, and time to death at baseline. Age was grand-mean centered and time to death was centered at two years before death (to avoid placing the intercept at a point in time when the measurement of cognition is not possible). Dichotomous covariates were effect-coded and continuous variables were centered. Baseline age was centered at 85 years, education at 9 years, and time to death at baseline at 5 years before death. To separate between-individual changes from within-individual changes in each model, baseline age and time to death from baseline were included in the models [6, 23, 38]. For each temporal index we also explored models describing change at a constant (linear trajectory) and changing rate (quadratic trajectory). That is, for each cognitive measure, four models were compared: (1) chronological aging linear change, (2) chronological aging quadratic change, (3) time to death linear change, and (4) time to death quadratic change. More detailed information and equations are shown in the Appendix. The Bayesian Information Criterion (BIC [39]), an index that combines information about model goodness of fit and parsimony, was used to compare the fit of the models. Models with lowest BIC are preferred and differences between models were compared based on Raftery's (1995) proposed criterion. Raftery (1995) reviewed model selection criterions using BIC index and proposed ranges of differences between BICs of nested models as grades of evidence of these differences, which were categorized as weak (0–2), positive (2–6), strong (6–10), and very strong (>10). We also calculated the proportional reduction in residual variance from unconditional means models, which has been conceptualized as a ΔPseudo R^2 [40]. When examining the association with individual characteristics variables, only significant parameter estimates were reported in order to facilitate the interpretation of the results.

3. Results

3.1. Time Metrics. For each cognitive measure, the BIC indices for the four models were compared. As can be seen in Table 1, for measures of cognitive status, quadratic time to death models fitted the data best. With regard to memory and visuospatial ability, linear time to death models were also the best fitting models. However, when crystallized abilities were explored, time to death was the model that provided a better fit for the Synonyms Test and the chronological age model was the best for Information Test. According Raftery's (1995) grades and considering the sample size of our study, the evidence of the differences between the models was very strong in all the cognitive measures. With regard to the random effects (Table 2), we found that in all the measures there was significant variability at intercept level but only significant variability at slope level was only found for the Prose Recall and Block Design Tests and crystallized cognitive abilities.

Table 1: BIC statistics for linear and quadratic chronological age and time to death models for each cognitive measure. These models wer adjusted for baseline age, sex, education, dementia diagnosis at any time point across the five measurement occasions, and time to death a baseline.

Time metric	Trajectory shape	MMSE	CLOCK	PROSE	MEMRECOG	MEMCORRESP	DIGSPAN	BLOCK	SYNUM	INFO
Age	Linear	11739.3	9922.2	7835.2	6998.5	7160.3	6473.4	9571.9	6966.7	11529.9
	Quadratic	11739	9961.1	7881.9	7051	7210.5	6536.9	9611.5	6974.4	11516.2*
Time to death	Linear	11662.7	9834.1	7799.2*	6871.2*	7122.4*	6435.8*	9555.6*	6947.1*	11549.6
	Quadratic	11589.5*	9820.1*	7830.7	6885.6	7161.2	6475.3	9580	6954.9	11526.3

Note. MMSE: Mini-Mental State Examination, CLOCK: Swedish Clock Test, PROSE: Prose Recall Test, MEMRECOG: Memory Recognition Test MEMCORRESP: Memory Correspondence Test, DIGSPAN: Digit Span Backward Test, BLOCK: Kohs Block Design Test, SYNUM: Synonyms Test, and INFO Information Test. * Indicating lowest BIC value.

3.2. Predictors of Change. Table 2 provides the significant parameter estimates for the intercept and slopes and the covariates associations identified for the best fitting models. On the one hand, a common pattern was found across all cognitive measures: (a) a significant decline over time; (b) dementia diagnosis which was negatively associated with the level and the slope; and (c) education which was positively associated with level but not with slope. On the other hand, some differences were found in age, sex, or time to death associations with the intercept and slope across the different measures of cognitive function.

With regard to baseline age, results showed that people older at study entry had lower initial scores on the MMSE and the Clock Test but only showed a faster decline in MMSE over time. For the memory tasks and visuospatial ability, older people also performed worse in the Memory Recognition, Memory Correspondence, and Block Design Tests, but age differences in rate of decline were only found for Digit Span. With respect to the crystalized abilities, there were no age differences at intercept or slope level.

Significant sex differences were found for Memory Correspondence and the Information Tests. Women performed better than men on Memory Correspondence but worse on the Information Test. No sex differences were found on the slope for any of the tests examined, except for the Information Test.

Time to death at the baseline was significantly positively associated with the level of MMSE, Clock, Memory Correspondence, and Digit Span Test and negatively associated with Prose Recall and the Information Test. Individuals who agreed to participate in the study when they were closer to death had higher cognitive scores than those who were further from death. Significant slope differences were found for all these variables, where individuals closer to death at study entry declined faster than individuals who entered the study further from death.

4. Discussion

The aim of this study was to explore the pattern of change in cognitive status and specific measures of cognitive abilities in a sample of oldest-old adults, comparing two different time metrics (chronological age and time to death) and therefore examining both underlying conceptual assumptions (age-related changes and terminal decline). Moreover, the association with individual characteristics as sex, education, and dementia diagnosis was also examined.

With respect to the time metrics, results showed that the time to death model provided a better representation of change for cognitive status, memory, and visuospatial ability. However, the results in the change in crystallized abilities did not follow such a consistent pattern. Although the trajectories of the scores in the Synonyms Test were better explained by a time to death model, the model that better described change in the Information Test was chronological age. Overall our results are consistent with those studies supporting the terminal decline hypothesis [11–13, 17, 18] and also provide some support to the distinction of the processes associated with decline in crystallized and other abilities suggested by previous research [11, 17]. Specifically, our findings suggest that in these oldest-old adults the changes in cognitive abilities can be better conceptualized within the framework of the terminal decline hypothesis and that there could be different underlying processes driving decline in some crystallized abilities. However, there is a still a need for further research to address which other processes might be underlying decline in other measures of crystallized abilities not considered here. In addition, it should be noted that terminal decline is part of normative aging and it is exceptionally complex to disentangle age-related changes, conceptualized as normative aging, and mortality-related changes, conceptualized as terminal decline. This complexity has been already discussed in previous research [18] (Steinerman et al., 2011) and future studies with cognitive data in previous developmental stages are needed to capture these complex interrelationships.

With respect to the predictors of change for each cognitive measure fitted to the time metric that provided the best fit, results showed a common pattern in all the studied variables. First, a significant decline in cognitive abilities over time was found regardless of the time metric used, consistent with previous research [19, 20]. Second, individuals diagnosed with dementia had lower scores in all the measures of cognition and showed a faster decline compared to individuals not diagnosed with dementia, also consistent with previous research [13, 20]. Third, more educated individuals performed better in all the measures of cognition

TABLE 2: Significant parameter estimates for models identified as best fitting in Table 1.

	Cognitive status		Memory				Visuospatial ability	Crystallized cognitive abilities	
	MMSE	CLOCK	PROSE	MEMRECOG	MEMCORRES	DIGSPAN	BLOCK	SYNUM	INFO
Intercept	25.84 (0.39)	13.49 (0.29)	8.66 (0.36)	9.54 (0.19)	6.86 (0.20)	3.21 (0.10)	10.35 (0.52)	17.67 (0.33)	32.04 (0.84)
Age L									−0.61 (0.10)
Age Q									−0.08 (0.02)
T Death L	−1.31 (0.13)	−0.29 (0.10)	−0.22 (0.08)	−0.10 (0.04)	−0.29 (0.04)	−0.10 (0.02)	−0.55 (0.11)	−0.19 (0.04)	
T Death Q	−0.16 (0.02)	−0.04 (0.01)							
Age (baseline)	−0.36 (0.06)	−0.18 (0.04)		−0.09 (0.03)	−0.12 (0.03)		−0.30 (0.09)		
Female					0.76 (0.21)				−3.64 (0.89)
Education	0.41 (0.08)	0.16 (0.06)	0.39 (0.06)	0.08 (0.04)	0.13 (0.04)	0.13 (0.02)	0.58 (0.11)		1.84 (0.18)
Dementia	−1.34 (0.43)	−6.70 (0.31)	−5.72 (0.33)	−5.22 (0.20)	−4.58 (0.22)	−1.32 (0.11)	−6.41 (0.56)	−2.89 (0.61)	−12.83 (0.95)
T Death (baseline)	0.41 (0.06)	0.14 (0.04)	−0.32 (0.04)		0.07 (0.02)	0.03 (0.01)			−0.58 (0.11)
Linear slope									
Age (baseline)	−0.04 (.02)					0.008 (0.001)			0.1 (0.03)
Dementia	−1.89 (0.13)	−1.26 (0.10)	−0.59 (0.07)	−0.65 (0.03)	−0.38 (0.04)	−0.15 (0.02)	−0.47 (0.09)	−0.19 (0.09)	−1.02 (0.14)
T Death (baseline)			−0.02 (0.01)	−0.01 (0.005)	−0.01 (0.005)	−0.007 (0.003)	−0.02 (0.01)		−0.06 (0.01)
Quadratic slope									
Female									−0.05 (0.02)
Dementia	−0.09 (0.01)	−0.07 (0.01)							0.06 (0.02)
T Death (baseline)	−0.01 (0.002)	−0.003 (0.001)							
Variances									
Intercept	16.92 (1.59)	8.17 (0.64)	7.32 (0.66)	2.88 (0.24)	3.12 (0.27)	0.63 (0.07)	26.48 (2.01)	20.14 (1.66)	28.95 (5.70)
Slope linear			0.04 (0.01)				0.16 (0.04)	0.06 (0.02)	0.57 (0.12)
Slope quadratic									
Residual	11.46 (0.74)	6.43 (0.25)	5.64 (0.29)	2.35 (0.10)	3.05 (0.13)	1.41 (0.05)	10.64 (0.54)	7.45 (0.44)	15.87 (0.91)
ΔPseudo R^2	.73	.23	.40	.48	.17	.08	.16	.02	.90

Note. MMSE: Mini-Mental State Examination, CLOCK: Swedish Clock Test, PROSE: Prose Recall Test, MEMRECOG: Memory Recognition Test, MEMCORRESP: Memory Correspondence Test, DIGSPAN: Digit Span Backward Test, BLOCK: Kohs Block Design Test, SYNUM: Synonyms Test, and INFO: Information Test.

than those with poorer education, but no differences in the rate of change by education were found. These findings were partially consistent with previous research. Education is generally significantly associated with level of performance but its association with rate of decline is not clear. Some studies have found an association only in some ranges of ages [41] or participants characteristics, for example, dementia [42]. A possible explanation could be found in the work of Muniz-Terrera et al. [13] which highlighted the differences in this association before and after the onset of terminal decline; however, further research is needed to address this possibility. Laukka et al. [17], within a single study, found that education was only related to rate of change for visuospatial ability. The variability of the findings about education and rate of decline in cognitive function could be due to the variations in study design or the different measures of education, as Anstey and Christensen [43] suggest, or the methods of analysis, as suggested by Piccinin et al. [42]. However, further research that integrates results from different studies using different measures of cognition and different measures of education should deepen our understanding of the association between education and rate of decline in cognitive function.

Associations with age, sex, and time to death differed across measures of cognitive abilities. On average, older people had poorer performance but baseline age associated differences in speed of decline were only found for MMSE and short-term memory. These results are partially consistent with previous research [12, 18, 42] and provide some evidence of the distinction between cognitive status measures and more domain-specific ones, which might have interesting implications from a psychometric point of view. With regard to sex, only intercept differences were found for Memory Correspondence and the Information Test. Women had better performance than men in the Memory Correspondence and lower scores in the Information Test on the initial level. These results are partially consistent with the findings of Johansson et al. [12] and could be explained because women have greater life expectancy [44]. Between-person proximity to death differences were found when comparing cognitive status measures and specific measures for crystallized ability, memory (except verbal memory), and visuospatial ability. A review on terminal change in cognition carried out by Bosworth and Siegler [11] highlighted that results vary depending on the measure of cognition studied. Indeed, Laukka et al. [17] indicated that further research on models including crystallized abilities measures is needed. Moreover, results showed that individuals who were closer to their death when they entered the study had a faster decline compared to those who were further from death, these results being consistent with previous studies [12, 13].

One of the strengths of our study is that it is one of the first, to our knowledge, to explore such a large number of measures of cognitive performance including measures widely used in clinical settings (MMSE and the Clock Test) and measures of memory, visuospatial, and crystallized abilities. The variety of cognitive measures considered does not only increase the comparability of our findings with previous research, which have only considered a single cognitive measure, but also enable us to address Bosworth and Siegler [11] and Laukka et al. [17] concerns on the potential variability of the results as a function of the measure of cognition examined. In addition, using linear mixed models with random intercepts and slopes allows us to capture between- and within-individual variability and to further separate between- and within-person chronology by including between-person differences in age and proximity to death at the first occasion [14, 23]. This point is especially relevant to avoid one of the potential causes for lack of convergence of the between- and within-person effects in longitudinal models of aging (for more details see [38]). Thus, the analytical strategy adopted in our study is suitable in order to meet our aim and consider terminal decline as a within-person process. However, some limitations should also be noted. First, although the sample of this study is one of the most representative of the oldest-old, these individuals may only represent a subset of survivors of their birth cohort at study entrance [45] and as they are relatively close to their death, their variability at slope level might be smaller than what we would expect from studies with younger populations and longer follow-ups. Therefore, research with different time metrics and different cognitive abilities should be carried out with younger samples. Second, in order to limit complexity of the models and obtain results that could be compared with previous research, only linear and quadratic models were examined. Further research with more measurements occasions should consider other nonlinear models as change point models, which are especially suitable models when researchers aim to estimate the point of onset of terminal decline. Third, there is an ongoing debate on the potential limitations of only including deceased individuals in these studies as the study becomes by its nature post facto and the generalization of our conclusions is limited to deceased population. Within this context, some studies have proposed using joint models for longitudinal and survival data in order to include surviving individuals in their samples (e.g., [46]). These joint models are especially appropriate to examine whether estimates of cognitive change are predictors of survival and allow the conclusions to be also generalized to surviving population. These models have not been adopted in the present study as there is still an ongoing debate on their suitability to study terminal decline as they do not specifically address Kleemeier's [8] operationalization of terminal decline [10]. It has been suggested that they mainly address a different research question as they explore whether those individuals who show decline or a faster decline compared to others show also a greater mortality risk as opposed to models that characterize cognitive decline in proximity to death and aim to examine whether those in close proximity to death are more likely to show greater cognitive decline. Further research including joint-survival models might contribute to detangling these issues.

In sum, our results support the fact that studying change according to terminal decline models might be the best option when compared to models that assume that changes are mainly driven by age-related changes [13, 17]. Moreover, our findings provide some evidence that there is a distinction between using cognitive status measures and domain-specific measures. As Steinerman et al. [7] suggested, cognitive status measures and domain-specific measures might not be equally

TABLE 3

	Level 1	Level 2
Age		
Linear	$y_{ij} = \pi_{0j} + \pi_{1j}\text{Age}_{ij} + r_{ij}$	$\pi_{0j} = \beta_{00} + \beta_{10}\,(\text{BaselineAge}) + \beta_{20}(\text{BaselineTimeToDeath}) + U_{0j}$ $\pi_{1j} = \beta_{10} + \beta_{11}\,(\text{BaselineAge}) + \beta_{21}\,(\text{BaselineTimeToDeath}) + U_{1j}$
Quadratic	$y_{ij} = \pi_{0j} + \pi_{1j}\text{Age}_{ij} + \pi_{2j}\text{Age}_{2j}^{2} + r_{ij}$	$\pi_{0j} = \beta_{00} + \beta_{10}\,(\text{BaselineAge}) + \beta_{20}(\text{BaselineTimeToDeath}) + U_{0j}$ $\pi_{1j} = \beta_{10} + \beta_{11}\,(\text{BaselineAge}) + \beta_{21}\,(\text{BaselineTimeToDeath}) + U_{1j}$ $\pi_{2j} = \beta_{20} + \beta_{21}\,(\text{BaselineAge}) + \beta_{21}\,(\text{BaselineTimeToDeath}) + U_{1j}$
Time to death		
Linear	$y_{ij} = \pi_{0j} + \pi_{1j}\text{TimeToDeath}_{ij} + r_{ij}$	$\pi_{0j} = \beta_{00} + \beta_{10}\,(\text{BaselineAge}) + \beta_{20}(\text{BaselineTimeToDeath}) + U_{0j}$ $\pi_{1j} = \beta_{10} + \beta_{11}\,(\text{BaselineAge}) + \beta_{21}\,(\text{BaselineTimeToDeath}) + U_{1j}$
Quadratic	$y_{ij} = \pi_{0j} + \pi_{1j}\text{TimeToDeath}_{ij} + \pi_{2j}\text{TimeToDeath}_{2j}^{2} + r_{ij}$	$\pi_{0j} = \beta_{00} + \beta_{10}\,(\text{BaselineAge}) + \beta_{20}(\text{BaselineTimeToDeath}) + U_{0j}$ $\pi_{1j} = \beta_{10} + \beta_{11}\,(\text{BaselineAge}) + \beta_{21}\,(\text{BaselineTimeToDeath}) + U_{1j}$ $\pi_{2j} = \beta_{20} + \beta_{21}\,(\text{BaselineAge}) + \beta_{21}\,(\text{BaselineTimeToDeath}) + U_{1j}$

appropriate for examining changes over time; and therefore, the type of measure used should be taken into account when choosing the time metric to model cognitive change. Future studies should replicate this one with younger populations and it would be extremely interesting to extend the present study including alternative theoretical time metrics as subjective or biological age.

Appendix

These models consist of two levels of analysis that allow researchers to explore how individuals change over time (Level 1) and how these changes vary across individuals (Level 2). Level 1 equation can be formulated as

$$y_{ij} = \pi_{0j} + \pi_{1j}\text{Time}_{ij} + r_{ij}, \quad \text{(A.1)}$$

where y_{ij} represents the value of the outcome variable for individual i at time j (a function of time in the previous equation); π_{0j} represents a person j performance level when time is equal to 0 (intercept); and π_{1j} represents the rate of change for each unit of time (slope). In this equation, Time_{ij}, is a metric of time over which change is structured.

Level 2 equations of an unconditional model can be formulated as

$$\begin{aligned} \pi_{0j} &= \beta_0 + U_{0j} \\ \pi_{1j} &= \beta_1 + U_{1j}, \end{aligned} \quad \text{(A.2)}$$

where π_{0j} and π_{1j} are considered as dependent variables, β_0 and β_1 being average level and rate of change, and U_{0j} and U_{1j} are each individual's deviation from the population average values, respectively. Specific equations for the present study are shown in Table 3.

Conflicts of Interest

The authors declare that they have no conflicts of interest.

Acknowledgments

Research reported in this publication was supported by the National Institute on Aging of the National Institutes of Health under Award no. P01AG043362 for the Integrative Analysis of Longitudinal Studies of Aging (IALSA) Research Network. The Origins of Variance in the Old-Old (OCTO Twin Study) was supported by a grant from the National Institute on Aging (NIA: AG 08861).

References

[1] S. M. Hofer and D. E. Alwin, Eds., *Handbook of Cognitive Aging. Interdisciplinary Perspectives*, SAGE Publications, 2008.

[2] C. Hertzog and J. R. Nesslroade, "Assessing Psychological change in adulthood: An overview of methodological issues," *Psychology and Aging*, vol. 18, no. 4, pp. 639–657, 2003.

[3] N. M. Laird and J. H. Ware, "Random effects models for longitudinal data," *Biometrics*, vol. 38, pp. 963–974, 1982.

[4] J. D. Singer and J. B. Willett, *Applied longitudinal data analysis: modeling change and event occurrence*, Oxford university press, 2003.

[5] L. Hoffman, "Considering alternative metrics of time: does anybody really know what, 'time', is?" in *Advances in Longitudinal Methods in the Social and Behavioral Sciences*, J. Harring and G. Hancock, Eds., pp. 255–287, Information Age Publishing, Charlotte, NC, USA, 2012.

[6] M. Sliwinski and J. Mogle, "Time-based and process-based approaches to the analysis of longitudinal data," in *Handbook of Cognitive Aging. Interdisciplinary Perspectives*, S. M. Hofer and D. E. Alwin, Eds., pp. 477–491, SAGE Publications Inc, 2008.

[7] J. Steinerman, C. B. Hall, M. J. Sliwinski, and R. B. Lipton, "Modeling cognitive trajectories within longitudinal studies: a focus on elders," *Journal of American Geriatric Society*, vol. 58, no. Sip 2, pp. S313–S318, 2010.

[8] R. W. Kleemeier, "Intellectual change in the senium," in *Proceedings of the social statistics section of the American statistical association*, vol. 1, pp. 290–295, Washington, DC, USA, 1962.

[9] K. F. Riegel and R. M. Riegel, "Development, drop, and death," *Developmental Psychology*, vol. 6, no. 2, p. 306, 1972.

[10] L. Bäckman and S. W. MacDonald, "Death and cognition: synthesis and outlook," *European Psychologist*, vol. 11, no. 3, pp. 224–235, 2006.

[11] H. B. Bosworth and I. C. Siegler, "Terminal change in cognitive function: An updated review of longitudinal studies," *Experimental Aging Research*, vol. 28, pp. 299–315, 2002.

[12] B. Johansson, S. M. Hofer, J. C. Allaire et al., "Change in cognitive capabilities in the oldest old: the effects of proximity to death in genetically related individuals over a 6-year period," *Psychology and Aging*, vol. 19, no. 1, p. 145, 2004.

[13] G. Muniz-Terrera, A. van den Hout, A. Piccinin, F. Mathews, and S. M. Hofer, "Investigating terminal decline: results from a UK population-based study of aging," *Psychology and Aging*, vol. 28, no. 2, pp. 377–385, 2013.

[14] A. M. Piccinin, G. Muniz, F. E. Matthews, and B. Johansson, "Terminal decline from within-and between-person perspectives, accounting for incident dementia," *The Journals of Gerontology Series B: Psychological Sciences and Social Sciences*, vol. 66, pp. 391–401, 2011.

[15] P. Ghisletta and U. Lindenberger, "Age-based structural dynamics between perceptual speed and knowledge in the berlin aging study: direct evidence for ability dedifferentiation in old age," *Psychology and Aging*, vol. 18, pp. 696–713, 2003.

[16] F. J. Infurna, D. Gerstorf, L. H. Ryan, and J. Smith, "Dynamic links between memory and functional limitations in old age Longitudinal evidence fo age-based structural dynamics from the AHEAD study," *Psychology and Aging*, vol. 26, no. 3, pp. 546–558, 2011.

[17] E. J. Laukka, S. W. McDonald, and L. Backman, "Terminal-decline effects for select cognitive tasks after controlling for preclinical dementia," *The American Journal of Geriatric Psychiatry*, vol. 16, pp. 355–365, 2008.

[18] D. Gerstorf, N. Ram, U. Lindenberger, and J. Smith, "Age and time-to-death trajectories of change in indicators of cognitive, sensory, physical, health, social, and self-related functions," *Developmental Psychology*, vol. 49, no. 10, pp. 1805–1821, 2013.

[19] N. Ram, D. Gerstorf, E. Fauth, S. Zarit, and B. Malmberg, "Aging, disablement, and dying: Using time-as-process and time-as resources metric to chart late-life change," *Research in Human Development*, vol. 7, no. 1, pp. 27–44, 2010.

[20] M. J. Sliwinski, S. M. Hofer, C. Hall, H. Bushke, and R. B. Lipton, "Modeling memory decline in older adults: The importance of preclinical dementia, attrition and chronological age," *Psychology and Aging*, vol. 18, pp. 658–671, 2003.

[21] V. Thorvaldsson, S. M. Hofer, and B. Johansson, "Aging and late-life terminal decline in perceptual speed," *European Psychologist*, vol. 11, no. 3, pp. 196–203, 2006.

[22] N. L. Pedersen, P. Lichtenstein, and P. Svedberg, "The Swedish twin registry in the third millennium," *Twin Research*, vol. 5, pp. 427–432, 2002.

[23] A. M. Piccinin, G. Muniz, C. Sparks, and D. E. Bontempo, "An evaluation of analytical approaches for understanding change in cognition in the context of aging and health," in *The Journals of Gerontology Series B: Psychological Sciences and Social Sciences*, vol. 66, 1, pp. i36–i49, 2011.

[24] B. Sheehan, "Assessment scales in dementia," *Therapeuti advances in neurological disorders*, vol. 5, no. 6, pp. 349–358 2012.

[25] M. F. Elias, A. Beiser, P. A. Wolf, R. Au, R. F. White, and R. B D'Agostino, "The preclinical phase of alzheimer disease: a 22 year prospective study of the framingham cohort," *Archives o Neurology*, vol. 57, no. 6, pp. 808–813, 2000.

[26] D. B. Howieson, A. Dame, R. Camicioli, G. Sexton, H. Payami and J. A. Kaye, "Cognitive markers preceding Alzheimer's dementia in the healthy oldest old," *Journal of the America Geriatrics Society*, vol. 45, no. 5, pp. 584–589, 1997.

[27] M. F. Folstein, S. E. Folstein, and P. R. McHugh, "'Mini-menta state', a practical method for grading the cognitive state of patients for the clinician," *Journal of Psychiatric Research*, vol 12, pp. 189–198, 1975.

[28] B. Johansson and S. H. Zarit, "Dementia and cognitive impairment in the oldest old: a comparison of two rating methods," *International Psychogeriatrics*, vol. 3, no. 1, pp. 29–38, 1991.

[29] B. Johansson, S. H. Zarit, and S. Berg, "Changes in cognitive functioning of the oldest old," in *Journals of Gerontology*, vol. 47 of *B Sciences and Social Sciences*, pp. 75–80, 1992.

[30] D. Wechsler, "A standardized memory scale for clinical use," *Journal of Psychology*, vol. 19, pp. 87–95, 1945.

[31] L. L. Thurstone and T. G. Thurstone, *Manual to SRA Primary Mental Abilities*, Chicago: Science Research Associates, 1949.

[32] D. Wechsler, *Manual for the Wechsler Adult Intelligence Scale-Revised*, New York: Psychological Corporation, 1991.

[33] I. Dureman and H. Salde, *Psykometriska och experimental-psychologiska metoder for klinisk tillampning*, Almqvist & Wiksell, Sweden, 1959.

[34] J. L. Horn, "Measurement of intellectual capabilities: a review of theory," in *WJ-R Technical Manual*, K. S. McGrew, J. K. Werder, and R. W. Woodcock, Eds., Chicago: Riverside, 1991.

[35] J. L. Horn and J. Noll, "Human cognitive capabilities: Gf-Gc theory," in *Contemporary Intellectual Assessment: Theories, Tests And Issues*, D. P. Flanagan, J. L. Genshaft, and P. L. Harrison, Eds., pp. 53–91, New York: Guilford, 1997.

[36] C. O. Jonsson and L. Molander, "Manual till CVB-Skalen [Manual of the CVB scales]," *Stockholm, Psykologi Forlaget*, 1964.

[37] R. C. Littell, G. A. Milliken, W. W. Stroup, and R. D. Wolfinger, 1996, SAS System for mixed models. Cary: SAS Institute Inc.

[38] M. Sliwinski, L. Hoffman, and S. M. Hofer, "Evaluating convergence of within-person change and between-person age differences in age heterogeneous longitudinal studies," *Research in Human Development*, vol. 7, no. 1, pp. 45–60, 2010.

[39] G. Schwarz, "Estimating the dimension of a model," *The Annals of Statistics*, vol. 6, no. 2, pp. 461–464, 1978.

[40] T. Snijders and R. Bosker, *Multilevel analysis: an introduction to basic and advanced multilevel modeling*, Sage, London, UK, 1999.

[41] C. Gale, M. Allerhand, and I. J. Deary, "Is there a bidirectional relationship between depressive symptoms and cognitive ability in older people? a prospective study using the english longitudinal study of ageing," *Psychological Medicine*, vol. 42, pp. 2057–2069, 2012.

[42] A. M. Piccinin, G. Muniz-Terrera, S. Clouston et al., "Coordinated analysis of age, sex and education effects on change in MMSE scores," *Journals of Gerontology Series B: Psychological and Social Sciences*, vol. 68, no. 3, pp. 374–2390, 2013.

[43] K. Anstey and H. Christensen, "Education, activity, health, blood pressure and apolipoprotein E as predictors of cognitive change in old age: a review," *Gerontology*, vol. 46, pp. 163–177, 2000.

[44] K. Anstey, M. A. Luszcz, L. C. Giles, and G. R. Andrews, "Demographic, health, cognitive and sensory variables as predictors of mortality in very old adults," *Psychology and Aging*, vol. 16, no. 1, pp. 3–11, 2001.

[45] S. M. Hofer and M. J. Sliwinski, "Design and analysis of longitudinal studies on aging," *Handbook of the Psychology of Aging*, vol. 6, pp. 15–37, 2006.

[46] P. Ghisletta, J. McArdle, and U. Lindenberger, "Longitudinal cognition-survival relations in old and very old age: 13-year data from the Berlin aging study," *European Psychologist*, vol. 11, pp. 204–223, 2006.

Effects of a 12-Week Exercise Training Program on Physical Function in Institutionalized Frail Elderly

Cristiane Batisti Ferreira,[1] Pâmela dos Santos Teixeira,[1] Geiane Alves dos Santos,[1] Athila Teles Dantas Maya,[1] Paula Americano do Brasil,[1] Vinícius Carolino Souza,[2] Cláudio Córdova,[3] Aparecido Pimentel Ferreira,[1,3] Ricardo Moreno Lima,[4] and Otávio de Toledo Nóbrega[2]

[1]*Interdisciplinary Center for Research Integrated Colleges Promove Brasília, Brasília, Brazil*
[2]*Medical Faculty, University of Brasília (UnB), Brasília, Brazil*
[3]*Physical Education Program, Catholic University of Brasília (UCB-DF), Brasília, Brazil*
[4]*Physical Education Program, University of Brasília (UnB), Brasília, Brazil*

Correspondence should be addressed to Aparecido Pimentel Ferreira; cidopimentel@gmail.com

Academic Editor: Adam B. Salmon

With the increase in life expectancy, the Brazilian elderly population has risen considerably. However, longevity is usually accompanied by problems such as the loss of functional capacity, cognitive decline, frailty syndrome, and deterioration in anthropometric parameters, particularly among those living in long-term care facilities. This randomized controlled trial aimed to verify the effects of exercise training on biochemical, inflammatory, and anthropometric indices and functional performance in institutionalized frail elderly. The sample consisted of 37 elderly people of both genders, aged 76.1 ± 7.7 years, who were randomly allocated into 2 groups: 13 individuals in the exercise group (EG) and 24 in the control group (CG). Anthropometrics, clinical history, functional tests, and biochemical evaluation were measured before and after the completion of a physical exercise program, which lasted for 12 weeks. The 12-week exercise program for frail elderly residents in a long-term care facility was efficient in improving muscle strength, speed, agility, and biochemical variables, with reversal of the frailty condition in a considerable number. However, no effects in anthropometric and inflammatory parameters were noted.

1. Introduction

Aging is a continuous process in which a progressive decline takes place in most physiological systems. This may expose the elderly to frailty, a syndrome characterized by a decrease in the homeostatic reserve and reduction of the body's ability to endure and perform, leading to a cumulative, vicious cycle of decline in multiple physiological systems and to vulnerability to adverse outcomes [1, 2].

In addition to physiological problems, aging is usually related to socioeconomic disadvantages. It is usually accompanied by an increase in expenditure, particularly with medications, in addition to decreasing income, since there is loss of production capacity and dependence almost exclusively of retirement income. On the other hand, the Brazilian family has changed significantly over the years, especially after the women's entry into the labor market, making home care difficult and increasing the demand for long-stay institutions. However, institutionalization may result in damage to functional decline and physical dependence, since older people living in the current models of long-term care facilities (LTCFs) do not seem to be properly stimulated [3].

Frailty decreases functional capacity by affecting the strength necessary to perform everyday activities [4] such as walking, raising from a chair, and reducing balance [5]. It is also insidiously related to a higher incidence of falls and disability as well as to hospitalization and mortality [1, 2, 6]. Consequently, frailty has healthcare cost implications, and its prevention could lead to a reduction in public costs and individual burden, which grows proportionally as the world population ages [7, 8].

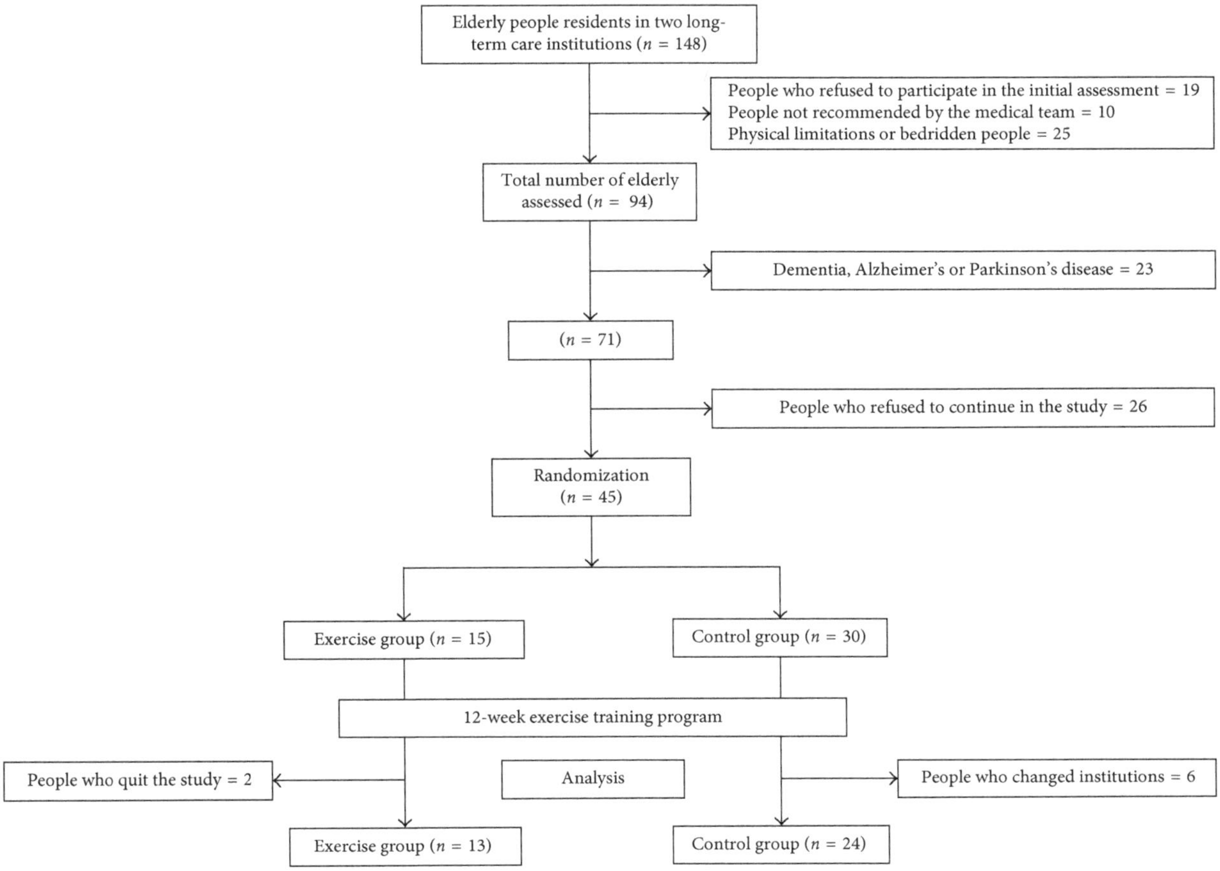

FIGURE 1: A schematic drawing of the sample.

Moreover, there is evidence that a decrease in physical capacity of older adults is related to an abnormal biochemical milieu such as insulin resistance, dyslipidemia, and systemic inflammation [9–12], but some controversy remains in this regard. Exercise training may represent a nonpharmacological strategy to prevent or treat frailty [13].

In terms of physical fitness, muscle strength seems to play a pivotal role in functional independence, with low muscle strength associated with a variety of comorbidities [14, 15] as well as with disability to perform everyday activities [16]. In addition to strength training, benefits for older adults have been observed in studies that evaluated multicomponent training programs [17–20]. However, an intervention capable of providing greater benefits has not been defined yet [20]. Also, physical exercise programs specific to the elderly population do not seem to be accessible, especially for institutionalized older people [18]. Thus, the aim of this study was to verify the effect of physical training on biochemical, inflammatory, and anthropometric traits as well as on functional performance of institutionalized frail elderly.

2. Materials and Methods

2.1. Study Characterization and Sample. This is a randomized experimental study conducted with institutionalized elderly volunteers. The sample consisted of 37 individuals of both genders, aged 60 years or older, who were residents of an LTCF in Brasília, Brazil. Subjects were randomly allocated to 2 groups after a series of recruitment steps as follows: 13 individuals in the exercise group (EG) and 24 in the control group (CG), according to a 2 : 1 ratio rationale between the CG and EG (Figure 1). Randomization was carried out by means of simple lottery applied to each subject in a process based on blindingly choosing cards which exhibited two options of letter (A or B), each representing one branch (CG or EG), with the amount of one letter in twofold excess compared to the other. The ratio of 2 : 1 between the CG and EG relies in the ethical premise of avoiding exposure of a vulnerable individual to a treatment arm of the study when efficacy is under consideration. This study was approved by the institutional research ethics committee, and the volunteers signed a consent form. Subjects aged over 60 years were diagnosed as prefrail or frail and who did not present limitations that precluded cognitive tests were recruited. Participants were declared fit by a medical doctor allowing them to undergo the exercise training program. The elderly diagnosed with dementia, Alzheimer's disease, or Parkinson's disease were excluded from the present study.

2.2. General Procedures of the Study. Experimental design of the study was based on data on anthropometric measurements, clinical history, functional tests, and biochemical evaluation assessed before and after the completion of a physical exercise program that lasted for 12 weeks.

The elderly in the EG participated in a training program performed 3 times a week, with sessions lasting 40 minutes, while subjects in the CG were instructed to maintain their usual activities of everyday life and to not change their physical activity habits during the study period.

2.3. Anthropometric Variables. To measure body mass, individuals stood on a Britannia® digital scale with a resolution of 0.1 kg wearing as few clothes as possible, immobile until the value was stable on the display. Height was assessed with a measuring tape with the subjects erected and arms relaxed, after deep inhalation. The body mass index (BMI) was determined as kg/m^2. The conicity index was determined by measures of weight, height, and waist circumference using the following mathematical equation:

$$\text{conicity index} = \frac{\text{waist circumference (m)}}{0.109\sqrt{\text{body weight (kg)}/\text{height (m)}}}. \tag{1}$$

2.4. Handgrip Strength. After participants became familiar with the equipment, they remained seated, with their shoulders in neutral position, elbows flexed at 90°, and fist in neutral position. Subjects were instructed to perform a maximum isometric contraction. Three attempts were made with alternate limbs, with a 60-second interval between attempts. The highest achieved reading was recorded for subsequent analyses. No verbal encouragement was offered during the test [21].

2.5. Timed Up and Go Test (TUG). A stopwatch was used to measure the time spent to get up from a chair, walk a 3-meter distance on habitual speed, go around an obstacle, and sit again. We used a chair with a 45-inch tall seat, a 65-inch tall armrest, and a full, straight backrest [22].

2.6. Sitting and Lift Test. The sitting and lift test was conducted in a chair with a 45 cm tall seat but with no lateral, armrest support and with a full, straight backrest leaning on a wall. Each time a participant stood up, it was counted out loud, and five repetitions were timed [23]. There was a period of familiarization to ensure that the participant's sitting position occupied the largest part of the seat.

2.7. Mini-Mental State Examination (MMSE). Answers were obtained from questions presented in the interview format, and a score cut was set based on the scores of 13 points for illiterate people, 18 points for people with 1 to 8 years of schooling, and 26 points for those with more than 8 years of schooling [24, 25].

2.8. Depression and Functionality Levels. The Katz scale was used to assess the autonomy of the elderly to perform the basic activities of daily living, with conditions classified according to scores achieved as total (0 point), severe (1 or 2 points), moderate (3 or 4 points), or light dependency (5 points) as well as independent (6 points). The scale of Yesavage was used for the screening of depression, assessing cognitive and behavioral aspects typically affected among older adults. In the present study, 11 to 15 points accounted for severe depression, whereas 6 to 10 points for mild depression and 0 to 5 as indicative of no depression. The Katz and Yesavage scales were implemented as described elsewhere [26].

2.9. Blood Drawing and Testing. Blood samples were obtained through a venous puncture. Serum triglycerides (TGs), high-density lipoprotein (HDL-c), total cholesterol (TC), and glucose were analyzed by enzyme-based colorimetric methods using commercially available kits (Advia 2400, SIEMENS Healthcare Diagnostics Inc., Tarrytown, USA). The Friedewald equation was used to yield low-density lipoprotein (LDL-c) and very low-density lipoprotein (VLDL-c) estimates [27]. Serum insulin was determined by fluoroimmunoassay using a commercially available kit (Immulite 2000, SIEMENS Healthcare Diagnostics Inc., UK). Vitamin D_3 (25 hydroxyvitamin D_3) was analyzed by double antibody radioimmunoassay using Vit D25 preextraction with acetonitrile (DiaSorin Inc., Stillwater, USA). Inflammatory mediators were analyzed using the enzyme-linked immunosorbent assay (ELISA) method with specific kits for each cytokine (eBioscience, USA). High-sensitivity C-reactive protein was determined by immunonephelometry (CardioPhase, Dade Behring, USA).

2.10. Identification of Frailty. Frailty was identified based on criteria described by Fried et al., which include unintentional weight loss, reports of exhaustion, reduction of walking speed, muscle weakness, and low level of physical activity. Elderly who did not display any of the criteria mentioned above were classified as nonfrail, whereas patients fitting in 1 or 2 criteria were considered prefrail. Only elderly displaying 3 or more criteria were classified as frail.

Loss of more than 4.5 kg or 10% of the body weight over the last year was considered as weight reduction. Exhaustion was identified when there was self-reported fatigue. Low walking speed was identified by measuring the time required to walk a distance of 4.0 meters forward and return. Males of height of <1.73 and ≥ 1.73 meters and females of height of <1.59 and ≥ 1.59 meters tested positive by reaching times of >7 and >6 seconds, respectively. Muscle weakness was defined on the basis of the handgrip strength test. Males scored positive by displayed strengths of <29.0 kgf for BMI < 24.0 kg/m^2, or <30.0 kgf for BMI 24.1–26.0 kg/m^2, or <32.0 kgf for BMI > 26.0 kg/m^2, while positive female patients were those with values of 17.0 < kgf for BMI < 23.0 kg/m^2, or <17.3 kgf for BMI 23.1–26.0 kg/m^2, or <18.0 kgf for BMI 26.1–29.0 kg/m^2, or <21.0 kgf for BMI > 29.0 kg/m^2. Patients scored for low level of physical activity when declared exercising with a frequency lower than twice a week.

2.11. Physical Exercise Program. The multiple component exercise program lasted 12 weeks, being performed 3 times

TABLE 1: Schematic demonstration of the weekly physical training program.

Variables	Physical training program (weeks/time)											
	1 W	2 W	3 W	4 W	5 W	6 W	7 W	8 W	9 W	10 W	11 W	12 W
Mobility	20′	20′	15′	15′	—	—	—	—	—	—	—	—
Flexibility	—	—	10′	10′	10′	10′	10′	10′	—	—	—	—
Aerobic resistance	20′	20′	15′	15′	15′	15′	10′	10′	15′	15′	10′	10′
Strength training	—	—	—	—	15′	15′	20′	20′	25′	25′	30′	30′
Total time	40′	40′	40′	40′	40′	40′	40′	40′	40′	40′	40′	40′

per week with each session lasting 40 minutes. Exercises were focused on improving mobility, flexibility, strength, and aerobic resistance (Table 1). Physical fitness and exercises for the training program were chosen after an initial assessment of the volunteers to gather variables to improve the independence of elderly people.

To implement the program, the EG was divided into 3 subgroups of approximately 5 elderly people in each group so that exercises were conducted in a personalized and individualized way. The subgroup was followed at all times by 2 physical educators and 3 monitors who did not know which elders were in each of the groups. The intensity and complexity of exercises were defined based on the initial assessment and adjusted weekly considering the subjective perception of effort (SPE) reported by each participant.

Owing to the clinical condition of participants, characterized by a high level of functional impairment, medical clearance was granted to perform up to moderate intensities of exercise, what resulted in exercises between 5 and 7 of SPE being selected according to an adapted Omni scale [28]. The intensity was collected during the exercise sessions during the 12 weeks.

2.12. Statistical Analysis. The sample size was estimated based on an "a priori" calculation, using the dependent variables "TUG" and "handgrip strength." After the analysis of preliminary data, with an alpha of 0.05 and a power of 0.80 for a two-tailed test, and assuming uneven groups, a sample of at least 12 participants for the EG and of 18 for the CG would be required to detect a significant difference in the order of 50% between treatment arms.

Clinical, anthropometric, biochemical, and inflammatory parameters on the postintervention moment were compared between the groups (intervention and control) using analysis of covariance (ANCOVA) models for variables with Gaussian distribution. Nevertheless, the nonparametric ANCOVA was employed for the variables that did not display Gaussian distribution in at least one of the groups. For ANCOVA models, measures obtained during postintervention were deemed dependent variables, whereas the groups (exercise and control) were deemed independent variables, with baseline measures as covariates. Intragroup comparisons of measurements were performed using the Student's t-test for paired samples or using a nonparametric Wilcoxon test whether measures displayed a Gaussian distribution or not, respectively. Comparisons of mean measurements between groups were conducted by the independent t-test. Comparisons of frequencies between groups used the chi-square test. A p value of less than 0.05 was considered significant. Analyses were carried out using SAS v 9.4 (SAS Institute, Inc., 1999).

3. Results

EG participants had a 61.5% attendance to exercise sessions and reported an average SPE of 5.2 during intervention. Tables 2 and 3 display descriptive statistics of clinical, anthropometric, biochemical, functional, and inflammatory variables observed in the sample, with their respective intragroup and intergroup comparisons.

Functional performance variables significantly improved in the EG when baseline and postintervention values were compared. The EG showed statistically superior left and right handgrip strength measures by 33 and 26%, respectively, in comparison to the CG endpoint levels. Regarding TUG and stand up/sit down tests, the EG had statistically lower values than the CG (38% for TUG and 29% for stand up/sit down). Also in the EG, anthropometric traits and MMSE exhibited no significant differences when baseline and postintervention were compared. None of these variables in the CG presented differences between the baseline and postintervention moments.

Regarding the biochemical and inflammatory traits, values checked for glucose, insulin, total cholesterol, triglycerides, vitamin D_3, and CRP showed significant differences when comparing baseline and postintervention moments in the EG, while only glucose values differed in the CG. No other changes were observed concerning biochemical and inflammatory variables among groups or moments.

Figure 2 shows the absolute prevalence of criteria for frailty as well as frequencies of elderly classified as frail and prefrail in pre- and postintervention moments. The EG showed $a \approx 34\%$ reduction in the prevalence of criteria for frailty, while the CG showed a reduction of ≈6% between evaluations conducted before and after the exercise program. A decrease of more than ≈73% in the number of elderly classified as frail was noted in the EG, with most participants migrating to a prefrail status. On the other hand, the CG remained similar between pre- and post-intervention periods.

4. Discussion

The main findings of this study showed an improvement in the biochemical and functional capacity (strength, speed, and agility) of residents of long-term care institutions after undertaking a 12-week exercise training program. Improvements

TABLE 2: Comparison of anthropometric, clinical, and functional performance variables between baseline and postintervention moments.

Variable	Exercise group ($n = 13$)		Control group ($n = 24$)	
	Baseline	Postintervention	Baseline	Postintervention
Age (years)	73.3 ± 6.4	—	77.8 ±8.0	—
Weight (kg)	67.4 ± 10.1	—	66.7 ± 11.9	—
Height (m)	1.59 ± 9.7	—	1.59 ± 8.6	—
Diseases (number)	2.2	—	1.7	—
Depression (%)	28.6%	18.2%*	24.0%	22.7%
Dependence (%)	36.4%	0.0%*‡	22.7%$	20.8%
MMSE (points)	17.4 (13.8; 20.9)	18.3 (15.8; 20.9)	18.1 (15.3; 21.0)	17.0 (15.1; 18.9)
BMI (kg/m^2)	26.4 (23.6; 29.2)	27.0 (26.4; 27.6)	26.8 (25.1; 28.6)	26.5 (26.1; 27.0)
Conicity index	1.36 (1.32; 1.40)	1.36 (1.34; 1.38)	1.38 (1.35; 1.41)	1.39 (1.37; 1.40)
Waist (cm)	95.8 (89.9; 101.6)	97.0 (95.2; 98.8)	97.96 (93.4; 102.5)	97.84 (96.4; 99.3)
LHS (kgf)	8.7 (3.7; 13.7)	16.7 (14.7; 18.7)†&	10.5 (8.1; 13.0)	11.2 (9.5; 12.9)
RHS (kgf)	10.1 (5.9; 14.4)	17.2 (15.2; 19.2)†#	11.0 (7.6; 14.4)	12.7 (11.0; 14.4)
TUG (s)	28.8 (20.4; 37.2)	20.9 (18.3; 23.4)†&	29.1 (21.3; 36.9)	28.9 (26.6; 31.2)
Stand/sit time (s)	33.5 (22.0; 45.0)	20.3 (17.2; 23.4)†#	27.7 (23.0; 32.5)	26.1 (23.6; 28.7)

*$p < 0.05$ for intragroup comparisons calculated using the chi-square test; ‡$p < 0.05$ for comparison of postintervention measurements between groups (exercise group versus control group) calculated using the chi-square test; $\$p < 0.05$ for comparison of baseline measurements between groups (exercise group versus control group) calculated using the chi-square test; †$p < 0.01$ for intragroup comparisons calculated using the paired t-test or Wilcoxon test. #$p < 0.01$; &$p < 0.01$ for comparison of postintervention measurements between groups (exercise group versus control group) calculated using ANCOVA or non-parametric ANCOVA, adjusted by base measurements as a covariate. MMSE = mini-mental state examination; BMI = body mass index; LHS = left handgrip strength; RHS = right handgrip strength; TUG = timed up and go test.

TABLE 3: Comparison of metabolic and inflammatory variables between baseline and postintervention moments.

Variable	Exercise group ($n = 13$)		Control group ($n = 24$)	
	Baseline	Postintervention	Baseline	Postintervention
Glycaemia (mg/dl)	100.9 (86.9; 115.0)	95.7 (88.3; 103.0)†	105.0 (84.6; 125.4)	94.3 (89.1; 99.5)‡
Insulin (μI/ml)	14.9 (10.1; 19.7)	11.3 (6.1; 16.4)†	16.0 (10.9; 21.1)	12.9 (9.3; 16.5)
TC (mg/dl)	168.5 (144.9; 192.0)	148.0 (132.9; 163.2)‡	166.4 (151.1; 181.7)	165.8 (155.1; 176.5)
TR (mg/dl)	151.7 (119.1; 184.3)	105.7 (83.7; 127.6)†	120.1 (93.0; 147.3)	120.7 (105.5; 136.0)
HDL (mg/dl)	48.6 (41.5; 55.7)	49.1 (44.4; 53.8)	50.3 (45.6; 54.9)	45.8 (42.5; 49.1)
LDL (mg/dl)	87.9 (72.8; 103.1)	83.5 (72.0; 95.0)	89.3 (76.4; 102.3)	93.7 (85.5; 101.8)
Vitamin D_3 (ng/ml)	21.7 (17.3; 26.2)	26.0 (22.6; 29.5)‡	22.2 (19.2; 25.1)	23.9 (21.4; 26.4)
CRP (mg/dl)	0.68 (0.46; 0.90)	2.41 (1.48; 3.35)‡	2.07 (−0.58; 4.7)	1.67 (0.98; 2.4)
IL6 (pg/ml)	14.0	17.1 (14.39; 19.86)	18.0 (14.7; 21.3)	16.1 (14.0; 18.2)
IL10 (pg/ml)	13.0	15.6 (11.4; 19.7)	17.9 (14.3; 21.5)	16.3 (13.0; 19.5)
IL1a (pg/ml)	14.6 (10.7; 18.4)	16.0 (14.0; 18.0)	17.6 (13.9; 21.4)	16.8 (15.23; 18.4)
IL1RAcP (pg/ml)	18.9 (12.9; 25.0)	16.1 (10.6; 21.6)	15.1 (10.7; 19.4)	16.7 (12.5; 21.0)

‡$p < 0.05$; †$p < 0.01$ for intragroup comparisons calculated by the paired t-test or Wilcoxon test. TC = total cholesterol; TR = triglycerides; HDL = high-density lipoprotein; LDL = low-density lipoprotein; CRP = C-reactive protein; IL = interleukin.

in biochemical, anthropometric, or inflammatory variables were not apparent when crude endpoints values of the exercise and control groups were compared. However, traits such as serum glucose, insulin, total cholesterol, triglycerides, vitamin D_3, and CRP showed significant improvements when baseline and postintervention stages of the EG are compared. Furthermore, a reduction in the absolute count of criteria elements for frailty was observed as well as in the proportion of the elderly considered frail in the EG after intervention.

The baseline physical status of the elderly participants presented extremely low performance scores when compared to studies conducted elsewhere, rending a sample with a major dysfunctional status [29–32]. Exercise-induced improvements in physical performance of institutionalized older adults are corroborated by previous reports [19], resulting in decreased risk of falls and attenuation of frailty. Nevertheless, Faber et al. reported the effects of 2 exercise programs with moderate intensity conducted in 15 long-term care institutions and found that both programs had positive effects on physical performance in prefrail elderly people but not in frail individuals [33]. On the other hand, the intervention described in the present study was successful in reversing the frailty phenotype in more than 70% of the frail elderly [34].

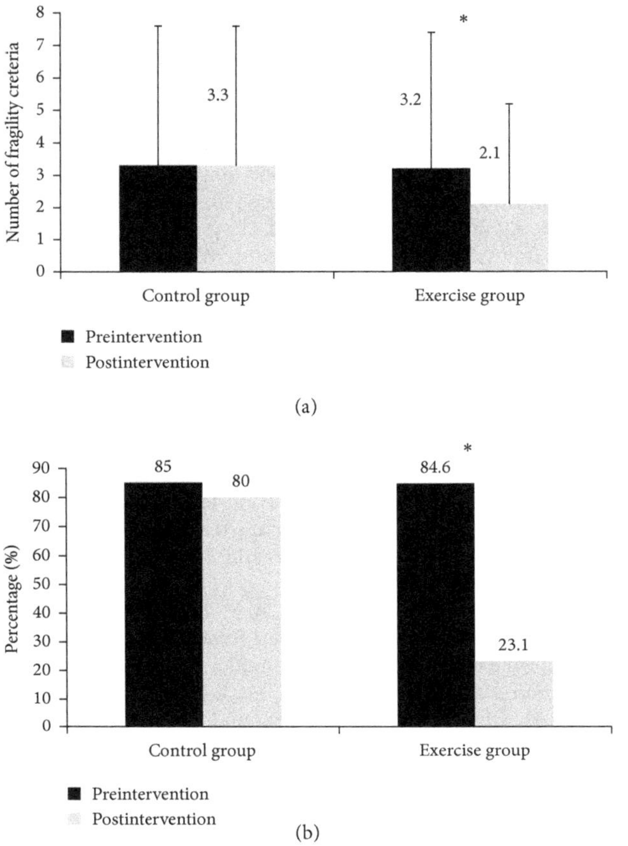

FIGURE 2: Absolute count of criteria for frailty (a) and proportion of elderly deemed frail and prefrail (b) in the control group and the exercise group. Black bar: preintervention moment; gray bar: postintervention moment. $^{*}p < 0.05$.

Also, a systematic review of randomized clinical trials with frail elderly patients showed contradictory data regarding improvements in risk for falls, mobility, balance, strength, functional capacity, and body composition [20]. Even among those who have shown improvements in functional capacity, it is not appropriate to attribute the success of these results to a specific element of the intervention protocol. Although most studies usually describe the intervention program in detail, some reports fail to describe appropriately load-related parameters, such as heart rate, lactate concentration, or SPE during interventions, and that might at least in part contribute to the contradictory results in the literature.

The mean PSE of 5.2 obtained herein renders the intensity of our exercise as moderate and supports a beneficial effect of this exercise intensity on functional parameters [35–37], risk of falling [33], balance [38], and self-reported health status [39]. Other studies show that exercise programs with higher intensity seem to generate better results [40, 41]. In this context, we believe that, besides intensity, other variables such as the duration, method, and type of the exercise may influence results in studies involving exercise programs in frail elderly, since responsiveness to training, time, and history of exposure cannot be neglected.

The literature shows that participation of the elderly population in regular physical activity is considered protective against various components of frailty [42]. Moreover, physical fitness among aged individuals is associated with better functioning of glucose and lipid metabolisms, with greater lean mass as well as with a lower, systemic inflammation [9, 11, 12, 43]. However, the physical training program conducted herein was not efficient in promoting improvements in the investigated interleukins and anthropometric variables. This suggests that the intervention was effective but limited to promoting adaptations on systems directly related to functionality (mainly neuromuscular effects) and on few metabolic traits (glucose, insulin, total cholesterol, triglycerides, vitamin D_3, and CRP). One possible explanation for such a narrowed repercussion can be based on the low adherence to our exercise program (61.5%). For instance, the Brazilian Guidelines for Cardiac Rehabilitation [44] affirm that patients who firmly adhere to programs display more pronounced adaptations in hemodynamic, metabolic, myocardial, vascular, and psychological parameters, not observed in the conditions herein. Another study analyzed the association between adherence and physiological changes in middle-aged adults, concluding that high adherence promoted improvements in physical parameters and quality of life [45]. In general, the literature presents consistent evidence that adherence to the exercise program associates with improved clinical outcomes, functional performance, and quality of life [46], and the levels of attendance described herein can be rendered as a limitation of the study.

Thus, more studies testing models of physical exercise with institutionalized elderly people are necessary to yield more beneficial protocols, having in mind protocols already in literature that were successful in reducing systemic inflammation and regulating the metabolic profile to boost anabolism and muscle protein synthesis [13]. But any intervention should take into consideration individual aspects. The type, intensity, and duration of the exercise program must be carefully chosen, and the frailty status, medical recommendations, history of diseases, and physical activity should be considered. In this case, programs based on multiple components, which address physical qualities such as mobility, balance, flexibility, aerobic capacity, and strength, similar to the model used in this study may be used. Part of literature supports this type of intervention, stating that these programs are more effective at improving general health of frail elderly people [19, 30, 47].

The present study is not without limitations. For example, a low participation rate in the exercise sessions was noted. Despite constant stimulation and customized work, adherence to the program was below expectations. Another limitation was the extremely low physical conditioning of the participants, as well as the elevated prevalence of depression, which explains greater social isolation and lower adherence to the exercise program, even though, at the end of the exercise program, there was a significant reduction in depression rates.

Nevertheless, our results corroborate that, regardless of physical limitations and frailty severity, elderly people are capable of participating in personalized training programs when their limits are considered. Additionally, strength training must be taken into account and should be carried out in an adapted, assisted way [32]. Training should offer benefits even when it is carried out in a nonintensive way. In addition, physical exercises can be a very effective strategy to implement beneficial routines to residents of long-term care institutions, particularly those with greater impairment as well as those diagnosed with frailty.

5. Conclusion

This study showed that a 12-week exercise training program in elderly patients with the syndrome of frailty living in long-term care institutions was efficient in improving aspects of their functional capacity, including muscle strength, speed, and agility, as well as glucose, insulin, total cholesterol, triglycerides, vitamin D_3, and CRP. Moreover, the intervention helped to reduce the amount of criteria for frailty syndrome, and there was a reversal of the frailty condition in a considerable number of elderly who attended the program. However, there was no repercussion regarding anthropometric, biochemical, and inflammatory features.

Conflicts of Interest

The authors declare that there are no conflicts of interest.

References

[1] L. P. Fried, C. M. Tangen, J. Walston et al., "Frailty in older adults: evidence for a phenotype," *Journals of Gerontology Series A: Biological Sciences and Medical Sciences*, vol. 56, no. 3, pp. M146–M156, 2001.

[2] K. Rockwood, "What would make a definition of frailty successful?," *Age and Ageing*, vol. 34, no. 5, pp. 432–434, 2005.

[3] K. Gonçalves Damascena, C. Batisti Ferreira, P. dos Santos Teixeira et al., "Functional capacity and obesity reflect the cognitive performance of older adults living in long-term care facilities," *Psychogeriatrics*, vol. 17, no. 6, pp. 439–445, 2017.

[4] C. H. Chou, C. L. Hwang, and Y. T. Wu, "Effect of exercise on physical function, daily living activities, and quality of life in the frail older adults: a meta-analysis," *Archives of Physical Medicine and Rehabilitation*, vol. 93, no. 2, pp. 237–244, 2012.

[5] R. J. Gobbens, K. G. Luijkx, M. T. Wijnen-Sponselee, and J. M. Schols, "Toward a conceptual definition of frail community dwelling older people," *Nursing Outlook*, vol. 58, no. 2, pp. 76–86, 2010.

[6] L. P. Fried, L. Ferrucci, J. Darer, J. D. Williamson, and G. Anderson, "Untangling the concepts of disability, frailty, and comorbidity: implications for improved targeting and care," *Journals of Gerontology Series A: Biological Sciences and Medical Sciences*, vol. 59, no. 3, pp. 255–263, 2004.

[7] D. M. Cutler, "Declining disability among the elderly," *Health Affairs*, vol. 20, no. 6, pp. 11–27, 2001.

[8] A. Kalache and A. Gatti, "Active ageing: a policy framework," *Advances in Gerontology*, vol. 11, pp. 7–18, 2003.

[9] M. A. Cabrera and W. Jacob Filho, "Obesidade em idosos: prevalência, distribuição e associação com hábitos e comorbidades," *Arquivos Brasileiros de Endocrinologia & Metabologia*, vol. 45, no. 5, pp. 494–501, 2001.

[10] A. P. Ferreira, C. B. Ferreira, V. C. Souza et al., "Risk of glycemic disorder in elderly women adjusted by anthropometric parameters and cytokine genotypes," *Revista da Associação Médica Brasileira*, vol. 57, no. 5, pp. 565–569, 2011.

[11] C. Cooper, W. Dere, W. Evans et al., "Frailty and sarcopenia: definitions and outcome parameters," *Osteoporosis International*, vol. 23, no. 7, pp. 1839–1848, 2012.

[12] M. Venturelli, F. Schena, and R. S. Richardson, "The role of exercise capacity in the health and longevity of centenarians," *Maturitas*, vol. 73, no. 2, pp. 115–120, 2012.

[13] L. E. Aguirre and D. T. Villareal, "Physical exercise as therapy for frailty," *Nestlé Nutrition Institute Workshop Series*, vol. 83, pp. 83–92, 2015.

[14] L. A. Schaap, A. Koster, and M. Visser, "Adiposity, muscle mass, and muscle strength in relation to functional decline in older persons," *Epidemiologic Reviews*, vol. 35, no. 1, pp. 51–65, 2013.

[15] A. L. Benedet, C. F. Moraes, E. F. Camargos et al., "Amerindian genetic ancestry protects against Alzheimer's disease," *Dementia and Geriatric Cognitive Disorders*, vol. 33, no. 5, pp. 311–317, 2012.

[16] E. Kennis, S. M. Verschueren, A. Bogaerts, E. Van Roie, S. Boonen, and C. Delecluse, "Long-term impact of strength training on muscle strength characteristics in older adults," *Archives of Physical Medicine and Rehabilitation*, vol. 94, no. 11, pp. 2054–2060, 2013.

[17] L. T. Fidelis, L. J. Patrizzi, and I. A. P. de Walsh, "Influência da prática de exercícios físicos sobre a flexibilidade, força muscular manual e mobilidade funcional em idosos," *Revista Brasileira de Geriatria e Gerontologia*, vol. 16, no. 1, pp. 109–116, 2013.

[18] R. M. Moreira, R. M. Teixeira, and K. O. Novaes, "Contribuições da atividade física na promoção da saúde, autonomia e independência de idosos," *Kairós Gerontologia, Revista da Faculdade de Ciências Humanas e Saúde*, ISSN 2176–901X, vol. 17, no. 1, pp. 201–217, 2014.

[19] E. L. Cadore, L. Rodríguez-Mañas, A. Sinclair, and M. Izquierdo, "Effects of different exercise interventions on risk of falls, gait ability, and balance in physically frail older adults: a systematic review," *Rejuvenation Research*, vol. 16, no. 2, pp. 105–114, 2013.

[20] C. de Labra, C. Guimaraes-Pinheiro, A. Maseda, T. Lorenzo, and J. C. Millán-Calenti, "Effects of physical exercise interventions in frail older adults: a systematic review of randomized controlled trials," *BMC Geriatrics*, vol. 15, no. 1, p. 154, 2015.

[21] A. P. Shiratori, R. da Rosa Iop, N. G. B. Júnior, S. C. Domenech, and M. da Silva Gevaerd, "Evaluation protocols of hand grip strength in individuals with rheumatoid arthritis: a systematic review," *Revista Brasileira de Reumatologia*, vol. 54, no. 2, pp. 140–147, 2014.

[22] J. Hyun, K. Hwangbo, and C. W. Lee, "The effects of pilates mat exercise on the balance ability of elderly females," *Journal of Physical Therapy Science*, vol. 26, no. 2, pp. 291–293, 2014.

[23] T. Yamauchi, M. M. Islam, D. Koizumi, M. E. Rogers, N. L. Rogers, and N. Takeshima, "Effect of home-based well-rounded exercise in community-dwelling older adults," *Journal of Sports Science & Medicine*, vol. 4, no. 4, pp. 563–571, 2005.

[24] L. S. Ferreira, M. do Socorro Pereira Pinho, M. W. de Macedo Pereira, and A. P. Ferreira, "Perfil cognitivo de idosos residentes em Instituições de Longa Permanência de Brasília-DF," *Revista Brasileira de Enfermagem*, vol. 67, no. 2, pp. 247–251, 2014.

[25] W. A. de Brito, L. Mendes, M. M. Sales et al., "Cognitive profile associated with functional and anthropometric aspects in elderly," *Revista Andaluza de Medicina del Deporte*, vol. 9, no. 4, pp. 154–159, 2016.

[26] P. dos Santos Teixeira, P. A. do Brasil, C. B. Ferreira, V. C. Souza, O. de Toledo Nóbrega, and A. F. Pimentel, "Obesidade e capacidade funcional podem estar associadas com diversas comorbidades em idosos residentes em

instituições de longa permanência," *Revista Brasileira de Pesquisa em Ciências da Saúde*, vol. 3, no. 2, pp. 01–09, 2016.

[27] A. P. Ferreira, C. B. Ferreira, C. J. Brito et al., "The effect of aerobic exercise intensity on attenuation of postprandial lipemia is dependent on apolipoprotein E genotype," *Atherosclerosis*, vol. 229, no. 1, pp. 139–144, 2013.

[28] R. F. Gearhart, K. M. Lagally, S. E. Riechman, R. D. Andrews, and R. J. Robertson, "Strength tracking using the OMNI resistance exercise scale in older men and women," *Journal of Strength and Conditioning Research*, vol. 23, no. 3, pp. 1011–1015, 2009.

[29] P. Szulc, C. Feyt, and R. Chapurlat, "High risk of fall, poor physical function, and low grip strength in men with fracture-the STRAMBO study," *Journal of Cachexia, Sarcopenia and Muscle*, vol. 7, no. 3, pp. 299–311, 2016.

[30] E. L. Cadore, A. Casas-Herrero, F. Zambom-Ferraresi et al., "Multicomponent exercises including muscle power training enhance muscle mass, power output, and functional outcomes in institutionalized frail nonagenarians," *Age*, vol. 36, no. 2, pp. 773–785, 2014.

[31] M. Giné-Garriga, M. Guerra, E. Pagès, T. M. Manini, R. Jiménez, and V. B. Unnithan, "The effect of functional circuit training on physical frailty in frail older adults: a randomized controlled trial," *Journal of Aging and Physical Activity*, vol. 18, no. 4, pp. 401–424, 2010.

[32] N. K. Latham, C. S. Anderson, A. Lee et al., "A randomized, controlled trial of quadriceps resistance exercise and vitamin D in frail older people: the Frailty Interventions Trial in Elderly Subjects (FITNESS)," *Journal of the American Geriatrics Society*, vol. 51, no. 3, pp. 291–299, 2003.

[33] M. J. Faber, R. J. Bosscher, M. J. C. A. Paw, and P. C. van Wieringen, "Effects of exercise programs on falls and mobility in frail and pre-frail older adults: a multicenter randomized controlled trial," *Archives of Physical Medicine and Rehabilitation*, vol. 87, no. 7, pp. 885–896, 2006.

[34] H. Kim, T. Suzuki, M. Kim et al., "Effects of exercise and milk fat globule membrane (MFGM) supplementation on body composition, physical function, and hematological parameters in community-dwelling frail Japanese women: a randomized double blind, placebo-controlled, follow-up trial," *PLoS One*, vol. 10, no. 2, article e0116256, 2015.

[35] L. P. Lustosa, J. P. Silva, F. M. Coelho, D. S. Pereira, A. N. Parentoni, and L. S. M. Pereira, "Impact of resistance exercise program on functional capacity and muscular strength of knee extensor in pre-frail community-dwelling older women: a randomized crossover trial," *Revista Brasileira de Fisioterapia*, vol. 15, no. 4, pp. 318–324, 2011.

[36] N. Fairhall, C. Sherrington, S. R. Lord et al., "Effect of a multifactorial, interdisciplinary intervention on risk factors for falls and fall rate in frail older people: a randomised controlled trial," *Age and Ageing*, vol. 43, no. 5, pp. 616–622, 2014.

[37] N. Fairhall, C. Sherrington, I. D. Cameron et al., "A multifactorial intervention for frail older people is more than twice as effective among those who are compliant: complier average causal effect analysis of a randomised trial," *Journal of Physiotherapy*, vol. 63, no. 1, pp. 40–44, 2017.

[38] M. N. S. dos Santos Lopes, C.G. Passerini, and C. de Fátima Travensolo, "Eficácia de um protocolo fisioterapêutico para equilíbrio em idosos institucionalizados," *Semina: Ciências Biológicas e da Saúde*, vol. 31, no. 2, pp. 143–152, 2010.

[39] M. Giné-Garriga, M. Guerra, and V. B. Unnithan, "The effect of functional circuit training on self-reported fear of falling and health status in a group of physically frail older individuals: a randomized controlled trial," *Aging Clinical and Experimental Research*, vol. 25, no. 3, pp. 329–336, 2013.

[40] D. R. Moore, K. A. Burgomaster, L. M. Schofield, M. J. Gibala, D. G. Sale, and S. M. Phillips, "Neuromuscular adaptations in human muscle following low intensity resistance training with vascular occlusion," *European Journal of Applied Physiology*, vol. 92, no. 4-5, pp. 399–406, 2004.

[41] F. C. Vechin, C. A. Libardi, M. S. Conceição et al., "Comparisons between low-intensity resistance training with blood flow restriction and high-intensity resistance training on quadriceps muscle mass and strength in elderly," *Journal of Strength and Conditioning Research*, vol. 29, no. 4, pp. 1071–1076, 2015.

[42] M. J. Peterson, C. Giuliani, M. C. Morey et al., "Physical activity as a preventative factor for frailty: the health, aging, and body composition study," *Journals of Gerontology Series A: Biological Sciences and Medical Sciences*, vol. 64, no. 1, pp. 61–68, 2009.

[43] B. J. Jeoung and Y. C. Lee, "A Study of relationship between frailty and physical performance in elderly women," *Journal of Exercise Rehabilitation*, vol. 11, no. 4, pp. 215–219, 2015.

[44] R. S. Moraes, A. C. L. da Nóbrega, R. R. T. de Castro et al., "Diretriz de reabilitação cardíaca," *Arquivos Brasileiros de Cardiologia*, vol. 84, no. 5, pp. 431–440, 2005.

[45] I. Imayama, C. M. Alfano, C. E. Mason et al., "Exercise adherence, cardiopulmonary fitness and anthropometric changes improve exercise self-efficacy and health-related quality of life," *Journal of Physical Activity and Health*, vol. 10, no. 5, pp. 676–689, 2013.

[46] L. S. Evangelista, M. A. Hamilton, G. C. Fonarow, and K. Dracup, "Is exercise adherence associated with clinical outcomes in patients with advanced heart failure?," *Physician and Sportsmedicine*, vol. 38, no. 1, pp. 28–36, 2010.

[47] D. T. Villareal, G. I. Smith, D. R. Sinacore, K. Shah, and B. Mittendorfer, "Regular multicomponent exercise increases physical fitness and muscle protein anabolism in frail, obese, older adults," *Obesity*, vol. 19, no. 2, pp. 312–318, 2011.

Correlates of Falls among Community-Dwelling Elderly in Thailand

Titaporn Worapanwisit,[1] Somkid Prabpai,[1] and Ed Rosenberg[2]

[1]Health Promotion and Health Education, Faculty of Education, Kasetsart University, Bangkok 10903, Thailand
[2]Department of Sociology, Appalachian State University, Boone, NC 28608, USA

Correspondence should be addressed to Ed Rosenberg; rosenberge@appstate.edu

Academic Editor: Barbara Shukitt-Hale

Nearly every nation is experiencing rapid population aging. One area of major concern is health; a major health risk for older adults is falling, and there are multiple negative consequences of falling. This is a global concern yet is underresearched in many nations. This study examines demographic, health, and environmental correlates of falling among community-dwelling Thai elderly. Data were collected from a sample of 406 adults aged 60–69. Significant ($p < 0.05$) fall correlates were urban residence, older age, greater BMI, impaired and uncorrected vision, chronic health conditions, medication use and medication side effects, poor muscle tone, and hazardous indoor and outdoor home environments. Results lead to recommendations for interventions to reduce fall risk that are both evidence-based and culturally acceptable.

1. Introduction

In the twenty-first century, most nations are experiencing rapid growth of their older populations, both in number and as a percent of the population. This growth is largely attributable to decreasing mortality due to advances in medicine and health promotion, and to fertility declines. The portion of the world's population aged 60+, 12% in 2015, is projected to rise to 22%, to 2.1 billion, by 2050.

The older adult growth rate is not uniform across nations: less-developed nations will experience more rapid growth. While those aged 60+ in developed countries grew by 29% from 2000 to 2015, less-developed countries can expect a 60–71% increase by 2030. By 2050 nearly 80% of the world's older population will live in these less-developed countries. Many Asian nations are in this latter category. By 2030, 60% of Asians will be 60+ and Asia will be home to more than half of the world's oldest-old persons (aged 80+) [1].

In this context, Thailand is typical of Asian nations. The World Health Organization [2] estimates that those aged 60+ will comprise 29.6% of the Thai population in 2050.

Population aging has serious implications for individuals, families, communities, and nations. The faster the aging, the more quickly and severely the challenges arrive, and the more difficult it is for governments to react effectively. Large-scale proactive initiatives, if and where they exist, seem the exception that proves the under-preparedness rule.

Adapting health care for an aging population is one such major challenge. As people live longer, all else equal, they will live longer with illness and other impairments. Extending healthy life expectancy is more difficult than extending life expectancy, and the "rectangularization of the survival curve" [3], where we live a long, healthy life ending in a brief, precipitous terminal drop, remains the Holy Grail of life extension.

One typology of causes of death is composed of noncommunicable diseases, communicable disease, and injuries. The World Health Organization [4] believes the distribution of noncommunicable disease deaths will remain relatively constant, while communicable disease deaths will decrease. In contrast, deaths due to injuries—the focus of this research—will grow through 2030. Injury-related deaths are large burden on society, financially and otherwise, but many of these deaths are preventable [5]. Unintentional-injury deaths, the five leading causes of which are falls, motor vehicle traffic crashes, suffocation, poisoning, and fire [6], focus the current study further.

A fall is "an unexpected event in which the participant comes to rest on the ground, floor, or lower level" [7]. Similarly, Bekibele and Gureje [8] described a fall as an unintentional loss of balance, causing one to make unexpected or unprepared contact with the ground or floor. Weir and Culmer [9] noted that a fall results from a complex combination of individual factors operating alone or in association with precipitating environmental factors.

Falls are by far the most common cause of injury and unintentional-injury death among older persons in the United States [10], accounting for more than one-half (55%) of the total; in contrast, the second most common cause, motor vehicle accidents, accounts for only 14% [11]. Both the NCHS and the Centers for Disease Control and Prevention [12] report that the rank of falls as a cause of unintentional-injury death rises with age, from tenth among those aged 25–34 to first for those aged 60+.

Falls also have greater consequences for older adults compared to younger adults. Elderly falls may cause serious, perhaps fatal injuries such as fractures, joint dislocation, and/or head trauma. But even if falls have no lasting impact on older adults' physical health, they can have significant effects on psychosocial health, including greater fear of falling that can lead to social isolation [13]. It is difficult to determine the definitive risk factors for falling [14]. Nonetheless, fall risk factors can be trichotomized as follows: (1) intrinsic risk factors related to normal age changes, gender, race, physical problems, medical conditions, cognitive impairment, and degree of physical inactivity, (2) extrinsic risk factors, such as outdated vision correction, taking multiple prescribed medications, improper footwear, and nonuse of assistive devices, and (3) environmental risk factors, such as loose carpet, lack of grab bars in the bathroom, poor lighting, unsafe stairs, and uneven or slippery surfaces. Over one-third of elderly fall at least once annually due to various intrinsic and extrinsic risk factors [15]; 30–50% of falls among community-dwelling elderly are due to environmental factors [16].

Each year, more than one-third of the American elderly fall, with outdoor falls comprising nearly half the total—about 45%—of all elderly falls [17]. Outdoor falls comprise nearly half the total—about 48%—of all elderly falls [18]. Since Americans spend only 7% of their time outdoors [19], this is greatly disproportionate. The same is true in Thailand, where the Health Insurance System Research Office (HISRO) [20] reported that Thai women and men aged 60–69 are more likely to fall in public settings than in the home.

Most outdoor falls are precipitated by environmental factors, such as uneven surfaces and tripping or slipping on objects and usually occur on sidewalks, curbs, and streets [21]. This finding has cross-cultural support from studies in Canada [22], England [23], Norway [24], Finland [25, 26], Israel [27], and Japan [28]. Several researchers [29–31] reported that prescription medications can contribute to fall risk. Jung et al. [32] found that mobility impairments (transferring, gait imbalance, and lack of equilibrium) increase fall risk. Guzman et al. [33] related nonuse of assistive devices to increased odds of falling. In a Thai study, Kuhirunyaratn et al. [34] reported that elderly who use psychotropic medications are almost twice as likely to fall as those who do not (see also [35, 36]). Gait disturbance, visual impairment, and depression also doubled fall risk, and inappropriate indoor environment (cluttered rooms, slippery floors, nonadapted bathrooms, and dim lighting) nearly tripled the risk of falling.

Still, measures to reduce fall risk can be taken, especially at the individual and community levels. Fall-reduction improvements can be made inside and outside the home [37], often inexpensively.

Since falls incidence and prevalence rise with age, since nearly every nation is experiencing rapid population aging, and since the health, economic, and quality of life impacts of falls are significant on both micro- and macrolevels, there is a need for evidence-based research on effective fall prevention strategies and programs that reduce fall risks. Fortunately, many such studies exist, looking at the efficacy of both single- and multi-factor interventions to reduce risk factors and fall incidence. Exercise is the most common intervention used to reduce fall risk factors in community-dwelling older adults. Balance, gait, and strength training have been shown to be effective methods to reduce and prevent falls among community-dwelling older adults [38]. For example, a study of older adults [39] found that fall evaluation, balance training, home hazard management, fall prevention education, exercise, and home visitations resulted in significant fall reduction. Other multifaceted interventions, such as exercise plus dietary supplements [40] and exercise plus fall prevention education [41], yielded reduced fall rates among older adults.

Overall, falls are the leading cause of unintentional-injury deaths and can result from multiple causes, either singly or in combination. The risk of such death rises with age. Even nonfatal falls have more serious consequences for older adults than younger age groups. Major findings include (1) compared to time spent outside the home, older adults are disproportionately likely to fall there, often due to lack of familiarity and uneven surfaces; (2) prescription medications, mobility impairments, and nonuse of assistive devices are associated with greater likelihood of falling; (3) lower perceived fall risk is related to higher likelihood of falling; and (4) many evidence-based fall-reduction interventions exist. Some of these findings have been demonstrated to have cross-cultural application.

It is utopian to believe fall-related injuries can be eradicated, but one can realistically hope to reduce fall incidence and prevalence, even as nations' population age and, as they do, the risk of falls increase. The aim of this research, by reporting demographic, health, and behavioral correlates of falls for community-dwelling Thai elderly, was to add to the knowledge base of universal versus culture-specific fall-reduction knowledge, attitudes, and practices. For older people, there seem to be cross-cultural commonalities in risk of falling. But there is likely variation in preventive or intervention activities; these can depend on aspects like a society's view of aging and older people and the cultural acceptability of a proposed intervention (thus the importance of properly framing the intervention).

Two types of relationships are of interest: those that support prior research and those that vary from prior research. The latter case may merely reflect methodological variance from prior studies but also could indicate the impact of cultural variation on the risk of falls. In both cases, the findings could help identify fall prevention strategies that could reduce falls among community-dwelling older adults, promote safe, independent, healthy aging, and be culturally appropriate.

2. Methods

2.1. Sampling, Sample, and Data Collection. Thailand, a country in Southeast Asia, comprises 77 provinces and is divided into four regions: North, Central, Northeast, and South. For this study, one province—Surat Thani—was randomly chosen from the Southern region due to the residence of the lead author ("researcher"). The province has 19 districts containing a total of 131 subdistricts. Ten districts were randomly selected, and from each, a convenience sample of one subdistrict was chosen. Convenience criteria were ease of access by the researcher (transportation and relative proximity), researcher safety, and ease of access to older adults. Each subdistrict has a hospital. The researcher met with each hospital's director; with the director's consent, the researcher then met with the hospital's Health Promotion Director to obtain a list of older adults. In each subdistrict, a list of all older adults was extracted from a database made available by public health officers. Each resulting list contained 80–200 older adults; the total for all ten subdistricts was 2203.

A random sample of 50 was drawn from each list. The 500 randomly selected Thai older adults then had to meet the following inclusion criteria: aged 60–69, voluntary participation, neither a current psychiatric diagnosis nor a history of such diagnoses, and sufficiently literate to complete a questionnaire with minimal assistance. Some were excluded due to being older than 69, and some chose not to participate. Nine older adults with a current psychiatric diagnosis or history of psychiatric diagnoses were excluded from the sample. No one was excluded due to illiteracy.

After exclusions, a sample contained 406 older adults. Demographic, health, and falls history data were collected via surveys administered at participants' homes or other convenient locations (e.g., senior clubs, temples) between 15 June and 31 October 2017. Demographic variables were age, gender, marital status, residential location, education, occupational status, residence type, number of family members in household, living arrangement, income, main source of income, and health service provider. Health variables were body mass index, vision, hearing, chronic condition diagnosis, medication use, and alcohol use. Fall history variables were falls since turning 60, falls in the past six months, falls in the past three months, general cause of falls (e.g., medication side effects, hazardous home environment), specific cause of falls (e.g., footwear, drowsiness, poor lighting), general (indoors and outdoors), and specific (e.g., kitchen, sidewalk, temple) locations of falls, fall-related health problems, and treatment (if any) after falling.

2.2. Data Analysis. Descriptive statistics (mean, median, standard deviation, frequency, and percentage distributions) were used to describe the demographic, health, and fall history data of the sample. Data were analyzed using SPSS version 17. Due to most variables being measured at the nominal level, including the dependent variable (fall measured as yes/no or never/ever), chi-square was calculated, and $p < 0.05$ was chosen to indicate statistical significance. In some cross tabulations, a cell had a frequency of zero; these instances related never/ever fall to muscle weakness, medical condition/lack of assistive devices, hazardous home environment, footwear/clothing, and indoor/outdoor area. In these cases, the Fisher Exact Test was calculated; $p < 0.001$ was chosen to indicate statistical significance [42].

2.3. Research Ethics. This study was approved by the ethics committee at Boromarajonani College of Nursing, Surat Thani, Thailand. It was also approved by the Ethics Committee of the Provincial Public Health Office in Thailand for the research involving human subjects. The purpose of the research was explained to participants, as were voluntary participation, identity protection (confidentiality), and researcher contact information. Informed consent was obtained from all participants. Survey data were entered into a password-protected database on the first author's secured computer.

3. Results

The demographic characteristics of the sample are presented in Table 1. There were 406 community-dwelling older adults aged 60–69 ($M = 64.60$, $SD = 3.20$), with slightly more (52.2%) in the older category. There were slightly more females (56.0%) than males. About two-thirds (63.85%) were living in towns, the rest in cities. Nearly half (46.8%) were married, with another 31% self-identifying as part of a couple; 12.1% were single, with smaller percentages separated or divorced. Over half (53.9%) had primary school education or less. Just over one-quarter (27.9%) considered themselves working (merchant or employee), with the rest reporting themselves as unemployed, pensioners, or gardeners. Four of five (80.5%) lived in their own homes, with another 12.3% living with relatives.

The number of family members in the household where the participant lived ranged from 1 to 9 persons, with two-thirds of participants living in households with 2–5 family members. Seventy percent lived with spouses and/or children; another 22% were living with nephews or nieces. Hardly any older Thais (1.2%) lived alone. Participants' mean income was 10,953 Thai baht per month

TABLE 1: Demographic characteristics of the sample.

Variable	Number ($n = 406$)	Percent
Age		
60–64	194	47.8
65–69	212	52.2
Mean: 64.6 years		
Standard deviation: 3.2 years		
Gender		
Male	175	43.1
Female	231	56.9
Residential location		
City	147	36.2
Town	259	63.8
Marital status		
Single	49	12.1
Couple	126	31.0
Married	190	46.8
Divorced	14	3.4
Separated	27	6.7
Education		
Uneducated	24	5.9
Primary school	195	48.0
Some secondary school	71	17.5
High school graduate	43	10.6
Vocational education	22	5.4
Bachelor's degree	6	1.5
Master's degree	45	11.1
Occupational status		
Unemployed	143	35.2
Pensioner	36	8.9
Merchant	62	15.3
Employee	51	12.6
Gardener	114	28.1
Residence		
Own house	327	80.5
Relative's house	50	12.3
Rental house	29	7.1
Number of family members in household		
Range: 1–9		
Mean: 3.51		
Standard deviation: 1.53		
Living arrangement		
Alone	9	1.2
Spouse	268	35.1
Children	265	34.9
Nephew/niece	168	22.0
Cousin	26	3.4
Others	26	3.4
Income (Thai baht per month, 1000 baht = US$ 30–31)		
Minimum: 500		
Maximum: 112,000		
Mean: 10,953		
Standard deviation: 12,520		
Main source of income		
Children	181	25.4
Spouse	68	9.5
Cousin	17	2.4
Pension	38	5.3
Government support	219	30.7
Working	190	26.6
Health service provider		
Government hospital	405	99.8
Private hospital	1	0.2

(about US$ 335). A bit less than one-third (30.7%) came from government support, followed by employment (26.6%) and children (25.4%). Thai elderly in the sample had, essentially, no savings. All but one of the 406 participants received health care from the government hospital.

Data on participants' health status are presented in Table 2. Body mass index (BMI) showed well over half (63.3%) to be overweight or obese. About three-fifths (61.3%) had normal vision. Of those with vision problems, more than four-fifths were diagnosed with presbyopia or blurry vision. Nine of ten participants had normal hearing; of those who did not, less than one in five used any type of hearing aid. The majority (60.1%) of participants had a diagnosed medical condition, with the primary ones being hypertension, hyperlipidemia, diabetes mellitus, benign prostate hypertrophy, or heart disease. Two-thirds (66.0%) used medications to help with their medical conditions, with the most common being antihypertensive drugs, antihyperlipidemia drugs, and antihyperglycemic drugs. Nine of ten participants (92.1%) reported not drinking alcohol.

Participants' fall history is described in Table 3. About three-quarters (73.9%) of the sample reported no falls since age 60, with the rest acknowledging one or more falls. Of the 26.1% reporting falls, most (21.1%) reported falling one or two times since turning 60. Only about one in ten had fallen in the six months preceding the study; even fewer had fallen in the preceding three months.

Although the great majority of the sample did not identify specific causes for their falls, some of the attributed causes, such as a hazardous home environment, were more common than others. Physical weakness, medication side effects, and lack of assistive devices were also reported. Regarding specific causes, improper footwear and "contact falls" (losing one's balance due to being jostled, bumping into furniture, etc.) were the most commonly mentioned.

More participants fell outdoors (65.1%) than indoors; about one in ten (11.3%) reported falls in both locations. As one might expect, the majority of outdoor falls (69.3%) occurred in the area surrounding the house. Indoor falls were most common in frequently used areas: kitchen, bedroom, and living room.

For Thai elderly, a fall comes with physical consequences; nearly all (97.2%) reported fall-related health problems. Of those reporting physical consequences, fortunately, most cited relatively minor problems: swelling/bruising, pain, and abrasions comprised 85.7% of reported consequences. More

TABLE 2: Health status of the sample.

Variable	Number (n = 406)	Percentage
Body mass index		
Underweight (<17.50 kg/m^2)	3	0.7
Normal weight (17.50–22.99 kg/m^2)	146	36.0
Overweight (23.00–27.99 kg/m^2)	192	47.3
Obese (≥28 kg/m^2)	65	16.0
Minimum: 15.56 kg/m^2		
Maximum: 43.75 kg/m^2		
Mean: 24.60 kg/m^2		
Standard deviation: 4.15 kg/m^2		
Vision		
Normal	249	61.3
Abnormal	157	38.7
Presbyopia	98	51.9
Blurry vision	64	33.9
Cataract	12	6.3
Glaucoma	3	1.6
Pterygium	12	6.3
Hearing		
Normal	367	90.4
Abnormal	39	9.6
Hearing aids	6	17.1
Deaf	29	82.9
Diagnosis of chronic condition		
No	162	39.9
Yes	244	60.1
Diabetes	76	19.2
Heart	18	4.6
Hypertension	167	42.3
Hyperlipidemia	99	25.1
Benign prostate hypertrophy	35	8.9
Medication use		
No	138	34.0
Yes	268	66.0
Antianalgesic drugs	51	11.0
Bone and joint medicine	15	3.21
Antidiuretic drugs	6	1.3
Antihyperglycemic drugs	77	16.6
Cardiac medications	16	3.4
Antihypertensive drugs	168	36.2
Antihyperlipidemia drugs	96	20.7
Antidepressive	1	0.2
Sleeping pill	14	3.0
Others	20	4.3
Alcohol drinking		
No	374	92.1
Yes	32	7.9

serious outcomes, such as lacerations, fractures, dislocations, or head injuries, were far less common, accounting for 14.3% of reported problems. Treatment behavior was quite varied: about one-quarter went to the hospital, another quarter obtained medications from a pharmacy, and another quarter used no treatment whatsoever.

Table 4 reports bivariate analyses of likelihood of falling and several independent variables. For community-dwelling Thais aged 60–69, falls are significantly more likely to occur among (1) city residents versus residents of towns; (2) older participants; (3) those with the least or the most education; (4) overweight and obese (measured by BMI) elderly compared to normal weight and underweight elderly; (5) those with visual impairment compared to those with normal vision; (6) those with a chronic health condition; (7) those using medications versus those who do not; (8) those reporting muscle weakness compared to those claiming no muscle weakness; (9) those reporting side effects from medications; (10) those with physical impairments who lack assistive devices; (11) those reporting a hazardous home environment; and (12) those using footwear or clothing that can contribute to falling.

4. Discussion

The sample of 406 community-dwelling Thai adults aged 60–69 had many traits that imply representativeness of the Thai population and, in fact, make this sample similar to those of other studies. There were more females than males, more in rural than urban areas, most were living in their own residences, and nearly all received health care from government facilities.

On the other hand, three-quarters of the Thai sample were married or cohabiting, educational attainment was low (over half had not attended secondary school), nearly all (about 19 of 20) lived with immediate or extended family, and over one-quarter reported their main source of income as their children (31% reported "government support").

In addition, nearly two-thirds (63.3%) were overweight or obese based on BMI; a solid majority (61.3%) reported normal vision, and 90.4% reported normal hearing. Six in ten had a chronic condition diagnosis, and two-thirds were taking one or more medications. As might be expected in a heavily Buddhist nation, over nine in ten (92.1%) reported not drinking alcohol.

Regarding falls history, only one-quarter (26.1%) of the sample reported one or more falls since turning 60 (compared to the one-third of American elderly who fall in a given year); however, the maximum age in the sample was 69, and it can be expected that falls incidence and prevalence will rise as the sample lives into its 70s, 80s, and 90s. Despite the disproportionate likelihood of falling outside (versus inside the home) based on percent of time spent outside, the most commonly attributed cause of falls was indoors: a "hazardous home environment."

Bivariate analyses found several factors were associated with higher fall risk: age, urban residence, low or high educational attainment, being overweight or obese, impaired vision, chronic health conditions, medication use and side effects, muscle weakness, nonuse of assistive devices, a hazardous home environment, and certain types of footwear/clothing.

One counterintuitive finding was the high percent (35.6%) of the sample with master's degrees (n = 45) reporting ever falling (Table 4). In general, the percent reporting a fall declined as education increased. This could result from increasing educational attainment leading to less physical and physically risky jobs, better health education and health promotion opportunities, and better overall health. The literature on the education-falls relationship reaches no

TABLE 3: Falls history.

Event	Number ($n = 406$)	Percentage
Falls since 60 years old		
None	300	73.9
Some	106	26.1
1 time	57	14.0
2 times	29	7.1
3 times	11	2.7
4 times	5	1.2
5 times	2	0.5
6 times	1	0.2
10 times	1	0.2
Falls in previous 6 months		
None	360	88.7
Some	46	11.3
1 time	33	8.1
2 times	9	2.2
3 times	3	0.7
4 times	1	0.2
Falls in previous 3 months		
None	376	92.6
Some	30	7.4
1 time	22	5.4
2 times	7	1.7
3 times	1	0.2
Attributed general causes of falls		
Muscle weakness		
No	339	83.5
Yes	67	16.5
Medication side effect		
No	334	82.3
Yes	72	17.7
Medical condition/lack of assistive devices		
No	357	87.9
Yes	49	12.1
Hazardous home environment		
No	309	76.1
Yes	97	23.9
Specific causes of falls		
Slippery shoes	51	10.8
Contact with other person/object	47	10.0
Slippery floor	40	8.5
Fatigue	39	8.3
Headache	25	5.3
Blurry vision	24	5.1
Muscle pain	24	5.1
Muscle weakness	22	4.7
Presbyopia	20	4.2
Dizziness	17	3.6
Slope/uneven ground	15	3.2
Cramp	13	2.8
Numb leg	13	2.8
Hard heeled shoes	13	2.8
Flushing toilet	12	2.5
Slippery bathroom	11	2.3
Foot abnormality	10	2.1
Long dress or sarong	10	2.1
Stumbling	9	1.9
Cesspool	9	1.9
Drowsiness	8	1.7

TABLE 3: Continued.

Event	Number ($n = 406$)	Percentage
In a hurry to void	8	1.7
Foot numbness	7	1.5
General numbness	6	1.3
Poor lighting	5	1.1
Stairs	5	1.1
Muscle tension	3	0.6
High-heeled shoes	3	0.6
Skewness	2	0.4
Falls location		
Outdoor	69	65.1
Indoor	25	23.6
Both	12	11.3
Indoor falls location		
Kitchen	22	30.6
Bedroom	14	19.4
Living room	11	15.3
Terraces	11	15.3
Bathroom	7	9.7
Stairs	6	8.3
Roof	1	1.4
Outdoor falls location		
House surroundings	52	69.3
Footpath/sidewalk	12	16.0
Street/road	4	5.3
Hospital/clinic	2	2.7
Sky walk/overpass	2	2.7
Mall/supermarket	1	1.3
Theatre	1	1.3
Temple	1	1.3
Falls-related health problems		
None	3	2.8
Some	103	97.2
Physical consequences		
Swelling/bruising	63	50.0
Pain	30	23.8
Abrasion	15	11.9
Fracture/dislocation	10	7.9
Laceration	6	4.8
Head injury	2	1.6
Treatment		
Buying drugs at pharmacy	29	27.4
Hospital	28	26.4
No treatment	26	24.5
Resting at home for 1-2 days	14	13.2
Resting for "a while"	6	5.7
Clinic	3	2.8

consensus: studies from Australia and Finland found the logically expected inverse relationship [26, 43], while other studies found a positive ([44], in America) or insignificant ([45], in Turkey) relationship between educational attainment and falls among older adults. Additional cross cultural and multivariate studies are needed to understand the relationship, if any, between educational attainment and falls among older adults.

In some ways, Thai culture can affect the risk and rate of elderly falls. Thai culture, historically and even today, is

Table 4: Likelihood of falling by selected factors.

Variable	Falling, number (%) Never	Ever	p value
Residential location			<0.001
City	88 (59.9)	59 (40.1)	
Town	212 (81.9)	47 (18.1)	
Gender			0.19
Male	135 (77.1)	40 (22.9)	
Female	165 (71.4)	66 (28.6)	
Age			0.029
60–64	153 (78.9)	41 (21.1)	
65–69	147 (69.3)	65 (30.7)	
Marital status			0.9
Single	34 (69.4)	15 (30.6)	
Couple	97 (77.0)	29 (23.0)	
Married	138 (72.6)	52 (27.4)	
Divorced	10 (71.4)	4 (28.6)	
Separated	21 (77.8)	6 (22.2)	
Education			0.009
Uneducated	19 (79.2)	5 (20.8)	
Primary school	137 (70.3)	58 (29.7)	
Secondary school	60 (84.5)	11 (15.5)	
High school graduate	38 (88.4)	5 (11.6)	
Vocational education	12 (54.5)	10 (16.7)	
Bachelor's degree	5 (83.3)	1 (16.7)	
Master's degree	29 (64.4)	16 (35.6)	
Residence			0.45
Own house	241 (73.7)	86 (26.3)	
Relative's house	35 (70.0)	15 (30.0)	
Rental house	24 (82.8)	5 (17.2)	
Number of family members in household			0.13
1 person	9 (52.9)	8 (47.1)	
2–4 persons	228 (75.0)	76 (25.0)	
5+ persons	63 (74.1)	22 (25.9)	
Living arrangement			0.08
Spouse	203 (75.7)	65 (24.3)	
Children	199 (74.8)	67 (25.2)	
Nephew/niece	118 (70.2)	50 (29.8)	
Cousin	16 (61.5)	10 (38.5)	
Others	20 (76.9)	6 (23.1)	
Alone	5 (55.6)	4 (44.4)	
Occupation			0.59
Unemployed	99 (69.2)	44 (30.8)	
Pensioner	27 (75.0)	9 (25.0)	
Merchant	48 (77.4)	14 (22.6)	
Employee	41 (80.4)	10 (19.6)	
Gardener	85 (74.6)	29 (25.4)	
Income			0.5
Below poverty line (<2,647 baht/month)	33 (70.2)	14 (29.8)	
Above poverty line (2,647+ baht/month)	267 (74.4)	92 (25.6)	
BMI			0.046
Underweight (<17.50 kg/m^2)	3 (100)	0	
Normal weight (17.50–22.99 kg/m^2)	115 (78.8)	31 (21.2)	
Overweight (23.00–27.99 kg/m^2)	142 (74.0)	50 (26.0)	
Obese (≥28 kg/m^2)	40 (61.5)	25 (38.5)	

Table 4: Continued.

Variable	Falling, number (%) Never	Ever	p value
Vision			0.001
Normal	198 (79.5)	51 (20.5)	
Abnormal	102 (65.0)	55 (35.0)	
Presbyopia	63 (64.3)	35 (35.7)	
Blurry vision	41 (64.1)	23 (35.9)	
Cataract	7 (58.3)	5 (41.7)	
Glaucoma	3 (100.0)	0	
Pterygium	7 (58.3)	5 (41.7)	
Hearing			0.065
Normal	276 (75.2)	91 (24.8)	
Abnormal	24 (61.5)	15 (38.5)	
Hearing aids	5 (83.3)	1 (16.7)	
Deaf	17 (58.6)	12 (41.4)	
Diagnosis of chronic condition			<0.001
No	144 (88.9)	18 (11.1)	
Yes	156 (63.9)	88 (36.1)	
Diabetes	53 (69.7)	23 (30.3)	
Heart	12 (66.7)	6 (33.3)	
Hypertension	105 (62.9)	62 (37.1)	
Hyperlipidemia	64 (64.6)	35 (35.4)	
Benign prostate hypertrophy	21 (60.0)	14 (40.0)	
Medication use			<0.001
No	125 (90.6)	13 (9.4)	
Yes	175 (65.3)	93 (34.7)	
Antianalgesic drugs	29 (56.9)	22 (43.1)	
Bone and joint medicine	5 (33.3)	10 (66.7)	
Antidiuretic drugs	1 (16.7)	5 (83.3)	
Antihyperglycemic drugs	53 (68.8)	24 (31.2)	
Cardiac medications	13 (81.3)	3 (18.8)	
Antihypertensive drugs	108 (64.3)	60 (35.7)	
Antihyperlipidemia drugs	62 (64.3)	34 (35.4)	
Antidepressive	1 (100.0)	0	
Sleeping pill	11 (78.6)	3 (21.4)	
Others	12 (60.0)	8 (40.0)	
Alcohol drinking			0.051
No	281 (75.1)	93 (24.9)	
Yes	19 (59.4)	13 (40.6)	
Muscle weakness			<0.001
No	300 (88.5)	39 (11.5)	
Yes	0	67 (100.0)	
Weak		22 (33.8)	
Fatigue		39 (60.0)	
Cramp		13 (20.0)	
Numb leg		13 (20.0)	
Numb foot		7 (10.8)	
Muscle tension		3 (4.6)	
Medication side effect			<0.001
No	319 (95.5)	15 (4.5)	
Yes	42 (58.3)	30 (41.7)	
Headaches		25 (34.2)	
Blurry vision		24 (32.9)	
Drowsiness		8 (11.0)	
Diuretic		8 (11.0)	
Muscle aches		24 (32.9)	
Numbness		6 (8.2)	
Dizziness		17 (23.3)	

TABLE 4: Continued.

Variable	Falling, number (%) Never	Ever	p value
Medical condition/lack of assistive devices			<0.001
No	300 (84.0)	57 (16.0)	
Yes	0	49 (100.0)	
Myopia		18 (36.7)	
Presbyopia		20 (40.8)	
Skewness		2 (4.1)	
Abnormal foot		10 (20.4)	
Home hazard environment			<0.001
No	300 (97.1)	9 (2.9)	
Yes	0	97 (100.0)	
Slippery floor		40 (41.2)	
Slope/uneven ground		15 (15.5)	
Stumbling		9 (9.3)	
Contact with other person/object		47 (48.5)	
Poor lighting		5 (5.2)	
Stairs		5 (5.2)	
Flushing toilet		12 (12.4)	
Cesspool		9 (9.3)	
Slippery bathroom		11 (11.3)	
Footwear/clothing			<.0001
No	300 (89.6)	35 (10.4)	
Yes	0	71 (100.0)	
Slippery shoes		51 (71.8)	
High-heeled shoes		3 (4.2)	
Hard-heeled shoes		13 (18.3)	
Long dress/sarong		10 (14.1)	
Indoor area			<0.001
No	300 (85.2)	52 (14.8)	
Yes	0	54 (100.0)	
Bedroom		14 (25.5)	
Kitchen		22 (40.0)	
Living room		11 (20.0)	
Terraces		11 (20.0)	
Stairs		6 (10.9)	
Bathroom		7 (12.7)	
Roof		1 (1.8)	
Outdoor area			<0.001
No	300 (86.7)	46 (13.3)	
Yes	0	60 (100.0)	
Home surrounding		52 (82.5)	
Foot path		12 (19.0)	
Department store		1 (1.6)	
Sky walk/overpass		2 (3.2)	
Street/road		4 (6.3)	
Theatre		1 (1.6)	
Temple		1 (1.6)	
Hospital/clinic		2 (3.3)	

collectivistic and family oriented. In a more individualistic and independent culture, such as in the United States, the government often provides economic, health care and other supports for older adults based on the assumption that the family will not or cannot do this. Within any given nation, this shift from a more communal to a more individualistic society tends to occur with modernization [46, 47]. However, the effects of modernization on the lived experience of older adults can be and are mediated by culture.

For example, in Thailand, China, and other Asian nations including highly modernized Japan, there is a strong cultural norm of filial piety that (adult) children will honor their aging parents by caring for them, even to the point of doing as much as they can for them. Regarding the focus of this research, this operationalization of filial piety can include activities the aging parents might still be quite capable of doing themselves, leading to less physical activity, less muscle tone, and thus increased fall risk.

The data suggest recommendations to reduce fall risk for older Thais. First, the interior home environment could be modified, often at little or no cost, to reduce the risk of falling. Examples include better lighting, nonskid flooring, and grab bars/handrails in the bathrooms and on stairs. Second, the external environment could be modified, given the disproportionate number of falls that occur outside and the 70% that occur on the "house surroundings." Smoothing/repairing uneven surfaces, and adding handrails on outside stairs or replacing stairs with ramps are examples of such modifications. Older adults could be strongly encouraged to maintain a healthy weight, to seek treatment for vision problems, to learn about and practice chronic disease self-management, and maintain regular physical activity. When it comes to clothing and footwear, safety should be a greater concern than vanity.

As is well known, the physical and psychosocial consequences of elderly falls are significant and negative, a drain on the time, energy, and resources of the older adult and his/her family. But these consequences, and thus the recommendations above, pertain to more macrolevels as well—the community and the nation. The World Health Organization, on a global level, and national organizations like AARP in the United States have developed guides to age-friendly homes, communities, and societies. Many of their assessments and recommendations are relevant and applicable cross culturally. New regulations for construction of home and business environments, subsidization of age-friendly renovations, and macrolevel initiatives to promote physical activity, fight obesity, and manage chronic health conditions can be implemented on community and national levels and adapted for cultural acceptability as necessary.

5. Conclusions

Globally and nationally, populations are aging. Rising life expectancy is due mainly to advances in medical science and technology (especially in reducing infant and child mortality). The rapid increase in the percent of older adults is due also to decades-long declines in fertility. The world and nations are aging, quickly and permanently, and this must be planned for.

Falling has significant and negative consequences for older adults and their families, communities, and societies. These consequences affect families, communities, and societies along several dimensions, including economic, psychosocial, and health care. Age is strongly related to falling; as populations age, it is more important than ever to take evidence-based steps to change knowledge, attitudes, and behaviors to reduce fall risk at home, in the community, and in society.

Data in this study came from a nonrepresentative sample of older Thai adults in one province of southern Thailand. Thus, generalizability is limited. Replication in the three other regions of Thailand would help assess both validity and reliability; more representative samples would also be advantageous.

Some results of this study of community-dwelling older Thais support prior research in other nations and thus add to the knowledge base of falls, fall risk, and fall-reduction strategies that have cross-cultural applicability. At the same time, some results vary from prior research and show the necessity of cultural awareness. It is only through such awareness that some questions—for example, why are the least- and most-educated Thai elderly more likely to fall?—will find answers, and only through such awareness can evidence-based interventions be developed to adapt to ensure cultural acceptability.

Conflicts of Interest

The authors declare that they have no conflicts of interest.

Authors' Contributions

All authors have contributed significantly to the research concept, literature review, and objectives. They all are in agreement with the content of the manuscript. All authors approved the manuscript and this submission.

Acknowledgments

This research was supported by the Institute for Health Workforce Development, Ministry of Public Health, Thailand; the Boromarajonani College of Nursing, Surat Thani, Thailand; and the Department of Physical Education, Kasetsart University, Thailand.

References

[1] United Nations, Department of Economic and Social Affairs, and Population Division, *World Population Ageing 2015*, Department of Economic and Social Affairs, and Population Division (UN), New York, NY, USA, 2015.

[2] World Health Organization, *What are the Main Risk Factors for Falls Amongst Older People and What are the Most Effective Interventions to Prevent These Falls?*, World Health Organization, Geneva, Switzerland, 2004.

[3] J. R. Wilmoth and S. Horiuchi, "Rectangularization Revisited: Variability of Age at Death within Human Populations," *Demography*, vol. 36, no. 4, pp. 475–495, 1999.

[4] World Health Organization, *The Global Burden of Disease: 2004 Update*, World Health Organization, Geneva, Switzerland, 2004.

[5] G. Bergen, L. H. Chen, M. Warner, and L. A. Fingerhut, *Injury in the United States: 2007*, National Center for Health Statistics, Hyattsville, MD, USA, 2008.

[6] Department of Health and Human Services, *Office of Disease Prevention and Health Promotion. Healthy People 2020*, 2013, http://www.healthypeople.gov/2020.

[7] L. D. Gillespie, M. Robertson, W. Gillespie et al., "Interventions for preventing falls in older people living in the community," *Cochrane Database of Systematic Reviews*, vol. 2, 2009.

[8] C. O. Bekibele and O. Gureje, "Fall incidence in a population of elderly persons in Nigeria," *Gerontology*, vol. 56, no. 3, pp. 278–283, 2010.

[9] E. Weir and L. Culmer, "Fall prevention in the elderly population," *CMAJ*, vol. 171, no. 7, p. 724, 2004.

[10] N. R. Hooyman and H. A. Kiyak, *Social Gerontology: A Multidisciplinary Perspective*, Allyn and Bacon, Boston, MA, USA, 9th edition, 2011.

[11] National Center for Health Statistics, *Mortality Multiple Cause Files, 2000–2013*, 2013, http://www.cdc.gov/nchs/data_access/vitalstatsonline.htm.

[12] Centers for Disease Control and Prevention, *Ten Leading Causes of Injury Deaths by Age Group Highlighting Unintentional Injury Death*, Centers for Disease Control and Prevention, Atlanta, GA, USA, 2014.

[13] M. Rogerson and C. Emes, "Fostering resilience within an adult day support program," *Activities, Adaptation and Aging*, vol. 32, no. 1, pp. 1–18, 2008.

[14] R. A. Newton, "Maximizing independence: reducing/preventing falls," *Geriatric Care Management Journal*, vol. 12, no. 2, pp. 16–19, 2002.

[15] K. Frick, J. Kung, J. Parrish, and M. Narrett, "Evaluating the cost-effectiveness of fall prevention programs that reduce fall-related hip fractures in older adults," *Journal of the American Geriatrics Society*, vol. 58, no. 1, pp. 136–141, 2010.

[16] G. Feder, C. Cryer, S. Donovan, and Y. Carter, "Guidelines for the prevention of falls in older people," *BMJ*, vol. 321, no. 7267, pp. 1007–1011, 2000.

[17] M. E. Tinetti, "Clinical practice. Preventing falls in elderly persons," *New England Journal of Medicine*, vol. 348, no. 1, pp. 42–49, 2003.

[18] T. Chippendale and V. Raveis, "Knowledge, behavioral practices, and experiences of outdoor fallers: Implications for prevention programs," *Archives of Gerontology and Geriatrics*, vol. 72, pp. 19–24, 2017.

[19] N. E. Klepeis, W. C. Nelson, W. R. Ott et al., "The National Human Activity Pattern Survey (NHAPS): a resource for assessing exposure to environmental pollutants," *Journal of Exposure Analysis and Environmental Epidemiology*, vol. 11, no. 3, pp. 231–252, 2001.

[20] Health Insurance System Research Office (HISRO), *Fall in Thai Elderly*, Mueang Nonthaburi, Thailand, 2010.

[21] W. Li, T. H. Keegan, B. Sternfeld, S. Sidney, C. P. Quesenberry, and J. L. Kelsey, "Outdoor falls among middle-aged and older adults: a neglected public health problem," *American Journal of Public Health*, vol. 96, no. 7, pp. 1192–1200, 2006.

[22] L. E. Weinberg and L. A. Strain, "Community-dwelling older adults' attributions about falls," *Archives of Physical Medicine and Rehabilitation*, vol. 76, no. 10, pp. 955–960, 1995.

[23] P. A. Bath and K. Morgan, "Differential risk factor profiles for indoor and outdoor falls in older people living at home in Nottingham, UK," *European Journal of Epidemiology*, vol. 15, no. 1, pp. 65–73, 1999.
[24] A. Bergland, G. B. Jarnlo, and K. Laake, "Predictors of falls in the elderly by location," *Aging Clinical and Experimental Research*, vol. 15, no. 1, pp. 43–50, 2003.
[25] O. P. Ryynanen, S. L. Kivela, and R. Honkanen, "Times, places, and mechanisms of falls among the elderly," *Zeitschrift Fur Gerontologie*, vol. 24, pp. 154–161, 1991.
[26] O. P. Ryynänen, S. L. Kivelä, and R. Honkanen, "Incidence of falling injuries leading to medical treatment in the elderly," *Public Health*, vol. 105, no. 5, pp. 373–386, 1991.
[27] J. Cwikel, "Falls among elderly people living at home: medical and social factors in a national sample," *Israel Journal of Medical Sciences*, vol. 28, pp. 446–453, 1992.
[28] S. Yasumura, H. Haga, and N. Niino, "Circumstances of injurious falls leading to medical care among elderly people living in a rural community," *Archives of Gerontology and Geriatrics*, vol. 23, no. 2, pp. 95–109, 1996.
[29] B. Resnick and P. Junlapeeya, "Falls in a community dwelling older adults: Findings and implications for practice," *Applied Nursing Research*, vol. 17, no. 2, pp. 81–91, 2004.
[30] M. Callisaya, J. E. Sharman, J. Close, S. R. Lord, and V. K. Srikanth, "Greater daily defined dose of antihypertensive medication increases the risk of falls in older people-a population-based study," *Journal of Gerontological Society*, vol. 62, pp. 1527–1533, 2014.
[31] H. Huang, M. Gau, C. Lin, and G. Kernohan, "Assessing risk of falling in older adults," *Public Health Nursing*, vol. 20, no. 5, pp. 399–411, 2003.
[32] Y. Jung, D. Shin, K. S. Chung, and S. E. Lee, "Health status and fall-related factors among older Korean women," *Journal of Gerontological Nursing*, vol. 33, no. 10, pp. 12–20, 2007.
[33] A. B. Guzman, J. M. Garcia, J. P. Garcia et al., "A multinomial regression model of risk for falls (RFF) factors among Filipino elderly in a community setting," *Educational Gerontology*, vol. 39, no. 9, pp. 669–683, 2013.
[34] P. Kuhirunyaratn, P. Prasomrak, and B. Jindawong, "Factor related to falls among community dwelling elderly," *Southeast Asian Journal of Tropical Medicine and Public Health*, vol. 44, no. 5, pp. 906–915, 2013.
[35] F. Baranzini, N. Poloni, and M. Diurni, "Polypharmacy and psychotropic drugs as risk factors for falls in long-term care setting for elderly patients in Lombardy," *Recenti Progressi in Medicina*, vol. 100, pp. 9–16, 2009.
[36] K. D. Hill and R. Wee, "Psychotropic drug-induced falls in older people: a review of interventions aimed at reducing the problem," *Drugs and Aging*, vol. 29, no. 1, pp. 15–30, 2012.
[37] J. Knodel, P. Vipan, and C. Napaporn, *The Changing Well-being of Thai Elderly: An Update from the 2011 Survey of Older Persons in Thailand. Chiang Mai*, Help Age International, London, UK, 2013.
[38] Panel on Prevention of Falls in Older Persons, American geriatrics society, and British Geriatrics Society, "Summary of the updated American Geriatrics Society/British Geriatrics Society clinical practice guideline for prevention of falls in older persons," *Journal of the American Geriatrics Society*, vol. 59, no. 1, pp. 148–157, 2011.
[39] P.-C. Sze, W.-H. Cheung, P.-S. Lam, H.-S. D. Lo, K.-S. Leung, and T. Chan, "The efficacy of a multidisciplinary falls prevention clinic with an extended step-down community program," *Archives of Physical Medicine of Rehabilitation*, vol. 89, no. 7, pp. 1329–1334, 2008.
[40] J. Swanenburg, E. D. de Bruin, M. Stauffacher, T. Mulder, and D Uebelhart, "Effects of exercise and nutrition on postural balance and risk of falling in elderly people with decreased bone mineral density: randomized controlled trial pilot study," *Clinical Rehabilitation*, vol. 21, no. 6, pp. 523–534, 2007.
[41] H.-C. Huang, C.-U. Liu, Y.-U. Huang, and W. G. Kernohan, "Community-based interventions to recede falls among older adults in Taiwan-long time follow-up randomized controlled study," *Journal of Clinical Nursing*, vol. 19, no. 7-8, pp. 959–968, 2010.
[42] J. Fleiss, *Statistical Methods for Rates and Proportions*, John Wiley and Sons, New York, NY, USA, 2nd edition, 1981.
[43] J. Dolinis, J. E. Harrison, and G. R. Andrews, "Factors associated with falling in older Adelaide residents," *Australian and New Zealand Journal of Public Health*, vol. 21, no. 5, pp. 462–468, 1997.
[44] J. T. Hanlon, L. R. Landerman, and G. G. Fillenbaum, "Falls in African American and white community-dwelling elderly residents," *Journals of Gerontology Series A: Biological Sciences and Medical Sciences*, vol. 577, no. 7, pp. M473–M478, 2002.
[45] T. C. Ozturk, R. Ak, U. A. Ebru, O. Onur, S. Eroglu, and S. Murat, "Factors associated with multiple falls among elderly patients admitted to emergency department," *International Journal of Gerontology*, vol. 11, no. 2, pp. 85–89, 2017.
[46] D. Cowgill, "Aging and modernization: a revision of the theory," in *Late Life Communities and Environmental Policy*, J. F. Gubrium, Ed., Charles C. Thomas, Springfield, IL, USA, 1974.
[47] M. Pipher, *Another Country*, Riverhead, New York, NY, USA, 1999.

22

The Influence of Education and Apolipoprotein ε4 on Mortality in Community-Dwelling Elderly Men and Women

Duke Appiah[1] **and Richard N. Baumgartner**[2]

[1]*Department of Public Health, Texas Tech University Health Sciences Center, 3601 4th Street, STOP 9403, Lubbock, TX 79430, USA*
[2]*Department of Epidemiology and Population Health, School of Public Health and Information Sciences, University of Louisville, 485 E. Gray St., Louisville, KY 40202, USA*

Correspondence should be addressed to Duke Appiah; duke.appiah@ttuhsc.edu

Academic Editor: Kathryn Peri

We investigated the risk of death in relation to the apolipoprotein ε4 allele and evaluated how it interacts with education in 50 elderly adults (mean age 73 years, 65.3% women) who were enrolled in 1993 into the New Mexico Aging Process Study. During years of follow-up, apolipoprotein ε2 appeared to be associated with a lower risk for all-cause mortality (hazard ratio (HR) = 0.73 95% confidence interval (CI): 0.30–1.71) compared to apolipoprotein ε3 carriers in models adjusted for age, sociodemographic variables, medical conditions, adiposity, and lifestyle factors. The apolipoprotein ε4 allele conferred almost a threefold elevated risk of mortality (HR = 2.76, CI: 1.42–5.37). An interaction between education and apolipoprotein e4 ($p = 0.027$) was observed with the HR of mortality among e4 carriers compared to noncarriers being 1.59 (0.64–3.96) for those with ≥college education; 6.6 (1.90–23.4) for those with some college or trade; and 14.1 (3.03–65.6) for participants with ≤high school education. No significant interaction was identified between apolipoprotein E genotype and cognitive function for mortality risk. These findings suggest that genetic (apolipoprotein ε4) and environmental (education) factors act interactively to influences survival in the elderly with higher education attenuating the adverse effect of apolipoprotein ε4 on mortality.

1. Introduction

Apolipoprotein E (APOE), with regard to longevity, can be said to be the most extensively studied gene [1]. APOE, a 299 amino acid plasma protein with its gene found on chromosome 19, plays a central role in lipid transport and metabolism and also possesses several immunomodulatory properties such as suppressing lymphocytic T cell proliferation [2–4]. It has three polymorphisms: ε2, ε3, and ε4 with the later being associated with increased susceptibility for several chronic diseases as well as mortality [5–7], while ε2 has been suggested to have a protective effect, compared to ε3 [8].

Reports on the association of APOE allelic variation with mortality has been equivocal with differences in estimates observed among different ethnic/racial populations [9–13]. Some of the possible explanations for the inconsistent results across studies is that APOE ε4 allele is associated with Alzheimer's and cardiovascular disease, two conditions that in themselves are among the most prevalent causes of mortality in the elderly, resulting in survival bias with reduced frequency of the e4 allele in persons aged 65 and older [8]. Additionally, secular trends and geographic variation in the rates of the aforementioned chronic diseases suggest that the risk of death conferred by APOE genotype may depend on complex interactions with various environmental or behavioral risk factors over the lifespan of an individual. In this regard, numerous reviews have raised the issue that most studies assessing the effect of APOE across populations and time ignore the effects of behavioral factors that predisposes people to disease [1].

A large body of research has demonstrated a positive association of educational attainment with better health outcomes [14, 15] as well as reduced mortality [16]. Accordingly, over the last decades, reports from numerous studies allude to a gene-environment interaction between APOE genotype and education on health outcomes, namely, dementia [17], brain structure and development [18, 19], and cognitive function [20–22]. However, observations concerning the possible modifying effect of educational status on mortality in the elderly, independent of chronic comorbidities, are limited. Therefore, we aimed to evaluate whether educational status would offset the adverse influence of the APOE ε4 allele on mortality among community-dwelling elderly adults.

2. Materials and Methods

The New Mexico Aging Process Study (NMAPS) was a longitudinal study conducted between 1979 and 2001 in Albuquerque, NM, to describe the nutritional status and factors associated with healthy aging in community-dwelling elderly persons. The study design, subject recruitment, and inclusion and exclusion criteria have been described in detail previously [23]. Briefly, to be enrolled in the study, a person had to be 60 years and older and have no preexisting medical conditions such as cancer (with the exception of non-melanoma skin cancer), recent myocardial infarction, type 2 diabetes mellitus, chronic obstructive pulmonary disease, or uncontrolled hypertension. About 90% of participants were non-Hispanic whites, 8% of Hispanic origin, and close to 2% being nonwhite. An annual visit was required for all participants in whom blood samples were obtained, and body composition, physical, functional, cognitive, and nutritional status were assessed. The yearly dropout rate for the study was approximately 3.6% with major chronic conditions and migration out of Albuquerque being the main reasons. The study was approved by the Human Subjects Research Review Committee of the University of the New Mexico School of Medicine with all participants providing informed consent in accordance with the Declaration of Helsinki, and all methods were carried out in accordance with the relevant guidelines and regulations. Participants who were alive at 1993, were followed up for 9 years (median, 7 years), and had genotype data together with measures of cognitive function were included in the current analysis.

APOE genotypes were assessed by restriction fragment length polymorphism analysis of polymerase chain reaction products, as previously developed [24, 25]. The assays were conducted in the Aging and Genetic Epidemiology (AGE) laboratory [23]. Of the 577 individuals who participated at baseline, 519 had APOE genotyped successfully. To distinguish unambiguously the effect of the APOE allele and genotype, we further excluded participants with APOE 2/4 (n = 15), resulting in an analytic sample of 504 participants.

Cognitive function was evaluated by using the modified version of the Mini-Mental State Examination (3MS) [26]. Depression was measured using the short form of the Geriatric Depression Scale [27], with a score of 5 or higher suggestive of depressive symptomatology.

Educational status was assessed using a questionnaire with possible responses being less than 12 years of education (high school), high school graduate or passed the tests of general educational development, some college or technical school, college degree, some grad school, masters degree, and doctorate. Other covariates of interest were sex, marital status, body mass index (BMI), bone mineral density, smoking status, diastolic blood pressure, and levels of total cholesterol and triglyceride. BMI was calculated by dividing weight in kilograms by the square of height in meters. Bone mineral density was measured by Lunar DPX DXA (GE/Lunar Radiation Corp., Madison, WI). Chronic conditions including cancer, nonvertebral or vertebral fracture, diabetes, ischemic heart disease, and cerebrovascular disease were all self-reported at each annual visit, verified against medical records, and coded according to the International Classification of Diseases, Ninth Revision (ICD-9) codes. ICD-9 codes used were 140–208 for cancer; 250 for diabetes (or fasting blood glucose level ≥ 7 mmol/L); 290, 294, and 331 for dementia; 430–438 for cerebrovascular disease; 410–414 and 428–429 for ischemic heart disease; and 800–829 nonvertebral or vertebral fracture. Deaths were ascertained using the National Death Index and verified whenever possible against state death certificates and local obituary reports.

2.1. Statistical Analysis. Differences in baseline characteristics by APOE genotype were assessed using chi-square for categorical variables and ANOVA for continuous variables that were normally distributed or the Kruskal–Wallis test for nonnormally distributed variables. In time-to-event analysis, the Kaplan–Meier method was used to evaluate the incidence of all-cause mortality in relation to APOE genotype groups with the censoring date being December 31, 2002. Attained age was used as the time scale for all analyses as this procedure offers the opportunity to account for the effect of survival bias (thus individual with the highest risk of mortality are not observed) [28]. Furthermore, the use of attained age as the time scale provides a more straight-forward interpretation of mortality since it is free of the confounding effect of age which is intrinsically taken into account as a measure of survival time [29]. Survival curves were then produced to graphically depict incident events with differences among groups assessed by means of the log-rank test. Adjusted hazard ratios (HRs) and 95% confidence intervals (CIs) for mortality were calculated using Cox proportional hazards regression. Four models with progressive adjustments were used. Model 1 was adjusted for demographic variables such as age, sex, education, and marital status. Model 2 comprised model 1 with further adjustment for levels of triglyceride, BMI, bone mineral density, and diastolic blood pressure. Model 3 further adjusted for psychological factors such as scores on both the Geriatric Depression Scale and the Modified Mini-Mental State Examination. Finally, model 4 also adjusted for incident medical conditions, including all cancers, nonvertebral or vertebral fractures, diabetes, ischemic heart disease, and cerebrovascular disease. APOE status was identified with dummy coded indicator variables with the 3/3 genotype used as the referent. Interactions of APOE ε4 allele and educational as well as other statistically significant covariates on the risk of mortality were explored using the likelihood ratio test to compare models with and without the interaction terms. The assumption of proportional hazards was assessed by graphical

Table 1: Baseline characteristics of participants in the New Mexico Aging Process Study.

Characteristics	Apolipoprotein E genotype group			p value
	APOE 2 carriers (N = 71)	APOE 3/3 (N = 336)	APOE 4 carriers (N = 97)	
Age, years	73.8 (6.4)	73.5 (6.5)	72.4 (5.8)	0.261
Sex, %				0.110
Male	45.1	32.1	36.1	
Female	54.9	67.9	63.9	
Education, %				0.642
High school or less	16.9	17.2	15.5	
Some college or trade	36.6	28.3	27.8	
College degree or higher	46.9	54.5	56.7	
Marital status, %				0.160
Single	30.4	42.9	40.4	
Married	69.6	57.1	59.6	
Current smoker, %	7.3	3.9	3.2	0.361
Depressive symptoms, %	4.2	4.5	4.1	0.988
Diastolic blood pressure (mmHg)	80.4 (10.2)	79.5 (11.3)	79.5 (10.8)	0.805
Total cholesterol (mmol/l)	5.10 (0.75)	5.47 (0.93)	5.49 (1.04)	0.008
Triglycerides (mmol/l)	1.61 (0.82)	1.62 (0.99)	1.55 (0.86)	0.820
Body mass index (kg/m^2)	25.4 (3.49)	25.5 (4.01)	24.7 (3.91)	0.252
Waist to hip ratio	0.92 (0.11)	0.88 (0.1)	0.89 (0.11)	0.062
Bone mineral density	1.10 (0.13)	1.07 (0.12)	1.09 (0.11)	0.145
Mini-Mental State Exam scores	94.6 (4.91)	95.2 (4.28)	94.1 (5.73)	0.107
Medical conditions at follow-up				
Diabetes	4.2	3.3	4.1	0.817
Fractures	12.7	13.4	11.3	0.867
Cancers	5.6	12.5	15.5	0.144
Ischemic heart disease	7.0	7.4	10.3	0.626
Cerebrovascular disease	5.6	4.5	9.3	0.190
Deceased at the end of study	9.9	11.0	17.5	0.183

Values are mean (standard deviation) for continuous variables and percentages for categorical variables; p values based on the chi-square test for categorical variables and ANOVA for normally distributed continuous variables or the Kruskal–Wallis test for nonnormally distributed continuous variables.

methods using Schoenfeld residuals. To assess the robustness of the estimates, we performed a sensitivity analysis which included information for the 15 participants with APOE ε2/4. A two-tailed probability value less than 0.05 was considered statistically significant, and all analyses were performed using SAS software, version 9.4 (SAS Institute, Inc., Cary, NC)

3. Results

The mean age of participants at baseline was 73.4 (range 61–91) with 65.3% being women. Approximately half of the participants reported having a college degree or higher and only 11.3% had a BMI of 30 or higher. Nearly 5% of the cohort was identified as having depressive symptomatology indicative of depression, and less than 2% of participants were classified as having dementia. Several differences in baseline characteristics were observed between men and women. Men were more likely than women to be older and have higher bone mineral density and higher body weight, with a significantly greater proportion reporting having graduated from college (66.3% versus 47.1%), currently married (86.2% versus 44.9%), diagnosed with ischemic heart disease (14.3% versus 4.6%), and cancer (16% versus 10%). Women were more likely to have higher levels of total cholesterol and triglyceride with a significantly greater proportion reporting fractures (15.5% versus 8%). A description of the cohort according to APOE genotype is shown in Table 1. The most common genotype was APOE 3/3 found in 66.7% of participants with 13.9% and 18.1% having ε2/3 and ε3/4 genotypes, respectively. Additionally, only 19.2% of participants had at least one ε4 allele. These percentages are consistent with other prospective population studies among the elderly, especially those 60 years and older. As expected, total cholesterol levels varied across APOE genotype groups ($p_{\text{for trend}} = 0.01$) with APOE ε2 carriers having the lowest levels of total cholesterol.

During follow-up, 61 (12%) deaths were recorded with fatal events occurring twice as often in men than women. Figure 1 shows unadjusted Kaplan–Meier cumulative incidence estimates for all-cause mortality according to APOE genotype and allele. The log-rank statistic suggests that APOE genotype and allele influenced mortality, with APOE ε4 carriers having a significantly higher number of deaths. In multivariable models (Table 2), participants with the APOE ε4/ε4 genotype had a greater risk of mortality (HR = 2.56, 95% CI: 1.33–4.94) compared to persons homozygous for ε3 allele (model 3). APOE ε4 carriers had a twofold elevated risk of mortality compared to non-APOE ε4 carriers (HR = 2.21, 95% CI: 1.20–4.09). These estimates increased in magnitude after further adjustment for chronic medical conditions yielding hazard ratios of 2.61 (CI: 1.33–5.14) and 2.76 (CI: 1.42–5.37) for APOE ε4/ε4 genotype and e4 allele carriers compared to persons homozygous for ε3 allele and non-APOE ε4 carriers, respectively.

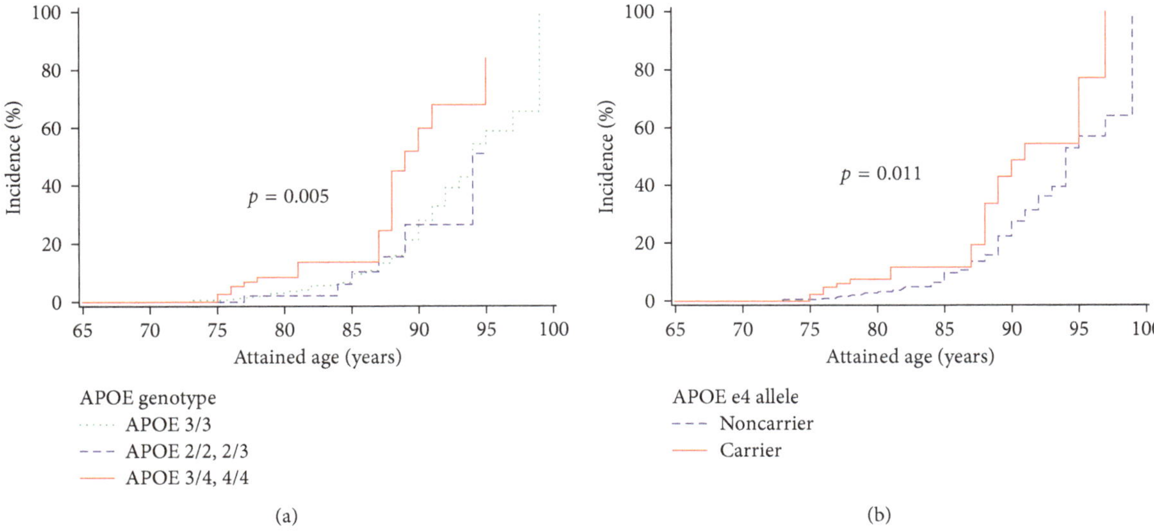

Figure 1: Kaplan–Meier cumulative incidence estimates for all-cause mortality by (a) APOE genotype and (b) APOE ε4 allele.

Table 2: APOE genotype and allele as predictors of all-cause mortality.

	Unadjusted	Model 1	Model 2	Model 3	Model 4
Apolipoprotein E genotype					
APOE ε3/3	1	1	1	1	1
APOE ε2/2, 2/3	0.80 (0.34–1.80)	0.73 (0.32–1.65)	0.73 (0.32–1.68)	0.75 (0.32–1.74)	0.73 (0.31–1.71)
APOE ε3/4, 4/4	2.38 (1.33–4.26)	2.34 (1.30–4.36)	2.53 (1.35–4.73)	2.56 (1.33–4.94)	2.61 (1.33–5.14)
Apolipoprotein E allele					
APOE ε4 noncarrier	1	1	1	1	1
APOE ε4 carrier	1.99 (1.17–3.38)	2.20 (1.25–3.86)	2.26 (1.24–4.13)	2.21 (1.20–4.09)	2.76 (1.42–5.37)

Model 1: adjusted for age, sex, education, and marital status; model 2: model 1 plus levels of triglyceride, body mass index, bone mineral density, and diastolic blood pressure; model 3: model 2 plus Geriatric Depression Scale and the Modified Mini-Mental State Examination scores; model 4: model 3 plus incident medical conditions occurring during follow-up (cancers, nonvertebral or vertebral fractures, diabetes, ischemic heart disease, and cerebrovascular disease).

Educational status appeared to be negatively associated with mortality with persons who had college education or more having lower risk of mortality compared to participants with high school education or less (HR = 0.79, 0.35–1.76). Howbeit, this did not approach statistical significance. Finally, we observed a significant interaction between educational status and APOE ε4 allele on the risk of mortality ($p = 0.027$). The HR of mortality among ε4 carriers compared to noncarriers was 1.59 (0.64–3.96) for those with ≥college education; 6.66 (1.90–23.4) for those with some college or trade; and 14.1 (3.03–65.6) for participants with ≤high school education. No significant interaction was identified between APOE genotype and cognitive function for mortality risk. These results remained unchanged when information from the 15 participants with APOE ε2/4 was included in the analysis, and APOE ε2/4 was not significantly associated with mortality which could possibly be attributed to the small sample size (data not shown).

4. Discussion

In this community-based sample of elderly adults, we observed that the APOE ε3/4 and ε4/4 genotypes were associated with higher incidence of all-cause mortality, independent of important confounders. However, this elevated mortality risk was offset by higher educational status. To our knowledge, this is the first study to report that APOE (genetic factor) and education (environmental factor) act interactively to influences survival in the elderly.

While the underlying mechanism by which education ameliorates the influence of APOE genotype on mortality among elderly adults is a topic of major interest, it is not fully understood. It is possible that education may exert some beneficial effects on survival through two main avenues. That is, either through increased socioeconomic resources over the life course that could aid in the prevention of chronic diseases or through neuroprotective mechanism involved in reducing age-related or pathological changes in the structure and function of the brain which in the long term might influence longevity [30, 31]. On the one hand, higher education, more often than not, provides numerous resources such as higher income, stable employment, better social networks, health-related self-efficacy, and access to safe neighborhoods [32]. Accordingly, a large body of evidence has shown that higher educational attainment, whether measured as years of education or degree completion, is associated with reduced incidence of chronic morbidities [33], delayed mortality [34], and improved overall health primarily due to better access and utilization of health care and the adaption of health-promoting behaviors and lifestyles [14].

On the other hand, education may moderate the expression of the APOE ε4 allele on the risk of mortality in the elderly by influencing age-related or pathological changes in brain-matter and cognitive reserve. Some [35], but not all [36, 37], neuroimaging studies of cognitively healthy elders have found higher education to be associated with low accumulation of amyloid-beta deposition [38]; physiologically increasing regional cortical thickness [39]; increasing white and gray matter volume [35] in the superior temporal gyrus, insula, and anterior cingulate cortex [18]; decreasing mean diffusivity in the bilateral hippocampus [40]; and influencing a greater metabolism in the anterior cingulate cortex [18]. Furthermore, higher education is reported to be positively related with anterior cingulate connectivity which in turn is associated with improved cognitive performances [18]. These results and several others provide profound evidence that brain and cognitive reserve delays the clinical manifestations of dementia [18]. Compared to persons without the APOE ε4 variant, those with two copies of the ε4 variant are known to have more than a sevenfold elevated risk of developing Alzheimer's disease [38], the 6th leading cause of mortality in the United States. Taken together, these results and that of the present study suggest that higher education may offset the negative effects of the APOE ε4 on mortality by increasing cerebral reserve capacity against Alzheimer's disease and other late-life cognitive-related diseases. Even among elderly adults with Alzheimer's disease, a history of higher education has been reported to aid in coping better with the effects of brain atrophy by increasing cognitive reserve [39].

There is a strong, positive, and well-documented relation between APOE genotype and morbidity and mortality, and our results are consistent with some [12, 41–46] but not other studies [2, 8–11, 13, 47, 48] conducted among the elderly. For instance, the Cache County study with 4701 participants aged 65 and older found a greater mortality risk in persons carrying the ε3/4 and ε4/4 genotype which persisted even after accounting for the effect of Alzheimer's and cardiovascular disease [42]. One of the several reasons for the diverging results for APOE and mortality may pertain to small samples. The improvement in statistical power offered by studies with longer follow-up, such as the NMAPS, is important because there is a greater chance of identifying an effect if it truly exists. The Rotterdam study which followed 6852 participants for a mean of 5.4 years [47] did not identify any association between APOE genotype and longevity. However, after follow-up was extended to a mean of 11.1 years [4], with improved risk factor adjustments, APOE ε2 carriers with normal weight were found to have a reduced risk of mortality. Other reasons for the divergent results could be due to the heterogeneity in the relative frequency of the APOE ε4 allele among ethnic/racial groups, as well as methodological issues including selection bias and inadequate adjustment for confounders, which can all potentially influence study results [49].

This study has several potential limitations. First, it was restricted to a sample of elderly community-dwelling persons who were predominantly Caucasians and generally in good health. Thus, the results may not be generalizable to other ethnic/racial groups or elderly community-dwelling persons. Second, not all participants enrolled in the study consented to give blood for genotyping. Although such participants were older, there was no difference with respect to mortality and chronic medical conditions between those who did and did not have genotype data. In any case, the effect of any difference on our results cannot be estimated. Because the distribution of APOE genotype was similar to that reported in other prospective cohort studies of elderly persons, we believe that our results are not seriously biased. Third, the sample size of the cohort was relatively smaller, and with the occurrence of fatal events not being common, the statistical power to detect very weak associations is limited. Nonetheless, the associations detected were strong and statistically significant. Finally, we did not observe any effect modification of chronic ailments such as cancer, impaired cognitive function, diabetes, ischemic heart disease, and cerebrovascular disease with APOE genotype on longevity. This may primarily be due to the low prevalence of these conditions in our cohort. Serious chronic medical conditions were the main reason for dropout from the NMAPS, followed by migration. However, persons who dropped out still contributed information to the analysis since they were censored at the last date known to be alive. Also, follow-up for mortality status in the cohort was nearly complete. Nonetheless, it remains possible that these medical conditions may play a moderating role in the relationship between APOE and mortality.

In summary, we observed that APOE ε4 allele is positively related to mortality risk with this elevated mortality offset by higher educational status; however, the mechanism underlying this association is not fully understood. Discovering candidate genes that influence longevity has great public health importance. With almost 15% of the general population known to have the APOE ε4 variant and this proportion increasing to about 40% among persons with Alzheimer's disease [38], the moderating effects of education, lifestyle, and behavioral factors on genes should be studied to achieve a better understanding of their influence on longevity. This will go a long way to aid in targeting interventions towards high-risk individuals which will in turn reduce morbidity and improve longevity as well as quality of life among such persons.

Conflicts of Interest

The authors declare that there are no conflicts of interest regarding the publication of this article.

Acknowledgments

The authors wish to acknowledge and thank Dr. Philip Garry who served as the Principal Investigator of the NMAPS and originally collected the data for APOE genotypes used in this analysis. This study was conducted within the New Mexico Aging Process Study which was supported by National Institute of Health Grants R01 AG10149 and AG02049.

References

[1] S. J. Lewis and E. J. Brunner, "Methodological problems in genetic association studies of longevity–the apolipoprotein E gene as an example," *International Journal of Epidemiology*, vol. 33, no. 5, pp. 962–970, 2004.

[2] K. Rockwood, B. Nassar, and A. Mitnitski, "Apolipoprotein E-polymorphism, frailty and mortality in older adults," *Journal of Cellular and Molecular Medicine*, vol. 12, no. 6, pp. 2754–2761, 2008.

[3] H. L. Zhang, J. Wu, and J. Zhu, "The role of apolipoprotein E in Guillain-Barre syndrome and experimental autoimmune neuritis," *Journal of Biomedicine and Biotechnology*, vol. 2010, Article ID 357412, 12 pages, 2010.

[4] M. C. Pardo Silva, A. C. J. W. Janssens, A. Hofman et al., "Apolipoprotein E gene is related to mortality only in normal weight individuals: the Rotterdam Study," *European Journal of Epidemiology*, vol. 23, no. 2, pp. 135–142, 2008.

[5] J. E. Eichner, "Apolipoprotein E polymorphism and cardiovascular disease: a HuGE review," *American Journal of Epidemiology*, vol. 155, no. 6, pp. 487–495, 2002.

[6] L. A. Farrer, "Effects of age, sex, and ethnicity on the association between apolipoprotein E genotype and Alzheimer disease. A meta-analysis. APOE and Alzheimer Disease Meta Analysis Consortium," *JAMA*, vol. 278, no. 16, pp. 1349–1356, 1997.

[7] C. Lahoz, E. J. Schaefer, L. A. Cupples et al., "Apolipoprotein E genotype and cardiovascular disease in the Framingham Heart Study," *Atherosclerosis*, vol. 154, no. 3, pp. 529–537, 2001.

[8] G. G. Fillenbaum, D. G. Blazer, B. M. Burchett, A. M. Saunders, and D. H. Taylor, "Apolipoprotein E ε4 and risk of mortality in African American and white older community residents," *Gerontologist*, vol. 42, no. 3, pp. 381–386, 2002.

[9] J. H. Lee, M.-X. Tang, N. Schupf et al., "Mortality and apolipoprotein E in Hispanic, African-American, and Caucasian elders," *American Journal of Medical Genetics*, vol. 103, no. 2, pp. 121–127, 2001.

[10] G. G. Fillenbaum, B. M. Burchett, J. H. Lee, and D. G. Blazer, "Mortality and apolipoprotein E in African-American, and White elders: an attempted replication," *American Journal of Medical Genetics*, vol. 119A, no. 2, pp. 141–146, 2003.

[11] K. A. Lane, S. Gao, S. L. Hui et al., "Apolipoprotein E and mortality in African-Americans and Yoruba," *Journal of Alzheimer's Disease*, vol. 5, no. 5, pp. 383–390, 2003.

[12] D. C. Ewbank, "Differences in the association between apolipoprotein E genotype and mortality across populations," *Journals of Gerontology Series A: Biological Sciences and Medical Sciences*, vol. 62, no. 8, pp. 899–907, 2007.

[13] M. F. Lima-Costa, S. V. Peixoto, M. Taufer, and E. H. Moriguchi, "Apolipoprotein e genotype does not predict 9-year all-cause mortality in brazilian older adults: the Bambui Cohort Study," *Journal of the American Geriatrics Society*, vol. 56, no. 12, pp. 2366–2368, 2008.

[14] J. D. Boardman, B. W. Domingue, and J. Daw, "What can genes tell us about the relationship between education and health?," *Social Science & Medicine*, vol. 127, pp. 171–180, 2015.

[15] C. E. Ross and J. Mirowsky, "Refining the association between education and health: the effects of quantity, credential, and selectivity," *Demography*, vol. 36, no. 4, pp. 445–460, 1999.

[16] R. A. Hummer and E. M. Hernandez, "The effect of educational attainment on adult mortality in the United States," *Population Bulletin*, vol. 68, no. 1, pp. 1–16, 2013.

[17] H. X. Wang, D. R. Gustafson, M. Kivipelto et al., "Education halves the risk of dementia due to apolipoprotein ε4 allele: a collaborative study from the Swedish brain power initiative," *Neurobiology of Aging*, vol. 33, no. 5, pp. 1007.e1–1007.e7, 2012.

[18] E. M. Arenaza-Urquijo, B. Landeau, R. La Joie et al., "Relationships between years of education and gray matter volume, metabolism and functional connectivity in healthy elders," *Neuroimage*, vol. 83, pp. 450–457, 2013.

[19] E. M. Arenaza-Urquijo, J. Gonneaud, M. Fouquet et al., "Interaction between years of education and APOE epsilon4 status on frontal and temporal metabolism," *Neurology*, vol. 85, no. 16, pp. 1392–1399, 2015.

[20] P. W. Van Gerven, M. P. J. Van Boxtel, E. E. B. Ausems, O. Bekers, and J. Jolles, "Do apolipoprotein E genotype and educational attainment predict the rate of cognitive decline in normal aging? A 12-year follow-up of the Maastricht Aging Study," *Neuropsychology*, vol. 26, no. 4, pp. 459–472, 2012.

[21] T. E. Strandberg, K. Pitkala, J. Eerola, R. Tilvis, and P. J. Tienari, "Interaction of herpesviridae, APOE gene, and education in cognitive impairment," *Neurobiology of Aging*, vol. 26, no. 7, pp. 1001–1004, 2005.

[22] Y. L. Ishioka, Y. Gondo, N. Fuku et al., "Effects of the APOE ε4 allele and education on cognitive function in Japanese centenarians," *Age*, vol. 38, no. 5-6, pp. 495–503, 2016.

[23] S. J. Wayne, B. J. Vellas, S. G. Brodie, P. J. Garry, and R. N. Baumgartner, "Apolipoprotein ε4 allele and problems with orientation are associated with a persistent decline in cognition in community-dwelling elderly persons," *Journals of Gerontology Series A: Biological Sciences and Medical Sciences*, vol. 60, no. 3, pp. 375–379, 2005.

[24] J. E. Hixson and D. T. Vernier, "Restriction isotyping of human apolipoprotein E by gene amplification and cleavage with HhaI," *Journal of Lipid Research*, vol. 31, no. 3, pp. 545–548, 1990.

[25] P. J. Garry, S. J. Wayne, and B. Vellas, "The New Mexico aging process study (1979–2003). A longitudinal study of nutrition, health and aging," *Journal of Nutrition, Health and Aging*, vol. 11, no. 2, pp. 125–130, 2007.

[26] E. L. Teng and H. C. Chui, "The Modified Mini-Mental State (3MS) examination," *Journal of Clinical Psychiatry*, vol. 48, no. 8, pp. 314–318, 1987.

[27] J. L. Sheikh and J. A. Yesavage, "Geriatric Depression Scale (GDS). Recent evidence and development of a shorter version," *Clinical Gerontologist*, vol. 5, pp. 165–173, 1986.

[28] K. C. Cain, S. D. Harlow, R. J. Little et al., "Bias due to left truncation and left censoring in longitudinal studies of developmental and disease processes," *American Journal of Epidemiology*, vol. 173, no. 9, pp. 1078–1084, 2011.

[29] R. Lamarca, J. Alonso, G. Gómez, and A. Muñoz, "Left-truncated data with age as time scale: an alternative for survival analysis in the elderly population," *Journals of Gerontology Series A: Biological Sciences and Medical Sciences*, vol. 53, no. 5, pp. M337–M343, 1998.

[30] C. J. Cook and J. M. Fletcher, "Can education rescue genetic liability for cognitive decline?," *Social Science & Medicine*, vol. 127, pp. 159–170, 2015.

[31] D. Bartres-Faz and E. M. Arenaza-Urquijo, "Structural and functional imaging correlates of cognitive and brain reserve hypotheses in healthy and pathological aging," *Brain Topography*, vol. 24, no. 3-4, pp. 340–357, 2011.

[32] J. K. Montez and L. F. Berkman, "Trends in the educational gradient of mortality among US adults aged 45 to 84 years:

bringing regional context into the explanation," *American Journal of Public Health*, vol. 104, no. 1, pp. e82–e90, 2014.
[33] A. I. Choi, C. C. Weekley, S.-C. Chen et al., "Association of educational attainment with chronic disease and mortality: the Kidney Early Evaluation Program (KEEP)," *American Journal of Kidney Diseases*, vol. 58, no. 2, pp. 228–234, 2011.
[34] J. P. Mackenbach, A. E. Kunst, F. Groenhof et al., "Socioeconomic inequalities in mortality among women and among men: an international study," *American Journal of Public Health*, vol. 89, no. 12, pp. 1800–1806, 1999.
[35] A. Foubert-Samier, G. Catheline, H. Amieva et al., "Education, occupation, leisure activities, and brain reserve: a population-based study," *Neurobiology of Aging*, vol. 33, no. 2, pp. 423 e15–423 e25, 2012.
[36] H. Christensen, P. J. Batterham, A. J. Mackinnon et al., "Education, atrophy, and cognitive change in an epidemiological sample in early old age," *American Journal of Geriatric Psychiatry*, vol. 17, no. 3, pp. 218–226, 2009.
[37] C. Bastin, I. Yakushev, M. A. Bahri et al., "Cognitive reserve impacts on inter-individual variability in resting-state cerebral metabolism in normal aging," *Neuroimage*, vol. 63, no. 2, pp. 713–722, 2012.
[38] E. H. Corder, A. Saunders, W. Strittmatter et al., "Gene dose of apolipoprotein E type 4 allele and the risk of Alzheimer's disease in late onset families," *Science*, vol. 261, no. 5123, pp. 921–923, 1993.
[39] Y. Liu, AddNeuroMed Consortium, V. Julkunen et al., "Education increases reserve against Alzheimer's disease–evidence from structural MRI analysis," *Neuroradiology*, vol. 54, no. 9, pp. 929–938, 2012.
[40] F. Piras, A. Cherubini, C. Caltagirone, and G. Spalletta, "Education mediates microstructural changes in bilateral hippocampus," *Human Brain Mapping*, vol. 32, no. 2, pp. 282–289, 2011.
[41] D. C. Ewbank, "Mortality differences by APOE genotype estimated from demographic synthesis," *Genetic Epidemiology*, vol. 22, no. 2, pp. 146–155, 2002.
[42] K. M. Hayden, P. P. Zandi, C. G. Lyketsos et al., "Apolipoprotein E genotype and mortality: findings from the Cache County Study," *Journal of the American Geriatrics Society*, vol. 53, no. 6, pp. 935–942, 2005.
[43] D. M. Little, V. C. Crooks, D. B. Petitti et al., "Mortality, dementia, and apolipoprotein E genotype in elderly white women in the United States," *Journal of the American Geriatrics Society*, vol. 57, no. 2, pp. 231–236, 2009.
[44] E. H. Corder, H. Basun, L. Lannfelt et al., "Attenuation of apolipoprotein E ε4 allele gene dose in late age," *The Lancet*, vol. 347, no. 9000, p. 542, 1996.
[45] E. H. Corder, L. Lannfelt, M. Viitanen et al., "Apolipoprotein E genotype determines survival in the oldest old (85 years or older) who have good cognition," *Archives of Neurology*, vol. 53, no. 5, pp. 418–422, 1996.
[46] B. T. Heijmans, P. E. Slagboom, J. Gussekloo et al., "Association of APOE ε2/ε3/ε4 and promoter gene variants with dementia but not cardiovascular mortality in old age," *American Journal of Medical Genetics*, vol. 107, no. 3, pp. 201–208, 2002.
[47] A. J. Slooter, M. Cruts, C. Van Broeckhoven, A. Hofman, and C. M. Van Duijin, "Apolipoprotein E and longevity: the Rotterdam Study," *Journal of the American Geriatrics Society*, vol. 49, no. 9, pp. 1258-1259, 2001.
[48] M. T. Vogt, J. A. Cauley, and L. H. Kuller, "Apolipoprotein E phenotype, arterial disease, and mortality among older women: the study of osteoporotic fractures," *Genetic Epidemiology*, vol. 14, no. 2, pp. 147–156, 1997.
[49] M. Eto, K. Watanabe, and K. Ishii, "A racial difference in apolipoprotein E allele frequencies between the Japanese and Caucasian populations," *Clinical Genetics*, vol. 30, no. 5, pp. 422–427, 1986.

Hypertension, Sarcopenia, and Global Cognitive Function in Community-Dwelling Older Women

Hélio José Coelho-Júnior,[1] Bruno Bavaresco Gambassi,[1] Maria-Claudia Irigoyen,[2] Ivan de Oliveira Gonçalves,[3] Paula de Lourdes Lauande Oliveira,[4] Paulo Adriano Schwingel,[5] Cândida Helena Lopes Alves,[6] Ricardo Yukio Asano,[3] Marco Carlos Uchida,[1] and Bruno Rodrigues[1]

[1]*Applied Kinesiology Laboratory (LCA), School of Physical Education, University of Campinas, Av. Érico Veríssimo, 701 Cidade Universitária "Zeferino Vaz", Barão Geraldo, 13083-851 Campinas, SP, Brazil*
[2]*Hypertension Unit, Heart Institute (InCor), Medical School of University of São Paulo, São Paulo, SP, Brazil*
[3]*Center of Health Sciences, University of Mogi das Cruzes, Av. Dr. Cândido Xavier de Almeida Souza, 200 Centro Cívico, 08780-911 Mogi das Cruzes, SP, Brazil*
[4]*Physical Education Department, Ceuma University, São Luis, MA, Brazil*
[5]*Laboratório de Pesquisas em Desempenho Humano (LAPEDH), Universidade de Pernambuco (UPE), Petrolina, PE, Brazil*
[6]*Departamento de Fisioterapia, Universidade Ceuma, São Luis, MA, Brazil*

Correspondence should be addressed to Hélio José Coelho-Júnior; coelhojunior@hotmail.com.br

Academic Editor: Antonello Lorenzini

The present study aimed to investigate whether sarcopenia interferes in the association between HTN and cognitive function in community-dwelling older women. One hundred and eleven older women were recruited and dichotomized in hypertensive ($n = 63$) and normotensive groups ($n = 48$). Volunteers underwent evaluations of the sarcopenic state (i.e., skeletal muscle mass, short physical performance battery (SPPB), balance), hemodynamic parameters, and global cognitive status (i.e., Mini-Mental State Examination (MMSE)). Data demonstrated that hypertensive patients had lower global cognitive status than normotensive subjects. When volunteers were divided according to sarcopenic status, data demonstrated that hypertensive patients with low performance on SPPB (0.006), low values of sarcopenic index (0.03), and low performance on sit-to-stand (0.09) demonstrated poor cognitive status compared with hypertensive patients with normal values of these variables. In conclusion, data of the current study indicate that the sarcopenic state might interfere in the association among hypertension and poor cognitive status, once a higher frequency of hypertensive patients with low lower limb muscle function (i.e., SPPB and sit-to-stand) and muscle mass index (i.e., Janssen index) was observed in the <24 MMSE segment, in comparison with hypertensive patients with normal results in these parameters.

1. Introduction

The worldwide projections have indicated an exponential increase in the elderly population in the next 40 years [1]. Indeed, the number of elderly people is expected to reach about 30% of the world population in 2050 [1].

The aging process is a continuous phenomenon accompanied by alterations in some physiological systems (e.g., cardiovascular, skeletal muscle, metabolism), collaborating to the development of geriatric syndromes and chronic diseases. Hypertension (HTN) is one of the most prevalent diseases in older people, affecting more than 70% of this population [2]. The main concern about this disease is its poor prognosis because patients with high blood pressure show an increased risk of stroke (i.e., hemorrhagic and ischemic) and myocardial infarction [2, 3].

However, in the last few years, an increasing number of studies have suggested that HTN is associated not only with elevated cardiovascular risk, but also with cognitive alterations [4–8]. In fact, cross-sectional studies have indicated that hypertensive patients show elevated odds to global and fragmented (e.g., executive function, memory) cognitive impairment than normotensive subjects [4–8]. In this sense, a recent report by the American Heart Association (AHA) shows that a considerable amount of studies have indicated that high blood pressure may promote several changes in the organic system that predispose the genesis of the dementia syndrome, such as Alzheimer's disease (AD) [8]. In addition, the researchers stated that despite recent remarkable progress about this issue, there is still much to know [8].

In turn, similar to HTN, an increased prevalence of sarcopenia—a neuromuscular disease characterized by a progressive muscular atrophy accompanied by low muscle strength and/or lower muscle limb function—is observed in older adults [9, 10]. Sarcopenia is known by its effects on muscular functionality, causing a marked decrease in mobility, transfer capacity, and, consequently, impairing the capacity to perform alone and effectively the activities of daily living [9–11]. Furthermore, besides its close association with impaired muscle functionality, sarcopenic people show elevated risk to present poor cognition [12].

Interestingly, data from population studies have demonstrated that the prevalence of HTN is increased in sarcopenic patients [13]. Moreover, it is worth mentioning that HTN and sarcopenia share several mechanisms present in the genesis of dementia, such as low-grade inflammation and arterial stiffness, which suggest that hypertensive patients with sarcopenia might present lower cognitive scores than nonsarcopenic hypertensive patients [8, 10, 12, 14–16]. However, to the best of our knowledge, no studies have been conducting to test this hypothesis.

Therefore, the present study aimed to investigate whether sarcopenia interferes in the association between HTN and cognitive function in community-dwelling older women.

2. Methods

This cross-sectional study was approved by the Research Ethics Committee of the University of Mogi das Cruzes (UMC) under protocol number 621-614 and was developed in accordance with the Declaration of Helsinki and with Resolution 196/96 revised in 2008 of the National Health Council. Since this study aimed at investigating the association between HTN, sarcopenic factors, and cognitive function in community-dwelling older women, volunteers were submitted to morphological, physical, cognitive, hemodynamic, and biochemical evaluations at rest.

2.1. Subjects. The study participants were recruited from two specialized healthcare centers for older adults in a town located in the metropolitan area of São Paulo, Brazil. Volunteers were recruited by convenience and asked verbally by the medical team and researchers about their participation in the study. All subjects provided informed consent before enrolment.

The exclusion criteria were use of hormone replacement and/or psychotropic drugs, cerebrovascular disease (e.g., stroke), endocrinal disease (e.g., diabetes), pulmonary disease, neurological or psychiatric disease (e.g., Parkinson's or Alzheimer's disease), musculoskeletal disorders, comorbidities associated with greater risk of falls, and any kind of dizziness, blurred vision, or lightheadedness when rise or remain standing for long, which could indicate orthostatic hypotension and/or labyrinthitis. The inclusion criteria were age ≥ 60 years, live in the community, 4–7 years of schooling, and be independent to perform the instrumental (IADL) and basic (ADL) activities of daily living. After the application of the exclusion and inclusion criteria, 111 older women were included in the analyses.

The volunteers were subdivided into normotensive and hypertensive groups according to the previous clinical diagnosis of HTN. Since both healthcare centers serve a large number of patients, and the medical team (i.e., nurse, physician and physical educator) is of limited size, the pathological conditions were simply recorded by the head physician and head nurse of each center. A specialist (i.e., cardiologist) who was not affiliated to and was outside the center then made the diagnosis of HTN, according to the guidelines [17].

3. Morphological, Physical, Hemodynamic, and Biochemical Evaluations

All subjects were instructed to refrain from physical exercise for 96 hours before the tests and to refrain from eating or drinking (including water) for 8 hours before the tests. All tests were conducted between 07:00 am and 10:00 am under a controlled temperature of 24°–26°C [18].

3.1. Assessment of Body Composition. A data acquisition system (Tanita InnerScan 50v, Tokyo, Japan) was used to measure the bioelectrical impedance. This system uses an electrical current to quantify the amount of intracellular and extracellular water in the body. The device has four electrodes: two are placed on the feet while the other two are placed in the hands of the volunteers. The device measures body mass index (BMI), total body mass, total muscle mass, and appendicular muscle mass. Janssen and Baumgartner muscle mass indexes were evaluated according to the following equations: Janssen index = absolute muscle mass/height^2; Baumgartner index = appendicular muscle mass/height^2 [10, 11, 18].

3.2. Short Physical Performance Battery. The SPPB includes three tests that evaluate lower-body function: a hierarchical test of standing balance, a 4-meter walk speed test, and a five repetitive chair stands. Each SPPB component test (balance, gait, and chair stand) is scored from 0 to 4 with a score of 0 representing the inability to perform the test and a score of 4 representing the highest category of performance. For the balance tasks, the participants were asked to stand with their feet side by side, followed by the semitandem (heel of one foot alongside the big toe of the other foot) and tandem (heel of one foot directly in front of and touching the other foot) positions for 10 s each. For gait speed, a 4-meter walk speed test at the participant's usual pace was timed. For the ability to rise from a chair, volunteers were requested to rise from a chair five times as fast as possible with their arms crossed in front of the body. The stopwatch was activated when the volunteer raised their buttocks off the chair and was stopped when the volunteer seated back. A summary performance score was obtained by adding the scores of each individual SPPB component test (range 0–12), with higher scores indicating better lower-body function [19–21].

3.3. Evaluation of Hemodynamic Parameters at Rest. The procedures for measurement of blood pressure were adapted from the VII Joint National Committee on Prevention, Detection, Evaluation, and Treatment of High Blood Pressure (JNC7) [22]. In summary, older women remained in a sitting position on a comfortable chair for 15 minutes in a quiet room. After this period, an appropriate cuff was placed at approximately the midpoint of the upper left arm (heart level). An automatic, noninvasive, and validated [23] arterial blood pressure monitor (Microlife-BP 3BT0A, Microlife, Widnau, Switzerland) was used to measure systolic blood pressure (SBP), diastolic blood pressure (DBP), and heart rate (HR). During blood pressure recording, volunteers remained relaxed in the sitting position, with parallel feet at one shoulder width, both forearm and hands on the table, supinated hands, back against the chair, without move or talk. The volunteer did not have access to blood pressure values during measurement. The evaluation lasted approximately 80 seconds and was performed three times with one minute of rest among the measurements. The mean of measurements of each volunteer was used in the final analysis. Mean arterial pressure (MAP), double product (DP), and pulse pressure (PP) were evaluated according to the following equations: $MAP = [SBP + (2 \times DBP)]/3$, $DP = SBP \times HR$, and $PP = SBP - DBP$. The size of the arm cuff was selected after measuring the arm circumference of each participant (Sanny, São Paulo, Brazil).

Table 1: Characteristics of older women according to hypertension.

Variables	Total (n = 111)	
	Normotensive (n = 48)	Hypertensive (n = 63)
Anthropometric characteristics		
Age (years)	65.5 ± 2.0	65.1 ± 1.9
Weight (kg)	63.8 ± 10.9	66.4 ± 10.4
BMI (kg/m^2)	26.0 ± 4.1	27.5 ± 4.5
Body fat (%)	32.7 ± 9.5	34.4 ± 7.3
Absolute muscle mass (kg)	41.4 ± 4.5	39.9 ± 7.6
Appendicular skeletal muscle mass (kg)	17.7 ± 4.6	17.4 ± 5.6
Janssen index (kg/m^2)	65.7 ± 6.5	63.0 ± 7.0
Baumgartner index (kg/m^2)	11.7 ± 1.6	11.9 ± 2.0
Physical functional tests		
Sit-to-stand (s)	15.2 ± 3.3	15.3 ± 3.3
Walking speed (m/s)	0.84 ± 0.33	0.72 ± 0.34
Side-by-side stand	9.7 ± 1.1	9.7 ± 1.1
Semitandem stand	9.7 ± 1.2	9.6 ± 1.4
Tandem stand	9.4 ± 1.6	8.7 ± 2.6
Short physical performance battery	9.6 ± 1.2	9.3 ± 1.5
Hemodynamic parameters		
SBP (mmHg)	126.0 ± 11.4	150.3 ± 18.0*
DBP (mmHg)	77.1 ± 9.0	87.5 ± 10.1
MAP (mmHg)	93.4 ± 8.3	106.6 ± 17.6*
HR (bpm)	75.3 ± 10.0	76.8 ± 11.5
DP (mmHg·bpm)	9508 ± 1561	11373 ± 2683*
PP (mmHg)	49.9 ± 11.7	62.4 ± 16.6*
Clinical parameters		
ADL	0.15 ± 0.36	0.10 ± 0.30
IADL	2.0 ± 2.1	2.8 ± 3.8
GDS	4.9 ± 6.4	4.0 ± 4.6
MMSE	25 ± 2	23 ± 3*
Average of drugs	0.31 ± 0.62	0.59 ± 0.79
Biochemical parameters		
Salivary NO (μM)	150.3 ± 97.0	110.5 ± 67.9

BMI = body mass index; SBP = systolic blood pressure; DBP = diastolic blood pressure; MAP = mean arterial pressure; HR = heart rate; DP = double product; PP = pulse pressure; ADL = activities of daily living; IADL = instrumental activities of daily living; GDS = geriatric depressive scale; MMSE = Mini-Mental State Examination; NO = nitric oxide. $^*P < 0.05$.

3.4. Saliva Collection. Saliva samples were collected at rest using a roller cotton (Cremer, São Paulo, Brazil). Researchers asked the participants to put a piece of cotton in their mouth and remove it when it became soggy. The samples were transferred to a Falcon tube and frozen immediately until the end of the experiment. In the laboratory, the samples were centrifuged and supernatants were stored at −80°C for posterior analyses using the Griess colorimetric method [24].

3.5. Measurement of Nitric Oxide (NO). The NO pool was considered the mensuration of nitrite (NO_2^-) levels in saliva. Briefly, a solution containing 0.1% N-(1-naphthyl)-ethylenediamine (NED) (Sigma) and 1.0% sulfanilamide (Sigma) was prepared in 2.5% phosphoric acid as the diluent. Saliva samples (50 μL) and Griess reagent (50 μL) were mixed and transferred to microplates. Absorbance was measured at 530 nm, and sodium nitrite ($NaNO_2$) was used as the standard. Nitrite quantification (μM) was achieved using a standard curve constructed with $NaNO_2$ at the concentrations of 100, 50, 25, 12.5, 6.25, 3.13, 1.66, and 0 μM [24]. Data were analysed using the Microplate software (CA, USA).

4. Questionnaires

All interviews were performed face to face, so that the application of the tests, along with their objectives, was explained individually to each participant. If a question was not understood, the interviewer repeated the question more slowly, up to three times.

4.1. Mini-Mental State Examination (MMSE). The participants' cognitive function was assessed using the MMSE,

Table 2: MMSE according to the presence of hypertension and high or low levels of variables related to sarcopenia.

	Total (n = 111)			
	Normotensive		Hypertensive	
Variables	High MMSE	Low MMSE	High MMSE	Low MMSE
Anthropometric characteristics				
Absolute muscle mass (kg)	25.7 ± 2.1	26.3 ± 2.7	21.8 ± 5.6	20.1 ± 8.8[a]
Appendicular skeletal muscle mass (kg)	25.6 ± 2.0	25.5 ± 3.5	20.3 ± 1.7[a]	23.3 ± 7.5
Janssen index (kg/m^2)	26.4 ± 2.4	26.0 ± 1.7	23.0 ± 3.8[a]	22.7 ± 2.8[a]
Baumgartner index (kg/m^2)	25.8 ± 2.4	25.2 ± 2.8	23.0 ± 3.2[a]	24.0 ± 3.4
Physical functional tests				
Sit-to-stand (s)	25 ± 2.9	26.1 ± 2.2	21.2 ± 7.1[a]	22.3 ± 6.8
Walking speed (m/s)	25 ± 2.6	25.0 ± 2.6	21.6 ± 6.7	21.7 ± 7.9
Short physical performance battery (points)	24.6 ± 3.6	25.7 ± 2.4	24.8 ± 2.9	22.9 ± 3.2[b]
Sarcopenia				
Absolute muscle mass plus walking speed	24.8 ± 2.3	28.0 ± 0.0	22.8 ± 2.4[b]	23.6 ± 0.5
Absolute muscle mass plus sit-to-stand	25.1 ± 1.7	27.1 ± 2.7	22.4 ± 3.5[b]	24.2 ± 3.5
Absolute muscle mass plus short physical performance battery	24.3 ± 3.2	24.2 ± 1.2	26.3 ± 2.7	—
Appendicular skeletal muscle mass plus walking speed	24.8 ± 2.3	24.3 ± 3.5	22.3 ± 2.3	25.3 ± 2.5
Appendicular skeletal muscle mass plus sit-to-stand	25.4 ± 1.8	27.0 ± 2.7	22.2 ± 3.3[ab]	24.3 ± 3.9
Appendicular skeletal mass plus short physical performance battery	25.0 ± 3.5	24.2 ± 1.2	26.0 ± 3.0	19.0 ± 0.0[ac]
Baumgartner index plus walking speed	24.7 ± 2.9	28.0 ± 00	23.1 ± 3.3	24.6 ± 3.7
Baumgartner index plus sit-to-stand	26.3 ± 2.6	27.0 ± 2.9	23.1 ± 2.9[a]	23.6 ± 2.8
Baumgartner index plus short physical performance battery	24.6 ± 3.3	24.2 ± 1.2	25.7 ± 2.4	25.0 ± 3.9
Janssen index plus walking speed	25.0 ± 2.7	26.3 ± 0.5	22.5 ± 2.2[b]	23.5 ± 1.4
Janssen index plus sit-to-stand	25.1 ± 1.7	25.2 ± 1.6	22.5 ± 3.5	21.8 ± 4.0
Janssen index plus short physical performance battery	23.4 ± 3.1	28.0 ± 0.0[a]	25.7 ± 1.5	24.0 ± 0.0

[a]$P < 0.05$ versus high NTS; [b]$P < 0.05$ versus low NTS; [c]$P < 0.05$ versus high HTS; [d]$P < 0.05$ versus low HTS; data are shown as mean ± SD; MMSE = Mini-Mental State Examination.

which is a standard test in cognitive aging research to assess mental status with a possible score of 0–30 [16]. MMSE evaluates orientation, registration, and short-term recall, attention and concentration, language (naming, sentence writing, and comprehension), and visuospatial abilities. Individual items are summed to generate the total score. If individuals decline or are unable to attempt a task, the value of that particular item would be missing. The MMSE was applied according to Brucki et al. [25].

4.2. Geriatric Depressive Scale (GDS). The quantification of depressive symptoms was evaluated by the short version of the geriatric depression scale (GDS). The scale comprises 15 questions about the feelings, or the frequency of the feelings, of the patient in front of some conditions of the life. The answers are based on a binary code: yes or no [26, 27].

4.3. Instrumental (IADL) and Basic (ADL) Activities of Daily Living. ADL and IADL were evaluated through Katz and Pfeffer index, respectively. The Katz ADL measures six self-care tasks using a dichotomous rating (dependent = 0; independent = 1) in the hierarchical order of decreasing difficulty as listed: bathing, dressing, toileting, transferring to and from a chair, maintaining continence, and feeding. A final score of six indicates *independency*, whereas a 0 score indicates a full dependence [28]. The Pfeffer questionnaire constitutes of a 10-item instrument. Each item is scored on a scale of 0 (independence) to 3 (dependence), where higher scores reflect greater dependency of the patient [29].

5. Statistical Analysis

To determine the differences in the continuous data between the groups (i.e., normotensive and hypertensive), Student's t-test for independent samples was performed. Comparisons between the groups according to the variables associated with sarcopenia were made using one-way analysis of variance (ANOVA) followed by Dunnett's post hoc test. A posteriori, chi-square test was performed to investigate the association between the dependent categorical variable (i.e., MMSE) and the independent categorical variables. The median values were chosen as the cutoff values. Multiple linear regression was applied to examine how the variability in MMSE could be explained by sarcopenic state and HTN. To be considered as an independent variable associated with HTN, the results were required to have a $P \leq 0.05$. All analyses were conducted using the IBM SPSS Statistics, version 20.0, software (IBM Corp., Armonk, NY, USA).

6. Results

Table 1 shows the characteristics of older women according to HTN. As expected, volunteers for both groups were elderly

>60 years old). BMI evaluation indicated that both groups showed an overweight phenotype. Regarding sarcopenia, groups demonstrated normal skeletal muscle indexes (i.e., Janssen and Baumgartner), as well as intermediate performance on SPPB [10]. However, walking speed values suggested a poor mobility in the hypertensive group (≤0.8 m/s), whereas normal results were found in the normotensive group (>0.8 m/s). Katz and Pfeffer's analyses indicated that volunteers for both groups showed an elevated level of independence to perform the ADL and IADL. Depressive symptoms were in an acceptable range of normality according to GDS. Lastly, suspected levels of dementia were found in the hypertensive group (<24 points) [30]. After application of Student's *t*-test, no significant differences were observed between normotensive and hypertensive older women regarding the anthropometric parameters and physical functional tests. However, the hypertensive group showed increased SBP, MAP, and DP, as well as reduced scores on the MMSE and salivary bioavailability of NO in comparison with normotensive volunteers.

Table 2 shows the dichotomized (i.e., *high* and *low*) results on MMSE according to the variables associated with sarcopenia. In line with the unadjusted analysis (i.e., Table 1), hypertensive patients showed lower results in MMSE, regardless of anthropometric characteristics, physical function tests, and sarcopenia. Moreover, analysis of *sarcopenic* domain indicated a possible association among hypertension, appendicular skeletal mass plus SPPB, and low scores in the MMSE.

The associations between the categorical variables using the chi-square test (χ^2) are shown in Table 3. Data demonstrated that hypertension plus low performance on SPPB (0.006), HTN (0.012), HTN plus low values on Janssen index (0.03), and HTN plus low performance on sit-to-stand (0.09) (tendency) were significantly associated with MMSE.

Table 4 shows the results from multiple linear regression to predict MMSE. Results indicate that MMSE variability was not explained by morphological (i.e., absolute muscle mass, appendicular skeletal muscle mass, Janssen index, and Baumgartner index) or functional (i.e., walking speed, SPPB, and sit-to-stand) parameters. On the other hand, variability in TUG was significantly explained by HTN (18%).

Table 3: Frequency (%) of the distribution of older women according to MMSE.

Variable	MMSE <24	MMSE ≥24	*P*
Hypertension			
Yes	24.4	29.7	0.012
No	8.1	37.8	
Hypertension plus low appendicular muscle mass			
Yes	19.2	30.8	0.650
No	11.5	38.5	
Hypertension plus low absolute muscle mass			
Yes	21.1	40.3	0.847
No	12.3	26.3	
Hypertension plus low sit-to-stand			
Yes	22.9	29.8	0.091
No	10.5	36.8	
Hypertension plus low walking speed			
Yes	20,4	44.4	0.991
No	11.1	24.1	
Hypertension plus low Janssen			
Yes	28.0	28.0	0.030
No	4.0	40.0	
Hypertension plus low Baumgartner			
Yes	13.2	23.5	0.363
No	16.2	47.1	
Hypertension plus low short physical performance battery			
Yes	24.6	26.3	0.006
No	7.0	42.1	

Data are shown as mean ± SD; MMSE = Mini-Mental State Examination.

7. Discussion

In the current study, hypertensive patients scored lower in the MMSE than normotensive patients. In addition, our findings indicate that sarcopenic state can interfere in this phenomenon, given that a higher frequency of hypertensive patients with reduced lower limb muscle function (i.e., SPPB and sit-to-stand (tendency)) and muscle mass index (i.e., Janssen index) was observed in the <24 MMSE segment when compared to hypertensive patients with normal results in these parameters.

Several experiments are in line with the findings of the present study and have demonstrated a negative association between HTN status and high blood pressure values with poor cognitive performance in older adults [4–7]. In the experiment of Obisesan [6], for example, the authors investigated the association between HTN status and cognitive performance using data from the Third National Health and Nutrition Examination Survey (NHANES III). As in the present study, results demonstrated that hypertensive patients showed a lower global cognitive score (i.e., MMSE) than normotensive patients. However, an increasing number of studies have extended these results and demonstrating that HTN is associated with a low functioning of numerous cognitive domains, such as executive function, praxis, learning, and memory [5, 7].

Unfortunately, we were unable to conduct cognitive-specific analysis to indicate what cognitive domains were associated with HTN and sarcopenia. It is noteworthy that MMSE is a global cognitive test, which does not contemplate the evaluation of some crucial cognitive domains to successful aging, such as executive function [8]. However, to the best of our knowledge, this is the first study aimed at investigating the association between HTN, sarcopenia, and cognitive performance, and future studies should be based on these seminal findings, along with the aforementioned data, and explore specific cognitive domains that demonstrate association with HTN (e.g., executive function).

In relation to sarcopenia, multiple linear regression results did not indicate a significant effect of sarcopenic parameters on MMSE variability. On the other hand, chi-square test showed that low lower limb muscle function (i.e., SPPB and sit-to-stand) and muscle mass index

Table 4: Results from multiple linear regression to predict MMSE.

Dependent variable	Predictor variable	Unstandardized beta	Standardized beta	P	sr^2
MMSE	Absolute muscle mass (kg)	0.045	0.078	0.729	0.02
	Appendicular skeletal muscle mass (kg)	−0.144	−0.133	0.577	−0.03
	Janssen index (kg/m^2)	0.065	0.146	0.322	0.05
	Baumgartner index (kg/m^2)	0.026	0.078	0.507	0.04
	Walking speed (m/s)	−0.317	−0.024	0.836	−0.01
	Short physical performance battery (points)	0.342	0.147	0.201	0.07
	Sit-to-stand (s)	0.008	0.043	0.703	0.02
	HTN	−2.255	−0.407	0.002	−0.18

MMSE = Mini-Mental State Examination; HTN = hypertension; sr^2 = square of semipartial correlation; $R = 0.528$, $R^2 = 0.279$; adjusted R^2.

(i.e., Janssen index) might interfere in the relation between HTN and cognitive function. These results are contradictory and should be interpreted with caution. Indeed, our sample is of limited size to perform a multiple linear regression analysis and our findings may be being underestimated, while a simple frequency of distribution of sarcopenic parameters, such as chi-square test, seems to be a better approach in this context.

Contrary to HTN, the association between sarcopenia and cognitive dysfunction has just recently begun to be demystified. In fact, only findings from 7 cross-sectional studies were analysed in a systematic review with meta-analytic regression, which demonstrated that the odds of poor global cognitive scores (i.e., MMSE) in sarcopenic patients were 2.6-fold higher than in non-sarcopenic patients [12]. In addition, longitudinal studies have demonstrated that sarcopenic patients showed an increased risk for the development of dementia in short-term follow-up periods (i.e., 1 year) [16, 31].

It is noteworthy that, in the study of Moon [31], low SPPB scores, but not low muscle mass, was associated with high risk of developing dementia. In the current study, volunteers with HTN and low performance on SPPB demonstrated a lower P value (0.0006) than those with HTN and low Janssen index (0.03) in the <24 MMSE segment, suggesting that lower limb muscle function might be more important than skeletal muscle mass in the context of HTN and cognitive function. Findings from Lee [32] support this hypothesis, given that low scores in physical tests were associated with cognitive impairment and atherosclerotic markers, while no significant associations were observed with low muscle mass.

Moreover, these findings indicate a possible biological process underlying the association between HTN, low lower limb muscle function, and poor cognition observed in the present study because atherosclerosis is one of the leading causes of dementia due to its strong association with vascular remodelling and stiffening [8, 33]. Interestingly, several studies performed by our group [11, 34] and other groups [14, 15, 35] have demonstrated that low muscle mass—combined or not with decreased muscle function—is associated with indirect measurements of arterial stiffness in older adults (e.g., pulse pressure), suggesting that the influence of the sarcopenic factors in the relationship between HTN and cognitive status is mediated by similar mechanisms. This hypothesis was recently confirmed in the elegant study performed by Kohara et al. [35] which observed that low muscle mass was strongly associated with poor cognitive scores and arterial stiffness.

In an attempt to understand whether these aforementioned mechanisms might be responsible for the results observed in the current study, we performed a new series of analyses (Supplementary Figure 1) evaluating PP levels and salivary NO bioavailability according to SPPB, sit-to-stand and SMI in the hypertensive volunteers. Our findings indicate that hypertensive patients with impaired performance in physical tests (i.e., SPPB and sit-to-stand) showed lower NO bioavailability than hypertensive patients with normal performance, but just sit-to-stand reached significant results ($P < 0.05$). On the other hand, P values were quite similar among the groups. Therefore, these findings indicate a possible mediation of NO in the results observed in the present study.

In fact, NO is an important vasoactive substance synthesized and released by the vascular endothelium affecting arterial morphology and functioning under physiological and physiopathological conditions [36–38]. However, its acute and chronic pharmacological (e.g., L-NAME, L-NMMA) or physiological inhibitions in humans and animals cause severe alterations in the vascular homeostasis, as, for example, reduction in the vascular cross-sectional area, compliance, as well as increase in pulse-wave velocity—a well-established marker of arterial stiffness [36–38]. Furthermore, numerous studies have argued a possible role of NO in the pathogenesis of dementia syndromes (e.g., Alzheimer's disease) through neurotoxicity and neuroprotective mechanisms [39].

Some limitations of the present study should be mentioned and addressed in future studies to a better understanding of the relation between HTN, sarcopenia, and cognitive function in community-dwelling older women, including our limited sample size and a number of cognitive evaluations, which avoid us to perform more robust statistical analysis, like logistic and multiple regressions. In addition, NO was the only possible mechanism investigated in the present study and several risk factors for the development of cognitive dysfunction are shared by HTN and sarcopenia, all of which may be responsible for the seminal results showed in the current study, such as inflammation, oxidative stress, and sedentary lifestyle.

Conflicts of Interest

The authors declare that there are no conflicts of interest regarding the publication of this paper.

Acknowledgments

This study was supported by Coordenação de Aperfeiçoamento de Pessoal de Nível Superior (CAPES) and Fundação de Amparo á Pesquisa do Estado de São Paulo (FAPESP) (2017/21320-4). Bruno Rodrigues received financial support from Conselho Nacional de Pesquisa e Desenvolvimento (CNPq-BPQ).

References

[1] U. Nations, *World Population Prospects, the 2017 Revision*, United Nations Publications, New York, NY, USA, 2017.

[2] D. Mozaffarian, E. J. Benjamin, A. S. Go et al., "Heart disease and stroke statistics—2016 update," *Circulation*, vol. 133, no. 4, pp. e38–e360, 2016.

[3] Organization, W.H., *Global Health Risks: Mortality and Burden of Disease Attributable to Selected Major Risks*, World Health Organization, Geneva, Switzerland, 2009.

[4] J. M. Starr, L. J. Whalley, S. Inch, and P. Ann Shering, "Blood pressure and cognitive function in healthy old people," *Journal of the American Geriatrics Society*, vol. 41, no. 7, pp. 753–756, 1993.

[5] H.-K. Kuo, F. Sorond, I. Iloputaife, M. Gagnon, W. Milberg, and L. A. Lipsitz, "Effect of blood pressure on cognitive functions in elderly persons," *Journals of Gerontology Series A: Biological Sciences and Medical Sciences*, vol. 59, no. 11, pp. 1191–1194, 2004.

[6] T. O. Obisesan, O. A. Obisesan, S. Martins et al., "High blood pressure, hypertension, and high pulse pressure are associated with poorer cognitive function in persons aged 60 and older: the Third National Health and Nutrition Examination Survey," *Journal of the American Geriatrics Society*, vol. 56, no. 3, pp. 501–509, 2008.

[7] J. M. D. Matoso, W. B. Santos, I. F. H. Moreira, R. A. Lourenço, and M. L. de Gusmão Correia, "Idosos hipertensos apresentam menor desempenho cognitivo do que idosos normotensos," *Arquivos Brasileiros de Cardiologia*, vol. 100, no. 5, pp. 444–451, 2013.

[8] C. Iadecola, K. Yaffe, J. Biller et al., "Impact of hypertension on cognitive function: a scientific statement from the American Heart Association," *Hypertension*, vol. 68, no. 6, pp. e67–e94, 2016.

[9] J. B. M. Diz, A. A. O. Leopoldino, B. S. Moreira et al., "Prevalence of sarcopenia in older Brazilians: a systematic review and meta-analysis," *Geriatrics and Gerontology international*, vol. 17, no. 1, pp. 5–16, 2017.

[10] A. J. Cruz-Jentoft, J. P. Baeyens, J. M. Bauer et al., "Sarcopenia: European consensus on definition and diagnosis Report of the European Working Group on Sarcopenia in Older People," *Age and ageing*, vol. 39, no. 4, pp. 412–423, 2010.

[11] H. J. Coelho Júnior, S. da Silva Aguiar, I. de Oliveira Gonçalves et al., "Sarcopenia is associated with high pulse pressure in older women," *Journal of Aging Research*, vol. 2015, Article ID 109824, 6 pages, 2015.

[12] K.-V. Chang, T.-H. Hsu, W.-T. Wu, K.-C. Huang, and D.-S. Han, "Association between sarcopenia and cognitive impairment: a systematic review and meta-analysis," *Journal of the American Medical Directors Association*, vol. 17, no. 12, pp. 1164.e7–1164.e15, 2016.

[13] K. Han, Y.-M. Park, H.-S. Kwon et al., "Sarcopenia as a determinant of blood pressure in older Koreans: findings from the Korea National Health and Nutrition Examination Surveys (KNHANES) 2008–2010," *PLoS One*, vol. 9, no. 1, Article ID e86902, 2014.

[14] A. M. Abbatecola, P. Chiodini, C. Gallo et al., "Pulse wave velocity is associated with muscle mass decline: health ABC study," *Age*, vol. 34, no. 2, pp. 469–478, 2012.

[15] M. Ochi, K. Kohara, Y. Tabara et al., "Arterial stiffness is associated with low thigh muscle mass in middle-aged to elderly men," *Atherosclerosis*, vol. 212, no. 1, pp. 327–332, 2010.

[16] S. Nishiguchi, M. Yamada, H. Shirooka et al., "Sarcopenia as a risk factor for cognitive deterioration in community-dwelling older adults: a 1-year prospective study," *Journal of the American Medical Directors Association*, vol. 17, no. 4, p. 372, 2016.

[17] B. D. H. Sociedade, S. B. D. Cardiologia, and S. B. D. Nefrologia, "VI Brazilian guidelines on hypertension," *Arquivos brasileiros de cardiologia*, vol. 95, no. 1, p. 1, 2010.

[18] H. J. Coelho Junior, B. Rodrigues, D. J. Feriani et al., "Effects of multicomponent exercise on functional and cognitive parameters of hypertensive patients: a Quasi-Experimental Study," *Journal of Aging Research*, vol. 2017, Article ID 1978670, 10 pages, 2017.

[19] A. N. Freire, R. O. Guerra, B. Alvarado, J. M. Guralnik, and M. V. Zunzunegui, "Validity and reliability of the short physical performance battery in two diverse older adult populations in Quebec and Brazil," *Journal of Aging and Health*, vol. 24, no. 5, pp. 863–878, 2012.

[20] J. M. Guralnik, L. Ferrucci, E. M. Simonsick, M. E. Salive, and R. B. Wallace, "Lower-extremity function in persons over the age of 70 years as a predictor of subsequent disability," *New England Journal of Medicine*, vol. 332, no. 9, pp. 556–562, 1995.

[21] J. M. Guralnik, E. M. Simonsick, L. Ferrucci et al., "A short physical performance battery assessing lower extremity function: association with self-reported disability and prediction of mortality and nursing home admission," *Journal of Gerontology*, vol. 49, no. 2, pp. M85–M94, 1994.

[22] A. V. Chobanian, G. L. Bakris, H. R. Black et al., "The seventh report of the joint national committee on prevention, detection, evaluation, and treatment of high blood pressure: the JNC 7 report," *JAMA*, vol. 289, no. 19, pp. 2560–2571, 2003.

[23] A. C. Cuckson, A. Reinders, H. Shabeeh, and A. H. Shennan, "Validation of the Microlife BP 3BTO-A oscillometric blood pressure monitoring device according to a modified British Hypertension Society protocol," *Blood Pressure Monitoring*, vol. 7, no. 6, pp. 319–324, 2002.

[24] H. J. Coelho-Júnior, M. Irigoyen, S. S. Aguiar et al., "Acute effects of power and resistance exercises on hemodynamic measurements of older women," *Clinical Interventions in Aging*, vol. 12, p. 1103, 2017.

[25] S. M. Brucki, R. Nitrini, P. Caramelli, P. H. F. Bertolucci, and I. H. Okamoto, "Sugestões para o uso do mini-exame do estado mental no Brasil," *Arquivos de Neuro-psiquiatria*, vol. 61, no. 3, pp. 777–781, 2003.

[26] O. P. Almeida and S. A. Almeida, "Short versions of the geriatric depression scale: a study of their validity for the diagnosis of a major depressive episode according to ICD-10 and DSM-IV," *International Journal of Geriatric Psychiatry*, vol. 14, no. 10, pp. 858–865, 1999.
[27] E. M. P. Paradela, R. A. Lourenço, and R. P. Veras, "Validação da escala de depressão geriátrica em um ambulatório geral," *Revista de saúde pública*, vol. 39, no. 6, pp. 918–923, 2005.
[28] R. E. D. L. Ferretti-Rebustini, M. A. A. Balbinotti, W. Jacob-Filho et al., "Validity of the Katz Index to assess activities of daily living by informants in neuropathological studies," *Revista da Escola de Enfermagem da USP*, vol. 49, no. 6, pp. 944–950, 2015.
[29] M. C. Dutra, R. D. S. Ribeiro, S. B. Pinheiro, G. F. de Melo, and G. A. Carvalho, "Accuracy and reliability of the Pfeffer Questionnaire for the Brazilian elderly population," *Dementia and Neuropsychologia*, vol. 9, no. 2, pp. 176–183, 2015.
[30] E. Herrera Jr., P. Caramelli, A. S. B. Silveira, and R. Nitrini, "Epidemiologic survey of dementia in a community-dwelling Brazilian population," *Alzheimer Disease and Associated Disorders*, vol. 16, no. 2, pp. 103–108, 2002.
[31] J. Moon, J. H. Moon, K. M. Kim et al., "Sarcopenia as a predictor of future cognitive impairment in older adults," *Journal of Nutrition, Health and Aging*, vol. 20, no. 5, p. 496, 2016.
[32] J. S. Lee, T.-W. Auyeung, J. Leung, T. Kwok, P.-C. Leung, and J. Woo, "Physical frailty in older adults is associated with metabolic and atherosclerotic risk factors and cognitive impairment independent of muscle mass," *Journal of Nutrition, Health and Aging*, vol. 15, no. 10, pp. 857–862, 2011.
[33] K. Ritz, N. P. Denswil, O. C. G. Stam, J. J. van Lieshout, and M. J. A. P. Daemen, "Cause and mechanisms of intracranial atherosclerosis," *Circulation*, vol. 130, no. 16, pp. 1407–1414, 2014.
[34] R. A. C. Sampaio, P. Y. S. Sampaio, M. Yamada et al., "Arterial stiffness is associated with low skeletal muscle mass in Japanese community-dwelling older adults," *Geriatrics and Gerontology International*, vol. 14, no. 1, pp. 109–114, 2014.
[35] K. Kohara, Y. Okada, M. Ochi et al., "Muscle mass decline, arterial stiffness, white matter hyperintensity, and cognitive impairment: Japan Shimanami Health Promoting Program study," *Journal of Cachexia, Sarcopenia and Muscle*, vol. 8, no. 4, pp. 557–566, 2017.
[36] R. M. Fitch, R. Vergona, M. E. Sullivan et al., "Nitric oxide synthase inhibition increases aortic stiffness measured by pulse wave velocity in rats," *Cardiovascular Research*, vol. 51, no. 2, pp. 351–358, 2001.
[37] S. Kinlay, M. A. Creager, M. Fukumoto et al., "Endothelium-derived nitric oxide regulates arterial elasticity in human arteries in vivo," *Hypertension*, vol. 38, no. 5, pp. 1049–1053, 2001.
[38] I. B. Wilkinson, S. S. Franklin, and J. R. Cockcroft, "Nitric oxide and the regulation of large artery stiffness," *Hypertension*, vol. 44, no. 2, pp. 112–116, 2004.
[39] A. Law, S. Gauthier, and R. Quirion, "Say NO to Alzheimer's disease: the putative links between nitric oxide and dementia of the Alzheimer's type," *Brain Research Reviews*, vol. 35, no. 1, pp. 73–96, 2001.

24

Muscle Strength, Physical Activity, and Functional Limitations in Older Adults with Central Obesity

Cassandra M. Germain,[1] John A. Batsis,[2] Elizabeth Vasquez,[3] and Douglas R. McQuoid[1]

[1]*Department of Psychiatry and Behavioral Sciences, Duke University Medical Center, P.O. Box 3119, Durham, NC 27710, USA*
[2]*Department of Medicine, Geisel School of Medicine at Dartmouth, Dartmouth-Hitchcock Medical Center, 1 Medical Center Drive, Lebanon, NH 03756, USA*
[3]*Department of Epidemiology and Biostatistics, School of Public Health, University at Albany (SUNY), One University Place, Albany, NY 12203, USA*

Correspondence should be addressed to Cassandra M. Germain; cassandra.germain@duke.edu

Academic Editor: F. R. Ferraro

Background. Obesity and muscle weakness are independently associated with increased risk of physical and functional impairment in older adults. It is unknown whether physical activity (PA) and muscle strength combined provide added protection against functional impairment. This study examines the association between muscle strength, PA, and functional outcomes in older adults with central obesity. *Methods.* Prevalence and odds of physical (PL), ADL, and IADL limitation were calculated for 6,388 community dwelling adults aged ≥ 60 with central obesity. Individuals were stratified by sex-specific hand grip tertiles and PA. Logistic models were adjusted for age, education, comorbidities, and body-mass index and weighted. *Results.* Overall prevalence of PL and ADL and IADL limitations were progressively lower by grip category. Within grip categories, prevalence was lower for individuals who were active than those who were inactive. Adjusted models showed significantly lower odds of PL OR 0.42 [0.31, 0.56]; ADL OR 0.60 [0.43, 0.84], and IADL OR 0.46 [0.35, 0.61] for those in the highest grip strength category as compared to those in the lowest grip category. *Conclusion.* Improving grip strength in obese elders who are not able to engage in traditional exercise is important for reducing odds of physical and functional impairment.

1. Introduction

Among those aged 60 and older, the combined prevalence of overweight and obesity, as assessed by body mass index (BMI), is estimated at over 70% [1]. The prevalence of central obesity is also rising among older adults in the US [2, 3] and is independently associated with functional impairment and disability [4, 5]. Central obesity is also associated with muscle weakness [6, 7], a known independent risk factor for physical disability [8] and mortality in older adults [9]. Thus, adults who carry excess weight *and* exhibit muscle weakness have a synergistic increased risk of functional impairment and subsequent disability than those who exhibit either symptom alone [10, 11].

Physical activity (PA) is associated with decreased risk of disability, delayed onset of functional impairment [12, 13], and recovery of function in older adults [14]. Physical activity is also associated with performance on key measures of physical performance including grip strength [15, 16]. Our group has previously demonstrated that PA moderates the risk of physical and functional limitations in normal weight and obese older adults [4, 17, 18]. Although previous work has demonstrated the association between grip strength and disability in middle and older adults [19, 20], whether higher levels of PA coupled with greater grip strength provides added benefits against physical and functional limitations in older adults who are obese is unknown. The current study extends our previous work to investigate the independent and combined effects of grip strength and physical activity on physical and functional outcomes in older adults with central adiposity. We examined (a) prevalence of physical and functional limitations by grip strength, (b) whether having higher grip strength was associated with reduced odds of physical and functional limitations, and (c) whether grip strength combined with PA is associated with additional reductions in physical and functional limitations. Given the compounded risk of disability among obese elders who also exhibit muscle weakness, it is important to identify ways of improving physical and functional outcomes within this particularly vulnerable group.

2. Methods

2.1. Data Source. This current study is a secondary analysis of existing data obtained from the 2006 and 2008 waves of the enhanced face-to-face interview of the Health and Retirement Study (HRS). HRS is a nationally representative panel survey of community dwelling adults aged 50 and older conducted by the University of Michigan and supported by the National Institute on Aging. The initial HRS sample was drawn in 1992 from a multistage, clustered area probability design of households, which targeted individuals born between 1931 and 1941. Follow-up interviews and new cohort additions have occurred at regular intervals and have resulted in a nationally representative sample of American adults over the age of 50. A random one-half of the larger HRS sample was preselected to complete an enhanced face-to-face interview in 2006, which included physical and biomarker measurements. The second half of the HRS sample received the enhanced face-to-face interview in 2008. Inclusion of both 2006 and 2008 waves ensures that all HRS respondents who were eligible for and consented to the enhanced face-to-face interviews are included in the analyses. Additional descriptions of sampling procedures and study design are available online at http://hrsonline.isr.umich.edu/.

2.2. Sample. A total of 6,555 community dwelling adults aged 60 years and older with clinically elevated waist circumference (WC ≥ 88 cm for women; WC ≥ 102 cm for men) [21, 22] and handgrip strength measurements were included in the sample. After eliminating respondents missing handgrip (n = 163) physical activity (n = 4), a total of 6,388 (2,364 men; 4,024 women) remained for analyses. Respondents of all races/ethnicities were included in the sample. Characteristics of those missing grip strength are provided in the Appendix. The study was exempted from Institutional Review Board review at all respective institutions due to the deidentified nature of the data used.

2.3. Measures

2.3.1. Muscle/Grip Strength. Participants' handgrip strength was measured using Smedley spring-type hand dynamometer (TTM®, Tokyo, Japan) in a standing position with their arm at their side at a 90-degree angle. Two measurements were taken with each hand (dominant and nondominant) and averaged across trials [23]. The highest averaged score from either hand was used as primary predictor in the current analyses. Sex-specific tertiles were determined using univariate analyses. Participants were then classified into three categories by sex-specific grip tertiles: low grip (LG), mid grip (MG), and high grp (HG).

2.3.2. Physical Activity. Physical activity (PA) was assessed using a self-report physical health questionnaire as part of the HRS interview. Respondents were asked *"How often do you take part in sports or activities that are vigorous, such as running or jogging, swimming, cycling, aerobics or gym, workout, tennis, or digging with a spade or shovel: more than once a week, once a week, one to three times a month, or hardly ever or never?"* and *"And how often do you take part in sports or activities that are moderately energetic such as, gardening, cleaning the car, walking at a moderate pace, dancing, floor or stretching exercises...?"* Frequency of engagement in HRS was reported as follows: more than once a week, once a week, one to three times a month, or hardly ever or never. Respondents reporting that they engaged in moderate or vigorous PA at least once per week were classified as active; those reporting activity less than once per week were classified as inactive (ref = 0).

2.3.3. Physical Limitations (PL). Physical limitations (PL) in HRS were assessed using a self-reported questionnaire. Respondents were asked to report whether they had difficulties *or* were unable to (yes/no) perform the following tasks because of a health or physical problem: walking several blocks, walking 1 block, sitting 2 hours, getting up from chair, climbing one flight of stairs, stooping, reaching arms, pulling/pushing large objects, lifting weights, and picking up a dime. All *yes* responses were compiled into a summary score in the HRS database ranging from 0 to 10. Univariate analyses revealed that 67% of our sample reported at least 1 limitation. For purposes of these analyses, respondents reporting difficulty or inability with performing two or more of the above tasks were classified as having physical limitations (0 = no limitations, 1 = limitation).

2.3.4. Functional Limitations. Activities of daily living (ADLs) and instrumental activities of daily living (IADLs) were used to assess functional limitations [24]. Respondents were classified as having ADL limitations if they reported difficulty *or* inability with one or more of the following: dressing, eating, or getting out of bed. Respondents were classified as having IADL limitations if they reported difficulty or inability with at least one of the following IADLs: preparing meals, managing money, or needing help with house/yard work. All limitations reported in this paper were measured in HRS using self-report. Respondents were instructed to exclude any difficulties that were expected to last less than three months.

3. Analyses

Overall prevalence and odds of physical, ADL, and IADL limitations was examined by grip strength category. Prevalence and odds of limitations were also examined within each grip category by activity level. Multivariate logistic

TABLE 1: Sample characteristics.

N	6,388
	M (SD)
Age, years	71.4 (7.48)
Education, years	12.2 (3.13)
Comorbidities	2.2 (1.21)
Waist circumference (cm)	108.0 (12.50)
Handgrip strength	28.6 (10.43)
Body mass index (kg/m)[a]	29.9 (5.14)
Sex, N (%)	
Female	4,024 (63.0)
Race, N (%)[b]	
White	5,325 (83.4)
Black	866 (13.6)
Other	1,96 (3.1)
Current smoker, N (%)	636 (10.0)
Physically active, N (%)	3,493 (54.7)
Handgrip tertile[b] N (%)	
Low	1,473 (23.1)
Mid	3,149 (49.3)
High	1,766 (27.7)
Physical limitations (PL)	3,803 (59.5)
Activities of daily living (ADL)	1,217 (28.2)
Instrumental activities of daily living (IADL)	2,404 (38.5)

[a]N = 6,279 with BMI measurements.
[b]Low grip ≤ 31.25 men, ≤ 18.5 women; high grip ≥ 43.5 men, ≥ 26.5 women.

were run using PROC SURVEYLOGISTIC (SAS Institute Cary, NC). Models were adjusted for age (at time of physical assessment), years of education, ethnicity (white, black, and other), sex, smoking status (yes, no), body mass index (bmi) kg/m^2, and number of medical comorbidities and weighted using the HRS respondent-level weights for physical measures, which includes adjustments for sample selection probability and nonresponse. Detailed documentation regarding HRS sample weight calculations is available at http://hrsonline.isr.umich.edu/sitedocs/wghtdoc.pdf. All data was examined using statistical tests that were two-sided with p values less than or equal to 0.05. Confidence intervals excluding 1.0 were considered statistically significant.

4. Results

Sample characteristics are presented in Table 1. The sample was predominantly white (83.4%) and female (63%). Overall prevalence of PL, ADL, and IADL limitations were 3,803 (59.5%), 1217 (28.2%), and 2404 (38.5%), respectively. Prevalence of PL, ADL, and IADL limitations was the highest in the lowest grip strength category, followed by MG, and was the lowest in the HG category. Prevalence of PL, ADL, and IADL limitations was also lower for those reporting engagement in physical activity within each grip category (Table 2).

Table 3 presents adjusted odds of PL, ADL, and IADL limitations by overall grip strength category and by activity level within each grip category. Overall odds of PL, ADL, and IADL limitation were significantly lower for those in MG category and the lowest in the HG category as compared to those in the LG grip category. In addition to increasing age, being female OR 2.00 [1.66, 2.42], $p \leq .001$, BMI 1.08 [1.06–1.11], $p \leq .001$, number of comorbidities 1.71 [1.57–1.85], $p < .001$, and being a current smoker 1.80 [1.30–2.48], $p \leq .01$, were independently associated with higher odds of PL. These risk factors were also associated with increased odds of IADL limitations: OR 1.80 [1.49–2.19], $p < .001$ for female status, OR 1.04 [1.02–1.06], $p \leq .001$ for BMI, OR 1.72 [1.58–1.87], $p < .001$ number of comorbidities, and OR 1.95 [1.42–2.67], $p \leq .001$, for current smokers. For ADL limitations, race OR 1.39 [1.08, 1.78], $p < .01$, higher BMI OR 1.04 [1.02, 1.07], $p < .01$, and comorbidities OR 1.38 [1.26, 1.52], $p \leq .001$, were associated with higher odds of limitation. Within grip categories, participating in physical activity did not appear to confer added benefits to reducing odds of disability or functional limitations.

5. Discussion

The current study examined the association between varying degrees of muscle strength, and odds of physical and functional limitations in older adults with central obesity who are physically active and inactive. We were primarily interested in (a) examining the prevalence of limitations by grip strength, (b) determining whether having higher grip strength was associated with reduced odds of physical and functional limitations, and (c) whether grip strength combined with PA is associated with additional reductions in physical and functional limitations. We found higher grip strength to be associated with lower prevalence of physical, ADL, and IADL limitations in elders with central obesity and increasing grip strength category to be significantly associated with progressively lower odds of physical, ADL, and IADL limitations after controlling for age, race, education, sex, BMI, medical comorbidities, and smoking status. This suggests that muscle strength is an important factor in preserving physical and functional impairment among those with central obesity independent of other known risk factors. Within grip categories, participating in physical activity was not associated with additional protection against odds of physical or functional limitations. In line with previous reports on risk factors for functional decline [25], we also found strong, independent associations between comorbidity and functional outcomes. These findings corroborate the need for targeted treatment and early intervention of chronic diseases among older adults, particularly the obese. Our findings extend the literature in that it provides supportive evidence to suggest that interventions aimed at improving muscle quality are beneficial even among obese elders with multiple health conditions.

Primary strengths of the current study include analyses of data from a nationally representative community dwelling sample of older adults with objective measures of grip strength and central adiposity (primary predictors). Limitations of the current analyses lie in the potential bias of self-reporting of physical outcomes and physical activity.

TABLE 2: Prevalence of physical, ADL and IADL limitations by grip tertiles and physical activity.

	Low grip			Mid grip			High grip		
	Overall	Low PA	High PA	Overall	Low PA	High PA	Overall	Low PA	High PA
Physical	1126 (76.4)	698 (84.8)	428 (65.9)	1839 (58.4)	1002 (70.9)	837 (48.2)	838 (47.5)	395 (59.9)	443 (40.0)
ADL	438 (37.4)	321 (45.6)	117 (25.1)	547 (25.6)	337 (30.7)	210 (20.1)	232 (23.0)	132 (28.2)	100 (18.5)
IADL	826 (57.6)	556 (69.3)	270 (42.8)	1141 (37.1)	689 (49.6)	452 (26.7)	437 (25.2)	237 (36.1)	200 (18.6)

Note. Low grip ≤ 31.25 men, ≤ 18.5 women; high grip ≥ 43.5 men, ≥ 26.5 women. ADL limitations difficulty or inability with ≥1 dressing, eating, or getting out of bed. IADL ≥1 preparing meals, managing money, house/yard work.

TABLE 3: Odds of physical and ADL limitations by grip tertile and activity level.

	N	Mid grip[ab]			High grip[ab]		
		Overall	Low activity	High activity	Overall	Low activity	High activity
Physical	6,388	0.54 (0.42, 0.69)	0.62 (0.42, 0.92)	0.54 (0.39, 0.75)	0.42 (0.31, 0.56)	0.40 (0.25, 0.63)	0.48 (0.33, 0.70)
ADL	4,320	0.58 (0.45, 0.76)	0.45 (0.32, 0.64)	0.91 (0.61, 1.37)	0.60 (0.43, 0.84)	0.50 (0.32, 0.79)	0.87 (0.53, 1.46)
IADL	6,248	0.59 (0.47, 0.75)	0.58 (0.41, 0.81)	0.69 (0.49, 0.97)	0.46 (0.34, 0.61)	0.40 (0.26, 0.61)	0.61 (0.40, 0.92)

Referent: low grip. ADL: activities of daily living, IADL: instrumental activities of daily living.
[a]Models are weighted and adjusted for age, sex, education, race, number of comorbidities, current smoking status, and body mass index.
[b]Observations with zero or negative weights do not contribute to estimates and were automatically eliminated from the analyses ($n = 3{,}028$).

In addition, the cross-sectional nature of the data limits our ability to make causal inferences regarding the association between muscle strength, physical activity, and functional outcomes in elders with central adiposity. We also cannot speak to the long-term impact of muscle strength on physical and functional outcomes in obese older adults. Additional research is needed to determine whether muscle strength and physical activity are protective against long-term functional decline in older adults with central obesity in the presence of other chronic health conditions.

6. Conclusion

Our results provide evidence that muscle strength is important for reducing odds of physical and functional limitations in obese elders. Among obese elders who are unable to engage in traditional aerobic activity, interventions that focus on preserving muscle strength are a viable means of reducing physical and functional limitations.

Appendix

See Table 4.

TABLE 4: Sample characteristics of missing grip.

N	163
Age, years	72.2 (7.80)
Education, years	11.22 (3.36)
Comorbidities	2.72 (1.23)
Waist circumference (cm)	108.0 (14.19)
Body mass index (kg/m)	29.9 (5.01)
Sex, *N* (%)	
Female	142 (89.0)
Race, *N* (%)	
White	115 (70.55)
Black	36 (22.09)
Other	12 (7.36)
Current smoker, *N* (%)	20 (12.27)
Physically active, *N* (%)	56 (34.366)

Conflict of Interests

Cassandra M. Germain, Ph.D. is supported in part by NHLBI IRS Diversity Supplement no. 3R01HL109219-02S1. Elizabeth Vasquez, Ph.D., has no financial disclosures. John A. Batsis, M.D., is partially supported by UB4HP19206-01-00 as a Medical Educator from the Health Resources and Services Administration, the Dartmouth Centers for Health and Aging, and has received support from the Department of Medicine, Dartmouth-Hitchcock Medical Center. He has served as a consultant to the legal firm Dinse, Knapp, McAndrew LLC, for a clinical case review in 2012. There is no other conflict of interests to report.

Authors' Contribution

Cassandra M. Germain, Ph.D., contributed to conceptualization, data analyses, and writing. John A. Batsis, M.D., contributed to conceptualization and writing. Elizabeth Vasquez, Ph.D., contributed to conceptualization and data analysis. Douglas R. McQuoid contributed to the analysis and final review of the paper.

Acknowledgments

The authors would like to acknowledge Rebecca Namenek Brouwer, from Duke University, Office of Clinical Research, for careful review and editing of earlier versions of this paper.

References

[1] Y. Wang and M. A. Beydoun, "The obesity epidemic in the United States—gender, age, socioeconomic, racial/ethnic, and geographic characteristics: a systematic review and meta-regression analysis," *Epidemiologic Reviews*, vol. 29, no. 1, pp. 6–28, 2007.

[2] S. B. Angleman, T. B. Harris, and D. Melzer, "The role of waist circumference in predicting disability in periretirement age adults," *International Journal of Obesity*, vol. 30, no. 2, pp. 364–373, 2006.

[3] L. Chaoyang, E. S. Ford, L. C. McGuire, and A. H. Mokdad, "Increasing trends in waist circumference and abdominal obesity among US adults," *Obesity*, vol. 15, no. 1, pp. 216–224, 2007.

[4] J. A. Batsis, C. M. Germain, E. Vásquez, F. Lopez-Jimenez, and S. J. Bartels, "Waist circumference, physical activity, and functional impairments in older U.S. adults: results from the NHANES 2005–2010," *Journal of Aging and Physical Activity*, vol. 23, no. 3, pp. 369–376, 2015.

[5] J. A. Batsis, A. J. Zbehlik, L. K. Barre, T. A. Mackenzie, and S. J. Bartels, "The impact of waist circumference on function and physical activity in older adults: longitudinal observational data from the osteoarthritis initiative," *Nutrition Journal*, vol. 13, no. 1, article 81, 2014.

[6] L. A. Schaap, A. Koster, and M. Visser, "Adiposity, muscle mass, and muscle strength in relation to functional decline in older persons," *Epidemiologic Reviews*, vol. 35, no. 1, pp. 51–65, 2013.

[7] V. L. Keevil, R. Luben, N. Dalzell et al., "Cross-sectional associations between different measures of obesity and muscle strength in men and women in a British cohort study," *The Journal of Nutrition, Health & Aging*, vol. 19, no. 1, pp. 3–11, 2015.

[8] N. N. Hairi, R. G. Cumming, V. Naganathan et al., "Loss of muscle strength, mass (sarcopenia), and quality (specific force) and its relationship with functional limitation and physical disability: the concord health and ageing in men project," *Journal of the American Geriatrics Society*, vol. 58, no. 11, pp. 2055–2062, 2010.

[9] C. R. Gale, C. N. Martyn, C. Cooper, and A. A. Sayer, "Grip strength, body composition, and mortality," *International Journal of Epidemiology*, vol. 36, no. 1, pp. 228–235, 2007.

[10] S. Stenholm, D. Alley, S. Bandinelli et al., "The effect of obesity combined with low muscle strength on decline in mobility in older persons: results from the InCHIANTI Study," *International Journal of Obesity*, vol. 33, no. 6, pp. 635–644, 2009.

[11] M. E. Bowen, "The relationship between body weight, frailty, and the disablement process," *The Journals of Gerontology, Series B: Psychological Sciences and Social Sciences*, vol. 67, no. 5, pp. 618–626, 2012.

[12] M. E. Miller, W. J. Rejeski, B. A. Reboussin, T. R. Have, and W. H. Ettinger, "Physical activity, functional limitations, and disability in older adults," *Journal of the American Geriatrics Society*, vol. 48, no. 10, pp. 1264–1272, 2000.

[13] D. H. Paterson and D. E. R. Warburton, "Physical activity and functional limitations in older adults: a systematic review related to Canada's Physical Activity Guidelines," *International Journal of Behavioral Nutrition and Physical Activity*, vol. 7, article 38, 2010.

[14] E. H. Ip, T. Church, S. A. Marshall et al., "Physical activity increases gains in and prevents loss of physical function: results from the lifestyle interventions and independence for elders pilot study," *Journals of Gerontology, Series A: Biological Sciences and Medical Sciences*, vol. 68, no. 4, pp. 426–432, 2013.

[15] T. Rantanen, J. M. Guralnik, R. Sakari-Rantala et al., "Disability, physical activity, and muscle strength in older women: the women's health and aging study," *Archives of Physical Medicine and Rehabilitation*, vol. 80, no. 2, pp. 130–135, 1999.

[16] D. Kuh, E. J. Bassey, S. Butterworth, R. Hardy, and M. E. J. Wadsworth, "Grip strength, postural control, and functional leg power in a representative cohort of British men and women: associations with physical activity, health status, and socioeconomic conditions," *Journals of Gerontology Series A: Biological Sciences and Medical Sciences*, vol. 60, no. 2, pp. 224–231, 2005.

[17] E. Vásquez, J. A. Batsis, C. M. Germain, and B. A. Shaw, "Impact of obesity and physical activity on functional outcomes in the elderly: data from NHANES 2005–2010," *Journal of Aging and Health*, vol. 26, no. 6, pp. 1032–1046, 2014.

[18] C. M. Germain, E. Vasquez, and J. A. Batsis, "Physical activity, central adiposity, and functional imitations in community-dwelling older adults," *Journal of Geriatric Physical Therapy*, In press.

[19] T. Rantanen, J. M. Guralnik, D. Foley et al., "Midlife hand grip strength as a predictor of old age disability," *The Journal of the American Medical Association*, vol. 281, no. 6, pp. 558–560, 1999.

[20] R. W. Bohannon, "Hand-grip dynamometry predicts future outcomes in aging adults," *Journal of Geriatric Physical Therapy*, vol. 31, no. 1, pp. 3–10, 2008.

[21] US Department of Health and Human Services: The Practical Guide to the Identification, Evaluation, and Treatment of Overweight and Obesity in Adult Bethesda: NIH–National Heart, Lung, and Blood Institute, 2000.

[22] M.-C. Pouliot, J.-P. Després, S. Lemieux et al., "Waist circumference and abdominal sagittal diameter: best simple anthropometric indexes of abdominal visceral adipose tissue accumulation and related cardiovascular risk in men and women," *The American Journal of Cardiology*, vol. 73, no. 7, pp. 460–468, 1994.

[23] A. M. Yorke, A. B. Curtis, M. Shoemaker, and E. Vangsnes, "Grip strength values stratified by age, gender, and chronic disease status in adults aged 50 years and older," *Journal of Geriatric Physical Therapy*, vol. 38, no. 3, pp. 115–121, 2015.

[24] D. Saliba, M. Orlando, N. S. Wenger, R. D. Hays, and L. Z. Rubenstein, "Identifying a short functional disability screen for older persons," *The Journals of Gerontology, Series A: Biological Sciences and Medical Sciences*, vol. 55, no. 12, pp. M750–M756, 2000.

[25] S. Stenholm, H. Westerlund, J. Head et al., "Comorbidity and functional trajectories from midlife to old age: the health and retirement study," *The Journals of Gerontology A: Biological Sciences and Medical Sciences*, vol. 70, no. 3, pp. 332–338, 2015.

Permissions

All chapters in this book were first published in JAR, by Hindawi Publishing Corporation; hereby published with permission under the Creative Commons Attribution License or equivalent. Every chapter published in this book has been scrutinized by our experts. Their significance has been extensively debated. The topics covered herein carry significant findings which will fuel the growth of the discipline. They may even be implemented as practical applications or may be referred to as a beginning point for another development.

The contributors of this book come from diverse backgrounds, making this book a truly international effort. This book will bring forth new frontiers with its revolutionizing research information and detailed analysis of the nascent developments around the world.

We would like to thank all the contributing authors for lending their expertise to make the book truly unique. They have played a crucial role in the development of this book. Without their invaluable contributions this book wouldn't have been possible. They have made vital efforts to compile up to date information on the varied aspects of this subject to make this book a valuable addition to the collection of many professionals and students.

This book was conceptualized with the vision of imparting up-to-date information and advanced data in this field. To ensure the same, a matchless editorial board was set up. Every individual on the board went through rigorous rounds of assessment to prove their worth. After which they invested a large part of their time researching and compiling the most relevant data for our readers.

The editorial board has been involved in producing this book since its inception. They have spent rigorous hours researching and exploring the diverse topics which have resulted in the successful publishing of this book. They have passed on their knowledge of decades through this book. To expedite this challenging task, the publisher supported the team at every step. A small team of assistant editors was also appointed to further simplify the editing procedure and attain best results for the readers.

Apart from the editorial board, the designing team has also invested a significant amount of their time in understanding the subject and creating the most relevant covers. They scrutinized every image to scout for the most suitable representation of the subject and create an appropriate cover for the book.

The publishing team has been an ardent support to the editorial, designing and production team. Their endless efforts to recruit the best for this project, has resulted in the accomplishment of this book. They are a veteran in the field of academics and their pool of knowledge is as vast as their experience in printing. Their expertise and guidance has proved useful at every step. Their uncompromising quality standards have made this book an exceptional effort. Their encouragement from time to time has been an inspiration for everyone.

The publisher and the editorial board hope that this book will prove to be a valuable piece of knowledge for researchers, students, practitioners and scholars across the globe.

List of Contributors

Amira Abou-Dest, Cédric T. Albinet, Geoffroy Boucard and Michel Audiffren
UMR CNRS 7295, University of Poitiers, Sport Sciences Faculty, Bat. A5, 5 rue Théodore Lefebvre, 86000 Poitiers, France

Hélio José Coelho Junior, Bruno Rodrigues, Daniele Jardim Feriani and Marco Carlos Uchida
School of Physical Education, University of Campinas, Campinas, SP, Brazil

Ivan de Oliveira Gonçalves
Center of Health Sciences, University of Mogi das Cruzes, Mogi das Cruzes, SP, Brazil

Ricardo Yukio Asano
School of Arts, Sciences and Humanities, University of São Paulo, São Paulo, SP, Brazil

Samuel da Silva Aguiar
Brazil School of Physical Education, Catholic University of Brasília, Brasília, DF, Brazil

Camila Bosquiero Papini, Priscila Missaki Nakamura, Amèrico Valdanha Netto, Lilian Teresa Bucken Gobbi and Eduardo Kokubun
Department of Physical Education, Universidade Estadual Paulista (UNESP), Avenida 24-A, 1515 Bela Vista, 13506-900 Rio Claro, SP, Brazil

Sebastião Gobbi
Department of Physical Education, Universidade Estadual Paulista (UNESP), Avenida 24-A, 1515 Bela Vista, 13506-900 Rio Claro, SP, Brazil
Department of Kinesiology and Community Health, University of Illinois at Urbana-Champaign, 906 South Goodwin Avenue, Urbana, IL 61801, USA

Emerson Sebastião
Department of Kinesiology and Community Health, University of Illinois at Urbana-Champaign, 906 South Goodwin Avenue, Urbana, IL 61801, USA

Prem S. Fry
Graduate Psychology Program, Trinity Western University, 7600 Glover Road, Langley, BC, Canada V2Y 1Y1

Dominique L. Debats
9711 RS 2E4 Groningen, The Netherlands

Timothy D. Verstynen
Department of Psychology, Carnegie Mellon University, Pittsburgh, PA 15213, USA
Center for the Neural Basis of Cognition, Carnegie Mellon University, Pittsburgh, PA 15213, USA

Brighid Lynch and Destiny L. Miller
Department of Psychology, University of Pittsburgh, 3107 Sennott Square, 210 South Bouquet Street, Pittsburgh, PA 15260, USA

Michelle W. Voss
Department of Psychology, University of Iowa, Iowa city, IA 52242, USA

Ruchika Shaurya Prakash
Department of Psychology, The Ohio State University City, Columbus, OH 43210, USA

Laura Chaddock
Department of Psychology, University of Illinois, Champaign-Urbana at Champaign, IL 61820, USA
Beckman Institute for Advanced Science and Technology, University of Illinois at Champaign-Urbana, Champaign, IL, USA

Chandramallika Basak
Department of Psychology, The University of Texas at Dallas, Dallas, TX 75080, USA

Amanda Szabo, Erin A. Olson, Thomas R. Wojcicki, Jason Fanning and Neha P. Gothe
Department of Kinesiology and Community Health, University of Illinois, Champaign-Urbana at Champaign, IL 61820, USA

Weihua Zhang
Nell Hodgson Woodruff School of Nursing Emory University, 1520 Clifton Road, Atlanta, GA 30322-4207, USA

Annlia Paganini-Hill
Department of Neurology, School of Medicine, University of California, Irvine, California, USA

Claudia H. Kawas
Department of Neurology, School of Medicine, University of California, Irvine, California, USA
Department of Neurobiology & Behavior, School of Biological Sciences, University of California, Irvine, California, USA
Institute for Memory Impairments and Neurological Disorders, University of California, Irvine, California, USA

María M. Corrada
Department of Neurology, School of Medicine, University of California, Irvine, California, USA
Institute for Memory Impairments and Neurological Disorders, University of California, Irvine, California, USA
Department of Epidemiology, School of Medicine, University of California, Irvine, California, USA

Kristy L. Smith, Kelly Carr, Alexandra Wiseman, Kelly Calhoun, Nancy H. McNevin and Patricia L. Weir
Department of Kinesiology, University of Windsor, Windsor, ON, Canada N9B 3P4

Michael A. Trujillo, Paul B. Perrin, Aaliah Elnasseh, Bradford S. Pierce and Melody Mickens
Virginia Commonwealth University, Richmond, VA, USA

Olga Theou
Geriatric Medicine, Dalhousie University, 5955 Veterans' Memorial Lane, Halifax, NS, Canada B3H 2E1

Darl Edwards
Medicine, University of Toronto, Toronto, ON, Canada M5S 1A8

Gareth R. Jones and Jennifer M. Jakobi
Health and Exercise Sciences, University of British Columbia Okanagan, 3333 University Way, Kelowna, BC, Canada V1V 1V7

Scott D. Wright
Gerontology Interdisciplinary Program, University of Utah, Salt Lake City, UT 84112-5880, USA

Amy Maida Wadsworth
Family and Consumer Studies Department, University of Utah, Salt Lake City, UT 84112, USA

Liza Stathokostas, Robert M. D. Little and Donald H. Paterson
Canadian Centre for Activity and Aging, Faculty of Health Sciences, 3M Centre 2225,The University of Western Ontario, London, ON, Canada N6A 3K7
School of Kinesiology, Faculty of Health Sciences, 3M Centre 2225,The University of Western Ontario, London, ON, Canada N6A 3K7

Matthew W. McDonald
School of Kinesiology, Faculty of Health Sciences, 3M Centre 2225,The University of Western Ontario, London, ON, Canada N6A 3K7

Elizabeth J. Johnson, Rohini Vishwanathan, Tammy M. Scott, Robert C. Green, Leonard W. Poon and Mary Ann Johnson
Jean Mayer US Department of Agriculture Human Nutrition Research Center on Aging at Tufts University, Boston, MA 02111, USA

Dorothy B. Hausman
University of Georgia-Athens, Athens, GA 30602, USA

Adam Davey
Temple University, Philadelphia, PA 19122, USA

L. Stephen Miller
Harvard University, Boston, MA 02115, USA

Marla Gearing
Emory University, Atlanta, GA 30322, USA

John Woodard
Wayne State University, Detroit, MI 48202, USA

Peter T. Nelson
University of Kentucky, Lexington, KY 40536, USA

Hae-Yun Chung
Yonsei University, Seoul 120-749, Republic of Korea

Wolfgang Schalch and Jonas Wittwer
DSM Nutritional Products, CH-4002 Basel, Switzerland

Louis Bherer
PERFORM Centre, Concordia University, Montreal, QC, Canada
Research Center, Institut Universitaire de Gériatrie de Montréal, Montreal, QC, Canada

Kirk I. Erickson,
Department of Psychology, University of Pittsburgh, Pittsburgh, PA, USA

Teresa Liu-Ambrose
Department of Physical Therapy, University of British Columbia, Vancouver, BC, Canada
Brain Research Centre, University of British Columbia, Vancouver Coastal Health Research Institute, Vancouver, BC, Canada

O. G. Geirsdottir and A. Ramel
The Icelandic Gerontological Research Center, Reykjavik, Iceland
Faculty of Food Science and Nutrition, University of Iceland, Reykjavik, Iceland

M. Chang
The Icelandic Gerontological Research Center, Reykjavik, Iceland
Department of Sport Science, School of Science and Engineering, Reykjavik University, Reykjavik, Iceland

K. Briem
The Icelandic Gerontological Research Center, Reykjavik, Iceland
Department of Physiotherapy, University of Iceland, Reykjavik, Iceland

P. V. Jonsson
The Icelandic Gerontological Research Center, Reykjavik, Iceland
Department of Geriatrics, National University Hospital of Iceland, Reykjavik, Iceland

I. Thorsdottir
School of Health Sciences, University of Iceland, Reykjavik, Iceland

Nathalie André and Michel Audiffren
Centre de Recherches sur la Cognition et l'Apprentissage, UMR CNRS 7295, Universitéde Poitiers, Poitiers, France
Maison des Sciences de l'Homme et de la Société, USR CNRS 3565, Université de Poitiers, Poitiers, France

Claude Ferrand
EA 2114, Psychologie desges de la vie, Université François Rabelais, Tours, France

Cédric Albinet
Centre de Recherches sur la Cognition et l'Apprentissage, UMR CNRS 7295, Universitéde Poitiers, Poitiers, France
Laboratoire Sciences de la Cognition, Technologie, Ergonomie (SCoTE), Université de Toulouse, INU Champollion, Albi, France

Titaporn Worapanwisit and Somkid Prabpai
Health Promotion and Health Education, Faculty of Education, Kasetsart University, Bangkok 10903, Thailand

Ed Rosenberg
Department of Sociology, Appalachian State University, Boone, NC 28608, USA

Duke Appiah
Department of Public Health, Texas Tech University Health Sciences Center, 3601 4th Street, STOP 9403, Lubbock, TX 79430, USA

Richard N. Baumgartner
Department of Epidemiology and Population Health, School of Public Health and Information Sciences, University of Louisville, 485 E. Gray St., Louisville, KY 40202, USA

Cassandra M. Germain and Douglas R. McQuoid
Department of Psychiatry and Behavioral Sciences, Duke University Medical Center, Durham, NC 27710, USA

John A. Batsis
Department of Medicine, Geisel School of Medicine at Dartmouth, Dartmouth-Hitchcock Medical Center, 1 Medical Center Drive, Lebanon, NH 03756, USA

Elizabeth Vasquez
Department of Epidemiology and Biostatistics, School of Public Health, University at Albany (SUNY), One University Place, Albany, NY 12203, USA

Index

www.ingramcontent.com/pod-product-compliance
Lightning Source LLC
LaVergne TN
LVHW060531210926
848485LV00005B/1183